Sixth Edition

OUR GLOBAL ENVIRONMENT

A Health Perspective

Anne Nadakavukaren

WAVELAND

PRESS, INC.

Long Grove, Illinois

For information about this book, contact:
Waveland Press, Inc.
4180 IL Route 83, Suite 101
Long Grove, IL 60047-9580
(847) 634-0081
info@waveland.com
www.waveland.com

Cover photo: NASA

10-digit ISBN 1-57766-402-7
13-digit ISBN 978-1-57766-402-4

Printed in the United States of America

9 8 7 6 5 4

CONTENTS

PART 2
OUR TOXIC ENVIRONMENT:
DOES EVERYTHING CAUSE CANCER?   159

PART 3
ENVIRONMENTAL DEGRADATION:
HOW WE FOUL OUR OWN NEST   355

16 Solid and Hazardous Wastes 536

PREFACE

Our Global Environment: A Health Perspective is intended as a text for introductory level courses in environmental health or human ecology, presenting a broad survey of the major environmental issues facing society early in the 21st century. The book combines an overall ecological concern with specific elements related to personal and community health, emphasizing the interrelatedness of the two and conveying to students an awareness of how current environmental issues directly affect their own lives.

Commencing with a rudimentary discussion of general ecological principles, the text focuses primarily on our present population-resources-pollution crisis and explains why human health and welfare depend on successful resolution of these challenges. Intended for a one-semester course, the text consists of 16 chapters and is divided into three main sections, each with its own introduction. Discussion within each chapter covers general aspects of the subject in question, while specific illustrative examples are treated in box inserts. The sixth edition updates information covered in previous editions and incorporates new issues of concern, including nuclear terrorism, genetically modified crop plants, mad cow disease, the obesity epidemic, and many others.

In order to give students a perspective on the kinds of actions being taken to deal with identified problems, a brief description of federal statutes dealing with particular environmental issues is included wherever appropriate. Moreover, the text reviews the latest developments in international efforts to negotiate binding treaties on issues of global concern, such as climate change, ozone-layer depletion, and tobacco use, and incorporates numerous examples of environmental problems and solutions from other nations. Appendices at the end of the book describe the various federal agencies dealing with environmental and health issues and provide names and Web addresses of major nongovernmental environmental organizations for the benefit of those students who wish to obtain further information or to become actively affiliated with such groups. The ability of citizens to influence public policy is stressed throughout the book, a basic purpose of the text being to provide students with sufficient information and insight into environmental problems to enable them to understand and participate in the public decision-making processes that will profoundly influence health and environmental quality in the decades ahead.

I would like to express my sincere gratitude to those who helped me make this book possible: to Heinz Russelmann, former Director of the Environmental Health Program at Illinois State University, whose encouragement, suggestions, and painstaking review of earlier editions of this text have been of invaluable assistance; to Dr. Sharron LaFollette for her careful review and comments on the chapters dealing with air pollution and toxic substances; to Dr. Kenneth Jesse, Professor of Physics (retired) at Illinois State University, for his thoughtful review and valuable suggestions on matters pertaining to ionizing radiation and noise pollution; to Dr. Anthony Otsuka, Professor in the Biological Sciences Department at Illinois State University, for his insightful comments on the sections dealing with mutations and cancer; to former colleague Phil Kneller, now at Western Carolina University, and to Tom Anderson of the McLean County Health Department for their suggestions and review of material on foodborne disease; to Linn Haramis at the Illinois Department of Public Health for his review of the passage on Lyme Disease; to Dr. Gregory Crouch, Associate Director of the Department of Environmental Health and Safety at Indiana University, for his valuable input on risk assessment and related topics; to Dr. Michelle Covi, Director of the Ecology Action Center in Normal-Bloomington for her review of the chapter on ecological principles; to Laurie Prossnitz, Waveland Press, whose friendly cooperation and painstaking editorial efforts have been sincerely appreciated; to Neil Rowe, publisher of Waveland Press, for his cooperation and help; and especially to my husband and daughters for their loving support and understanding during the course of this project.

Anne Nadakavukaren

PEOPLE, PROGRESS, AND NATURE

IS CONFLICT INEVITABLE?

Wangari Maathai, Kenyan environmentalist and Nobel Peace Prize winner for her efforts to reverse deforestation in her home country. [© *Micheline Pelletier / Corbis*]

In nature there are neither rewards nor punishments—
there are consequences.

—R. G. Ingersoll

1

Human beings, as a species, are unquestionably the dominant form of life on earth today. Inhabiting every continent, roaming the seas, exploring space, creating glittering cities and festering slums, taming rivers, bringing water to the desert, harnessing the atom, tinkering with the gene—people often deceive themselves into believing they are all powerful creatures, apart from the rest of nature. Yet a half-million years of cultural evolution cannot alter the fact that humans, like all other living organisms, are inextricably bound up in the web of interdependency and interrelationships that characterize life on this planet. Human health, well-being, and indeed survival are ultimately dependent on the health and integrity of the whole environment in which we live. Today the natural world that we share with all other forms of life on this planet is under unprecedented attack, not by outside forces of evil, as in a science fiction movie, but rather by a wide range of human activities and the sheer pressure of human numbers. Sometimes unwittingly, sometimes with full awareness of the consequences of our actions, we are rapidly altering the basic foundations of the environment that sustains us.

Although the destructive impact of human activities on the natural environment is nothing new—as the extinction of wooly mammoths by Prehistoric hunters or the deforestation of ancient Greece bears witness—the "human footprint" has expanded exponentially during the past two centuries, particularly in the years since World War II. What were once local or regional problems have now become issues of global concern, demanding unprecedented international cooperation if they are ever to be resolved. Achieving such cooperation and commitment requires a fundamental understanding of the nature of the problems facing society and a realization by policymakers and the public of the consequences of inaction.

In the United States, attitudes regarding humanity's relationship to the natural world have changed radically during the past 100 years. Reflecting prevailing beliefs in the "Old World" countries from which they came, most pre-20th century American immigrants considered themselves "above nature" and viewed the seemingly infinite resources of a sparsely populated continent simply as "things" to be exploited for human benefit. Though a few early American writers like Thoreau extolled the value of unspoiled surroundings, most of his contemporaries viewed wilderness as an enemy to be conquered and proceeded to do so. After the Civil War, destruction of America's natural heritage accelerated, as railroads connected the far-flung regions of a vast continent and millions of settlers streamed westward. By the end of the 1800s, the "frontier" was no more; most of the virgin forests east of the Mississippi had been felled, the enormous herds of bison that once blanketed the Great Plains had been reduced to a pitiful remnant, and the passenger pigeon was about to become extinct.

At the dawn of the 20th century, attitudes toward the natural world began to change, slowly but inexorably. At first concerns focused almost exclusively on the rate at which Americans were depleting what had once seemed an inexhaustible supply of natural resources. The so-called Progressive Conservation Movement was led not by citizen activists but by scientific professionals—experts in forestry, botany, geology, hydrology—and championed by a young, intelligent, and energetic president, Theodore Roosevelt. Influenced by his conservationist friend, John Muir, Roosevelt set aside land for national forest reserves and national monuments and by the time he left office in 1909, national forest acreage had nearly tripled to 100 million acres. Early 20th-century conservationists like Roosevelt, Muir, and forestry expert Gifford Pinchot bore little resemblance to present-day environmentalists, however; most were wealthy sportsmen, primarily interested in saving resources for use by future generations; the integrity of ecosystems or the human health impact of pollutants had not yet entered the consciousness of those who called themselves "conservationists." Nevertheless, our modern concern for wilderness, biodiversity, and natural beauty was born from the collective thinking of these pioneers of the movement.

Following Teddy Roosevelt, a succession of presidents, both uninformed and uninterested in the conservation issues so enthusiastically addressed by their predecessor, largely ignored such matters. Not until the Dust Bowl days of the 1930s was the conservation theme revived by President Franklin Roosevelt, whose administration first tackled the all-too-obvious problem of soil erosion by creating the Soil Conservation Service.

World War II brought an end to the Great Depression and spawned momentous new forces that radically altered life on this planet, greatly accelerating the pace and expanding the scope of environmentally destructive forces. WW II marked an epochal environmental turning point in numerous ways. Exposure to ionizing radiation in the form of fallout from nuclear bomb testing made the post-war generation of children the first ever to grow up with strontium-90 in their bones. The fruits of wartime research on DDT ushered in a new "Age of Chemicals" that promised to end the scourge of insect-borne disease and famine but subsequently proved to have a darker side as well. In the immediate post-war years, wartime austerity receded into memory, succeeded by a period of booming prosperity and reckless optimism regarding the benefits of growth. Industrial and agricultural production soared and Americans rushed forward in a feverish quest for the "good life" through rampant consumerism. While a few scientists fretted that the environmental life-support systems undergirding national prosperity were being undermined, most citizens subscribed to the belief that no price was too great to pay for economic growth.

The public's comfortable assumption that everything was rosy was irreversibly shattered in 1962 by an unassuming middle-aged woman, Rachel Carson, whose best-selling book, *Silent Spring*, constituted a scathing indictment of humanity's war against nature, especially the indiscriminate use of chemical pesticides. It's difficult for young people today to comprehend the impact *Silent Spring* had in 1962. To a large extent, the book's publication marked the opening salvo of the environmental revolution (in fact, Carson was the first to popularize the word "environment") because *Silent Spring* succeeded, where earlier efforts had fallen short, in opening the public's eyes to the full extent of a problem they had hitherto ignored. *Silent Spring* expanded the earlier elitist focus on wilderness preservation and resource conservation to include toxics issues and human health—concerns to which the vast middle class of Americans could whole-heartedly relate. During the 1960s, "ecology" became a household word, introduced by career biologists who, having identified environmental abuses, raised the alarm at what they saw. By the late 1960s the public, too, had become aware of what was happening, reacting with dismay to pollution-choked rivers and smoggy skies, and demanding the policy actions that characterized the following decades.

The fledgling environmental movement "took off" in 1969, thanks to a series of eco-disasters that convinced ordinary citizens "enough is enough!" Key events that year included an offshore oil rig blowout at Santa Barbara, fouling scenic California beaches with sticky crude and dying seabirds; a spectacular fire raging across the surface of Cleveland's grossly polluted Cuyahoga River; and an application by giant oil companies for permission to build an oil pipeline across Alaska.

These and other mounting environmental insults prompted Wisconsin Senator Gaylord Nelson to suggest the nation hold an "Environmental Teach-In," an idea that quickly caught on and culminated in a coast-to-coast public relations event held on April 22, 1970—the first national celebration of Earth Day. Acclaimed as the "largest one-day outpouring of public support for any social cause in American history," Earth

Day 1970 attracted participants from all walks of life—biologists, bureaucrats, home-makers, farmers, economists, educators, and millions upon millions of students. Older Americans protesting the gradual uglification of "America the Beautiful" also offered strong support, as did many existing national environmental organizations such as the Sierra Club, National Wildlife Federation, Audubon Society, and others. Not surprisingly, the burgeoning environmental movement had opponents as well, particularly among those who viewed activists' demands as a threat to corporate profits. Many observers at the time downplayed the significance of environmentalism, assuming it was simply the latest fad among white, liberal "flower children." But they were wrong. Environmentalism didn't fade away after April 1970 but rather was institution-alized in the form of an impressive array of far-reaching new laws enacted by Congress during the 1970s. These laws today constitute the legal framework for America's war against pollution and ecological degradation. Earth Day made environmentalism a permanent issue in U.S. political dialogue.

Over the years since the first Earth Day, the U.S. has devoted an enormous amount of time, money, and people power to solving the environmental problems highlighted by that event. Many of those efforts are still ongoing and some have met with a considerable degree of success—certainly the air Americans breathe today and the waterways in which they recreate are far cleaner than they were in the late 1960s and early 1970s. However, as in so many aspects of life, it seems that no sooner do we solve one problem than several more emerge to take its place. As U.S. air quality, water quality, and the management of solid and hazardous wastes gradually improved, concerns regarding global-scale challenges such as ozone-layer depletion, desertification, loss of biodiversity, and climate change took center stage—but have proven much more difficult to resolve. Solutions to these problems require far more than a quick technological "fix" like installing scrubbers on polluting power plants. Instead, success ultimately depends on halting population growth, devising new energy and transportation strategies, making fundamental changes in how the world's agricultural and forest lands are managed, and so forth.

The contrast between the public's response to the relatively straightforward environmental problems focused upon by activists in the early 1970s and those confronting society today has been aptly described by Gus Speth, founder of the World Resources Institute and author of the thought-provoking book *Red Sky at Morning* (2004). Whereas the pollution/toxics problems evoking protests in the 1970s were close to home and easy to understand (what's confusing about a toxic waste dump in your backyard?!), those now on the global agenda are scientifically complex and still subject to a degree of uncertainty. The earlier problems were highly visible and imme-diate—robins dying of pesticide poisoning—but climatologists' warnings of the dire consequences associated with global warming a century hence strike many people as too theoretical and too far in the future to worry about today. Similarly, since the major impacts of climate change, tropical deforestation, and species loss will be on people and places far away rather than on our own communities, we're less motivated to take potentially painful policy actions than was the case three decades ago. All of these factors have diluted the once-emphatic demand that government "do something right now!" to address these issues, even though polls continue to show that most Americans still consider themselves "environmentalists."

Organized political opposition from vested interests who feel threatened by spe-cific policies or actions proposed to address global environmental challenges have also increasingly blocked adoption of major new initiatives comparable to those enacted in the 1970s. Political leadership at the highest levels of government, such as that exem-plified by Teddy Roosevelt a century ago, has largely been lacking in recent years, especially in the United States. Though once the undisputed leader in cutting-edge environmental initiatives, the U.S. today is widely criticized both at home and abroad for obstructing international efforts to deal meaningfully with a wide array of global environmental problems, most notably that of climate change. The European Union, largely indifferent to such issues until the mid-1980s, has become the leading environmental actor on the world stage; nevertheless, without active cooperation from the world's largest economy and third most populous nation (i.e., the U.S.), future progress in resolving global environmental issues will be problematic at best.

In spite of these challenges, however, there are reasons for optimism about humanity's chances of reversing the current downward spiral of environmental degradation. Perhaps the most hopeful trend is the worldwide proliferation of small grassroots organizations made up of committed citizens like Wangari Maathai, Kenyan environmentalist and founder of the Green Belt Movement, who in 2004 became the first African woman to win the Nobel Peace Prize. Maathai was cited for her tireless work to reverse deforestation in her home country by mobilizing thousands of rural women to plant over 30 million trees, thereby protecting soil resources and rehabilitating degraded land. Maathai and millions of others like her, working independently on their own local problems but united in their determination to save our planet's natural heritage for future generations to enjoy, have recognized that we don't have to sit back as passive spectators to the despoliation of our environment and the impoverishment of our society. They realize that much can be done to limit the impact of advanced technology on the natural world and to incorporate environmental considerations into national policy making. These activists, ordinary people from all walks of life, have an important message for the rest of us: to a great extent the technical know-how to prevent further deterioration exists—what is needed most is a societal commitment to get the job done.

The most important decisions being made in the environmental health arena today are political decisions, balancing ecological concerns with economic and social considerations. Individuals wishing to become involved in protecting and enhancing environmental quality will find their efforts most effective when directed toward influencing environmental policy-making bodies at every level of government. To be a successful eco-advocate, however, requires a thorough understanding of the nature of our environmental crisis, how the present situation developed, what the human impact of these threats may be, and what actions have already been taken in an attempt to restore and maintain a quality environment. These are the issues this book will attempt to address in the belief that a well-informed, politically active citizenry is an essential ingredient for staving off eco-catastrophe and embracing programs of sustainable development. A firm conviction that global security in the years ahead is intimately related to the success of such efforts was movingly expressed by Maathai who, upon learning she had been awarded the Nobel Prize, responded:

> . . . protecting the global environment is directly related to securing peace . . . those of us who understand the complex concept of the environment have the burden to act. We must not tire, we must not give up, we must persist.

INTRODUCTION TO ECOLOGICAL PRINCIPLES

> Hurt not the earth, neither the sea, nor the trees.
>
> —Bible, Revelations 7:3

In July of 1969, when astronauts Neil Armstrong and "Buzz" Aldrin became the first humans to land on the moon and gazed back at their home planet more than 200,000 miles away, they were filled with a sense of wonder at the beauty and uniqueness of Earth. Of all the heavenly bodies of which we are aware, our planet is neither the largest nor the smallest, the hottest nor the coldest, yet it *is* extraordinary in one vital respect—in all the universe Earth is the only planet known to support life. Within the narrow film of air, soil, and water that envelops the surface of the globe, extending vertically from the deepest ocean trenches more than 36,000 feet below sea level to about 30,000 or more feet above sea level, exists what ecologists call the **biosphere**—that portion of Earth where life occurs.

The known limits of the biosphere have been steadily expanding as scientific discoveries over the past several decades have revealed an astonishing array of species thriving in habitats once regarded as too extreme to support life. Such surprises include heat-loving bacteria living near deep-sea hydrothermal vents where water temperatures may reach 250°F (121°C) and microbes feasting on sulfur compounds in oil deposits more than 5,000 feet below the earth's surface (Smil, 2002; Kashefi and Lovely, 2003). Nevertheless, even though a number of bizarre aquatic species inhabit the ocean depths and bioaerosols such as microbial spores and pollen grains may be found floating in the upper reaches of the atmosphere, by far the greatest number of living things are found in the region extending from the permanent snow line of tropical and subtropical mountain ranges (about 20,000 feet above sea level) to the limit of light penetration in the clearest oceans (about 600 feet deep). Here a vast assemblage of plant, animal, and microbial life can be found—approximately 1.75 million known species, with a likely 11–12 million more yet to be discovered (Heywood and Watson, 1995). These species interact both with each other and with their physical environment; over very long periods of time they become modified in response to environmental pressures and, in turn, they themselves modify their physical surroundings.

The first living organisms on Earth (probably forms similar to bacteria) are now thought to have arisen more than 3.5 billion years ago on a planet whose environment was considerably different from that of the present-day world. The life activities of those early organisms, feeding upon and reacting with the chemical compounds in the waters where they first arose, were responsible for the creation of the modern atmosphere, which made possible the emergence of higher forms of life. The first primitive organisms evolved in a world devoid of atmospheric oxygen but rich in carbon dioxide. This carbon dioxide in turn provided a carbon source for the evolutionarily more advanced photosynthetic organisms that could produce their own food by utilizing the sun's energy to convert carbon dioxide and water into carbohydrates, releasing oxygen as a waste product. It was through the action of such photosynthetic organisms that the earth's atmosphere gradually became an oxygen-rich one, permitting the development of the types of life with which we are familiar today. In this way, the life activities of one group of organisms profoundly altered the environment and created conditions that facilitated the emergence of other forms of life. The ability of living things to modify their surroundings and the tendency of other organisms to respond positively or negatively to such changes have been constant features of evolutionary progression throughout the ages and remain so today.

Ecosystems

The concept of nature as divided into basic functional units called **ecosystems** reflects scientists' recognition of the complex manner in which living organisms interact with each other and with the nonliving (or abiotic) components of their environment to process energy and cycle nutrients. The concept is admittedly imprecise, since few ecosystems have definitive spatial boundaries or exist in splendid isolation. Adjacent ecosystems commonly influence each other, as when a pond ecosystem is altered by materials washing into it from surrounding terrestrial ecosystems, and certain components (e.g., water birds, insects) may be moving in and out on a regular basis (Smith, 1986). Similarly, the concept of ecosystems is a broad one, its main usefulness being to emphasize the interdependence of the biotic and abiotic components of an area. An ecosystem has no defining size limitations: an abandoned tire casing containing trapped rainwater, microorganisms, and swarms of mosquito larvae can be regarded as an ecosystem; so can a family-room aquarium, a city park, a cornfield, a tidepool, a cow pasture, or, indeed, the entire planet Earth. Any of these widely diverse situations can be considered an ecosystem so long as living and nonliving elements are present and interacting to process energy and cycle materials (Stiling, 1992).

Biotic Community

The most familiar classification system used for grouping plants and animals is one based upon presumed evolutionary relationships—lions, tigers, and leopards being grouped in the cat family; wheat, corn, and rice in the grass family; and so forth. However, ecologists tend to arrange species on the basis of their functional association with each other. A natural grouping of different kinds of plants and animals within any given habitat is termed by ecologists a **biotic community.**

"Biotic community," like "ecosystem," is a broad term that can be used to describe natural groupings of widely differing sizes, from the various microscopic diatoms and zooplankton swimming in a drop of pond water to the hundreds of species of trees, wildflowers, ferns, insects, birds, mammals, and so forth, found in an Appalachian forest. Biotic communities have characteristic trophic structures and energy flow patterns and also have a certain taxonomic unity, in the sense that certain species tend to exist together.

Box 1-1   Of Orcas and Otters

Nature is full of surprises, one of the latest being the near-disappearance of sea otters from Alaska's western coastline. Equally surprising is the identity of the agent responsible for the unexpected population crash and the demonstration that only a few members of a transient species can have a profound impact in linking interactions across ecosystems.

Playful marine mammals once hunted almost to extinction by fur traders, sea otters (*Enhydra lutris*) experienced a dramatic comeback following adoption in 1911 of an international treaty that prohibited killing of these animals. By the 1970s sea otter populations had recovered to pre-hunting levels in many parts of their historic range, giving conservationists reason to assume that their long-term survival was assured. Rebounding sea otter populations were regarded as good news for coastal marine ecosystems; as a "keystone species" of its biotic community, the sea otter plays a pivotal role in maintaining the health of the near-shore kelp "forests" on which a diverse assemblage of plant and animal species depend. As voracious predators of kelp-eating sea urchins, the otters prevent overgrazing of the giant algae, thereby contributing to overall ecosystem stability.

Until the late 1980s, sea otter populations along Alaska's Aleutian archipelago appeared healthy and thriving, but by 1990 the picture there suddenly and inexplicably began to change. Along a 500-mile stretch of western Alaska, the number of sea otters, which had been estimated at 53,000 in the 1970s, plummeted to just 6,000 in 1997—a 90% decline in population size. Scientists who had been studying the ecology of the area for several decades were initially at a loss to explain what was happening. They knew the animals weren't experiencing reproductive failure because studies of radio-tagged otters showed that birth and survival rates of otter pups remained at normal levels. Aerial surveys conducted by the U.S. Fish and Wildlife Service in 1965 and again in 1992 confirmed that the recent decline in the otter population was widespread throughout the island chain—the otters weren't simply relocating from one area to another. Consequently, the only explanation for the animals' drastic decline

was increased mortality—but why? If otters were falling victim to disease or toxic pollutants, then researchers should have observed carcasses washing up onshore, but not even one had been sighted. Starvation was an unlikely explanation, since sea urchins, the otters' favorite food, were in plentiful supply. That left predation as the only plausible cause for rising otter death rates.

In 1991 when one member of the research team observed an otter being attacked and eaten by an orca, or killer whale (*Orcinus orca*), the sighting was regarded as an anomaly; orcas and sea otters had always shared the same waters and no one had ever seen the whales preying on their small, furry neighbors. However, over the next several years more such attacks were documented and gradually the scientists became convinced that a fundamental change in orca behavior was responsible for the dwindling number of otters. Gradually the case against the whales grew more persuasive; on Adak Island, observations revealed that 65% of the otters in easily accessible Kulak Bay disappeared over the course of one year, while in Clam Lagoon, whose entrance from the sea was too shallow and narrow for the orcas to enter, the otter population decline was only 12%. Finally, statistical analyses of what the rate of observed orca attacks was likely to be if killer whales were responsible for the 90% observed decrease in otter numbers yielded a figure almost identical to the number of attacks actually witnessed. The verdict now was beyond doubt—orca predation was the cause of the otter population crash.

Again, however, the question was why? Why would orcas, whose preferred food had always been the much larger, more nutritious harbor seals and sea lions, suddenly begin eating sea otters? As one ecologist studying the phenomenon remarked, it's like "eating popcorn instead of steaks."

The answer to the riddle demonstrates how truly complex are the workings of nature. Since the late 1970s, populations of sea lions and seals have collapsed across the western North Pacific. While the cause of this event remains controversial, the most likely explanation is overfishing by commercial trawlers in the Bering Sea. The decline in perch and herring led directly to the crash in seal and sea lion populations which, in turn, forced killer whales to resort to a diet of otters. Considering the large energy requirements of orcas and the minimal caloric value of an otter, researchers calculate that a single killer whale may consume 1,825 otters per year, a figure which suggests that as few as four orcas may be responsible for the observed otter depopulation along more than 2,000 miles of shoreline!

Unfortunately, the ecological implications of this sad story don't end with the near-disappearance of Alaskan sea otters. With populations of their main predator so depleted, sea urchins in the affected areas are now experiencing a population explosion; hordes of hungry urchins are gobbling up the kelp beds, reducing the density of these underwater "forests" 12-fold in just ten years. If the kelp forest ecosystem collapses, as it is likely to do now that its keystone species (the sea otters) has been removed, many other components of this biotic community will be affected. Populations of rockfishes, sculpins, and greenlings—fish that live within the kelp beds—are likely to decline as their habitat vanishes; starfish, living in the open ocean

beyond the kelp but also preyed upon by otters, will probably increase in numbers; seagull populations may remain stable, since those birds can turn to a diet of invertebrates as their preferred fish species dwindle; but less versatile bald eagles—totally dependent on fish—will either starve or go elsewhere as their food supply disappears.

It requires quite a stretch of the imagination to comprehend how catching too many herring in the North Pacific could result in the destruction of kelp forests and the loss of eagles along the Alaskan coast. Nevertheless, the fact that just such a scenario is now unfolding vividly demonstrates the complexity and interconnectedness of biotic communities and illustrates how human activities can set in motion a series of cascading events, culminating in the demise of species we never intended to harm.

References

Estes, J. A., M. T. Tinker, T. M. Williams, and D. F. Doak. 1998. "Killer Whale Predation on Sea Otters Linking Oceanic and Nearshore Ecosystems"; Kaiser, Jocelyn. "Sea Otter Declines Blamed on Hungry Killers." *Science* 282, no. 5388 (Oct. 16):390, 473–476.

Individuals of the same species living together within a given area are collectively referred to as a **population.** Such populations constitute groups more or less isolated from other populations of the same species. A population within the biotic community of a region is not a static entity but is continually changing in size and reshuffling its hereditary characteristics in response to environmental changes and to fluctuations in the populations of other members of the community.

The community concept is one of the most important ecological principles because (1) it emphasizes the fact that different organisms are not arbitrarily scattered around the earth with no particular reason as to why they live where they do, but rather that they dwell together in an orderly manner; and (2) by illuminating the importance of the community as a whole to any of its individual parts, the community concept can be used by humans to manage a particular organism, in the sense of increasing or decreasing its numbers. Emphasizing biotic communities as a whole, rather than focusing on their constituent species, is helpful also in demonstrating why removing one species from a community (or, conversely, introducing a nonnative species into a community) can often have unintended—and sometimes disastrous—consequences.

European settlement of the sparsely populated North American continent launched a gigantic experiment in human interference with natural ecosystems. The sad tale of beaver exploitation provides one dramatic example of how a stable biotic community can unravel simply by eliminating one of its members. In the late seventeenth century, French traders began trapping these once-abundant mammals, shipping enormous numbers of valuable pelts back to Europe to accommodate the insatiable demands of the hat-making industry. So extensively and heavily were they hunted that within 150 years beavers faced extinction from the Great Lakes region all the way to Oregon and California. Only as their numbers plummeted did the beavers' role within their biotic community become apparent. With the demise of their architects, beaver dams were no longer maintained and eventually washed away. As a result, rates of stream flow sharply accelerated, destroying the spawning beds of fish species that relied on the quiet waters behind the dams for breeding. Marshy areas created by the dams were either drained or flooded, depending on location, and waterfowl populations declined as nesting sites were lost. Flooding increased in frequency and intensity, streamside erosion worsened, and siltation of river channels accelerated. Disappearance of the beaver, perceived by the trappers as a creature that was "going to waste" in the wilderness, thus led to surprisingly far-reaching effects (Ashworth, 1986).

The brown tree snake, native to Australia, Papua New Guinea, and the Solomon Islands, is notorious for having nearly wiped out the native forest birds of Guam, where it appeared in the late 1940s or early 1950s, most likely having hitchhiked aboard military aircraft. [*USGS photo by G. Rodda*]

Introducing a nonnative species (i.e., an exotic) into an established biotic community can be every bit as destabilizing as removing a component species. Time and again, accidentally or deliberately, humans have released plants or animals into a new environment only to see them quickly attain major pest status, usually due to the absence of natural predators that could keep their numbers under control. In the United States, West Nile encephalitis virus, zebra mussels, Asian longhorned beetles, and northern snakeheads (the "pit bull" of fish) are but the most recent in a host of unwanted aliens to invade our shores—gypsy moths, European starlings, carp, kudzu, purple loosestrife, water hyacinths, sea lampreys, Formosan termites—to mention but a few of the most notorious. Elsewhere in the world, exotic species have been equally disruptive; in the Netherlands, six North American muskrats brought to that country in 1906 have, in the absence of natural enemies, multiplied into the millions. Spreading throughout the country via the hundreds of thousands of miles of canals that characterize Holland, the muskrats have become major pests by burrowing into and weakening the vital dikes that protect the low-lying country from devastating floods. Along the Mediterranean coast, a Pacific seaweed, *Caulerpa taxifolia*, accidentally released from aquarium tanks at Monaco's Oceanographic Museum, has proliferated from the French Riviera to the shores of Croatia. Wherever it goes, *Caulerpa* crowds out native plant and animal species, producing a monoculture that threatens to destroy the entire Mediterranean ecosystem. Another uninvited migrant native to the east coast of North America, Leidy's comb jelly, was discharged with ships' ballast water into the Black Sea where it has multiplied so rapidly since the late 1980s that a single cubic meter of seawater now contains as many as 500 of the tiny animals. Because the jellyfish out-competes native fish for the zooplankton both eat, popula-

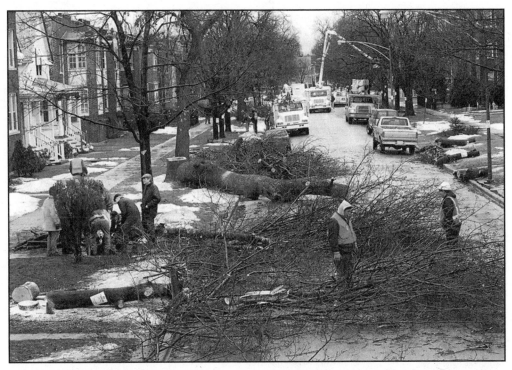

In 1999 more than 20 trees were cut down in one neighborhood on Chicago's North Side to prevent further spread of the Asian longhorned beetle. [*Chicago Tribune photo by Carl Wagner. All rights reserved. Used with permission.*]

tions of indigenous fish species have plummeted and the entire Black Sea ecosystem is now on the verge of collapse (Baskin, 2002; Bright, 1998).

In our attempts to "control nature" we must never forget that the intricate interdependencies that have evolved over the millennia among the biotic communities of the earth cannot be altered without provoking a corresponding change somewhere else in the ecosystem.

Ecological Dominants

Although all members of a biotic community have a role to play in the life of that community, it is obvious that certain plants or animals exert more of an influence on the ecosystem as a whole than do others. As George Orwell might have put it, "All animals are equal, but some animals are more equal than others." Those organisms which exert a major modifying influence on the community are known as **ecological dominants.** Such dominants generally comprise those species that control the flow of energy through the community; if they were removed from the community, much greater changes in the ecosystem would result than if a nondominant species were removed. For example, when farmers chop down the dominant hardwood trees in an eastern forest to clear the land for cultivation, the changes produced by this removal (i.e., loss of animal species that depend on the trees for food and shelter, loss of shade-loving plants that proliferate under the canopy, change in soil microbiota, raising of soil temperature, increase in soil erosion, and so forth) are much more pronounced than would be the changes brought about when the farmers' children wander into the

Table 1-1 100 of the World's Worst Invasive Alien Species

Micro-Organisms
avian malaria
banana bunchy top virus
rinderpest virus

Macro-Fungi
chestnut blight
crayfish plague
Dutch elm disease
frog chytrid fungus
phytophthora root rot

Aquatic Plants
caulerpa seaweed
common cord-grass
wakame seaweed
water hyacinth

Land Plants
African tulip tree
black wattle
Brazilian pepper tree
cogon grass
cluster pine
erect pricklypear
fire tree
giant reed
gorse
hiptage
Japanese knotweed
Kahili ginger
Koster's curse
kudzu
lantana
leafy spurge
leucaena
melaleuca
mesquite
miconia
mile-a-minute weed
mimosa

Land Plants *(cont'd.)*
privet
pumpwood
purple loosestrife
quinine tree
shoebutton ardisia
Siam weed
strawberry guava
tamarisk
wedelia
yellow Himalayan raspberry

Aquatic Invertebrates
Chinese mitten crab
comb jelly fish
book flea
golden apple snail
green crab
marine clam
Mediterranean mussel
Northern Pacific seastar
zebra mussel

Land Invertebrates
Argentine ant
Asian longhorned beetle
Asian tiger mosquito
big-headed ant
common malaria mosquito
common wasp
crazy ant
cypress aphid
flatworm
Formosan subterranean termite
giant African snail
gypsy moth
khapra beetle
little fire ant
red imported fire ant

Land Invertebrates *(cont'd.)*
rosy wolfsnail
sweet potato whitefly

Amphibians
bullfrog
cane toad
Caribbean tree frog

Fish
brown trout
carp
large-mouth bass
Mozambique tilapia
Nile perch
rainbow trout
walking catfish
Western mosquito fish

Birds
Indian myna bird
red-vented bulbul
starling

Reptiles
brown tree snake
red-eared slider

Mammals
brushtail possum
domestic cat
goat
grey squirrel
macaque
monkey mouse
nutria
pig
rabbit
red deer
red fox
ship rat
small Indian mongoose
stoat

Source: Courtesy of the Invasive Species Specialist Group, www. issg.org/database.

forest and pick all of the trilliums and lady slippers they find growing there. In either case, the stability of the ecosystem is upset, but the loss of several species of spring wildflowers, while unfortunate, has much less effect on the forest community as a whole than does the loss of the dominant oaks, maples, and beeches.

In most terrestrial biotic communities certain plants comprise the dominant species because they not only provide food and shelter for other organisms, but also directly affect and modify their physical environment. That is, they contribute to a build-up of topsoil, moderate fluctuations of temperature, improve moisture retention, affect the pH of the soil, and so on. As a general rule, the number of dominant species within a community becomes progressively fewer as one moves toward the poles and greater the closer the community is to the tropics. While a northern coniferous forest may consist of only spruces or firs, a jungle in Sumatra may have a dozen or more tree species that could be considered dominants. In addition to the effects of latitude, one can also generalize that dominant species are fewer in regions where climatic conditions are extreme, like tundra and deserts (Odum, 1959).

Among animal species in a biotic community, certain **keystone predators** help maintain greater biotic diversity than would exist in their absence. Keystone, or dominant, predators moderate competition among the species upon which they prey, reducing the density of strong competitors and thereby allowing less aggressive competitors to maintain their populations within the community. As described earlier in box 1-1, stability of the kelp "forest" ecosystem along Alaska's Pacific Coast had long been maintained by sea otters preying heavily on kelp-eating sea urchins. With urchin populations kept at tolerable levels by otter predation, a food supply for other herbivores in that biotic community was maintained and a diverse range of species flourished. When otter numbers suddenly dropped, the population of sea urchins exploded, overwhelming their competitors and resulting in a sharp decline in the biodiversity of the kelp forest community.

Biomes

The species composition of any particular biotic community is profoundly affected by the physical characteristics of the environment, particularly temperature and rainfall. The kinds of plants and animals one would see while touring Yellowstone National Park would differ significantly from those found on a trek through the Amazon. Ecologists have divided the terrestrial communities of the world into general groupings called **biomes,** areas that can be recognized by the distinctive life forms of their dominant species. In most cases, the key characteristic of a biome is its dominant type of vegetation. We might define a biome as a complex of communities characteristic of a regional climatic zone. Each biome has its own pattern of rainfall, its own seasons, its own maximum and minimum temperatures, and its own changes of day length, all of which combine to support a certain kind of vegetation. Since climatic zones change in a relatively uniform pattern as one moves from the poles toward the equator, the earth's biomes form more or less continuous latitudinal bands around the globe. Starting at the polar regions, let's take a brief look at the major biomes of the earth (note: ecologists list numerous subdivisions of the biomes described here, but for our purposes these general groupings will suffice).

Tundra

The northernmost of the world's land masses, tundra is characterized by permanently frozen subsoil called **permafrost.** In this biome rainfall is quite low, about 8 inches annually, but because the permafrost doesn't allow moisture to penetrate beyond the upper few inches of soil, the tundra in summer is dotted with numerous lakes and bogs—and probably the world's most voracious mosquitoes! The tundra is windy, with only a few stunted trees. The dominant vegetation here consists of moss, lichens, grass, and some small perennials. Animal life is limited in the number of species but very abundant in the number of individuals. These include caribou or reindeer, birds, insects, polar bears, lemmings, foxes, rabbits, and fish. Reptiles and amphibians are absent. The tundra is basically a very fragile environment. Because of the slow rates at which tundra plants grow and decompose (due to the low temperatures and the characteristics of permafrost), the thick, spongy matting of lichens, grasses, and sedges that typify tundra is especially slow to recover from disturbance. Tracks of vehicles or animals can remain visible for decades. Great care must be taken in building on tundra because heat from structures will melt the permafrost and cause uneven settling, which often badly distorts the buildings. Until the 1960s the tundra was relatively unexploited, but with the construction of the Alaska oil pipeline and similar kinds of mineral development in Canada and Siberia, that situation has changed.

Taiga

A Russian word for "swamp forest," the taiga is sometimes called the **boreal forest.** This biome covers much of Canada, Scandinavia, and Russia. The Canadian taiga alone constitutes fully 10% of all forests worldwide and 25% of intact virgin forests. Here the dominant vegetation consists of conifer trees—mainly spruces, firs, and pines—that have needlelike leaves that stay on the trees for three to five years. Some deciduous trees such as aspens, alders, and larches are also prominent. In general, the trees are much less diverse in number of species than those in the deciduous forests farther south and the soils have a different kind of humus and are more acid. Precipitation in the taiga is only moderate but, because drainage is poor, lakes, ponds, and bogs are common here. Animals of the taiga include bears, moose, lynxes, weasels, wolverines, and 186 species of land birds; indeed, 30% of all land birds in Canada and the United States nest and raise their young in the boreal forest, though most migrate south as winter approaches (Blancher, 2002). Because of the huge stands of just one or two species of conifers, the taiga provides an opportunity for periodic outbreaks of pests like the spruce budworm, which can defoliate huge areas of forest. Perhaps because of the lack of diversity of species, taiga populations tend to undergo "boom or bust" cycles fairly regularly.

Temperate Deciduous Forest

This biome occurs in a belt south of the taiga where climate is milder and where rainfall is abundant relative to the amount of evaporation. This is the biome familiar to most of us because it is the one in which Western, as well as Chinese and Japanese, civilization developed. Soil types and elevations vary widely within this biome. Maples, beech, oaks, and hickories are common trees; many species of ferns and flowering herbaceous plants are also found. The deciduous forest has a great variety of mammals, birds, and insects, as well as a modest number of reptiles and amphibians. Because of the annual leaf drop, deciduous forests generate soils rich in nutrients, which in turn support a multitude of soil microbes. When such forests are cleared, the richness of the soils can be maintained if great care is taken to see that their supplies of nutrients and decaying organic matter are preserved (in a sense, raising crops or grazing animals is akin to mining the soil, since the nutrients leave along with the crops, meat, wool, or whatever is removed). All too often, however, short-term careless exploiters have allowed soils to deteriorate or have ignored opportunities to improve them. Unfortunately, economic considerations often lead individuals who are exploiting an ecosystem to use short-term strategies that are disastrous for humanity in the long run.

Grasslands

In regions where annual rainfall is not sufficient to sustain the growth of trees and evaporation rates are high, we find the grasslands of the world. These may be called by different names in various countries: prairie, veldt, savannah, steppe, pampas, llanos. All are characterized by the dominance of grasses and herds of grazing animals. Carnivores also abound, such as coyotes and lions, as do rodents and many species of reptiles. The grassland biome has a higher concentration of organic matter in its soil than does any other biome, the amount of humus in grassland soil being about 12 times greater than that in forest soils. The extraordinary richness of grassland soil has led to the establishment of extremely successful agricultural ecosystems in the grassland areas. These systems can break down rapidly, however, if careful soil conservation is not practiced. The interlaced roots and creeping underground stems of grasses form a turf that prevents erosion of the soil. When the turf is broken with a plow or overgrazed, the soil is exposed to the erosive influences of wind and water, resulting in such calamities as the "Dust Bowl" of the Great Plains in the 1930s. In temperate regions the widespread conversion of natural grasslands to cropland has greatly reduced the geographical extent of this biome. In the tropics, however, grasslands have expanded considerably as a result of deforestation; today tropical grasslands constitute the world's most extensive ecosystem (Smil, 2002).

Desert

Areas receiving less than 10 inches annual precipitation and featuring high daytime temperatures are classified as deserts. These areas are concentrated in the vicinity of 30° north and 30° south latitude. Lack of moisture is the essential factor shaping the desert biome. Most deserts are quite hot in the daytime and, because of the sparse vegetation and resultant rapid reradiation of heat, quite cold at night. Desert plants and animals are characterized by species that can withstand prolonged drought. Among plants such adaptations include waxy cuticle on stems or leaves, reduction in leaf size, and spiny growths to repel moisture-seeking animals. Plants may appear to be widely spaced, but if their roots were visible, the ground between them would be seen to be laced with a shallow root system to take maximum advantage of any rain that does fall. Proportionately more annual plants are found in the desert biome than in any other; because their seeds often require abrasion or a rain heavy enough to leach out inhibiting chemicals, the desert appears to bloom almost overnight after a heavy rain. For the most part, desert animals are active at night, remaining under cover during the heat of the day. Desert soils contain little organic matter and must ordinarily be supplied with both water and nitrogen fertilizer if they are to be cultivated. Human activities have already produced a great increase in the amount of desert and wasteland, removing many once-productive acres from cultivation. Occasional years of good rainfall cause people to forget that the desert is inherently a very fragile environment.

Tropical Rain Forest

This biome is found in Central and South America, central Africa, and South and Southeast Asia. It is characterized by high temperatures and high annual rainfall; 100 inches or more of annual precipitation is common in this biome. Year-round temperature variation is slight. Tropical rain forests are characterized by a great diversity of plant and animal species and by four distinct layers of plant growth—the top canopy of trees reaching 200 feet or more, a lower canopy of densely intertwined treetops at about 100 feet, a sparse understory, and only a very few plants growing at ground level. A wide variety of epiphytic plants can be found. Both plant and animal species exist in greater diversity in the tropical rain forest than anywhere else in the world, though numbers of individuals of a particular species are usually limited. To most people, the luxuriant growth of a tropical jungle implies a rich soil, and one hears many glowing promises of the agricultural riches to be reaped by turning the Amazon or Congo River basins into farmland. The truth of the situation is far different, however. Tropical forest soils in general are exceedingly thin and nutrient-poor. They cannot maintain large reserves of minerals needed for plant growth, primarily because heavy rainfall and a high rate of water flow through the ground to the water table leach them from the soil. The leaching process leaves large residues of insoluble iron and aluminum oxides in the upper levels of tropical forest soils, a process termed "laterization." With the exception of certain fertile river valleys, primitive slash-and-burn agriculture is the only type suitable to most areas of the tropical rain forest. Unfortunately, this fragile ecosystem is being destroyed more rapidly than any other biome due to human population growth and in some cases, such as in Brazil, as a direct consequence of governmental actions.

It should be noted that in areas where there are substantial variations in altitude, the biomes differ at different elevations. This is primarily because air temperature decreases about 6°C for every 1,000-meter increase in altitude and because, especially in desert areas, rainfall increases with altitude.

This brief survey of biome characteristics should make it obvious that various regions differ in their ability to return to an ecologically stable condition once they have been disrupted by human activities. Thus it should not be surprising that certain practices are far more devastating to the local ecology in some areas than they are in others. For example, strip mining in the flat or gently rolling lands of Illinois, Indiana, and Ohio is certainly disruptive to the environment, yet with proper soil reclamation practices the land can be restored to productive uses once mining has ceased. In the arid regions of the High Plains and Southwest, however, exploitation of fossil fuel reserves by strip mining presents a real threat that the acres thus despoiled could never recover and would remain permanent wastelands.

Ecological Niches

Within any biotic community each species is defined by its own unique position, or **niche,** different from that of any other member of the community and determined largely by its size and food habits. Through the processes of evolution and natural selection, plants and animals have become increasingly better adapted to the specific environments in which they live. In order to reduce competition among species for food and living space, organisms have become more specialized in terms of the foods they utilize, period of the day or night during which they are active, and/or the types of microhabitats they exploit. Thus, in an ecological context, the term niche denotes not simply the physical space that a species occupies but, more importantly, what that species *does* (Pianka, 1988). The **Principle of Competitive Exclusion,** basic to ecological theory, holds that when two species are competing for the same limited resources, only one will survive. Only when the environmental resources in a given community are partitioned among the coinhabiting species by means of niche diversification is direct competition minimized, thus permitting coexistence of species.

The benefits of niche diversification can be well illustrated by several species of lice, which peacefully coexist on a human host by restricting their activities to different anatomical regions. The body louse, notorious in history as the vector of typhus fever, feeds on parts of the body below the neck; the closely related head louse confines its activities to the head and neck. The fact that the two are quite similar in appearance and occasionally interbreed indicates their close relationship, but niche diversification is quite apparent in their different behavioral patterns. Head lice cement their eggs ("nits") to hairs of the scalp, while body lice usually glue theirs to fibers of clothing; in fact, body

Box 1-2   Pets, People, and Public Health

The health threat posed by imported exotic animals—the subject of frequent warnings by concerned biologists—became starkly evident in the early summer of 2003. In June of that year more than 70 midwesterners fell victim to a rare viral disease endemic to the rainforests of central and west Africa. "Monkeypox," so-named because it was first described in an outbreak among a group of laboratory monkeys, most commonly infects several species of tropical rodents and has occasionally broken out among human populations in remote areas of Africa—but never before in the United States. Suddenly, a little-known exotic disease erupted in the American heartland and alarmed public health officials hastily mobilized to determine where it had come from and how to contain it.

Since all the confirmed human cases were individuals who had been in direct contact with recently purchased native or imported wild mammals, the search for the source of the problem rapidly focused on the pet industry. Traceback investigations based on victim interviews quickly solved the mystery. In April 2003, a shipment of approximately 800 small mammals, mostly various species of rodents, had arrived in Texas from the West African nation of Ghana. Some of these animals, including several Gambian rats, were shipped by the importer to a vendor in the Chicago area who lodged these animals adjacent to cages housing prairie dogs, wild native rodents whose popularity as house pets has been steadily growing in recent years. Laboratory testing by the national Centers for Disease Control and Prevention (CDC) revealed that at least one of the Gambian rats was harboring the monkeypox virus and concluded that it had transmitted the pathogen to its prairie dog neighbors. Shipments of the now-infected prairie dogs from this vendor to other pet dealers in Illinois, Indiana, Wisconsin, and elsewhere in the Midwest resulted in monkeypox disease among pet store employees and customers who inadvertently purchased infected animals. Transmission of the virus across the species barrier occurred when victims came into direct contact with body fluids or blood from infected prairie dogs or were bitten by the animals. Fortunately, none of the monkeypox cases in this outbreak proved fatal (past outbreaks of monkeypox in Africa have killed up to 10% of people infected), though 18 required hospitalization.

The monkeypox scare, happily of short duration, highlights the serious danger posed by the massive—and growing—international trade in exotic animals. In recent years, shifting consumer preferences for "unusual" animal companions such as pygmy hedgehogs, African dormice, fat-tailed gerbils, ferrets, bushbabies, and many other small, furry "pocket pets"—as well as tropical fish, reptiles, and birds—have resulted in a booming market for the largely unregulated importation of wild animals from far-flung corners of the globe. Today millions of such animals reside in households all over the U.S. and, indeed, in homes all over the world, since the desire to possess a nontraditional pet seems to be universal. Unfortunately, aside from the fact that some exotics could themselves become invasive pests if they escape or are released, these new arrivals, like the Gambian rat, may be carriers of disease organisms that could wreak havoc in their new environment. Such threats are not theoretical; past outbreaks of infectious human diseases such as salmonellosis and tularemia have been linked to the commercial trade in imported reptiles and native prairie dogs, respectively. As the search for unusual pet species extends ever-deeper into formerly isolated regions of the world, it is nearly inevitable that pathogens once restricted to animal hosts will jump the species barrier to infect humans.

In spite of the seriousness of the threat, few governments have acted to regulate trade in exotic pets. In the U.S., some states—most notably California, Hawaii, and Florida—prohibit the sale of animals, especially small predators, that might become invasive if they were to escape into the wild. Elsewhere, unless an exotic animal eats plants or is on the list of endangered species banned from international trade, it's likely that its entry as an article of commerce will go unchallenged. Even where attempts are being made to control the cross-border trade in exotic species, Internet sales and transactions conducted at large trade shows and pet fairs make enforcement of existing regulations easy to circumvent. In 2001 the federal National Invasive Species Council proposed a far-reaching plan to curb importation of harmful species, but few of its recommendations have yet been acted upon by Congress.

Congressional approval wasn't necessary, however, for federal agencies to take prompt action following the monkeypox outbreak. Within days of determining the source of infection, the CDC and the Food and Drug Administration (FDA) issued a joint order prohibiting importation into the U.S. of any African rodents. The same order bans the sale and transport of both prairie dogs and of six genera of African rodents already in this country. The release of any of these animals into the wild is also prohibited. All the rodents in the April 2003 shipment from Ghana, as well as any prairie dogs that had been exposed to these ani-

mals, were immediately quarantined and CDC issued guidelines on how they should be euthanized, specifying that their bodies should be incinerated, not buried.

Thanks to quick action on the part of health authorities and the cooperation of the pet industry, the monkeypox outbreak was effectively contained with no loss of human life. Experts caution, however, that as long as exotic species continue to flood into the country to meet consumer demand, future emerging disease outbreaks are virtually inevitable. Perhaps it's time for pet lovers to resolve to stick with cats and dogs.

References

Baskin, Yvonne. 2002. *A Plague of Rats and Rubbervines*. Washington, DC: Island Press/Shearwater Books.

CDC. 2003. "Update: Multistate Outbreak of Monkeypox." *Morbidity & Mortality Weekly Report,* July 2.

lice spend most of their time on clothing, coming into contact with the human body only when taking a blood meal. A third type, the crab louse, is morphologically specialized for life among the widely spaced, coarse hairs of the pubic areas. Unlike body and head lice that constantly move about, crab lice tend to settle in one spot and feed off and on for many hours at a time. Through behavioral and territorial specialization, these species avoid competition and thrive in their own unique ecological niche.

In other situations, species may utilize the same physical space but minimize competition by restricting their feeding activities to different times of the day. Within any given area one can find some species that are diurnal (active during the day), such as most birds, grazing animals, primates, and so on; other species that are nocturnal (active at night), including most snakes, many predators such as lions, foxes, owls, and so on; and still others such as deer and rabbits that prefer the in-between hours of dawn and dusk. Structural modifications among species allow animals inhabiting the same general area to utilize different foods. The finches of the Galapagos Islands, immortalized by Charles Darwin, were very similar in appearance and obviously evolved from the same parental stock, but modifications in their beak structure permitted each species to utilize a different type of food—insects, small seeds, medium-sized seeds, or large seeds, depending on the size and shape of beak—and thus to coexist within the same geographic area.

Examples of niche diversification illustrate the fact that throughout evolutionary history ecosystems have become exceedingly complex through increasingly effective adaptation of organisms within any natural community. Such a complex ecosystem is generally quite stable unless something happens to change that environment to which the organisms have become so well adapted. The processes of natural selection and adaptation are too slow to permit the vast majority of organisms to adjust quickly to radical changes in their surroundings. When such changes occur, the animal and plant populations generally die out or move elsewhere and the previously stable ecosystem collapses or, at a minimum, becomes less varied and less stable.

Limiting Factors

Most of us intuitively realize that a specific plant, animal, or microbe can live in some places but not others. Corn plants, for example, thrive in central Illinois but not in Norway; ferns are abundant in Appalachian forests but not in the Mohave Desert; the bacterium responsible for botulism (*Clostridium botulinum*) may produce its poison in home-canned green beans but never in fresh ones. The reason why living things occur and thrive where they do depends upon a variety of conditions. Sometimes those conditions are quite obvious: summer temperatures in Norway are not hot enough nor is the growing season long enough to produce a bountiful corn harvest; lack of water and shade make survival of ferns impossible in a desert environment. In some cases the factors that control where a plant or animal lives are not quite so apparent: *Clostridium botulinum* can multiply and produce its deadly toxin only in an environment where oxygen is absent; hence it may present a threat in improperly canned foods, but seldom in fresh ones.

Environmental conditions that limit or control where an organism can live are called **limiting factors.** Obviously not every factor in an organism's environment is equally important in determining where that plant or animal can live. Components that are relatively constant in amount and moderately abundant are seldom limiting factors, particularly if the individual in question has a wide limit of tolerance. On the other hand, if an individual has a narrow limit of tolerance for a factor that exists in low or variable amounts, then that factor might indeed be the crucial determinant in where the organism can live. For example, most higher forms of life require a plentiful supply of oxygen to carry out their metabolic activities. Nevertheless, even though oxygen is essential, because it is so abundantly present and readily available to most land plants and animals it is almost never a limiting factor in terrestrial communities. On the other hand, lack of oxygen can definitely be a limiting factor for a number of aquatic organisms. The larvae of certain insects such as mayflies and caddisflies, as well as important game fish such as brook trout, simply die or move elsewhere when levels of dissolved oxygen in a waterway drop below a critical point.

Although the Native Americans who taught the Pilgrims to bury a dead fish in each hill of corn must have intuitively understood the concept, the idea of limiting factors was first formulated in 1840 by the German biochemist Justus Liebig while studying problems of fertility in agricultural soils. Liebig was experimenting with the use of inorganic chemical fertilizers in place of manures then currently in use and found that crop yields were affected not so much by the nutrients needed in large quantities—such as carbon dioxide and water, since these were generally present in plentiful supply—but by some mineral, such as copper, needed in minute amounts but lacking from particular soils. From this observation he proclaimed his famous **Law of the Minimum**, stating that "the growth of a plant is dependent on the amount of foodstuff which is presented to it in a minimum quantity." Succeeding generations of ecologists have expanded Liebig's concept to include not only mineral nutrients but also such things as light, temperature, pH, water, oxygen supply, and soil type as possible limiting factors to the distribution of organisms.

Further investigations revealed a complicating fact: when some factor other than the minimum one is available in very high concentrations, this may moderate the rate at which the critical one is used. For example, plants growing in the shade require less zinc than those growing in the sun. Thus shade-grown plants are less affected by a zinc-deficient soil than are plants of the same species growing in full sunlight. Also, some organisms can substitute a chemically similar nutrient for one that is deficient, as can be seen in certain mollusks that partially substitute strontium for calcium in their shells when amounts of calcium are low.

To make matters more complex, by the early 20th century it became clear that the old adage, "If a little bit is good, then more must be better," was quite untrue so far as the needs of living things were concerned. The concept of the Law of the Minimum was broadened by the American ecologist Victor Shelford, who demonstrated that too much of a limiting factor can be just as harmful as not enough. Organisms have both an ecological maximum and minimum, the range in between these two extremes representing that organism's limits of tolerance.

Limits of Tolerance

Subsequent investigations in regard to tolerance ranges have revealed a great deal about why certain species live where they do. Not surprisingly, those plants and animals that have a wide range of tolerance for all factors are the ones that have the widest distribution. However, some organisms can have a wide tolerance range for some factors but a narrow range for others, and thus their distribution will be accordingly more limited. Not all stages of an animal's or plant's life cycle are equally sensitive to the effect of limiting factors. Among many spore-forming bacteria, for example, high temperatures that would be almost instantly fatal for actively growing cells have no effect on the spore stage unless the duration of exposure is fairly long. In general, the most critical period when environmental factors are most likely to be limiting (i.e., when the range of tolerance is narrowest) is during the reproductive period. Susceptibility of the young to conditions that adult organisms could tolerate with little difficulty is well established in regard to acid rainfall. The low pH levels that are blamed for the near-total disappearance of many species of fish in lakes throughout eastern Canada, northeastern United States, and parts of Scandinavia have been shown to be lethal to fish eggs and fingerlings, but not to adult fish. Thus the effects of acid rain on aquatic life are much less dramatic than the effects of, for example, a chemical spill into a river. Rather than a massive, immediately visible (and smelly!) fish kill, the fish in an acidifying lake simply fail to reproduce and become less and less abundant, older and older, until they die out completely.

Other examples of the vulnerability of the reproductive stage include the observations that while adult cypress trees can grow either on dry ground or with their bases continually submerged in water, cypress seedlings can only develop in moist, unflooded soil. Similarly, some adult marine animals such as blue crabs can tolerate fresh water that is slightly salty and so are frequently found in rivers some distance upstream from the sea. Their young, however, can thrive only in salt water, so reproduction and permanent establishment of these organisms in rivers cannot occur. Among humans, the very young also display less tolerance to environmental extremes than do adults. Many widespread environmental toxins have been shown, some in tragic ways, to have a much more devastating effect on developing fetuses and young children than on adults. The drug thalidomide and organic mercury are just two substances that have been ingested by pregnant women with no harmful effects on themselves but with disastrous results on their unborn children. Levels of air pollution that are largely ignored by the adult population can cause severe respiratory distress in infants and children. It's important for us to keep in mind the qualifications to the range of tolerance concept when we hear official assurances that exposure to this or that substance is "safe." What is safe for one segment of the population may be far from safe for others.

Energy Flow Through the Biosphere

Living things are dependent for their existence not only on proper soil and c. conditions but also on some form of energy. A basic understanding of the flow energy through an ecosystem is fundamental to the study of how that system function.

The ultimate source of all life activities, from the unfolding of a flower bud to the 100-meter dash of an Olympic athlete is, of course, the sun. Some 93 million miles (150 million km) from the earth, the sun emits vast amounts of electromagnetic radiation which, traveling through space at a rate of 186,000 miles (300,000 km) per second, takes about nine minutes to reach the earth's surface. There is no energy loss as the sun's radiation travels through space, but since its intensity decreases inversely as the square of the distance from the sun, the amount of solar radiation intercepted by the earth is but one two-billionth of the sun's total energy output. On this seemingly tiny portion all life on earth depends. More than half the incoming radiation is unusable by living things, however. Electromagnetic radiation consists of several different wavelengths. Of the total amount of energy received from the sun, 9% is in the form of short-wave, high-energy ultraviolet rays; 53% is in the form of long-wave, infrared waves (heat waves); and 38% is visible light (Smil, 2002). Only those wavelengths within the visible spectrum, particularly those in the red and blue range, can be absorbed and utilized by green plants. These, through the process of photosynthesis, convert solar energy into the energy of chemical bonds. The complex and still not fully understood mechanism whereby plants harness certain wavelengths of sunlight and use this energy to join molecules of carbon dioxide and water to form the simple sugar glucose, releasing oxygen in the process, makes possible the existence of all higher forms of life. The transfer of this captured energy from organism to organism is basic to the functioning of ecosystems. Before examining the paths of energy flow, however, let us take a brief look at some physical laws that control and limit the amount of energy available to living things.

Laws of Thermodynamics

An understanding of many problems in both environmental science and energy technology depends on a basic conception of the principles that govern how energy is changed from one form into another. Known as the first and second laws of thermodynamics, these principles can be summarized as follows.

The First Law of Thermodynamics. Sometimes called the Law of Conservation of Energy, it states that energy can neither be created nor destroyed, even though it may be changed from one form into another. **Solar energy** that is absorbed by rocks or soil or water on the earth's surface is converted into **heat energy** which, because of temperature differentials and the earth's rotation, gives rise to winds and water currents that are a form of **kinetic energy.** When such kinetic energy accomplishes work such as the raising of water by wind, then it has been changed into **potential energy,** so-called because the latent energy of a water droplet in a cloud or at the top of a dam can be converted into some other kind of energy when it falls. In the same way, light energy absorbed by the chlorophyll molecules in a leaf is converted into the potential energy of chemical bonds within carbohydrates, proteins, and fats. As light energy passes from one form to another, it may appear that most of it is eventually lost or consumed (how often have we heard references to that misnomer, "energy consumption"?). This is a misconception, however, for if one maintained a global balance sheet it would show that all the energy that enters the biosphere as light is reradiated and leaves the earth's surface in the form of invisible heat waves. The form of energy leaving the system is different from the incoming radiation, but no energy has been either created or destroyed during its passage through the biosphere.

The Second Law of Thermodynamics. This law states that with every energy transformation there is a loss of usable energy (that is, energy that can be used to do work). Put another way, all physical processes proceed in such a way that the availability of the energy involved decreases (note that the availability, not the total amount, of energy is what decreases—the latter would be a violation of the First Law). The Second Law introduces the concept of **entropy,** the idea that all energy is moving toward an ever less available and more dispersed state. This process will continue until all energy has been transformed to heat distributed at a uniform temperature throughout the solar system—at which point the stable state will have been achieved.

The Second Law has some interesting implications concerning ecological relationships. Perhaps the most important of these is the fact that no type of energy transformation is ever 100% efficient—there will always be a significant loss of usable energy whenever energy is transferred from one organism to another. This explains why we need a continued input of energy to maintain ourselves and why we must consume substantially more than a pound of food in order to gain a pound of weight. In addition, because a given quantity of energy can be used only once, the ability to convert energy into useful work cannot be "recycled." Thus energy, unlike the essential minerals and gases, moves in a unidirectional way through ecosystems, becoming ever more dispersed and eventually being degraded to heat. Bearing these fundamental physical laws in mind, let's now take a more detailed look at the flow of energy through the biotic community.

Food Chains

Although overly simplistic, the concept of a **food chain** is useful for conveying a general understanding of how energy moves through ecosystems. Basically, a food chain involves the transfer of food energy from a given source through a series of organisms, each of which eats the next lower individual in the chain. In terms of energy flow, the living components of the ecosystem can be subdivided into three broad categories:

1. *Producers*—the green plants that convert the sun's energy into food energy. On land the major producers are the flowering plants and the conifers; in water they are mainly the diatoms, microflagellates, and green algae.

2. *Consumers*—animals; primary consumers are the herbivores and secondary consumers are the carnivores.

3. *Decomposers*—primarily bacteria and fungi, some insects. Decomposers are essential for recycling detritus back into the soil where it is once again available for use by producer organisms. No community could exist very long without decomposers.

There are basically three types of food chains. The most familiar of these, called a **grazing food chain** (or "predator chain"), may be typified by a grass → rabbit → fox association that starts with a plant base and proceeds from smaller to larger animals. Less conspicuous but equally important is the **detritus food chain,** where dead organic matter (detritus) is broken down by microorganisms, primarily bacteria. Small animals eat particles of this detritus, securing energy largely from assimilation of the energy-rich bacteria. The small animals, in turn, become a source of energy for larger consumers. A prime example of a detritus food chain accounting for a substantial portion of an ecosystem's energy flow can be found in the salt marsh habitat of many coastal areas. Here plants such as marsh grass die and are washed into estuaries where they are decomposed by microbes into finely divided particles which are then consumed by such primary consumers as fiddler crabs and mollusks. These, in turn, may be eaten by secondary consumers such as raccoons, water birds, or other crabs.

A variation on grazing food chains can be seen in certain **parasitic chains,** in which energy flows from larger to smaller animals (e.g., dogs that provide an energy source for fleas that in turn are fed upon by parasitic protozoans). In energy terms, however, there is no fundamental difference between a parasitic food chain and a grazing food chain, since a parasite is basically a "consumer."

Ecological Pyramids

Through the interactions of the community, a unidirectional flow of energy occurs from producers to primary consumers to secondary consumers, and so on. Each of these stages in a food chain is called a **trophic level.** It should be noted that placement of an organism into one trophic level or another depends on what that organism *does,* not to which species it belongs, since individuals of the same species may feed at different trophic levels, depending on factors such as age or sex. A male mosquito, for example, is an herbivore (primary consumer), dining on plant juices and nectar, while his mate would be classified as a carnivore (secondary consumer) when she takes the blood meal essential for egg laying. Similarly, while grazing animals such as cattle and horses are strict vegetarians as adults, their young thrive on a diet of mother's milk, making them, in effect, secondary consumers.

To describe the relationships among members of various trophic levels, ecologists frequently use the concept of **ecological pyramids.** If we examine a food chain in terms of its animal and plant constituents, it becomes apparent that these forms can be arranged into what is called a "pyramid of numbers." At the bottom of the pyramid are multitudes of energy-producing plants, then a smaller number of herbivores that feed upon them, then a still smaller number of primary carnivores, followed by an even smaller number of secondary carnivores. The animals at the top of the heap, the final consumers, are usually the largest in the community, while those organisms at the bottom of the pyramid, the producers, are usually the smallest, but much more abundant. In addition, the organisms at the lower trophic levels usually reproduce more rapidly and more prolifically than those higher up, so there is seldom danger of a predator eating itself out of its food supply. It should be noted, however, that in those cases where the size of the producer organisms is very large and the size of the primary consumers is small (e.g., a cherry tree being munched upon by hundreds of caterpillars), the shape of the pyramid of numbers may be inverted.

Just as the number of individual organisms in a community is generally greatest at the lower trophic levels, so the living weight, or **biomass** (measured as dry weight per unit area), is generally greatest at the producer trophic level. In the same way, biomass of the primary consumers will be greater than that of the secondary consumers, so the ecological biomass pyramids used to portray weight relationships among trophic levels will often look identical to numbers pyramids. Biomass, which in effect is an indicator of the amount of energy stored within an ecosystem, varies widely from one type of biotic community to another. For example, the amount of biomass in a tropical rain forest far exceeds that in a comparable area of abandoned field, while open ocean water is relatively poor in terms of biomass.

Although biomass pyramids, like numbers pyramids, usually have a broad base and tapered apex, in those situations where the organisms at the producer level are much smaller than the consumers, the shape of the biomass pyramid may be upside-down. This occurs because the "standing crop biomass" (the total dry weight of

Box 1-3   Tourism: Environmental Boon or Bane?

Tourism has been a mixed blessing for nations striving to diversify local economies by marketing the charms of their sun-swept beaches, verdant rain forests, or native wildlife. Tourist dollars (and euros and yen) have been pouring into exotic locales from Belize to Bali as developing countries vigorously promote international tourism as a means to stimulate investment and earn foreign currency. At first glance, their efforts appear stunningly successful. Travel and tourism is estimated to be the world's largest industry, employing one out of every 12 people. In the least-developed countries, tourism ranks second only to oil as a source of foreign exchange, while in some small island nations in the Caribbean and South Pacific, fully 40% of total earnings comes from international tourism. Yet such gains come at a price. The foreign investment needed to create the tourism infrastructure (e.g., upscale hotels, recreational facilities, modern airports) has increased the overall cost-of-living for local residents while providing mainly low-wage service jobs. Governments themselves frequently reap fewer benefits than expected because the foreign operators who control the tourist industry in many developing nations send most profits back to their home countries.

More obvious are tourism's negative environmental impacts. Some of the world's most unique and scenic tourist destinations are increasingly at risk of being "loved to death," degraded and polluted by the very visitors who come to enjoy their natural beauty. In many poor countries where public services such as sewage treatment, garbage collection, and provision of safe drinking water were already inadequate, the upsurge in demand posed by tourists who take such amenities for granted has only made matters worse. In tourist locales throughout the developing world, discarded plastic bottles and bags, soda cans, and food containers litter beaches and other tourist attractions. Untreated wastewater discharges from cruise ships and hotels add to the burden of pollution in coastal waters and local streams. In some chronically water-short regions, available supplies are diverted to fill resort swimming pools, launder tourists' clothes and bedding, or main-

tain lush golf courses, while local people may experience water shortages and rising utility prices. Excessive water demand can cause long-term ecological damage as well. In Israel, water levels in the Dead Sea have dropped more than 100 feet in the last 50 years, due in part to withdrawals to serve the tourist industry; some observers predict that if present trends continue, the famous inland sea could dry up completely by 2050. In numerous tropical seaside resorts such as Cancún, Mexico, construction of resort hotels, marinas, and docking facilities has destroyed coastal mangrove forests, salt marshes, and other wildlife habitats. Coral reefs are being crushed by the massive anchors of cruise ships, while careless breakage (or deliberate looting) by the rubber fins and hands of an estimated six million snorkelers and scuba divers adds to reef destruction. At many prime tourist destinations, the sheer number of visitors is the main problem. Some governments have tried to minimize human pressures on ecologically fragile sites by limiting the number of tourists permitted at any given time, but whether the limits set are sufficiently protective is open to debate.

Reacting against the despoilation and commercialization so evident at many of the currently popular vacation spots, a growing segment of the traveling public has begun to reject the more conventional "fun-in-the-sun" sites in favor of less-frequented, more pristine locations where efforts are being made to keep the "human footprint" as light as possible. Since the mid-1990s, "**ecotourism**," as this new trend is called, has become the fastest-growing segment of the travel and tourism industry. Defined by the International Ecotourism Society as "responsible travel to natural areas that conserves the environment and sustains the well-being of local people," ecotourism is closely related to the concept of sustainable development, requiring that the impact of travel on the environment and people of the host country be a positive one. Genuine ecotourism seeks to practice what it preaches, striving to minimize energy use, waste, and pollution. It also involves local people in the management of tourist enterprises, thereby channeling a substantial portion of tourism earnings back to the community. Doing so gives local people a sound economic reason to protect the land and wildlife they might otherwise exploit, since they see they can earn more money guiding tour groups or catering to other tourist needs than they ever could by hunting, poaching, or subsistence farming.

Today ecotourists can be found trekking in the mountains of Nepal, bird-watching in a Costa Rican rain forest, taking lessons in reef ecology while scuba diving off Australia, or cruising to Antarctica to view penguins in their icy habitat. The burgeoning interest in ecotourism has already prompted environmentally positive governmental actions, such as giving protected status to valuable natural areas threatened by logging, mining, or agricultural development and has created employment opportunities and training for people living nearby.

The growing popularity—and profitability—of ecotourism has resulted, predictably, in a watering-down or outright corruption of the concept by some operators. Claiming adherence to the principles of ecotourism, some providers limit their environmental commitment to using low-flow shower heads and refraining from laundering visitors' sheets and towels on a daily basis. Others stress their "green" values in promotional advertising but not in their facilities and programs. The situation has prompted a growing demand for a clear set of codified standards—a green certification program—that prospective ecotourists can rely upon to choose a travel package or resort destination that does, in fact, provide

the environmentally friendly experience they seek. Currently there are over 100 tourism certification programs worldwide, but they are based on widely differing standards, with no international guidelines to provide tourists with trustworthy, reliable information. A move is now underway to create a global accreditation body to certify the green tourism certification programs. Once such a system is in place, environmentally conscious travelers will have a valuable tool for assessing the plethora of "green tourism" claims currently confronting vacationers.

In the meantime, would-be ecotourists can make a personal contribution to environmental preservation by choosing to stay in lodgings that minimize use of electricity, water consumption, and waste generation; they can scrupulously follow rules and regulations for visitors, refrain from buying souvenirs made from endangered species, and respect local customs and manners. Tourists can be a positive force for safeguarding the world's remaining natural areas if they travel with a keen awareness of their impact on natural ecosystems and a commitment to "tread lightly on the Earth."

References

Honey, Martha. 2003. "Protecting Eden: Green Standards for the Tourism Industry." *Environment* 45, no. 6 (July/Aug).

Mastny, Lisa. 2002. "Redirecting International Tourism." *State of the World 2002*. New York: The Worldwatch Institute/ W.W. Norton.

organisms present at any one moment in time) that can be maintained by a steady flow of energy in a food chain depends to a large extent on the size of the individual organisms. The smaller the organisms, the greater their metabolic rate per gram of biomass. Thus the smaller the organism, the smaller the biomass that can be supported at a given trophic level; in the same way, the larger the organism, the larger the amount of biomass at any one point in time. This is why in, say, an aquatic ecosystem the biomass of the blue whale would be far greater than the biomass of the microscopic diatoms and zooplankton on which it feeds. The biomass pyramid that illustrates the energy relationships in such a situation would be an inverted one. This doesn't mean that the producer organisms are defying the laws of nature; it simply reflects the fact that the tiny phytoplankton have very high metabolic rates and that they reproduce much more rapidly than do whales, having complete turnovers in their populations within very short time periods.

Whereas pyramids of numbers tend to exaggerate the importance of small organisms and pyramids of biomass often understate their role, pyramids of energy give the

A tour boat carries visitors to view the tropical rain forest in Tortuguero National Park, on Costa Rica's Caribbean coast. Such "ecotourists" are the fastest-growing segment of the travel industry. [*Mathew Nadakavukaren*]

best picture of energy flow through a food chain, showing what actually is happening within the biotic community. As was mentioned earlier, light energy from the sun is captured by green plants and stored in the form of chemical bonds in the molecules of starch, glucose, fats, and so forth. However, as the Second Law of Thermodynamics states, only a portion of the energy stored by one trophic level is available to the next higher one, since a considerable amount is lost at every stage of transformation. Thus when cows graze in a pasture, some of the chemical bond energy in the grass is converted into the muscle tissue that represents stored food in the cow. The largest portion of energy derived from the grass, however, is lost in the form of waste heat during respiration. A lesser amount is lost as unassimilated food materials in feces or urine and as organic material that is not eaten by the next higher trophic level (i.e., just as people do not eat every part of a cow or pig, so many animals leave certain parts of their prey unconsumed; such "rejects" constitute an energy loss to the food chain).

At each transfer within a food chain, most of the chemical energy stored in organisms of the lower level is lost and therefore unavailable to those at the higher level. The magnitude of such energy losses ranges from a high of 99% (i.e., an energy transfer efficiency of just 1%) for most warm-blooded animals to approximately 85% for many species of insects and other small invertebrates (Bush, 2000). Since the total amount of energy entering the food chain is fixed by the photosynthetic activities of plants (and plants are less than 1% efficient, on the average, in converting solar energy into chemical energy), obviously more usable energy is available to organisms occupying lower positions in the food chain than to those at higher trophic levels. This basic fact of life explains why countries like China and India are largely vegetarian. In order to produce enough food to sustain many millions of people, such nations cannot afford the luxury of wasting the amount of energy involved in raising animals for meat. The constraints of energy transfer also explain why populations which, because of where they live, are almost exclusively dependent on meat as a food source cannot permit their numbers to grow very large. One important factor contributing to the small population size of Eskimo groups is that these people exist as top carnivores of a relatively long food chain:

diatoms ⟶ zooplankton ⟶ fish ⟶ seals ⟶ Eskimos

The preceding observations should make it readily apparent that food chains are limited by energy considerations to no more than four or five trophic levels. A food chain of unlimited length is a physical impossibility, because the higher the feeding level, the less energy there is available within a given area. An animal that is a high-level consumer must range over wide areas in order to find enough food to support itself. Eventually the point is reached where the energy required to secure the food is greater than the energy obtained by eating it. At such a point no more organisms can be supported and the upper limits of the food chain have been reached.

Of course in most real communities the actual structure of trophic levels is much more complex than the food chain concept portrays. A "food web" would be a more accurate depiction, since many organisms feed on many different species and in some cases on more than one trophic level. Humans, for example, can be quaternary or tertiary consumers by eating fish, secondary consumers when dining on roast turkey, or primary consumers when munching on peanut-butter sandwiches. The many interlocking food chains tend to promote stability for organisms at the higher levels, providing them with alternative food sources should one or more of the prey species become less abundant. In general, the more complex the food web, the more stable the ecosystem is likely to be.

Biogeochemical Cycling

Every home gardener who maintains a compost pile in the backyard intuitively understands the basic principles of biogeochemical cycling. All living organisms are dependent not only on a source of energy, but also on a number of inorganic materials that are continuously being circulated throughout the ecosystem. These materials provide both the physical framework that supports life activities and the inorganic chemical building blocks from which living molecules are formed. When such molecules are synthesized or broken down, changed from one form into another as they move through the ecosystem, their components are not lost or degraded in the same way in which energy moving through a food chain becomes unusable. Indeed, the manner in which inorganic materials move through ecosystems differs fundamentally from the movement of energy through those same systems in that matter, unlike energy, is conserved within the ecosystem, its atoms and molecules being used and reused indefinitely.

The cycling of earth materials through living systems and back to the earth is called **biogeochemical cycling.** Of the 92 naturally occurring chemical elements, about 40 are essential to the existence of living organisms and hence are known as **nutrients.** Some of these nutrients are fairly abundant and are needed in relatively large quantities by plants and animals. Such substances are termed **macronutrients** and include carbon, hydrogen, oxygen, nitrogen, phosphorus, potassium, calcium, magnesium, and sulfur. Others that are equally necessary but are required in much smaller amounts are called **trace elements.** These include such substances as iron, copper, manganese, zinc, chlorine, and iodine. The perpetuation of life on this planet is ultimately dependent on the repeated recycling of these inorganic materials in more or less circular paths from the abiotic environment to living things and back to the environment again. Such cycling involves a change in the elements from an inorganic form to an organic molecule and back again. Biogeochemical cycles are important because they help retain vital nutrients in forms usable by plants and animals and help maintain the stability of ecosystems.

Organisms have developed various adaptations to enable them to capture and retain nutrients. As we have seen in our discussion of biomes, plants in both the tropical rain forest and in desert regions have widespread, shallow root systems that permit them quickly to absorb water and the mineral nutrients that it carries in dissolved form before these can be lost through rapid runoff, competition from other organisms, or evaporation. In the tropical rain forest, for example, virtually all the mineral nutrients are retained in plant tissues and the topsoil of this biome is extremely nutrient-poor. If nutrient cycling did not occur, amounts of necessary elements would constantly decrease and would make the development of stable plant and animal populations impossible, since there is no constant addition to the source of nutrients from outside (as there is of energy in the form of sunlight).

There are basically two types of biogeochemical cycles—gaseous and sedimentary—depending on whether the primary source for the nutrient involved happens to be air and water (gaseous cycle) or soil and rocks (sedimentary cycle).

Gaseous Cycles

The elements moved about by gaseous cycles, primarily through the atmosphere but to a lesser degree in water, recycle much more quickly and efficiently than do those in the sedimentary cycle. Gaseous cycles pertain to only four elements: carbon, hydrogen, oxygen, and nitrogen. These four constitute about 97.2% of the bulk of protoplasm and so are of vital importance to life. An examination of two of these, the carbon and nitrogen cycles, gives an idea of the complexity of gaseous cycles.

Carbon cycle. Carbon atoms are the basic units of all organic compounds and hence, along with water, could be considered the most important component of biological systems. The principal inorganic source of carbon is the carbon dioxide found in the atmosphere and dissolved in bodies of water (the concentration of carbon dioxide dissolved in water is about 100 times greater than the amount present in the atmosphere; for this reason, carbon dioxide is much more accessible to aquatic organisms than to species living on land). Another large source of inorganic carbon lies in storage within deposits of fossil fuels—coal, oil, gas—but the largest amount of all occurs in the form of carbonate sediments such as limestone, formed under the seas and gradually uplifted during slow geologic processes.

Carbon is made available to living organisms through the process of photosynthesis, whereby green plants utilize solar energy to combine carbon dioxide and water, ultimately producing carbon-containing simple sugars. These constitute the basic building blocks for the synthesis of all other organic molecules. Animals obtain the carbon they need by eating plants and resynthesizing these into new carbon-containing compounds. Completion of the cycle, the breakdown of organic molecules to release inorganic carbon dioxide, is accomplished by several different pathways: (1) through the processes of respiration, whereby plants and animals take in oxygen and release carbon dioxide as a waste product; (2) through the decay of dead organisms or animal wastes, whereby bacteria and fungi decompose the carbon-containing organic molecules, releasing large amounts of carbon dioxide through their respiratory activities; (3) natural weathering of limestone; and (4) by the combustion of organic fuels (coal, oil, gas, wood). The last of these sources of inorganic carbon is causing growing concern among scientists who note that while the amount of atmospheric carbon remained relatively stable for millions of years, it has been rising significantly since the onset of the Industrial Revolution. Accelerating rates of increase in atmospheric carbon levels, especially during the past half century, have prompted warnings of world-wide climate change as the so-called "Greenhouse Effect" intensifies (see chapter 11).

Nitrogen cycle.   The major reservoirs of nitrogen in the ecosystem are the 78% of free nitrogen gas that makes up our atmosphere and the nitrogen stored in rock-forming minerals. Atmospheric nitrogen, however, is biologically inert and cannot be utilized as such by most green plants. In nature, gaseous nitrogen is returned to the soil and converted to a form accessible to plants in one of two ways.

1. Lightning passing through the atmosphere can convert nitrogen to nitrogen oxide; when nitrogen oxide is dissolved in water it can be acted upon by certain bacteria in the soil which convert it into nitrate ions that can be absorbed by plant roots.

2. Fixation of atmospheric nitrogen by *Rhizobium sp.* bacteria that live in symbiotic association with leguminous plants inside root nodules, converting nitrogen to nitrates; certain species of free-living soil bacteria (*Azobacter, Clostridium*) and some cyanobacteria (*Anabaena, Calothrix, Nostoc*) also have the ability to fix free nitrogen into nitrates.

Of these two methods, fixation of atmospheric nitrogen by bacteria is by far the most significant way of making nitrogen available to other organisms. To complete the nitrogen cycle, nitrogenous wastes in the form of dead organisms, feces, urine, and so forth, are decomposed to ammonia by other types of soil bacteria; ammonia in turn is acted upon by nitrifying bacteria that form more nitrates. Such nitrates may be taken up again by plants or further broken down by another group of microorganisms called de-nitrifying bacteria, which act upon nitrates to produce free nitrogen that is once again returned to the atmosphere.

Since the early 20th century, natural processes of cycling nitrogen have been supplemented by human activities, which have more than doubled the annual rate at which fixed nitrogen enters the land-based nitrogen cycle (little is known about nitrogen cycling in the oceans). Industrial nitrogen fixation for fertilizer production constitutes the largest human addition of new nitrogen to the global nitrogen cycle; burning of fossil fuels releases gaseous forms of nitrogen into the atmosphere from their long-term storage in geological formations; and still-expanding cultivation of such leguminous crops as soybeans and alfalfa further increases nitrogen releases to the global environment (Vitousek et al., 1997). The adverse ecological consequences of such massive new additions of nitrogen will be discussed in subsequent chapters.

Sedimentary Cycles

Many of the elements that are essential for plant and animal life occur most commonly in the form of sedimentary rocks from which recycling takes place very slowly. Indeed, such sedimentary cycles may extend across long periods of geologic time and for all practical purposes constitute what are essentially one-way flows. In comparison with gaseous cycles, sedimentary cycles seem relatively simple. Iron, calcium, and phosphorus are examples of nutrients whose cycling occurs via the basic sedimentary pattern. A brief look at the phosphorus cycle will give an idea of the transformations involved.

Phosphorus cycle.   Phosphorus, a key element in the nucleic acids DNA and RNA, as well as a component of the organic molecules that govern energy transfer within living organisms, occurs principally in the form of phosphate rock deposits. Smaller, though locally significant, amounts occur where quantities of excrement from fish-eating birds accumulate or in deposits of fossil bones. When such phosphate reservoirs are exposed to rainfall, phosphorus ions dissolve and can be absorbed by plant roots and incorporated into vegetative tissue. At the same time, much phosphorus is effectively lost from the ecosystem through runoff to the sea. Animals obtain the phosphorus they need by eating plants. When animals excrete waste products or when they die and decay, phosphates are returned to the soil where they once again become available for uptake by plants or are lost by downhill transport into the sea. Within shallow coastal areas some of this phosphorus is taken up by marine phytoplankton, which constitute the ultimate source of phosphorus for fish and sea birds. However, much of the phosphorus entering the sea is carried by currents to the deeper marine sediments where it is inaccessible to living organisms and may remain locked up for millions of years until future geologic upheavals. The large amounts of phosphate being produced commercially today for use as fertilizers come from the mining of phosphate rock. Unfortunately, much as in the case of oil or coal, such phosphate deposits constitute an essentially nonrenewable resource, since the processes responsible for their creation occurred millions of years in the past.

The fact that the general pattern in sedimentary cycling is a downhill one, where materials tend to move through ecosystems into relatively inaccessible geologic pools, poses some interesting implications for the stability of ecosystems. The loss of soluble mineral nutrients from upland areas to the lowlands and oceans is curbed only by local biological recycling mechanisms that prevent downhill loss from outpacing the release of new materials from underlying rocks. Such local recycling depends upon the return of dead organic material to the soil where breakdown and reuse of materials can occur. Human disruption of this process through widescale removal of potential nutrients (e.g., by logging, which removes trees that would otherwise have died and decayed in place; grazing of livestock that consume local resources but whose flesh, wool, bones, and so on will be disposed of elsewhere) accelerates the impoverishment of certain ecosystems where essential mineral nutrients are already in short supply. In such situations the lowlands have not benefited either, for the increased flow of materials they receive generally pass into the sea and out of biological circulation before they can be assimilated. Concern about the long-range stability of ecosystems demands that we begin to pay more careful attention to the biological recycling of inorganic materials that move in sedimentary cycles.

Change in Ecosystems

The fact that ecosystems undergo dramatic change over vast periods of time is now well accepted. Geologists have shown us how mountains are worn down and washed to the seas, forming thick layers of underwater sediments that eons later may be uplifted by immense tectonic pressures to form new mountains; deserts expand and retreat as rainfall patterns shift; and periodically great glacial ice sheets move southward, changing the face of the earth. As land forms and climate change, it is not surprising that the biotic communities within the affected ecosystems change also. It is now recognized that the biotic communities in past geologic eras differed greatly from those existing today. What is less well understood is that present ecosystems have a dynamic quality of their own, their component communities changing in an orderly sequence within a given area, a process known as **ecological succession.**

Succession

On May 18, 1980, Mount St. Helens volcano in southwestern Washington State exploded in a blast that obliterated the lush fir and hemlock forests that had blanketed

Box 1-4   Unnatural Disaster: The Aral Sea and Human Folly

A "quiet Chernobyl" is the term some use to describe the ecological catastrophe that has befallen the Aral Sea—a situation not as immediately deadly and dramatic as the infamous 1986 nuclear power plant meltdown, but equally devastating to the long-term habitability of the region. Today the former Soviet republics that border the Aral, Kazakhstan and Uzbekistan, are beset with declining harvests, powerful dust storms, climate change, and diminishing biodiversity. Their economies have collapsed and public health is plummeting, all due to misguided Soviet-era agricultural policies that are slowly destroying Central Asia's key natural resource.

A vast inland body of fresh water fed by the Syr Darya and Amu Darya rivers, the Aral Sea was once the fourth largest lake in the world. For centuries the influx of river water was just sufficient to offset water losses from the lake due to high evaporation rates, and the size of the Aral remained relatively stable. However, in the early 1960s Soviet leaders ordered the rapid expansion of irrigated agriculture throughout the Aral basin in an all-out effort to boost production of the region's "white gold"—cotton. As increasing amounts of water from the Syr Darya, Amu Darya, and their tributaries were diverted to cotton fields, the amount of inflow available to replace water losses in this naturally arid region steadily declined. Today every drop of the Amu Darya, which formerly had twice the flow of the Syr Darya, is lost before reaching the Aral. By 1989 parts of the sea had become so shallow that its basin divided into two separate parts; by the late 1990s the Aral had shrunk by 50% of its pre-1960 area, the water level had dropped 72 feet, and volume of flow into the sea was down 75%.

The Aral's water quality, as well as its quantity, also has steadily deteriorated. Salt-laden runoff from improperly irrigated farmlands has increased the salinity of the lake to the point where most of its native fish species have disappeared and a once-thriving commercial fishing industry has collapsed. The lake's environment has now been so adversely altered that experts fear the damage may be irreversible. Indeed, by 1997 the salt content of Aral water was so high

that the World Bank pronounced the sea "biologically dead."

Surrounding land areas also have suffered. As the margins of the sea recede, 20,000 square miles of salt-encrusted exposed sea bottom have provided a seemingly inexhaustible source of toxic sand—an estimated 40,000 tons annually—that is feeding dust storms so large and powerful that they are regularly tracked by Russian cosmonauts in orbit. Some of these storms may deposit their load as far as 1,200 miles away, but the greatest amount falls on areas within the Aral basin where up to half a ton per acre of salts and sand poison farmlands—and farmers' lungs—each year.

The moderating effect the Aral has long exerted on regional climate is also diminishing as the sea shrinks. Rainfall has become less frequent, temperature extremes more pronounced. The frost-free growing season in parts of the basin has now diminished to less than the minimum 200 days essential for cotton cultivation, threatening the region's economic viability. Irrigation diversions and faulty drainage practices have adversely impacted the Aral watershed far from the sea itself. Wetlands adjacent to the rivers, as well as floodplain forests, have dried up and vanished, as have many of the wildlife species that inhabited them. Salinization of soils, caused by excessive application of water without adequate drainage, has brought dissolved salts to the soil surface and significantly reduced crop yields.

The quality of the water remaining in the rivers has deteriorated to the point that it threatens the well-being of humans as well as wildlife. Runoff of phosphates, nitrates, and ammonia due to heavy fertilizer applications and contamination of drinking water supplies with toxic pesticides, chemical defoliants, and sewage is blamed in part for the scandalously high rates of infant mortality, maternal deaths, psychological disorders, and general poor state of health throughout the region. In one of the poorest areas of Uzbekistan, 97% of the women are now suffering from anemia—the highest rate in the world. The incidence of tuberculosis, an indicator of poor living conditions, is higher in this area than anywhere in Europe or the former Soviet Union. Thyroid and kidney problems, as well as liver cancer, have risen sharply since the early 1980s. Some observers warn that unless immediate steps are taken to halt the use of dangerous pesticides, provide safe drinking water, and reverse pollution of the rivers, the region may become uninhabitable.

Can the Aral be saved? In 1988 the USSR's top hydraulic engineer incautiously remarked that "it is time for all the wailing to stop. The case is closed, and the people here will have to learn to live without the sea." While the situation is dire, a recent World Bank-financed project has raised hopes of reversing at least some of the damage. In 2003 construction began on a dike intended to prevent Syr Darya water entering the Aral's small northern portion, known as the Small Sea, from flowing into its larger southern basin, regarded as hopelessly doomed due to high evaporation rates. By raising water levels in the Small Sea, engineers hope to reduce salinity levels there and submerge much of the now-exposed seabed. Improvements to waterworks along the Syr Darya that would increase the river's volume of flow are planned as well. If successful, both the local environment and the economy will benefit.

Critics of the World Bank's efforts in the region are skeptical that this latest initiative will do much to meet the most urgent needs of the 5 million people most affected. Since 1992 when international agencies first stepped in to address the Aral Sea disaster, plans for projects that would improve deplorable health and sanitation conditions have repeatedly been shelved in favor of more grandiose economic development plans for the wider region. After more than 10 years, the expenditure of millions of dollars for preparatory studies and pilot projects (many of which were discontinued or never even begun), and numerous visits by foreign advisory groups, virtually nothing has been accomplished. Living conditions have become so bad that the Peace Corps will no longer station representatives in the area and the United Nations has reduced the number of its personnel. Local people wryly joke that if everyone visiting the region to advise on how to solve its problems brought a bucket of water with them, the Aral Sea would be full again—a sad commentary on the mood of hopelessness and disillusionment prevailing in a human-made disaster area.

References

Becker, P. J. 1999. Peace Corps Volunteer, Kazakhstan, personal communication.

Feshbach, Murray, and Alfred Friendly, Jr. 1992. *Ecocide in the USSR*. New York: Basic Books.

Pala, Christopher. 2003. "$85 Million Project Begins for Revival of the Aral Sea." *New York Times*, Aug 5, D3.

Small, Ian, and Noah Bunce. 2003. "The Aral Sea Disaster and the Disaster of International Assistance." *Journal of International Affairs* 56, no. 2 (Spring).

its slopes for centuries. The collapse of the mountain's north face triggered an avalanche of mud and rocks that swept 15 miles down the Toutle River Valley, burying everything in its path under a 140-foot layer of volcanic debris. Observers surveying the scene at the time might understandably have wondered whether life could ever return to a scene of such devastation, yet within a year perennial wildflowers such as fireweed were blooming on the ash-laden mountainside. Year by year, the avalanche-affected area has become progressively greener. By the early 1990s, ecologists studying the area reported that 83 of the 256 plant species known to have been present prior to the eruption were once again thriving. While researchers concede that a return to anything resembling normal conditions will take more than a century (the area in the vicinity of the crater itself still remains virtually barren), the process of regeneration is well underway (Wilford, 1991).

The gradual, step-by-step changes over time in the relative abundance of dominant species within a biotic community following a disturbance are termed **succession** (Huston and Smith, 1987). While the sequence of events following the Mount St. Helens eruption provides one of the most dramatic recent illustrations of the process,

May 29, 1973

August 19, 1987

July 29, 2000

This series of images depicts the dramatic shrinking of the Aral Sea, once the fourth largest lake in the world. By 1989 parts of the sea had become so shallow its basin divided into two parts. [*Courtesy of USGS Eros Data Center, based on data provided by the Landsat science team*] numerous examples of succession in action can be seen all around us. While a casual glance at the plants and animals living together on a vacant city lot or an abandoned pasture may suggest an environmentally stable situation, such an impression is deceptive. If one could observe the same scene over a period of many years, it would be obvious that the composition of the area's biotic community, as well as the physical environment itself, is slowly changing in a directional manner toward a relatively stable, self-perpetuating stage called the **climax community.** Depending on the particular location involved, the changes might take thousands of years or be completed within decades, but in any case the process of change would follow a definite sequence.

The concept can be more easily understood by examining, step by step, the mechanisms of succession in a specific situation. Imagine that a retreating glacier has left behind a barren landscape of scoured bedrock or glacial till. Will the surface of the rock remain lifeless forever? Of course not; over a period of time, perhaps thousands of years if the climate is cold and dry, faster if it is warm and wet, changes in the biotic community occupying the surface of the rock will change it beyond recognition.

At first the only factors that can change the nature of the rock's surface are physical ones. Rain falls, combining with carbon dioxide in the air to form a dilute solution of carbonic acid. Bit by bit, this gradually begins to wear down the rocky surface. If the climate is a northern or temperate one, freezing and thawing may occur, helping to split the rock further. Wind erosion may also play a part. Algal and fungal spores or plant seeds will be carried to the site by air currents or by animals passing through the area, and colonies of lichens or other hardy plants establish themselves on the rock surface. The life processes of these organisms hasten the deterioration of the rock, and when the plants die, their dead organic matter contributes toward building up a thin layer of soil. These **pioneer plants** of the first stage of succession generally are small, low-growing species that can tolerate severe climatic conditions (e.g., intense sunlight, wide fluctuations in daily temperature, periodic wetting and drying), produce large numbers of spores or seeds annually, grow rapidly, and have short life cycles. While pioneer plants are quite tolerant of adverse physical conditions, they are generally intolerant of other organisms. For example, once lichens have helped to corrode rock, create a small amount of soil, and maintain better moisture conditions, mosses take over and crowd out the lichens. These may form a dense cover, attracting insects and other small invertebrates. The mosses continue to build up deposits of organic matter and soil as more rock is broken away and as the old mosses and lichens die. The most significant change these organisms can produce in an environment is that created by their own dead bodies. As decayed organic material accumulates, erosion of the rock slows down, but herbaceous plants move in and assume dominance. Insects and other arthropods will be the main form of animal life at this stage, but some small mammals and reptiles may be present also.

As succession continues, shrubs and tree saplings eventually establish themselves, and since the taller plants furnish shade and act as a windbreak, the moisture conditions of the soil and near-soil atmosphere improve and temperature fluctuations at soil level become less extreme. Gradually the shrubs become the dominant plants, shading out many of the annual herbaceous species. Corresponding animal types change also, insects perhaps becoming fewer but bird species increasing in number. As the shrub stage matures, sapling trees begin to predominate. Shade-loving plants proliferate under the canopy. The large trees that characterize the late stages of succession in forest ecosystems are long-lived species that grow slowly and tend to persist for an indefinite period of time if environmental conditions of the area remain more or less constant. This relatively stable, self-perpetuating assemblage of species represents the climax community. Of course in reality a change in environmental conditions, especially climate, is not unusual, and natural events such as fires, high winds, earthquakes, or pest outbreaks (or unnatural events such as lumbering or grazing) can create a mosaic of successional stages within a given region. It is important to note that during the successional process it is not only the composition of the biotic community that is constantly changing through time—the physical environment is being substantially altered as well. Thus succession represents a dynamic process in which abiotic factors influence the plants and animals of the community, and these, in turn, modify the physical habitat.

The preceding example of succession beginning when pioneer organisms colonize an area formerly devoid of life is referred to as **primary succession.** A less extreme but far more common situation is that of **secondary succession.** In this case, succession proceeds from a state in which other organisms are still present; new life doesn't have to start from scratch, so to speak. Even in cases where the disturbed area may appear quite barren, roots, rhizomes, or dormant seeds lying underneath the soil surface quickly initiate the process of revegetation, joined by migrant species from outside the area taking advantage of the altered conditions. In the case of Mount St. Helens, for example, buried seeds and roots gave rise to new shoots pushing through the volcanic debris as erosion thinned the overlying ash. Examples of secondary succession are legion—abandoned Vermont farmland reverting to forest, revegetation of Yellowstone National Park after the devastating fires of 1988, untended suburban lawns growing up in weeds. In such cases succession begins at a more advanced stage but proceeds, like primary succession, in a directional, more or less predictable manner toward the climax community (Stiling, 1992).

Thus far we have only referred to terrestrial succession, but the same concept applies to most enclosed bodies of water as well. A newly formed lake (e.g., one left behind by a retreating glacier) will generally have clear water with little or no vegetation or debris. Gradually silt and dead materials are deposited on the lake bottom. The sides of the lake may also be eroded by wave action and thus help fill in the deeper parts of the basin. Around the edges of the lake rooted aquatic plants such as water lilies and pickerel weed, rushes, cattails, and so forth, become established. With the accumulation of dead organic material, the supply of nutrients necessary for the growth of algae and microorganisms is increased and they flourish accordingly, providing a food source for fish and other large animals. This process of nutrient enrichment is called **eutrophication.** The speed with which this phenomenon occurs is greatly accelerated when human-produced substances such as phosphate detergents, chemical fertilizers, or sewage is introduced. Eventually, as the lake becomes more completely filled with sediment, the whole area is converted into a marsh. Terrestrial grasses and moisture-tolerant plants subsequently move in, converting the marsh into a meadow, and finally the grasses are displaced by trees, resulting in a climax community. The length of time required for such succession to take place varies widely, depending on such variables as the original depth of the basin, the rate of sedimentation, and other physical conditions that affect the growth of organisms. It should be mentioned in passing, however, that not all aquatic succession results in the establishment of a terrestrial climax community. In cases where the body of water is very large and deep or where there is strong wave action, a stable aquatic community may form and undergo no further change.

Although the later stages of succession are characterized by biotic communities better able to withstand adverse environmental conditions and more stable in terms of species composition and population, humans have generally preferred to utilize the types of communities characterized by the earlier stages of succession. In aquatic ecosystems, for example, the desirable food and game fish such as trout, bass, and perch

Figure 1-1   Primary Succession

rain weathers rock

airborne spores

"pioneer plants" (lichens)

mosses displace lichens; attract small insects

herb stage; erosion of rock almost halted now

shrubs replace herbs

climax community established

Figure 1-2 Aquatic Succession

newly-formed lake

clear water

silt and debris accumulate

sediment deepens; water becomes shallower

marsh replaces lake

marsh meadow forms

climax forest →

are all found in the clear, well-oxygenated water of deep, non-eutrophic lakes or in swiftly flowing streams. The carp that thrive in waters at a more advanced successional stage are less highly regarded. In relation to land communities, the development of agriculture and pastoralism has resulted in humans exerting increasingly effective efforts to maintain succession at an early, simplified stage. By replacing natural biotic communities with large expanses of just a few species of crop plants and through the attempt to eliminate such competitors as insects, rodents, and birds, agricultural humans have further simplified biotic communities, often undermining the stability of ecosystems in the process.

The stresses that humans are today imposing upon natural ecosystems extend far beyond the biological simplification of agricultural communities, however. The toxic pollutants being discharged into the air and water in unprecedented amounts are subjecting biotic communities to pressures with which they are evolutionarily unequipped to cope. Perhaps even more serious, the sheer increase in numbers of humans and their domestic animals is creating physical pressures that in many parts of the world are changing ecosystems in ways that are severely detrimental, not only to the biological communities which inhabit them but to human long-term interests as well.

References

Ashworth, William. 1986. *The Late Great Lakes: An Environmental History.* New York: Alfred A. Knopf.

Baskin, Yvonne. 2002. *A Plague of Rats and Rubbervines: The Growing Threat of Species Invasions.* Washington, DC: Island Press/Shearwater Books.

Blancher, Peter. 2002. "Importance of Canada's Boreal Forest to Land Birds Final Report." *Bird Studies Canada* (Dec).

Bright, Chris. 1998. *Life Out of Bounds: Bioinvasion in a Borderless World.* New York and London: W.W. Norton.

Bush, Mark. 2000. *Ecology of a Changing Planet.* 2nd ed. Upper Saddle River, NJ: Prentice Hall.

Heywood, V. H., and R. T. Watson, eds. 1995. *Global Biodiversity Assessment.* Cambridge: Cambridge Univ. Press.

Huston, M., and T. Smith. 1987. "Plant Succession: Life History and Competition." *American Naturalist* 130:168–198.

Kashefi, Kazem, and Dereck L. Lovely. 2003. "Extending the Upper Temperature for Life." *Science* 301, no. 5635 (Aug. 15).

Odum, Eugene P. 1959. *Fundamentals of Ecology.* Philadelphia: W. B. Saunders.

Pianka, Eric R. 1988. *Evolutionary Ecology.* 4th ed. New York: Harper & Row.

Smil, Vaclav. 2002. *The Earth's Biosphere: Evolution, Dynamics, and Change.* Cambridge, MA: The MIT Press.

Smith, Robert L. 1986. *Elements of Ecology.* 2nd ed. New York: Harper & Row.

Stiling, Peter D. 1992. *Introductory Ecology.* Upper Saddle River, NJ: Prentice Hall.

Vitousek, P. M., J. Aber, R. W. Howarth, G. E. Likens, P. A. Matson, D. W. Schindler, W. H. Schlesinger, and G. D. Tilman. 1997. "Human Alteration of the Global Nitrogen Cycle: Cases and Consequences." *Issues in Ecology,* no. 1 (Spring). Ecological Society of America.

Wilford, John Noble. 1991. "The Gradual Greening of Mt. St. Helens." *New York Times,* Oct. 8, B9.

POPULATION DYNAMICS

The command "Be fruitful and multiply" was promulgated, according to our authorities, when the population of the world consisted of two people.
—William R. Inge (1931)

"**S**tanding room only" is a phrase used only half in jest to describe the possible human predicament on this finite planet if present growth rates continue unchecked indefinitely into the future. Population projections based on a continuation of current growth rates reveal that within a few centuries, every human on the planet would have just one square meter of land, excluding polar ice caps, on which to live; if the world's present population size were to double twenty times, each individual would have to make do with just 0.7 millionth of an acre of arable land (Rohe, 1998). Obviously such figures represent an exercise in the absurd. Common sense observation of the world around us reveals that when populations of any organism explode, be they swarms of migratory locusts, tent caterpillars, or lemmings marching toward the sea, something, sooner or later, brings that population back into a state of relative equilibrium with its environment. There is no reason to suppose that humans, any more than locusts, caterpillars, or lemmings, can defy the laws of nature by multiplying indefinitely. Certain ecological principles govern the ways in which populations change in size. The study of such changes, or population dynamics, is of great practical importance to those who wish to predict or control the population size of other organisms or, even more important today, to forecast trends in human population growth and, if possible, guide such growth into ecologically sustainable patterns.

Population Attributes

As we saw in chapter 1, a biotic community is made up of populations of a number of different species that are bound together by an intricate web of relationships, interacting with each other and with the physical environment. Any population exhibits certain measurable group attributes that are unique to that population. Such group attributes include birth and death rates, age structure, population density, spatial distribution, and so forth. Knowing what these characteristics are for any given population is helpful in predicting how that population will change in response to changes in the environment.

Basically, assessing dynamic changes within a population largely revolves around keeping track of additions to that population from births and immigration and of losses from the same group due to deaths and emigration. Age structure of the population also must be taken into account in those species, such as *Homo sapiens*, where generations tend to overlap.

Limits to Growth

Nearly 150 years ago Charles Darwin observed in his *Origin of Species* that all organisms have a tendency to produce many more offspring than will survive to maturity. Indeed, in nature a given population of organisms tends to maintain relatively stable numbers over a long period of time. Although a single oyster may produce up to 100 million eggs at one spawning, an orchid may release a million seeds, or one mushroom may be responsible for hundreds of thousands of fungal spores drifting through the air, nevertheless, the world has not yet been overwhelmed with oysters, orchids, or mushrooms. Even much less prolific species theoretically could give rise to staggering numbers of offspring. Darwin himself cited the example of the slow-breeding elephant (gestation period of 600–630 days), showing that the progeny from a single pair would number 19 million after 750 years, assuming that all survived to reproductive age.

Obviously the increase of populations as described above could only occur in a situation where no forces act to slow the growth rate—a scenario that is virtually nonexistent in the real world, at least for any extended period of time.

The maximum growth rate that a population could achieve in an unlimited environment is referred to as that population's **biotic potential.** In reality, of course, no organism ever reaches its biotic potential because one or more factors limit its growth. Such limiting factors include food shortages, overcrowding, disease, predation, and accumulation of toxic wastes. Taken together, the environmental pressures that limit a population's inherent capacity for growth are termed **environmental resistance.** Environmental resistance is generally measured as the difference between the biotic potential of a population and the actual rate of increase as observed under laboratory or field conditions (Odum, 1959).

Population Growth Forms

In the early 1900s a number of population biologists were curious to discover what would happen to a population if most of the usual factors of environmental resistance were removed. They devised carefully controlled laboratory experiments to chart growth curves for populations where limitation of resources, predation, parasites, and other factors that normally contribute to high death rates would not come into play. Their findings revealed that populations exhibit characteristic patterns of increase that biologists call **population growth forms.** Experimentation with a wide variety of organisms has revealed two basic patterns, described as the S-curve and the J-curve.

S-Curve

A classic study in population dynamics was carried out by Russian biologist G. F. Gause in 1932 using a population of the protozoan, *Paramecium caudatum.* Gause placed one paramecium into an aquarium with a broth of bacterial cells suspended in water to provide a food supply and then carefully observed the subsequent growth of that population. He found that numbers of paramecia increased rather slowly for the first few days, then increased very rapidly for a period; finally the rate of increase began to slow and gradually leveled off as the upper limits of growth were reached and a steady-state equilibrium was achieved. The growth pattern thus revealed is that of an S-curve (sigmoid curve). The upper limit of such a curve, called the **upper asymptote,** indicates that point at which increased mortality has brought birth and death rates into balance once again (in the case of Gause's paramecia, increased mortality was due to overcrowding in the culture and the inability of the constant food supply to support all the organisms). The population density at the upper asymptote thus represents an equilibrium level between the biotic potential of that population

Figure 2-1

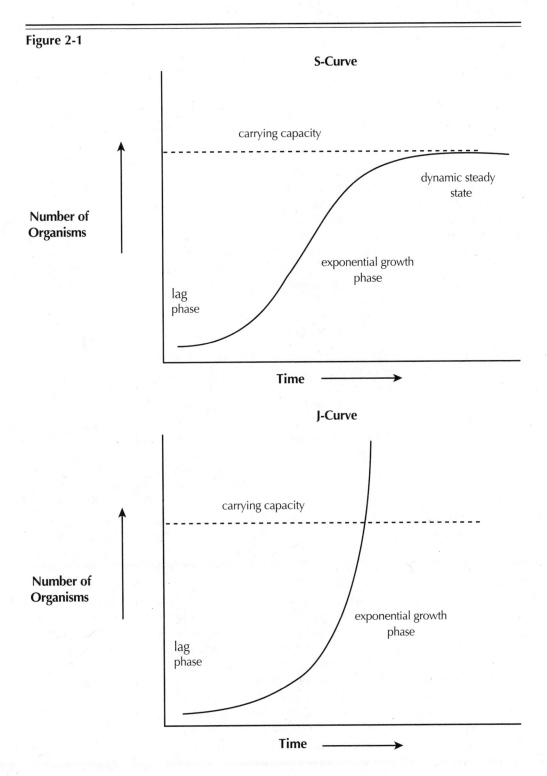

and the environmental resistance. Thus the upper asymptote of the S-curve is often referred to as the **carrying capacity** of that environment—the limit at which that environment can support a population.

J-Curve

The sigmoid growth pattern discussed above, typical of populations as diverse as microorganisms, plants, and many types of birds and mammals as well, results from the gradually increasing pressures of environmental resistance as the population density increases. Another type of population growth form, more dramatic because it frequently results in the population "crashes" that attract widespread journalistic attention, can be represented by a J-curve. In this situation population growth increases at rapid exponential rates up to or even beyond the carrying capacity of the environment. The environmental resistance becomes effective only at the last moment, so to speak, and as a result populations that have overshot the carrying capacity suffer severe diebacks. This pattern is frequently seen in many natural populations such as lemmings, algal blooms, and certain insects. It should be apparent that the early phases of growth represented by S-and J-curves are identical: a preliminary "lag" phase, during which time the rate of increase is relatively slow, followed by a logarithmic, or exponential, growth phase during which not only do the actual numbers grow rapidly, but the rate of increase also increases (in the manner of compound interest). Thus, a J-curve basically can be considered an incomplete S-curve since the sudden imposition of limiting effects halts growth before the self-limiting effects within a population become apparent.

Homeostatic Controls

Food shortage, excess predation, and disease are not the only factors that can cause populations to decline. Extensive research has shown that a number of self-regulating factors, or **homeostatic controls,** in the form of behavioral, physiological, and social responses within a population are also very important in controlling its size. Each population appears to have an optimal density, and if this optimum is exceeded a number of stress-related responses become evident. For example, it has been observed that among the snowshoe hares of northern Canada, population crashes occur at regular 9–10 year intervals even in the absence of predators, disease, or human hunting pressures. Researchers have found that during the rapid die-off phase of these oscillations, large numbers of hares suffer a stress-induced degeneration of their livers, resulting in inadequate glycogen reserves. The animals may then exhibit "shock disease," lapsing into convulsions, coma, and ultimately death (Farb, 1963).

Classic studies on the effects of overcrowding in rats have shown that even when abundant food is present, self-regulating mechanisms induce population crashes when rat populations exceed a certain density. When crowded, rats begin to exhibit abnormally hostile behavior; social interactions become pathological and fighting intensifies, often with fatal results to one of the combatants. Some individual males become hyperactive and hypersexual, attempting to mate without the customary courtship rituals and often mounting males, nonreceptive females, and juveniles indiscriminately. Pregnant females under crowded conditions frequently abort; if the young are born alive they are frequently killed by the mother or die as a consequence of neglect. It has been suggested that the cause of such deviant behavior can be traced to the effects of crowding-induced stress on the functioning of the endocrine system, which regulates hormone levels in animals. Whether the rats' response to crowding is indicative of what we can expect among human populations as our species continues to increase is open to question, but there are those who point to rising levels of violence and aggression in many parts of the world as ominous portents.

Human Population Growth

Insights gained from laboratory studies of microbial populations have an importance far transcending mere academic interest. The exponential curves tracking the growth of paramecia in biologists' aquaria or of migratory locusts in the Sahel have a parallel in the growth patterns that typify many human societies today. The fact is that

Figure 2-2

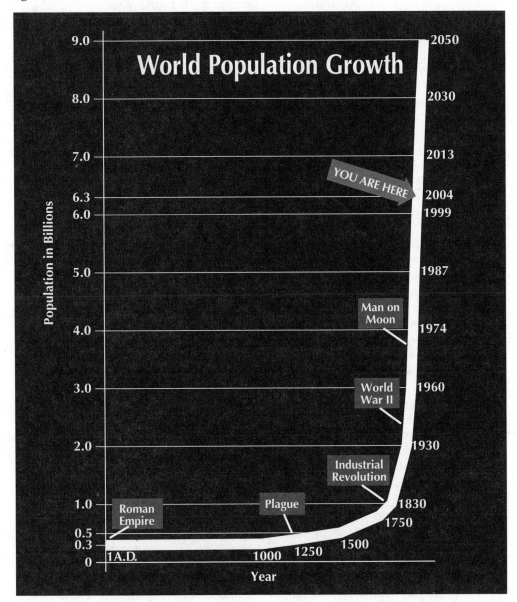

Source: Population Connection. Used with permission.

during the 20th century—and particularly during the last 50 years—the human species has experienced an unprecedented population explosion, with growth rates resembling those depicted on a J-curve. Although the average *rate* of growth is now decreasing after reaching a peak in the early 1970s (perhaps indicating that humans are S-curve rather than J-curve organisms?), in terms of absolute numbers the annual increase to the world's total population is now approximately 77 million, considerably more than the 70 million or so added each year when the "population explosion" was headline news (UNFPA, 2002). Many informed observers strongly contend that the most critical environmental issue facing humanity today—and perhaps the most difficult to tackle—is overpopulation. The explosive growth of the human species is arguably the most significant development of the past million years. No other event, geological or biological, has posed a threat to earthly life comparable to that of human overpopulation. We have little hope of significantly reducing other types of environmental degradation if present rates of population increase are not reversed.

Until recently, people who warned of an impending population/resource crunch or advocated even the mildest measures to restrain birth rates were either ridiculed, castigated, or ignored. One of the earliest to voice alarm was British clergyman-economist Thomas Malthus who, some two hundred years ago, argued that the rapid population growth his country was then experiencing was a prelude to mass misery. Demonstrating that population grows geometrically (2, 4, 8, 16, 32) while agricultural production increases only arithmetically (1, 2, 3, 4, 5), Malthus contended that population would always tend to outpace additions to the food supply, thereby condemning the bulk of humanity to a marginal standard of living and frequent bouts of famine, war, and disease. Although Malthus' "dismal theorem" stimulated a great deal of discussion at the time, his views were soon discounted when improvements in British agricultural technology and the opening of the American prairies to grain production resulted in food supply increases far exceeding the number of new mouths to be fed. As a result, Malthus' warnings were largely dismissed and forgotten. The prevailing attitude throughout the 19th century and well into the 20th viewed population growth as a desirable phenomenon, enhancing a nation's productivity, wealth, and power. Indeed, as late as the 1930s, the main population concern in the United States was that the temporary dip in the American birth rate experienced during the Depression years might indicate a worrisome *shrinking* of U.S. population size!

However, after World War II, and especially since the 1960s, concerns that population growth rates were excessive began to be expressed, first by a handful of farsighted individuals and private organizations, later by national governments and international agencies. Such concern was precipitated by the awareness that intensive efforts to improve living standards and ensure national stability in the newly independent developing nations were largely being nullified by the rapid population growth they were experiencing. Today the governments of most developing countries regard their rate of population increase as too high and have adopted policies aimed at stabilizing numbers as quickly as possible. Unfortunately, such efforts should have been launched decades earlier; the momentum of growth is now so enormous and the existing population base so large, that the ability of some countries to curb growth before national carrying capacity is surpassed is very much in doubt. In order to understand why the seriousness of our current population crisis was recognized so belatedly and why there's such a sense of urgency now, we need to look at some demographic facts.

Historical Trends in Human Population Growth

Assuming that the first humans appeared on earth between 1.5 million and 600,000 years ago, we can estimate that somewhere between 60 and 100 billion people have inhabited the planet at some time. Today the earth supports over 6 billion human inhabitants—close to 6% of all who have ever lived. We don't have enough information to estimate accurately what populations were before AD 1650, but we can make some educated guesses based on circumstantial evidence (e.g., number of people who could be supported on X square miles by hunting and gathering, by primitive agriculture, and so on). On this basis, it's been calculated that the total human population in 8000 BC was about five million people. By the beginning of the Christian Era, when agricultural settlements had become widespread, world population is estimated to have risen to about 200–300 million, and increased to about 500 million by 1650. It then doubled to one billion by 1850, to two billion by 1930, and to four billion by 1975; by 1987 world population passed the 5 billion mark, hit 6 billion late in 1999, and continues to climb. Thus not only has world population been increasing steadily (with minor irregularities) for the past million years, but the rate of growth also has increased.

Doubling Time

Perhaps the best way to describe growth rate is in terms of **doubling time**—the time required for a population to double in size. During the period from 8000 BC to AD 1650, the population doubled about every 1,500 years. The next doubling took 200 years, the next 80 years, and the next, 45 years.

Historical evidence indicates that the increase in human numbers did not occur at a steady, even pace but rather that three main surges occurred. The first took place about 600,000 years ago with the evolution of culture (developing and learn-

Table 2-1   Doubling Time of World Population

Date	Estimated Human Population	Doubling Time (in years)
8000 BC	5 million	1500
AD 1650	500 million	200
AD 1850	1 billion	80
AD 1930	2 billion	45
AD 1975	4 billion	36

ing techniques of social organization and group and individual survival); the next occurred about 8000 BC with the agricultural revolution; and the most recent began about 200 years ago with the onset of the industrial-medical-scientific revolution (Ehrlich, Ehrlich, and Holdren, 1977). Bearing in mind that changes in the size of populations occur when birth and death rates are out of balance, one can reasonably conclude that each of these spurts indicates that the story of human population growth is not primarily a story of changes in birth rates, but of changes in death rates. Let's now take a closer look at some of the demographic facts that help to explain our current population dilemma.

Birth Rates, Death Rates, and Fertility Rates

Birth rates are generally expressed as the number of babies born per 1,000 people per year. Prior to the Industrial Revolution, birth rates in every society typically were in the 40–50 per thousand range. Today the birth-rate gap between nations has widened dramatically, exemplified by Germany and Japan's 9, among the world's lowest, compared to 55, the highest, in the West African nation of Niger. Indeed, in recent years a nation's birth rate can be looked at as a crude barometer of its level of economic development, since the most prosperous, most technologically advanced countries generally are characterized by low birth rates.

Box 2-1   Is an AIDS-Induced Population Crash Likely?

Current statistics are horrifying enough: by 2004 there were almost 40 million people worldwide infected with the human immunodeficiency virus (HIV), the virus that causes AIDS; another 20 million had already died of the disease. In the absence of a massive, well-coordinated response to the epidemic, 45 million more people will be infected by 2010. Adding to the human tragedy are the 13 million AIDS orphans, children who have lost a mother or both parents to AIDS before they reached 15 and whose numbers are projected to reach 25 million by 2010. Sadly, public health officials fear that the grim toll exacted since HIV/AIDS was first described in 1981 represents but the "tip of the iceberg," warning that the epidemic is still in its early stages and continues to "spiral out of control."

Indeed, HIV/AIDS has become a **pandemic**—global in scope—affecting almost every country in the world. In regions such as the Caribbean, North America, and central Africa where the disease has been well established since the early 1980s, the infection continues to rage; in areas previously spared, HIV/AIDS is now spreading rapidly. In sub-Saharan Africa, currently home to more than 70% of the world's AIDS victims, the early focus of infection along major truck routes has now broadened to include both urban centers and rural hinterlands of all the countries in the region. Recently eastern Europe, most notably Russia and Ukraine, has witnessed a more rapid increase in HIV-infection rates than anywhere else in the world, due primarily to intravenous drug use. The AIDS threat is most explosive in the world's two demographic giants, India and China. By 2004 the number of HIV-positive Indians was estimated at 5.1 million—second only to South Africa—while China, until recently largely unaffected, is now believed to have close to a million. Health officials predict that in the decades ahead there will be more AIDS cases in these two countries than anywhere else in the world.

Just as the geography of HIV/AIDS is expanding, the sociology of the pandemic is volatile and dynamic as well. Population subgroups formerly thought to be at low risk of infection are now experiencing an alarming increase in disease rates. Once confined primarily to homosexual men and intravenous drug abusers, HIV/AIDS prevalence is rising dramatically among women and infants as heterosexual contact becomes the main route of transmission in many countries; indeed, within the last few years more women than men have become infected. Increased infection rates among women means that more children are born HIV-positive. In many African countries 5% or more of pregnant women attending prenatal classes test HIV-positive; as many as 4 out of 10 of these women will transmit the infection to their infants. UNAIDS (Joint United Nations Programme on HIV/AIDS) estimated that in 2002 three million children were suffering from HIV/AIDS.

These realities have health experts forecasting an explosion in the number of HIV infections in the years immediately ahead, with young men and women—particularly the latter—under the age of 25 destined to comprise more than half of all new victims.

While no country can afford to be complacent about AIDS, to date the disease has been most devastating to the nations of sub-Saharan Africa, all of which have infection rates of 5% or more among the adult population (2001 regional average of 8.4%). In several nations of southern Africa, infection rates are significantly higher than the regional average—over 20% of those in the 15–49 age group in South Africa, Botswana, Zambia, and Zimbabwe are now HIV-positive. The fact that HIV prevalence among young and pregnant women is well above these national averages (e.g., in the cities of Botswana, 45% of expectant mothers in 2001 were infected) suggests that overall infection rates are likely to rise further.

As the epidemic in Africa continues to rage, spreading into countries largely unaffected a decade ago, it seems relevant to question whether AIDS may provide an example of one of those forces of environmental resistance acting to bring a halt to what seems to be a runaway rate of population increase in Africa. Since heterosexual relations constitute the major route of transmission in African countries, AIDS' demographic implications are a subject of considerable speculation. If women of childbearing age sicken and die while still relatively young, total fertility rates obviously will be lower than they would have been in the absence of AIDS. Similarly, if child mortality rises because HIV-positive mothers are transmitting the virus to their babies *in utero* or in breast milk, overall growth rates should be affected.

Whether AIDS-influenced declines in growth rates will be large enough to cause an actual decrease in population size—or even a leveling off—in African countries that are currently growing at rates averaging 2.5% annually is doubtful, however. Data from Uganda, one of the first countries to be hard-hit by the HIV/AIDS epidemic, yield no evidence that the disease is having any noticeable influence yet on fertility rates. Indeed, in 2004 Uganda reported a 3% growth rate, a figure which, if maintained, would lead to a doubling of the population in just 24 years. This situation can be explained, at least in part, by the fact that death due to AIDS generally doesn't occur until 8–10 years after infection with the HIV virus. If a woman acquired her infection soon after becoming sexually active in her late teens or early twenties, she could still live long enough to bear a number of children. Although AIDS may reduce fertility to some extent (i.e., AIDS may prevent the additional births that would have occurred

were the woman to live a normal life span), researchers predict that the impact of such a decline will simply be to lower present growth rates in certain African countries to somewhere between 0.5 to 2%—rates that still represent relatively rapid growth. South Africa and several neighboring countries, however, may be exceptions to the general rule. South Africa's very high infection rate prompted the U.S. Census Bureau to project a population decline in that country, from its current 44 million to just 31 million in 2050, about half what it would have been without AIDS. Botswana already has a negative growth rate due to AIDS mortality.

While much remains to be learned about the association between HIV/AIDS and fertility, population experts generally agree that in spite of the tragic humanitarian aspects of the disease, African populations will continue to grow for the foreseeable future—not as rapidly as they would in the absence of AIDS, but grow nevertheless.

References

Barnett, Tony, and Alan Whiteside. 2002. *AIDS in the Twenty-first Century*. Palgrave MacMillan.

Lampty, Peter, et al. 2002. "Facing the HIV/AIDS Pandemic." *Population Bulletin* 57, no. 3 (Sept).

Death rates are calculated in the same way as birth rates, representing the annual number of deaths per 1,000 population. Birth and death rates are frequently referred to as "crude" rates because they don't reflect the wide variations in age distribution within a population—a fact that might result in misleading conclusions when comparing statistics from different countries. For example, the fact that the Palestinian Territory has a death rate of 4 per 1,000 population while the death rate in Italy is 10 might lead one to assume that Palestinians enjoy better health care and a higher standard of living than do Italians. Such an assumption would be erroneous, however, since the reason for the Palestinian Territory's apparent advantage is that 46% of the Palestinian population is under the age of 15—an age cohort everywhere typified by a low likelihood of death. Italy, on the other hand, is characterized by an aging population; only 14% of Italians are under 15, while 19% are over age 65 (compared to just 3% among Palestinians). Even with excellent medical care, death rates are bound to be higher in a predominantly middle-aged to elderly population than in one primarily composed of the very young.

Total fertility rates (TFR), representing the average number of children each woman within a given population is likely to bear during her reproductive lifetime (assuming that current age-specific birth rates remain constant), perhaps give a clearer picture of reproductive behavior than do crude birth rates. Although *world* TFR has

Figure 2-3   Adults and Children Estimated to be Living with HIV as of Late 2004

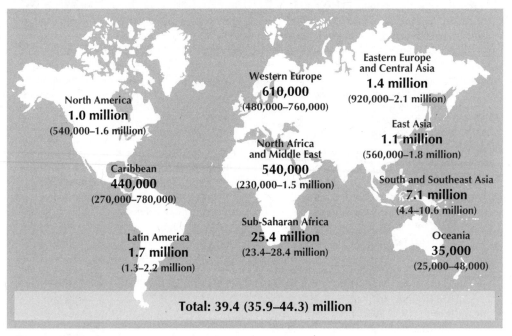

Western Europe
610,000
(480,000–760,000)

Eastern Europe
and Central Asia
1.4 million
(920,000–2.1 million)

North America
1.0 million
(540,000–1.6 million)

East Asia
1.1 million
(560,000–1.8 million)

North Africa
and Middle East
540,000
(230,000–1.5 million)

Caribbean
440,000
(270,000–780,000)

South and Southeast Asia
7.1 million
(4.4–10.6 million)

Latin America
1.7 million
(1.3–2.2 million)

Sub-Saharan Africa
25.4 million
(23.4–28.4 million)

Oceania
35,000
(25,000–48,000)

Total: 39.4 (35.9–44.3) million

Source: *AIDS Epidemic Update: December 2004*, UNAIDS. Reproduced with kind permission of UNAIDS, www.unaids.org.

been gradually falling in recent decades to its present level of 2.8, the wide discrepancies in national fertility rates are illustrated by countries such as Niger, whose total fertility rate of 8 is currently the world's highest, and by Hong Kong, whose total fertility rate of 0.9 suggests a preference for one-child families on that crowded island (Population Reference Bureau, 2004).

Growth Rates

Since birth rates represent additions to a population and death rates represent subtractions, a change in population size is represented by the difference between the two, that is, the **growth rate** (sometimes called the **rate of natural increase**). Growth rates, which do not take migration into account, can be calculated quite simply by subtracting the death rate from the birth rate. Take the case of Pakistan, for example: with a 2004 birth rate of 34 and a death rate of 10, the growth rate of Pakistan's population will be 34 minus 10, or 24 per 1,000 population. However, because growth rate is expressed as a percentage (i.e., per 100), not per 1,000 as in birth and death rates, Pakistan has an annual growth of 2.4%.

Growth rate is the critical factor to look at to get a quick impression of what is happening to a particular population. It is entirely possible that a country could have a traditionally high birth rate and still have a relatively low growth rate if the death rate is high also. In fact, just such a situation was characteristic of most human societies in the world until only a few hundred years ago.

When the average person hears that Pakistan has a population growth rate of 2.4%, the number may fail to make an appropriate impact, since most of us find it difficult to conceptualize what a 2.4% growth rate means in human terms. Besides, 2.4% really doesn't sound like very much! However, when expressed in terms of doubling time, the importance of growth rates takes on a new perspective. By calculating the annual growth rate of a population and then referring to a conversion table, we can learn what the doubling time of that population will be:

Table 2-2   2004 Population Data for Selected Countries

Region or Country	Population* (millions)	Birth Rate	Death Rate	Growth Rate, %	Doubling Time–yrs.
World	6,396	21	9	1.3	54
AFRICA	885	38	14	2.4	29
Egypt	73.4	26	6	2.0	35
Ethiopia	72.4	41	18	2.4	29
Ghana	21.4	33	10	2.2	31
Niger	12.4	55	20	3.5	20
Nigeria	137.3	42	13	2.9	24
South Africa	46.9	24	13	1.0	70
Kenya	32.4	38	15	2.3	30
Congo, Dem. Rep. of	58.3	46	15	3.1	23
ASIA	3,875	20	7	1.3	54
Bangladesh	141.3	30	9	2.1	33
China	1,300.1	12	6	0.6	120
India	1,086.6	25	8	1.7	41
Iraq	25.9	36	9	2.7	26
Japan	127.6	9	8	0.1	630
Philippines	83.7	26	6	2.0	35
Thailand	63.8	14	7	0.8	92
Turkey	71.3	21	7	1.4	50
Vietnam	81.5	18	6	1.2	58
LATIN AMERICA	549	22	6	1.6	45
Argentina	37.9	19	8	1.1	66
Brazil	179.1	20	7	1.3	54
Colombia	45.3	23	6	1.7	41
Cuba	11.3	11	7	0.5	144
Mexico	106.2	25	5	2.1	33
Panama	3.2	23	5	1.8	38
Peru	27.5	23	6	1.7	41
Venezuela	26.2	24	5	1.9	36
NORTH AMERICA	326	14	8	0.6	114
Canada	31.9	11	7	0.4	162
United States	293.6	14	8	0.6	114
EUROPE	728	10	12	–0.2	—
France	60.0	13	9	0.4	180
Germany	82.6	9	10	–0.2	—
Ireland	4.1	16	7	0.8	84
Italy	57.8	10	10	–0.1	—
Poland	38.2	9	9	–0.0	—
Russia	144.1	10	17	–0.6	—
Spain	42.5	10	9	0.1	716
United Kingdom	59.7	12	10	0.1	716
Ukraine	47.4	9	16	–0.8	—

*(mid-2004)
Source: Population Reference Bureau, 2004 World Population Data Sheet.

Growth Rate	Doubling Time
0.5%	140 years
0.8%	87 years
1.0%	70 years
2.0%	35 years
3.0%	24 years
4.0%	17 years

Thus, with an annual growth rate of 2.4%, the population of Pakistan, already at 159 million, will double in just 29 years. In human terms this means that *just to maintain present standards of living* everything in Pakistan needs to be doubled in 29 years—food production, provision of jobs, educational facilities, medical personnel, public services, and so forth. Whether such a Herculean task can be accomplished remains to be seen; certainly the leaders of Pakistan (and of a great many other nations whose doubling times are similarly brief) face a formidable challenge in the decades ahead, especially at a time when the "revolution of rising expectations" has created a grassroots demand for improved living standards, not just maintenance of the status quo.

Population Explosion

With a basic understanding of what birth, death, and growth rates imply, let us now turn our attention to the crucial question of why growth rates have so accelerated during the past several generations. Surveying the history of human population growth (an admittedly risky enterprise, particularly for the prehistoric period), we can say with a fair degree of certainty that birth rates throughout the world were uniformly high until relatively modern times. (Some anthropologists doing research among contemporary hunter-gatherer societies have forwarded the idea that, prior to the agricultural revolution, birth rates among primitive peoples were lower than among subsequent agricultural societies. This they attribute to environmental restraints causing such groups to attempt to space the births of their children.) Even today, while birth rates in most parts of the world are gradually declining, women in most sub-Saharan African nations continue to bear children at traditionally high levels.

With birth rates having apparently held steady during most of human history, we must look then to changes in death rates to explain why growth rates have shot upwards. Each of the three major changes in human lifestyle mentioned earlier effected a decline in the death rate. Cultural advances among prehistoric humans probably reduced the death rate to some slight degree, but the consequences of this cultural evolution were minor compared with the changes wrought by the agricultural revolution. The increase in food supply, the more settled mode of existence, and the general rise in living standards are thought to have reduced mortality rates and increased life expectancy to some degree over that of primitive peoples.

Even so, the gains were gradual until about 200–300 years ago when improvements in public sanitation, advances in agriculture, and the control of infectious disease resulted in a precipitous decline in death rates, particularly in regard to infant and child mortality.

The growth in human numbers that resulted from these improved conditions was not, of course, a steady, uninterrupted rise. Wars, famine, and disease provoked periods of sharp population declines among localized groups. Certainly the most spectacular reversal of the overall growth trend was the impact of bubonic plague (the notorious "Black Death" of the Middle Ages) on the societies of Europe. Plague first reached the Continent in AD 1348 and within two years had killed approximately

India's population crisis is fueled by a growth rate that could lead to a doubling of its current size in just 41 years. [*Agency for International Development*]

25% of the total population. Successive outbreaks of the disease continued to sweep across Europe during the next several decades, during which time the population of England dropped by nearly one-half (two-thirds of the student body at Oxford University died during one episode of plague), and many regions in both Europe and Asia were similarly decimated. Nearly constant warfare and the disease and famine that frequently accompanied such conflict also had a negative influence on population growth. Particularly devastating in terms of civilian suffering was the Thirty Years' War (1618–1648), during which time it is estimated that as many as one-third of the inhabitants of Germany and Bohemia died as a direct result of the war. Outside of Europe, warfare, even prior to the World Wars of the 20th century, resulted in enormous loss of life. Conquest and subjugation of Native American civilizations by European colonizers, tribal warfare in Africa, the Moghul invasion of Hindu India, and centuries of internal strife in China resulted in high death rates and sometimes severe depopulation within the affected groups. Perhaps the most extreme example of a population being decimated by warfare involves the most bloody, savage war ever fought in South America. This five-year conflict, which ended in 1870, pitted the combined forces of Brazil, Uruguay, and Argentina against those of Paraguay. The result was virtual extinction for the Paraguayans, whose army was outnumbered 10 to 1 and included 12-year-old boys fighting alongside their grandfathers. Within a five-year period, the population of Paraguay dropped from an estimated 525,000 to 221,000, of whom slightly less than 29,000 were men. A new generation of Paraguayans was sired courtesy of the Brazilian army of occupation (Herring, 1960).

Such examples, while tragic in terms of individual suffering, and occasionally disastrous to certain ethnic groups or nationalities (e.g., the total extermination of native Tasmanians by white settlers), nevertheless represented only minor aberrations from the general upward trend. In general, world population has increased more or less steadily, at first quite slowly but subsequently faster and faster from ancient times right up to the present.

Demographic Transition

By the latter half of the 19th century, western Europe began to witness a demographic phenomenon unlike any that had occurred previously anywhere in the world. Toward the end of the 1700s and early in the 1800s, as the Industrial Revolution began transforming an entire way of life, death rates started to fall gradually in response to a more adequate food supply, improved medical knowledge, better public sanitation, and so forth. As a result, growth rates predictably accelerated, and during the early years of the 19th century western Europe experienced a population boom. This led, among other things, to massive emigration to the Western Hemisphere. By approximately 1850 another rather surprising trend became apparent: throughout the industrializing nations of that era, birth rates began to fall for the first time since the agricultural revolution. The Scandinavian countries (which were among the first to compile accurate demographic records) provide a good example of the changes that were occurring. In Denmark, Norway, and Sweden the combined birth rate was about 32 in 1850; by 1900 it had dropped to 28 and today stands at 12, among the lowest in the world. Elsewhere in western Europe similar declines were becoming apparent. This phenomenon—the falling of both birth and death rates that has characteristically followed industrialization—marked the onset of the **demographic transition**, a trend that accelerated throughout the 20th century. By the 1930s, decreases in the birth rates in some countries had outpaced decreases in death rates, though actual birth rates remained somewhat higher than death rates.

Reasons for the demographic transition are still being debated, but the cause for declining birth rates probably centers on the realization by married couples that in an industrial society children are an economic liability; they are expensive to feed, clothe,

Figure 2-4 The Classic Stages of Demographic Transition

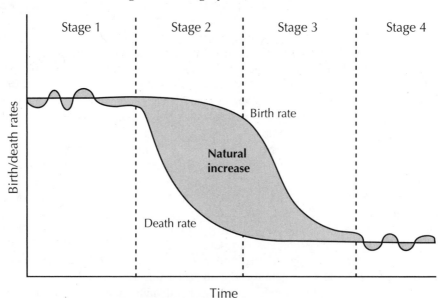

Source: "Population: A Lively Introduction" by Joseph A. McFalls, Jr., *Population Bulletin* 58, no. 4 (Dec. 2003). Used with permission of the Population Reference Bureau.

and educate; they reduce family mobility and make capital accumulation more difficult. In rural areas of Europe, population pressures on a finite amount of land and the modernization and mechanization of farming techniques, which reduced the amount of manual labor needed, combined to bring about a reduction in rural birth rates also. In addition, during the late 1800s and into the 20th century, a trend toward marrying at a later age undoubtedly contributed to the decreasing birth rates.

The decline in both birth and death rates that marked the demographic transition in western Europe became noticeable in both eastern Europe and North America several decades later. Today Russia and most of the formerly Communist nations of eastern Europe have some of the lowest birth rates in the world, attributed in large part to poor economic conditions that have convinced young women that now is not the time to start a family. Recently, however, in Russia and several other former Soviet republics, the decline in mortality rates experienced almost everywhere else in the world has been reversed. Due largely to rampant alcoholism and a deteriorating health care system, death rates, especially for Russian men, have risen dramatically since the mid-1960s; infant mortality has increased also, far surpassing that of other industrialized countries. By 2004, 13 out of every 1,000 Russian babies were dying before their first birthday, compared to 6.7 in the United States and just 3 in Japan. This situation of falling birth rates and rising death rates has resulted in an unprecedented population decline in that region of the world. In North America today, Canada's demographic statistics mirror those of western Europe. The United States, by contrast, outpaces all other industrialized countries in its rate of population growth, in part due to a slightly higher birth rate and record-high levels of immigration.

In the nations of Asia, Africa, and Latin America where traditional societies were only marginally influenced by the dynamic economic and social changes occurring in Europe and North America, demographic patterns changed very little until early in the 20th century. In the areas under the control of imperial powers, improvements in public sanitation and an imposed peace between formerly warring factions within the subject nations permitted a gradual increase in population levels. This gradual decline in death rates took a quantum leap in the years immediately following World War II as modern drugs and public health measures were exported from the industrialized nations to the developing countries. Virtually overnight, the widely applauded introduction of "death control" into traditional cultures produced the most rapid, widespread change known in the history of population dynamics. The situation in Sri Lanka (formerly Ceylon) is a good case in point.

Prior to World War II, a major killer in many tropical countries was the mosquito-borne parasitic disease, malaria. In Sri Lanka a malaria epidemic during 1934–1935 may have been responsible for half the deaths occurring in the country that year (Sri Lanka had a death rate of 34 during that time period). Not only did many victims die outright, but many others were so debilitated by their bouts with the recurring cycles of chills and fever that they became more susceptible to other illnesses. Thus malaria was a contributory cause of death in some cases and a primary cause in others. In 1945, at the end of World War II, the death rate in Sri Lanka stood at 22. One of the great technological innovations to rise out of the war was introduced into Sri Lanka—the synthetic chemical insecticide DDT. Wide-scale spraying with DDT brought rapid control over the mosquitoes, with a corresponding plunge in the incidence of malaria. As a result, the death rate on the island was cut by more than half within a decade and has continued to drop since then to its present low of 6. Thus, the number of Sri Lankans has soared upwards.

Victory over malaria, yellow fever, smallpox, cholera, and other infectious diseases has been responsible for similar decreases in death rates throughout most of the underdeveloped world. This trend has been most pronounced among children and

Box 2-2   Seeking Greener Pastures: International Migration

In late June 2000, customs officials at the British port of Dover were horrified to discover the bodies of 58 Chinese stowaways amidst a cargo of tomatoes in a sealed truck container just arrived from Zeebrugge, Belgium. One of just two survivors told authorities of the desperate migrants' futile efforts to attract attention to their plight after the truck's refrigeration unit was turned off, leaving them to suffocate slowly on one of Europe's hottest days.

This shocking incident of human trafficking was neither the first nor the last in an ongoing saga of human willingness to take desperate, sometimes fatal, gambles in an effort to find employment and a better life far from an impoverished homeland. From U.S.-bound Mexicans risking death in the Arizona desert to Afghanis on floundering boats seeking illegal entry to Australia, the large-scale movement of economic migrants and refugees across national borders is a demographic phenomenon of growing importance.

Historically, up-or-down changes in birth or death rates have been the main determinants of fluctuations in population size over time. In recent decades, however, international migration has become a key factor as well. By the first decade of the 21st century, approximately 3 million people each year were leaving their native lands to settle elsewhere. In doing so, they have a profound impact on the demographic situation of the receiving country, not only in terms of age structure (most migrants are young adults) and gender balance (primarily male in such receiving areas as the Persian Gulf oil sheikdoms and the mining areas of southern Africa), but also in terms of sheer population size.

Not counting refugees, the United Nations estimates that by 2000 at least 168 million people were living outside their country of birth, up from 75 million in the mid-1960s. While approximately half of all international migrants move from one developing country to another, the impact of international migration is most keenly felt in the nations of the developed world. Today only five major countries officially welcome migrants from other countries as permanent residents: the United States, Canada, Australia, New Zealand, and Israel.

Collectively, these nations admit 1.2 million legal immigrants annually. However, since the 1960s Europe—once a major exporter of migrants—has become a prime destination for millions of guest workers, refugees, and immigrants from Asia, Africa, the Middle East, and, most recently, eastern Europe and the lands of the former Soviet Union. Even Japan—probably the world's most homogenous nation—currently hosts almost 700,000 foreign workers.

Reasons for the vast population shift are numerous, but can be roughly divided between economic and noneconomic considerations, further influenced by the interaction among "push," "pull," and network factors. The millions of Mexicans and Central Americans leaving their native lands for "El Norte" are attracted by the prospects of higher wages and a more secure economic future. Similarly, the mass migration of Turks to Germany to take advantage of that nation's guest worker program or of Filipina nurses to fill urgently needed staff positions in hospitals throughout the U.S. and Canada were prompted by the "push" generated by poor economic conditions at home and the "pull" of worker-recruitment efforts in the receiving countries. Over time, migrant flows to specific foreign destinations are reinforced by networking, whereby earlier emigrants facilitate the later migration of family members and friends by providing them with information, temporary lodging, even financial assistance.

Noneconomic forces encouraging international migration include, most notably, war and political or religious persecution. The influx of Vietnamese into the U.S. following the Communist takeover of South Vietnam in 1975 is a classic example. Fear of political repression and persecution has sent Cubans to Miami, Sri Lankan Tamils to Switzerland, and Hong Kong Chinese to Canada. Its promise as a haven from religious persecution of Jews has resulted in Israel's having one of the world's highest annual net immigration rates.

International migration has begun to have a marked impact on the ethnic composition of several receiving nations, provoking worries that the influx of alien newcomers may have a deleterious impact on local economies and culture. Immigration has become a hot domestic policy issue in several European countries and has given rise to far-right political movements with a distinctly antiforeign flavor. Anxieties have grown with the increasing percentage of foreign-born residents within populations that until recently were largely homogeneous. Today 9% of the residents of Germany, Austria, and Belgium are foreign-born; that percentage rises to 19% in Switzerland and fully 36% in tiny Luxembourg. Immigration is changing the ethnic composition of the U.S. as well. During most of the 19th and 20th centuries, immigrants to the U.S. were overwhelmingly of European origin; since the 1990s, however, over 80% came from either Latin America (51%) or Asia (30%).

Perhaps the most profound consequence of high immigration rates will be the long-term effect on the ultimate population size of the receiving nations. Already the impact is becoming apparent in low-birth-rate western European countries where immigration has been the major force restraining population decline. Some European leaders argue that new immigration policies welcoming foreign residents are urgently needed to bolster the labor force and save social welfare programs for the burgeoning elderly population. Research carried out by the UN Population Division, however, indicates that unless the annual influx of immigrants increases threefold (from 237,000 to 677,000), the populations of Germany, France, Italy, and the U.K. (the four countries that attract 88% of all immigrants to Europe) will continue to decline. To retain current labor force levels in those countries, the number of immigrants admitted annually would have to exceed 1 million, and to "save social security" that fig-

ure would have to rise to almost 9 million. Given existing attitudes, few expect that European policymakers will agree to such a drastic increase in immigration even to avert inevitable population decline. Nevertheless, in Europe as well as in all the other countries of destination, migrants have augmented the population base and kept national fertility rates higher than they would have been otherwise, postponing eventual population stabilization or decline.

In the United States, where fertility rates among native-born citizens hover around replacement level, 40% of total population growth by the early 21st century was due to immigration, with over a million new residents entering the country each year. Projections indicate that by 2050, fully 15% of the U.S. population—60 million people— will be foreign-born. Past assumptions that U.S. population growth rates would soon mirror those of Europe and that zero population growth would be achieved early in the 21st century have now been abandoned, thanks largely to the impact of immigration.

In many countries around the world, governments now view their immigration levels as too high; nevertheless, given a likely intensification of push/pull factors in the years ahead, transboundary migration seems certain to continue.

References
Martin, Philip, and Elizabeth Midgley. 2003. "Immigration: Shaping and Reshaping America." *Population Bulletin* 58, no. 2 (June).
Martin, Philip, and Jonas Widgren. 2002. "International Migration: Facing the Challenge." *Population Bulletin* 57, no. 1 (March).

young adults. Since 1960, according to a World Bank report, the number of children who die before reaching their fifth birthday has declined by two-thirds, thanks to greater public access to standard immunizations and oral rehydration therapy for treating diarrheal diseases (Altman, 1993).

This decline in death rates was qualitatively different from the slow, long-term decline that occurred throughout most of the world following the agricultural revolution. It was also different in kind from the comparatively more rapid decline in death rates in the Western world over the past century. The difference is that it came about in response to a spectacular environmental change in the nations of Asia, Africa, and Latin America largely through the control of infectious diseases, not through a fundamental change in their institutions or way of life. Furthermore, the change did not originate in these countries themselves, but was introduced from the outside. The importation of death control without corresponding adoption of birth control in the mid-20th century resulted in a large portion of humanity moving rapidly from a situation of high birth and death rates to one of low death rates but still-high birth rates— and a corresponding explosive increase in total population size. By the 1960s and 1970s, alarmed observers like population biologist Paul Ehrlich were referring to this phenomenon as the "population bomb" and forecast dire consequences for scores of developing nations apparently stymied by cultural and economic realities that suggested their fertility rates would remain well above replacement level indefinitely. However, by the 1980s and 1990s, a steady decline in fertility in almost all developing nations—except those in sub-Saharan Africa—was well underway, signaling that the demographic transition was indeed a near-universal phenomenon. Today, even in nations where levels of economic development remain low, access to modern contraceptives and greater employment opportunities for women have resulted in larger-than-expected fertility declines within the past two decades. Nevertheless, it will take at least another generation or two for most developing nations to complete their demographic transition, characterized by replacement-level fertility and a stable population size. In the meantime, the demographic gap between developed and developing nations continues to widen. According to the United Nations Population Division (UNFPA, 2002), fully 97% of world population growth is occurring in developing countries that already are finding it difficult to support current numbers, let alone the additional millions projected for the decades immediately ahead.

Age Structure

It's relatively easy to comprehend the significance of birth and death rates so far as population growth is concerned, but there are other characteristics of a population that are important also. Age structure refers to the number of people in different age categories within a given population. In countries where populations are growing rapidly because of high birth rates and declining death rates, a large percentage of the population is made up of young people; in many African and Asian countries, 40% or more of the population is under the age of 15. In western Europe, by contrast, there are proportionately many more people in the middle and older age groups. In countries where children comprise a large segment of the population, there hasn't been time yet for individuals born during the period of "death control" to reach the older age groups where death rates are higher than those of the younger age categories. In most of these countries the greatest decreases in death rates among infants and children occurred in the late 1940s and the large numbers of children born in that period reached their peak reproductive years in the 1970s. Their children, in turn, are further inflating the lower tiers of the population structure. The extraordinarily large percentage of children that characterizes the current population of most developing countries accounts for the fact that their death rates today are as low as, or lower than, death rates in the industrialized countries where a significantly larger percentage of the population is elderly.

One of the most significant features of age structure in a population is the proportion of people who are economically productive (arbitrarily considered to be those persons between 15 and 59) in relation to those who are dependent on them. The proportion of dependents in the underdeveloped countries is much higher than in the developed nations, presenting an additional heavy burden to those countries as they struggle for economic development. The high percentage of people under 15 is also indicative of the explosive growth potential of their populations. In most developing nations this percentage is 35–40%, while in Uganda children comprise fully 51% of the population! By contrast, the percentage under 15 in most industrialized countries

Box 2-3 Global Graying

While leaders of the developing nations struggle to meet the needs of still-growing populations, their counterparts in the industrialized world are facing an entirely different problem: a disproportionate and rapidly increasing percentage of elderly citizens as the "baby bust" generates ever-smaller cohorts of young people. Thanks to improved health care, nutrition, and general standard of living, today's elderly are experiencing a degree of longevity unprecedented in human history. Indeed, it's estimated that in all of human history, two-thirds of all the people who have ever reached age 65 are living today. Global life expectancy has lengthened more in the last 50 years than it did throughout the previous 5,000. Until the onset of the industrial era, only 2–3% of people born lived beyond age 65; today in developed countries that figure is 15% and rising. By 2030, the United Nations estimates that fully one-quarter of the planet's population will be in the "senior" category.

While "global graying" is underway in virtually every country, nowhere are the effects more acutely felt at present than in Japan and Europe. Characterized by plummeting birth rates and excellent health care, those countries have been witnessing a steady decline in the proportion of young people and a simultaneous swelling of the ranks of the elderly. The statistics are truly astounding: Italy now has more citizens over 60 years old than it has under the age of 20—the first nation in history to experience such a transformation in age structure. In what one commentator refers to as the "Floridazation" of the developed world, many countries have or will soon attain the 19% elderly population that already characterizes the "Sunshine State." Italy, Greece, and Japan have already reached that benchmark and will soon be joined by Germany, Belgium, and Spain; by 2016 France and the United Kingdom will be added to the list (higher fertility rates in the U.S. and Canada should postpone their year of reckoning until 2021 and 2023, respectively).

So why should these trends cause any concern? After all, humans have always considered long life among the greatest of blessings, and for years environmentalists and population control advocates have preached the virtues of small family size. Now that these goals have been attained, at least in some countries, why isn't there universal rejoicing? Certainly from an ecological standpoint the news *is* good, since all of the countries in question could be considered overpopulated in terms of their environmental impact. Any reduction in population size can only improve congestion, levels of pollution and consumption, and impact on ecosystems. Worries about global aging trends focus primarily on economic and socio-political considerations, with some analysts predicting that this unprecedented demographic age shift promises to become the overriding economic and political issue of the 21st century.

Paramount among the issues involved is the impact on retirement benefit systems. Like the U.S. Social Security System, the "safety net" social programs in place in most industrialized nations were created at a time when average life expectancy was less than the legal retirement age and when the ratio of young workers to retired persons was heavily weighted toward the former group. Most social security schemes, in essence, borrow from today's workers to support today's retirees. However, as the retired population grows larger and the proportion of young people in the population shrinks, the economic burden on working-age men and women will become increasingly heavy. Today throughout the industrialized world there are three working taxpayers for every retired person. However, unless national retirement systems are radically reformed, by 2030 there will be only 1.5 workers for every pensioner. In negative-growth countries like Italy and Germany the ratio will be just 1:1. While American politicians debate how to "Save Social Security," the dilemmas confronting leaders in Europe and Japan are even more urgent. With lower birth rates, more rapidly aging populations, larger public pension benefits, and weaker private pension systems than in the U.S., Europeans and Japanese will be hard pressed to preserve social programs and a high standard of living. Health care costs in an aging world will be even more burdensome than pensions. Since the elderly consume three to five times more health care services per person than do younger citizens, health care spending is likely to soar. Experts predict that to meet existing old-age benefit commitments, within the next 30 years developed nations cumulatively will have to spend an extra 12–13% of GDP. Fears are that this unprecedented burden could destabilize the global economy, threatening financial and political institutions worldwide.

Global graying presents national security concerns as well. Whether developed countries remain able to maintain their military commitments in light of a shrinking pool of potential soldiers and sailors is as yet an unanswered question. Pressure to relax immigration restrictions to ease worker shortages could mount in some countries, in turn creating more strife and political turmoil in areas where an ethnic imbalance is already provoking nationalistic resentment.

In an effort to forestall such problems, several European nations, most notably France and Sweden, have implemented economically costly incentives to encourage childbearing. For the most part, however, such programs have had minimal long-term effects on fertility in societies where young women frequently view children as impediments to a career and an expensive inconvenience.

Whether or not current developed-world attitudes become more pronatalist in the future (and there's no indication they will), global graying is inevitable in the decades ahead because the elderly of 2050 have already been born. The implications of this trend—for society, the economy, and for the environment—will be profound in ways we can now only dimly foresee. As Nicholas Eberstadt, a demographer at the American Enterprise Institute remarked: "What is happening now has simply never happened before in the history of the world. . . . If these trends continue, in a generation or two there may be countries where most people's only blood relatives will be their parents."

References

Peterson, Peter G. 2002. "The Shape of Things to Come: Global Aging in the Twenty-First Century." *Journal of International Affairs* 56, no. 1 (Fall): 189–210.

———. 1999. "Gray Dawn: The Global Aging Crisis." *Foreign Affairs* 78, no. 1 (Jan/Feb): 42–55.

is 20%. In the United States, for example, there are two people of working age for every one who is too young or too old to work; in Mexico and Nigeria there is only one. Thus, underdeveloped countries have a much greater proportion of people in their pre-reproductive years. As they grow up and marry, the size of the childbearing fraction of the population will increase tremendously and their children will further inflate the size of the youngest age groups. The existence of such large numbers of young people means that even if great progress were made immediately in reducing the number of births per female in those countries, it would still be some 30 years before such birth control could significantly slow down population growth.

For those nations that have recently experienced rapidly declining fertility, there may be some positive short-term economic consequences resulting from their shifting demographic profile. As their large current crop of youngsters enters the workforce and is replaced at the bottom of the age structure pyramid by a much smaller cohort of "baby-busters," economic development could soar, just as it did in South Korea, Taiwan, and Thailand when their fertility rates began a free-fall a few decades ago. Economists are urging leaders in these countries to take advantage of this "demographic dividend"—a narrow window in time when the working-age population will be at an all-time high in relation to the number of young children and elderly citizens. A lower dependency load during this once-only opportunity will facilitate higher savings and investment, providing that governments develop wise economic policies and invest adequate resources to improve education, health care, and the status of women. If they let this opportunity pass, the "window" will close as the ranks of the elderly steadily climb (Sheehan, 2003; "Economics Focus," 2002).

Figure 2-5   Age and Sex Distribution in More and Less Developed Regions

More developed regions

Less developed regions

Least developed countries

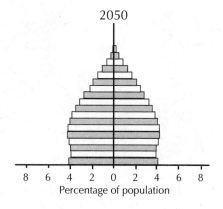

Source: The Sex and Age Distribution of the World Populations: 1998 Revision, Vol. II: Sex and Age. United Nations (medium variant projections). Used with permission.

In many Third World countries children make up nearly 50% of the population, indicative of the explosive growth potential in those nations least able to provide for a rapidly growing population. [*Agency for International Development*]

Urbanization

The "urban explosion," referring to the tremendous population increase in metropolitan areas, has been one of the most marked phenomena related to the overall growth of human populations during the past century. Urbanization is, of course, one of the oldest of demographic trends, having its roots in the small settled communities made possible by an agricultural way of life. The first true cities are believed to have arisen in Mesopotamia about five or six thousand years ago, but growth of urban areas proceeded rather slowly during the millennia that followed. Increase in urban populations depended almost entirely on an influx of new residents from the surrounding countryside. Due to extremely poor sanitary conditions and crowded living conditions, mortality rates in these urban centers were higher than birth rates, and not until recent times have urban centers become self-sustaining in terms of population growth.

The advent of the Industrial Revolution gave a tremendous impetus to the growth of cities, and the rate of increase has continued to accelerate ever since. As an example of the great population shift that has occurred, consider the change in rural-urban ratios in the United States: in 1800 a mere 6% of all Americans lived in an urban area; the number of city dwellers increased to 15% by 1850 and to 40% by 1900. In 2004, 79% of the U.S. population lived in cities. [Note: in the United States, "urban" is defined as any community with a population of 2,500 or more. Different countries use different cutoff points to distinguish "urban" from "rural" populations, complicating the comparison of urbanization statistics from various parts of the world. For example, while American demographers utilize the 2,500 figure, their colleagues in Iceland consider a village of 200 as "urban"; in Italy the corresponding number is 10,000, while in densely populated Japan, a community is considered "urban" only when its population surpasses 50,000! (Haub, 1993).]

In the world as a whole, population increased by a factor of 2.6 during the years between 1800 and 1950; during that same time period the number of people living in cities over 20,000 population grew from 22 million to over half a billion—a factor of 23. In the largest cities (100,000 or more) of the industrialized countries, the growth was even more rapid, increasing by a factor of 35. By 1950, 29% of the world's people lived in cities; by 2004 the percentage of urban dwellers in the world had risen to 48 and is expected to reach 50% by 2007 (UNFPA, 2002).

In recent years this urban expansion in the developed world has slowed somewhat, but since 1900 has accelerated at a great rate in the nations of Asia, Africa, and Latin America, fueled in equal measure by natural population growth within cities and by in-migration from rural hinterlands. While the annual urban growth rate was just 0.7% between 1990–1995 in the more developed regions of the world, cities in the developing nations grew by 3.4% each year during the same period. That *rate* of growth is now declining and is projected to average 2.4% annually until 2025. However, since the base size of today's urban population is so much larger than it was a decade or two ago, the yearly increase in *numbers* of people living in cities, estimated by the UN Centre for Human Settlements at 64 million, will continue to rise. By 2030, according to United Nations projections, the percentage of the world's population classified as "urban" will reach 60% (84% in the industrialized countries vs. 56% in the developing world). Virtually all the growth in human numbers during the next 25 years will occur in urban areas, particularly in the larger cities of Asia and sub-Saharan Africa (O'Neil and Balk, 2001; Brockerhoff, 2000). Latin American populations, already 75% urbanized, will exhibit continued growth in the number of city dwellers, but at a much slower pace than previously (Brea, 2003).

Box 2-4 The "Urban Penalty"

For the Third World's urban poor, city life can be downright hazardous to one's health. In a situation reminiscent of the early years of the Industrial Revolution in England, where deplorable living conditions in the new factory towns were reflected in strikingly higher mortality rates in urban slums than in the countryside, rural migrants to the megacities of Africa, Asia, and Latin America are paying a high penalty in death and disease in their quest for a better life. Among the urban poor in most developing countries, the number of underweight children and the prevalence of malnutrition is greater than it is among rural populations. Infectious and parasitic diseases, usually associated with life in the medically underserved countryside, also take a heavy toll among slum dwellers. In many respects the urban poor can be said to suffer the "worst of both worlds," afflicted not only by the pathogenic ailments and nutritional deficiencies characteristic of poor living conditions anywhere, but also, increasingly, by the chronic diseases associated with more sedentary urban lifestyles: obesity due to increased sugar consumption, circulatory problems, stress, and mental illness.

To a large extent, the health problems suffered by the urban poor are provoked by the substandard environmental conditions in their homes and neighborhoods. Whether living in an illegal squatter settlement or a teeming tenement, impoverished city dwellers cope daily with grossly overcrowded conditions and close proximity to pathogen-laden human wastes. The latter situation, a result of too-few public toilets and the lack of sewers, is a major cause of the high incidence of diarrheal diseases—typhoid, cholera, dysentery—that occur when fecal pathogens contaminate food or drinking water. Limited supplies of treated water force many of the urban poor to draw their drinking water from nearby streams or drainage ditches heavily polluted with sewage or industrial wastes. Not surprisingly, waterborne diseases remain a leading cause of child mortality in Third World cities.

Inadequate or nonexistent garbage collection constitutes another health problem, as decaying wastes and piles of rubbish provide both food and shelter for hordes of disease-carrying rodents and flies. In the absence of sewers to drain off stormwater and human excrement, many slum areas are plagued by constantly wet soil and stagnant pools of water. This situation, along with the slum dwellers' common practice of defecating directly on the ground, creates ideal breeding conditions for parasitic worms and disease-carrying mosquitoes. Hookworms thrive in such environments, their eggs passing in human excrement to the damp soil where they hatch into larvae that penetrate through the bare feet of victims to perpetuate the cycle of infection. Inside the human body, hookworms feed on the host's blood; severe anemia may develop if the infestation is heavy, leaving the victim susceptible to other infections as well. Hookworm-infected slum children often suffer stunted growth, lack of energy, and diminished mental capacity, reducing their prospects for productive employment as they grow older. Mosquito-borne ailments such as malaria, yellow fever, dengue, and filariasis are also common in this environment; malaria in particular is a leading cause of death among children in illegal settlements.

While many of the health problems experienced by the urban poor exist in rural areas as well, they are greatly exacerbated by the overcrowded, cramped conditions in megacity shantytowns. Acute respiratory infections, tuberculosis, influenza, mumps, and measles all spread much more readily in densely packed urban slums than elsewhere, facilitated by the constant influx of susceptible new rural-to-city migrants (who themselves may be carriers of virulent new disease strains) and by the larger-than-average proportion of the very young among urban poor populations. Since these people generally lack sufficient income to pay for vaccines or medical care and often lack means of transportation to reach a distant hospital or clinic, they frequently have no greater access to health care facilities in the city than they did in their home villages. This can be particularly problematic when accidents or fires cause serious injury. In the overcrowded, substandard housing conditions that characterize poor neighborhoods, open cooking fires or kerosene heaters are a frequent cause of burns, especially among women and girls. Other hazards within slum dwellings include accidental poisonings caused by medicines, pesticides, or other toxic products left accessible to children for lack of secure storage space.

High levels of violence plague urban squatter areas to a far greater extent than in the countryside or in more affluent sections of the same city. This problem is particularly grim in Latin America and the Caribbean, where the stresses of daily life in low-income urban areas is reflected in a murder rate of 7.7 per 1,000 people—more than double the world average of 3.5 per 1,000. Traffic accidents cause many deaths and injuries among slum residents, not surprising since many illegal settlements are located along the sides of busy roadways. When accidents or fires occur, ambulances or fire trucks may be slow in arriving (if they arrive at all), due to absence of paved roads or to the settlement's location on an inaccessible steep hillside or waterlogged area.

The siting of illegal settlements in itself may constitute a major obstacle to residents' health. Lack of income forces squatters to choose land that others would find undesirable. Such locations include precariously steep slopes subject to mudslides during the rainy season; desert land plagued by dust storms; floodplains that are periodically inundated; empty areas adjacent to municipal garbage dumps or chemical waste sites; land next to polluting industries or noisy airports. Such settlements seldom enjoy the amenities taken for granted elsewhere—sewers, paved roads, utilities, public transportation, garbage collection. Impoverished migrants live there because they can't afford anything better, accepting trade-offs in health and quality of living for other items they deem more urgent for survival—like food, children's education, or a piece of equipment (e.g., a bicycle or a sewing machine) that will help them earn a living. As growth in the developing world's megacities continues to soar, urban planners and municipal officials need to redouble their efforts to attack the environmental and infrastructure problems that currently condemn their poorest citizens to a life of poor health and limited opportunity.

References

Hardoy, Jorge E., and David Satterthwaite. 1989. *Squatter Citizen*. London: Earthscan Publications Ltd.

United Nations Centre for Human Settlements. 2001. *Cities in a Globalizing World: Global Report on Human Settlements 2001*. London: Earthscan Publications Ltd.

The phenomenal rate of urban growth over the past century has given rise to a new term—**megacity**—coined to describe any urban area with a population of 10 million or more. In 1900 there were none; at that time London, with a population of 5 million, was the world's largest city. One hundred years later, the United Nations estimates there are now 19 megacities, 13 of them in the developing world. Fifteen more will be added to the list by 2015, all of them in less-developed countries (Brockerhoff, 2000). Such growth is already having a staggering impact on the ability of those municipalities to provide even the rudiments of a decent standard of living. Much of the population growth in Third World cities occurs in so-called "illegal settlements"— slum areas and shantytowns built without regard to local regulations, often on land illegally occupied or illegally subdivided. These squatter settlements continue to spread like ugly cancerous growths around the periphery of almost every large city in the developing world. Estimates indicate that between 30–60% of the people in developing world cities currently live in substandard housing (World Resources Institute, 1996). These uncontrolled settlements are growing even faster than the urban areas as a whole, with the consequence that in the years ahead an ever-larger segment of Third World urban populations will be living in the squalor and hopelessness that characterize these shantytowns.

In most cases the urbanization trend seems to be caused by the hope for a better, more comfortable life, and though most migrants continue to live in abject poverty,

Figure 2-6   The 15 Largest Cities of the World in 2015

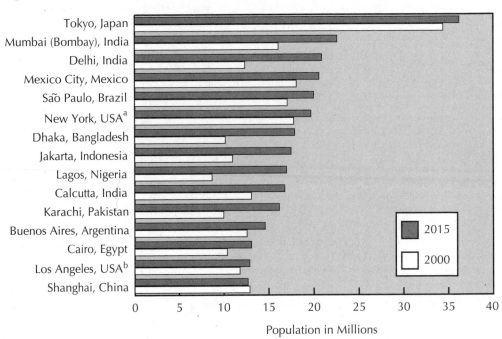

ª Refers to the New York-Newark urbanized area.

ᵇ Refers to the Los Angeles-Long Beach, Santa Ana urbanized area.

Source: Adapted from Table 8 in *World Urbanization Prospects: The 2003 Revision*, United Nations Population Division.

nearly all seem to prefer to remain there rather than return to the deprivation of their rural home villages. Ironically, recent studies have shown that, contrary to migrant expectations, the quality of life in many developing world cities today is worse than it is in the rural areas they left behind (Brockerhoff and Brennan, 1998). Throughout the developing world, poverty is increasingly becoming an urban phenomenon. At the beginning of the 21st century, approximately half of the world's poorest people are living in urban settlements and the World Bank predicts that by 2025 most people in developing world cities will be living in poverty. Historically, urbanization seems to have the universal effect of breaking down the traditional cultures of those who migrate to the cities, where anonymity is the main feature. The overwhelming majority of urban dwellers in developing countries are migrants who have brought their peasant culture with them. They generally lack the specialized education and skills required to penetrate the city's complex social web. Migrants inevitably find that their limited skills make them incapable of contributing to the economy and consequently they are scarcely any better off than before.

The rapid increase in the populations of Third World cities presents a number of very serious problems that government officials are going to find extremely difficult to manage. Two of the most pressing needs, if disease outbreaks are to be prevented, will be the provision of safe drinking water and sewage disposal. During the 1980s impressive gains were made in bringing water and sanitation services to urban residents in the developing nations. By 1990, according to official statistics, approximately 500 million more city dwellers worldwide had access to adequate drinking water than was

Figure 2-7   World Urban and Rural Population, 1950–2030

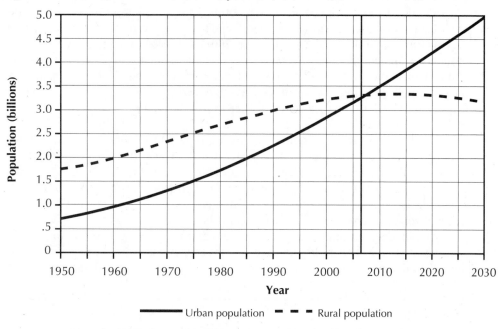

Urban population — — — Rural population

Note: In 2007, the world will have more urban dwellers than rural ones.

Source: Figure 4, *Population Newsletter* (June 2004), United Nations Population Division. Used with permission.

the case in 1980; similarly, those served by sewerage projects increased by close to 300 million (Briscoe, 1993). This apparent improvement may be overstated, however. Not only are questionable criteria used for determining what constitutes "adequate" provision of safe drinking water and sanitation services, but the accuracy of the statistics provided by many developing country governments to international agencies such as the United Nations is highly questionable and often contradicted by detailed studies of specific cities. For example, in Ghana's second-largest city, Kumasi, where official figures indicate that 99% of the population has an adequate piped water supply, a large percentage of residents obtain that water from shared standpipes, necessitating long waits for their turn at the tap. The situation is even worse in Luanda, capital of Angola, where one standpipe serves 600–1,000 people, or in Nouakchott, Mauritania, where 2,500 residents are dependent on a single standpipe. In many other Third World cities the fact that a water tap is present within the home doesn't guarantee dependable access to water because the flow through distribution pipes can be cut off at any time. In Chennai (formerly Madras), India's fourth-largest city, a prolonged drought during the early 1990s resulted in the restriction of tap water provision to just two hours every two days. Even under normal conditions, residents of many cities throughout the developing world must cope with an intermittent water supply on a daily basis, utilizing the few hours when water is flowing to fill every available storage vessel before the tap runs dry once again.

Just as official figures exaggerate improvements in urban water supply, so do they paint an overly optimistic picture of gains in sanitary services. In 1994, the World Health Organization reported that more than half of urban Africans, two-thirds of Asian city dwellers, and three-quarters of those in Latin America and the Caribbean enjoyed adequate sanitation. However, the determination of "adequate" was based largely on residents' access to a public latrine, regardless of the number of people sharing the same facility. Many families share poorly maintained, often overflowing privies with 100 or more neighbors. Millions of urban residents in developing countries don't have access even to simple latrines, having to resort to roadside ditches or open spaces (Hardoy, Mitlin, and Satterthwaite, 2001). Exposed, untreated human wastes in the midst of densely populated areas pose a direct public health threat, but ongoing efforts to meet the sanitary needs of developing world cities are being overwhelmed by the continually growing number of residents to be served. Municipal officials might be forgiven for wondering if they were on a treadmill—having to run faster and faster just to remain in place!

As urban populations continue to expand, provision of such basic services will undoubtedly lag even further behind, increasing the threat of epidemic disease and worsening already serious problems of water pollution. Air quality is already at dangerous levels in many Third World cities; of the 15 urban areas ranked as "most polluted," 13 are in Asia where the health of millions of residents is impaired by choking levels of vehicular emissions. This situation is likely to worsen as the number of old, poorly maintained automobiles and pollutant-emitting trucks, buses, and motorbikes rises exponentially. The proliferation of motor vehicles has spawned a new hazard to life in Third World cities; due to nonexistent or poorly enforced driving regulations,

Much of the urban population growth in Third World cities occurs in slum areas that lack even the most basic rudiments of a decent standard of living.

traffic accidents have become a leading cause of death and disability in urban areas, taking an even greater toll among pedestrians than motorists (Brockerhoff, 2000). Pressures on municipal authorities to provide jobs, housing, transportation, and social facilities will mount inexorably within the coming years and will present those societies with economic and environmental challenges which may prove impossible to meet.

Population Projections

The obvious question to anyone looking at a graphic representation of population growth such as that in figure 2-2 is "How long will growth continue?" and "At what level will population ultimately stabilize?" The implicit assumption, and one that is validated by the results of numerous animal experiments, is that human population growth cannot continue indefinitely. Statistical evidence indicates, in fact, that the world population annual growth rate peaked at about 2% in the early 1970s, declining gradually since then to its present 1.3%. Nevertheless, although a growth rate decrease is good news, in terms of absolute numbers population size will continue to increase for many decades, due to the world's enormous population base and the large proportion of young people in developing countries. Talk of a population "explosion," common during the 1970s and 1980s, has been replaced by the metaphor of a giant freight train, slowing a bit, but still traveling dangerously fast with heavy momentum.

Optimists see the booth as half empty. [*Toles © 1999 The Washington Post. Reprinted with permission of Universal Press Syndicate. All rights reserved.*]

The United Nations, an organization logically quite interested in future world growth patterns, regularly publishes projections of population size for the next several decades. Such projections are not just extrapolations of present trends, but take into consideration trends in fertility, mortality, migration, and so on (they do not consider the possibility of major disasters such as a nuclear war, however). The United Nations Population Division presents several sets of projections, all of which assume that there will be some lowering of fertility rates (a substantial drop in fertility is assumed for the low projection, a less significant decline for the high projection) in regions where these are currently quite high. The most widely used medium range projection antici-pates a world population of 8.9 billion by 2050, a figure that reflects a drop in fertility rates to replacement level or below in most countries (a group of high-fertility African nations, plus Afghanistan and Yemen, are exceptions to the general downward trend) and a rise in HIV/AIDS-related mortality rates in a number of severely impacted countries. Given these assumptions, the United Nations' "best guess" for ultimate world population size is 9.5 billion to be reached around 2100. However, if fertility rates deviate even slightly from the replacement level figure presumed for the medium-range estimate, the size of world population at the time of stabilization will be dramatically different from the 9.5 billion figure cited above. For example, if fertil-ity were to remain constant everywhere at current levels (2.8), world population would more than double by 2050, to 12.8 billion. If the anticipated fertility decline is 2.5 children per woman instead of the assumed 2.0, world population size in 2050 would be approximately 10.6 billion. Conversely, greater-than-anticipated fertility declines, such as an average of 1.5 children per woman worldwide, would reduce the world total in 2050 to 7.4 billion (UNFPA, 2002). Quite obviously, the childbearing decisions of millions of individual couples will have an enormous impact on total world population size at the time growth eventually levels off. While both the United Nations and the World Bank are proceeding on the debatable assumption that world population growth will stabilize approximately a century from now, widely divergent fertility patterns in different areas of the world guarantee that some regions will achieve population stability long before others do. Poland, Austria, Greece, Slovakia, and Sweden have already reached zero population growth (ZPG), while several coun-tries, including Germany, Russia, Ukraine, Italy, and Bulgaria actually have negative growth rates. By 2050 the UN projects that the populations of 30 developed nations, including Japan and most of the European countries, will be smaller than they are today, as deaths among the large cohorts of elderly outnumber births.

Looking at population projections on a regional basis, Asia, thanks to its already huge population base, will experience the largest increase in total numbers, in spite of declining fertility levels. India alone, growing by about 20 million annually, is expected to surpass China to become the world's most populous country within the next few decades. Africa currently boasts the world's highest growth rates and will more than double its current population by 2050. Together, Africa and Asia will account for fully 80% of the world's total population at the time of stabilization. Latin America and the Caribbean nations continue to grow at a rate second only to Africa. In 1960 there were approximately equal numbers of Latin Americans and North Americans; by 2050 there will be almost 800 million people living south of the Rio Grande, 457 million to the north. Only Europe, among major geographical regions, is projected to experience population decline in the years ahead, falling from 728 million in 2004 to 668 million in 2050 (Population Reference Bureau, 2004).

Obviously, making global population projections is a risky business, with accu-racy of forecasts depending not only on the childbearing decisions of millions of indi-vidual couples but also on trends in mortality rates. While most long-range

Box 2-5 Population Pressures Spur Mideast Tension

The "Arab street" is angry—and crowded. From Iraq to Morocco, annual population growth in the Middle East and North Africa (MENA), currently 2%, is more rapid than anywhere else in the world except for sub-Saharan Africa (2.5%). Within the region, several countries currently boast growth rates comparable to those of the fastest-growing African nations: the Palestinian Territory's 3.5% growth rate is equal to that of Niger, while Yemen, at 3.3%, isn't far behind. While media reports of violence and instability in MENA countries tend to focus on repressive political regimes, religious fanaticism, or long-standing territorial disputes, stress due to over-population and competition for increasingly scarce resources undoubtedly contribute to the present turmoil throughout the region.

Severe population pressure in the Middle East and North Africa is a relatively recent phenomenon. Throughout much of recorded history, numbers remained relatively stable around 30 million. By the early 20th century, population had grown to an estimated 60 million, rising gradually to about 100 million by mid-century. Only in the latter half of the 20th century did the region's population growth explode, fueled by rapid improvements in sanitation and medical care that sharply reduced infant and child mortality. Between 1950 and 2000, the region's population size soared to 380 million, nearly four times the number inhabiting the region just 50 years earlier.

Although fertility in most MENA nations has declined in recent decades, dropping from an average of 7 children per woman in 1960 to 3.6 in 2001, striking differences exist from one country to another. Most successful in rapidly lowering birth rates has been Iran, where government leaders, alarmed that runaway population growth was hindering economic development, launched a family-planning program that succeeded in reducing fertility from an average of 6.6 children per woman in the early 1990s to just 2.5 in 2003. Turkey, Lebanon, and several of the Persian Gulf sheikdoms have also experienced notable declines in population growth rates during that same period. At the opposite extreme, fertility decline has been minimal or nonexistent in

Iraq, Saudi Arabia, Yemen, and the Palestinian Territory, where 5 or more children per woman continues to be the norm (in densely overcrowded and tumultuous Gaza, family size averages 7 children). Several cultural factors make stabilization of population size in these countries a distant prospect: the pivotal importance of family, customs that favor early marriage and stigmatize women who remain single, the low educational status of many women, and the near-exclusion of women from paid employment—all reinforce the traditional preference for many children.

High fertility is reflected in the predominantly youthful age structure of the region. Over one-third of all people living in the Middle East and North Africa (fully 48% of Yemenis, 47% of Iraqis, and 46% of Palestinians) are under the age of 15. This huge cohort of children and young adolescents ensures continued population growth for at least another generation or two. The number of women of childbearing age is projected to double by 2030 and the population of the region as a whole will be nearly twice its present size by 2050. The demands of a youthful society are already straining the ability of governments in the region to provide the high quality educational and medical facilities so essential in a modern society.

In the years immediately ahead, as millions of young Arabs, Turks, and Iranians reach working age, pressure on national governments to provide adequate employment opportunities will grow more acute. Already the region has the world's highest unemployment rates—about 14% of the working-age population is jobless, with an even higher percentage of young people and women so affected. Fully half of the young Arab men polled by a UN team preparing the "Arab Human Development Report 2002" told interviewers they hoped to emigrate because they had little hope of finding work in their homeland. Just to maintain current levels of employment, by 2010 MENA countries need to create 50% more jobs than existed in the mid-1990s. A case in point is Egypt, where an additional half-million new jobs each year are required to absorb the army of young people entering the workforce. Doing so will prove daunting, given the stagnant economic conditions in many Middle Eastern nations; failure to do so, however, will increase popular discontent and could precipitate social and political strife.

Population pressures also are having a serious impact on water supplies. Living in a largely desert environment, MENA residents are confronted by the world's most acute water shortages. Exploding population growth during the last quarter of the 20th century resulted in per capita renewable freshwater supplies declining by more than 50%, to 1,500 cubic meters per year. By 2025, that amount is projected to drop to just 1,000 cubic meters per person, a figure widely regarded as the threshold for water scarcity. Even these figures are misleadingly optimistic, because the lion's share of renewable freshwater in the region is located in just a few countries: Turkey, Syria, Iraq, and Iran. Elsewhere, average per capita water availability is already far below the 1,000-cubic-meter threshold; in Saudi Arabia, Jordan, Yemen, Israel, and the Palestinian Territory, among others, the figure is below 250 cubic meters per year. Unfortunately, this group includes several of the countries where populations are growing most rapidly and whose economies are least able to deal effectively with water scarcity issues.

In the Internet Age, hundreds of millions of Middle Easterners and North Africans, all too aware of the opportunities and comfortable lifestyle enjoyed by citizens in more developed lands, will inevitably demand the same for themselves and their children. Unfortunately, the sheer pressure of their numbers on available resources will likely make such demands difficult, if not impossible, to fulfill. Those attempting to understand the political and social ferment, the violence and anger that so often dominate news stories about the Middle East and North Africa, must take into account the growing demographic pressures that make such turmoil inevitable.

Reference

Population Reference Bureau. 2001. "Population Trends and Challenges in the Middle East and North Africa." (Oct).

projections show global population growth halting between 2050–2100, the ability of natural ecosystems to support additional billions of people has been questioned. Since almost all of the expected increase will occur in the poorest countries where people are most dependent on natural ecosystems for their survival and well-being, many observers insist that population growth needs to be stabilized long before it reaches the theoretical levels projected by the United Nations. Recognizing the enormous cooperative effort needed to resolve humanity's demographic dilemma, 1,670 scientists from 70 countries have signed a population stabilization statement drafted by the Union of Concerned Scientists, declaring that:

> Fundamental changes are urgent if we are to avoid the collision our present course will bring about. . . if vast human misery is to be avoided and our global home on this planet is not to be irretrievably mutilated. (Tobias, 1998)

References

Altman, Lawrence K. 1993. "Big Health Gains Found in Developing Countries." *New York Times*, July 7.

Brea, Jorge A. 2003. "Population Dynamics in Latin America." *Population Bulletin* 58, no. 1 (March).

Briscoe, John. 1993. "When the Cup Is Half Full: Improving Water and Sanitation Services in the Developing World." *Environment* 35, no. 4 (May).

Brockerhoff, Martin P. 2000. "An Urbanizing World." *Population Bulletin* 55, no. 3 (Sept).

Brockerhoff, Martin, and Ellen Brennan. 1998. "The Poverty of Cities in Developing Regions." *Population and Development Review* 24, no. 1 (March): 75–114.

"Economics Focus: Does Population Matter?" 2002. *The Economist*, December 7.

Ehrlich, Paul R., Anne H. Ehrlich, and John P. Holdren. 1977. *Ecoscience: Population, Resources, Environment*. New York: W. H. Freeman and Co.

Farb, Peter. 1963. *Ecology, Life Nature Library*. Time Inc.

Hardoy, Jorge E., Diana Mitlin, and David Satterthwaite. 2001. *Environmental Problems in an Urbanizing World*. London: Earthscan Publications, Ltd.

Haub, Carl. 1993. "Tokyo Now Recognized as World's Largest City." *Population Today* 21, no. 3 (March).

Herring, Herbert. 1960. *A History of Latin America*. New York: Alfred A. Knopf.

Odum, Eugene P. 1959. *Fundamentals of Ecology*. Philadelphia: W. B. Saunders Company.

O'Neil, Brian, and Deborah Balk. 2001. "World Population Futures." *Population Bulletin* 58, no. 1 (Sept).

Population Reference Bureau. 2004. *World Population Data Sheet*.

Rohe, John F. 1998. *A Bicentennial Malthusian Essay: Conservation, Population and the Indifference to Limits*. Traverse City, MI: Rhodes & Easton.

Sheehan, Molly O. 2003. "Population Growth Slows." *Vital Signs 2003*. New York: Worldwatch/W.W. Norton.

Tobias, Michael. 1998. *World War III: Population and the Biosphere at the End of the Millennium*. New York: Continuum.

UN Population Division (UNFPA). 2002. *World Population Prospects: The 2002 Revision*.

World Resources Institute (WRI). 1996. *World Resources 1996–97*. New York: Oxford Univ. Press.

POPULATION CONTROL

> We want better reasons for having children than not knowing how to prevent them.
> —Dora Russell, English feminist (1925)

Apocalyptic visions of a planet imploding under the sheer weight of human numbers, so prevalent just a few decades ago, are now giving way to the realization that the "population bomb" has largely been de-fused. Thanks in part to the alarms raised during the 1960s and 1970s when the world population growth rate was at its peak, the introduction of family-planning programs and modern means of contraception into high-fertility Third World nations has had a profound impact in reducing runaway population growth. Indeed, a number of developing countries are now close to achieving population stability, having completed their demographic transition far more rapidly than experts had predicted. However, media reports alleging that overpopulation is no longer a problem mistakenly assume that the decline in growth rates implies a leveling-off in total population size. In fact, owing to an already-enormous population base, today's 1.3% population growth rate, down from the 2% prevailing at the peak of the "population explosion," translates to a world population increase of 77 million annually—about the same as the yearly increment in the early 1970s when alarm bells were ringing. Also, as mentioned in the preceding chapter, high fertility and correspondingly high rates of population growth continue to be the norm in most nations of Africa and the Middle East. These countries, among the world's poorest, could see their populations more than double in size by 2050. Even in the Asian and Latin American nations hailed as success stories for rapidly reducing birth rates, fertility remains well above replacement level; these countries will continue to experience significant population increase in the decades immediately ahead.

As described in chapter 2, studies of population dynamics clearly demonstrate that no species can sustain limitless growth. Just as declining *death* rates caused the population explosion, it is widely assumed that a decrease in *birth* rates will humanely bring a halt to future growth. The accuracy of that assumption hinges on the success of both governments and the private sector in providing family-planning services to all who desire them and on the childbearing decisions of millions of individual couples.

Early Attempts at Family Limitation

Although most traditional cultures have consistently encouraged prolific childbearing, records indicate that during stressful periods of famine, war, or civil upheaval many couples throughout history have attempted in various ways to prevent unwanted births. While some of the methods employed were based on nothing more than superstition, others were moderately effective and continue to be used today.

One of the oldest documented means of contraception, referred to in the Old Testament story of Onan (Genesis 38:9), is that of withdrawal (*coitus interruptus*), whereby the man withdraws his penis from the vagina prior to ejaculation. Since a keen sense of timing is essential to the success of this method, withdrawal has the highest failure rate of any major method of birth control, but it does have the advantage of requiring no drugs or devices nor access to medical personnel for its use—and it costs nothing. Where couples are highly motivated not to have children, it can be fairly successful and, in fact, is believed to be the method by which European couples substantially reduced birth rates in that part of the world during the early years of the demographic transition. Even today, millions of couples worldwide continue to rely on withdrawal as a means of preventing unwanted births. In several countries of eastern Europe and the Middle East—Ukraine, Romania, Albania, Bosnia, Armenia, Azerbaijan, and Turkey—it remains the most common means of birth control even today, with 20%–30% of contracepting couples relying on this age-old method (PRB, 2002). In the past, the popularity of withdrawal prompted numerous attacks on the method by certain disapproving segments of society. Some doctors declared that the practice would lead to both physical and mental illness, but such admonitions fell largely on deaf ears. One 40-year-old German farmer, warned of the dire consequences of indulging in *coitus interruptus,* calmly retorted, "I don't believe that. Otherwise everybody would be sick."

Crude barriers to the cervix, similar in concept to the modern diaphragm or cervical cap, were used by women in ancient Egypt who fashioned such devices out of leaves, cloth, wads of cotton fibers, or even crocodile dung!

Herbal concoctions have been used for both contraceptive and abortive purposes for thousands of years. The modern era's contraceptive pill, along with hormonal patches and injectables, are but the most recent in a venerable line of antifertility drugs widely employed in ancient and medieval societies as well as in folk cultures right up to the present time. Although it long was fashionable to dismiss such brews as totally useless, recent research has found that some of the plants used are, in fact, remarkably effective in preventing pregnancy, while others are powerful abortifacients. The contraceptive properties of drugs extracted from such plant materials as pomegranate rind, black pepper, ivy, cabbage flowers, and willow bark were described in Greek and Roman medical literature almost two thousand years ago. Pennyroyal (*Mentha pulegium*), a member of the mint family, was widely used for centuries to induce abortions, as was rue (*Ruta graveolans*), which has both abortifacient and contraceptive properties. In recent decades the results of a number of studies and field observations confirm that certain plant substances do indeed exert an antifertility effect (a phenomenon first noticed in relation to spontaneous abortions or a failure of ovulation among grazing animals when feeding on certain plants). Preliminary research has confirmed many of the claims made by ancient medical authorities and efforts are now ongoing in a number of countries, especially India and China, to conduct clinical and laboratory tests of traditional drugs believed to possess contraceptive properties (McLaren, 1990; Riddle, 1992).

The use of condoms dates back at least to the 16th century when a fine linen sheath worn on the penis during intercourse was recommended as a means of preventing the spread of venereal disease. By the 17th century condoms made of lamb intestines, tied shut at the end with a ribbon, were introduced for the express purpose of preventing conception and by the 18th century were reportedly available for use by patrons at all the finer houses of prostitution in Europe (some versions were also made of silk!). With the advent of vulcanized rubber in 1844, a truly effective and relatively cheap (advertised at $5 per dozen in 1850) male contraceptive became available for the masses. Nevertheless, rubber condoms were not widely used until World War I when they were distributed among the troops as protection against venereal disease (Stokes, 1980; McLaren, 1990).

Other birth control practices with a similarly long history include douching (flushing out the vagina with a water solution immediately after intercourse), almost totally ineffective in spite of its popularity; and breast-feeding of infants, quite an effective means of suppressing the onset of ovulation following childbirth and thereby helpful in spacing pregnancies. In fact, prior to the advent of modern contraceptives, breast-feeding was the chief tactic employed by women to prevent an unwanted second pregnancy soon after childbirth. A survey conducted in Bangladesh revealed that, on average, each month of breast-feeding increases the birth interval between babies by about 0.4 months (Weiss, 1993; Kleinman and Senanayake, 1984).

When such birth control methods failed, as they frequently did, women commonly resorted to abortion, a very ancient practice believed to have been the most prevalent method of family limitation throughout history.

As a last resort, unwanted children in past centuries frequently fell victim to infanticide—the deliberate killing of babies, particularly girl babies, immediately after birth. This practice was quite common in ancient Greece and in several Asian countries up until fairly recent times, especially during periods of famine or civil upheaval.

Modern Family-Planning Movement

The origins of the modern family-planning movement in the United States can be traced to the publication in 1832 of a contraceptive textbook, *Fruits of Philosophy,* written by Dr. Charles Knowlton. Dr. Knowlton won renown as the first person in the United States to be jailed for advocating birth control. The development of the diaphragm in the 1840s further stimulated public interest in contraceptive techniques and although proponents of birth control were viciously persecuted by so-called "societies for the suppression of vice," the resultant notoriety only enhanced sales of birth control literature. Open discussion of sex or reproductive matters was still taboo during those years of Victorian morality, however, and an "establishment" backlash against the growing birth control movement was reflected in the passage in 1873 of the Comstock Law, a federal mandate that prohibited sending birth control information or devices through the mail, such items being defined as "obscene."

Toward the end of the 19th century, the burgeoning feminist movement lent support to the concept of family planning, stressing the health burdens imposed on women by too many children born too close together. An outstanding pioneer of family planning in America was Margaret Sanger, a nurse in New York City who was appalled by the extent of poverty due to over-large families and the rate of maternal death due to abortion among the people with whom she worked. Recognizing that the Comstock Law prevented such people from obtaining the contraceptive information they so badly needed, she launched a personal crusade to overturn that legislation. In 1914 Sanger founded the National Birth Control League and began publishing a monthly magazine, *The Woman Rebel,* containing birth control information—which the Post Office therefore refused to distribute. The following year she circulated a more comprehensive birth control pamphlet, *Family Limitation,* which also violated the Comstock Law. Sanger was indicted for this action, but the indictment was subsequently dropped. In 1916 Mrs. Sanger opened the first birth control clinic in America, in a section of Brooklyn, New York. For this offense she was arrested and served 30

Box 3-1   When All Else Fails . . .

When contraceptives are unavailable, not used, or fail, abortion remains today, as it has for millennia, the birth control method of last resort. Even in this modern age of the Pill and the Patch, accidents still happen; as a result, more than one out of five pregnancies in the United States ends in abortion, a reflection of the reality that close to half of all American pregnancies are unplanned.

Controversy over the legalization of abortion has been raging in the U.S. for more than a century and shows no signs of mellowing. By the mid-1800s American physicians had launched a vigorous lobbying effort to outlaw abortion, a practice unaddressed by either state or federal laws up to that time. Motivated in part by a belief that abortion was morally wrong, but also by a desire to put "quack" doctors out of business and by opposition to new social roles for women, anti-abortion lobbyists had succeeded in making the procedure illegal everywhere in the U.S. by 1900 (outlawing abortions didn't end them of course—it simply made them more dangerous).

This situation prevailed until the 1960s, when public attitudes toward abortion began to shift. Concerns about the "quality of life" as opposed to mere biological existence were voiced, as was the view that anti-abortion statutes discriminated against poor women, since the wealthy could, and did, travel abroad to obtain a desired abortion. By 1970, the states of Alaska, Hawaii, New York, and Washington had completely legalized first-trimester abortions and one-third of all states permitted first-trimester abortions in situations where (1) continuation of the pregnancy might endanger the life or health of the mother; (2) when the child might be born severely deformed or mentally retarded; or (3) when an unmarried girl under 16 became pregnant due to rape or incest. In 1973 the U.S. Supreme Court stunned the nation by issuing its historic *Roe v. Wade* decision, ruling that states cannot place any restrictions on abortion during the first trimester other than to require that the procedure be performed by a physician. During the second trimester the state can regulate abortion only in ways to protect maternal health; only during the last trimester, said the Court, may the state prohibit abortion unless the life of the mother is in danger.

The Court's 1973 landmark ruling invalidated all remaining state anti-abortion laws but it did nothing to end the controversy surrounding the issue. If anything, the debate has only grown more heated during the thirty-odd years since *Roe v. Wade*, polarizing both society and politics.

During the 1980s the number of abortions in the U.S. held relatively steady at about 1.6 million annually. However, by the early 1990s surgical abortions began a gradual decline, down to 1.31 million in 2000—the lowest level since the 1970s. A number of factors have contributed to this trend, among them a decline in sexual activity among adolescents; that, plus more consistent and effective use of contraceptives by those teens who do engage in sex has cut the number of unwanted teenage pregnancies, thereby reducing the demand for abortions. Changes on the "supply side" are significant as well. For the past several decades "Right to Life" groups vehemently opposed to women's "Right to Choose" have lobbied vigorously at every level of government to make legal abortion more difficult to obtain and have pressured hospitals and health care providers not to offer abortion services. As a result, by 2000 the number of abortion providers in the U.S. had declined to approximately 1,800—down from a high of 2,900 in 1982.

The vast majority of all abortions (93%) are now being performed in clinics rather than hospitals, primarily in large metropolitan areas; in rural areas, only 3% of all counties have an abortion provider. Laws in various states mandating waiting periods prior to obtaining an abortion, as well as restrictions on minors' access to abortion and on insurance coverage for the procedure, have also had their intended effect of discouraging women from seeking services. The near-total ban on federal funding to poor women wanting abortions similarly has made legal abortion unaffordable for many who would otherwise have opted for the procedure. It is impossible to say how many abortions these restrictions have prevented, but there is no question that they have had a disproportionate impact on women living in poverty, women in under-served rural areas, and on young women.

To some extent, the decline in *surgical* abortions reflects a rise in *medical* abortions. In September 2000, after years of controversy as to whether its use should be permitted in the U.S., the so-called "French abortion pill," originally known as RU-486 but now referred to as **mifepristone**, was approved by the FDA. Used in combination with a prostaglandin, mifepristone has been shown to be both safe and 96.97% effective when taken within 7 weeks after a woman's last menstrual period. A woman opting for medical abortion must visit a doctor to receive counseling and a dose of mifepristone; two days later an oral dose of prostaglandin is taken, either at the doctor's office or clinic or at home. For most women, bleeding and expulsion of the fetus then occurs within four hours. In the small percentage of cases that fail, a standard suction procedure must be performed to complete the abortion. In 2001, only six months after FDA approved its use, mifepristone accounted for 6% of all U.S. abortions. The fact that medical abortion is noninvasive, removing any risk of uterine perforation, and that it requires no anesthesia makes it more appealing than surgical abortion to many women.

Most recently, a significant factor in reducing abortion demand in the U.S. has been the growing use of **emergency contraception**; estimates indicate that approximately 51,000 pregnancies were prevented in 2000 alone, thanks to use of the "morning-after pill." By 2003, surveys indicated that 6% of all American women reported having used either Preven™ or Plan B™, with sales of these products increasing exponentially each year. Unlike mifepristone, "morning-after pills" are not abortifacients; instead, they work by preventing or delaying ovulation or by inhibiting the implantation of a fertilized egg. Essentially high-dose birth control pills, emergency

contraception consists, in the case of Preven™, of four pills containing progestin and estrogen, or, with Plan B™, two pills containing progestin only. Accompanying the pills are a patient information booklet and a urine pregnancy test. The patient is instructed to take the pregnancy test and, if the results are negative, to take two pills (one in the case of Plan B™) immediately, following with the remaining dosage 12 hours later. When used within three days of sexual intercourse (the sooner, the better!), the pills' effectiveness in preventing pregnancy is estimated at 75–89%; not as good as conventional contraceptives used before or during intercourse, but certainly better than nothing (manufacturers of Plan B™ claim 95% effectiveness of their product if taken within 24 hours of having sex). In the U.S., as of mid-2005 morning-after pills were available by prescription only, a problematic situation when time is of the essence. Women's advocacy groups and the makers of Plan B™ were bitterly disappointed when the acting director of the FDA, disregarding the recommendations of an advisory panel and his own staff, vetoed a request to allow morning-after pills to be sold over the counter, as they are in several European countries. Such a move would have substantially increased prompt access and further reduced the number of unintended pregnancies—and abortions—experienced by American women each year.

References

Finer, Lawrence B., and Stanley K. Henshaw. 2003. "Abortion Incidence and Services in the United States in 2000." *Perspectives on Sexual and Reproductive Health* 35, no. 1 (Jan/Feb): 6–15.

Planned Parenthood Federation of America. 2003. *"Mifepristone: Expanding Women's Options for Early Abortion."* http://www.plannedparenthood.org/library/ABORTION. Accessed Nov. 12, 2003.

days in prison, but the resulting public outcry led to a gradual easing of legal restrictions against the family-planning movement.

Mrs. Sanger traveled extensively throughout the country, seeking to persuade both the medical profession and the public at large of the importance of facilitating access to birth control. By 1932 the Birth Control League had established 80 clinics throughout the United States; in 1937 the American Medical Association officially endorsed birth control; finally, by 1938, two major court cases resulted in the overthrow of the Comstock Law and, in effect, made it possible for doctors to prescribe contraceptives to patients (except in Connecticut and Massachusetts where contraceptives remained illegal under state law until the 1960s). In 1942 the National Birth Control League and its affiliated clinics became Planned Parenthood Federation, with Margaret Sanger as honorary chairperson (League of Women Voters Education Fund, 1982).

Birth Control—Its Health Impact

Over the years the services offered by Planned Parenthood have expanded to include premarital counseling and fertility assistance in addition to the original intent of providing birth control information to married women. However, the basic rationale of all family planning work in America—today as in 1916 when the first clinic opened its doors—is to promote the health and well-being of mothers and children by preventing unwanted births. Because of the threat that uncontrolled fertility poses, both to maternal health and to that of infants, it is generally accepted today that no community health program can be considered complete if it fails to provide ready access to birth control devices and information.

Enhancement of maternal and child health through family planning is largely related to one of three basic parameters: (1) age of the mother, (2) interval between births, and (3) total number of births during a woman's reproductive lifetime. A brief examination of each of these factors reveals how uncontrolled fertility has a major impact on mortality and morbidity rates among both women and infants.

Age of Mother

Although the average woman is fertile from her early teens until her late 40s, the biologically optimum period for childbearing is much shorter, extending from approximately 20 to 30 years of age. In fact, research suggests that becoming pregnant is increasingly difficult as women approach middle age. The ability to conceive appears to peak at age 31 and declines steadily every year thereafter. From a safety standpoint, mothers either younger or older than this optimum age span run an increased risk of difficulties or death during pregnancy and childbirth, and their infants are statistically more likely to die than are babies of mothers in their 20s.

Girls in their early teens whose pelvic bones and reproductive organs are not yet fully developed are more likely to suffer obstructed or prolonged labor and to die during childbirth than are women in their prime reproductive years. In addition, babies of young mothers have a tendency to be born premature or underweight, factors that greatly increase their susceptibility to infectious diseases and malnutrition. Studies have revealed consistently higher infant mortality rates among babies born to mothers under age 20 as compared to those born to mothers in their late 20s. In addition, even when healthy at birth, babies born to mothers 15 or under are much more likely to die before their first birthday than are babies whose mothers are in their 20s. Reasons for this discrepancy are unclear, but may be due to neglect, abuse, or inadequate parenting skills on the part of very young mothers (Phipps, Blume, and DeMonner, 2002).

Among women over 35, pregnancy poses an increased risk of complications during childbirth. Studies of pregnant women aged 44 and older reveal considerably higher rates of medical complications such as high blood pressure and diabetes compared to women in their 20s and 30s; women in the over-44 cohort also are much more likely than younger mothers to have a Caesarean delivery (Dulitzki et al., 1998). Mothers over

Box 3-2 The Perils of Pregnancy

While motherhood can be a woman's greatest blessing, it also entails serious health risks, particularly if the woman is young, poor, and living in a developing nation. Each year an estimated half-million Third World women die as a result of pregnancy or childbirth; another 15–20 million survive but incur injuries or illness that seriously affect their health and well-being for years afterwards. Childbirth-related disabilities are tragic for many reasons: they blight the lives of young women during what should be their most productive years; they impose serious financial and psychological stress on the affected families; they affect the quality of care the sick mother is able to give her children; and they are largely preventable.

For the most part, maternal death or disability is a result of inadequate or nonexistent medical care during pregnancy, labor, and immediately following childbirth. While most women in rich nations have regular prenatal checkups, poor Third World women may never see a doctor prior to delivery—and half don't have medical care even then. In Africa and Asia, many pregnant women see no reason to visit a doctor unless they have a specific complaint, not realizing the importance of good prenatal care. Others live in remote areas where no doctor is available, while some simply can't afford medical care. In Muslim countries, scarcity of female physicians may prevent women from accessing health care, since cultural taboos forbid a female patient being examined by a male doctor.

Dilapidated, poor-quality medical facilities in many parts of the developing world constitute another obstacle to adequate medical attention. Women who arrive at such hospitals or clinics in urgent need of emergency obstetric care often fail to receive proper or timely treatment because of inadequate staffing, lack of equipment, and a chronic shortage of surgical supplies. Unsafe abortions pose yet another health hazard to Third World women. Though accurate figures are hard to come by, the World Health Organization estimates that as many as one out of every ten pregnancies in developing countries is terminated by abortion, many of them self-induced or performed by unskilled providers, and all-too-frequently ending in death or disability for the desperate woman.

Among the more tragic consequences of pregnancy and childbirth in areas where good prenatal health care is lacking is a condition known as **obstetric fistula**, one of several potential consequences of obstructed labor. Occurring most commonly among young women who marry and conceive a child before their pelvic bones are fully grown, fistula constitutes what one physician calls "a comprehensive social and psychological disaster." Once common worldwide, obstetric fistula today is virtually unknown in developed countries where high-quality medical services are widely available and marriage of very young girls is illegal. Among impoverished communities in Asia and sub-Saharan Africa, however, the lives of an estimated two million or more women are blighted by obstetric fistulas and another 50,000–100,000 join their ranks each year.

A fistula, or hole, in the birth canal forms as a result of prolonged labor, caused by constant pressure of the baby's head against the mother's pelvis. This pressure gradually cuts off the blood supply to the surrounding tissue, causing it to rot away and leaving a hole between the vagina and the bladder, the vagina and rectum, or both. As a consequence, the woman experiences uncontrollable leakage of urine and feces and becomes a social pariah, constantly wet and foul-smelling. Frequently rejected by their husbands, avoided by friends and relatives, and plagued by feelings of self-loathing and depression, women suffering from fistula often die prematurely due to infection-induced kidney failure.

Ironically, obstetric fistula is both preventable and curable. Postponing marriage and pregnancy for very young girls and ensuring access to facilities providing Caesarean sections could largely eliminate the problem of obstructed labor that gives rise to obstetric fistulas. For women already suffering from this condition, reconstructive surgery is successful for approximately 90% of women seeking such treatment. Unfortunately, most sufferers are unaware that treatment exists; those who *do* know often cannot afford the $100–$400 cost of the operation, plus the approximately two weeks of post-operative care needed to prevent subsequent infection. Recently a United Nations-sponsored team of experts visited nine African countries in an effort to assess the extent of the obstetric fistula problem and the ability of hospitals to treat those afflicted. Information gathered will be used to develop an action plan for preventing and treating fistula in sub-Saharan Africa.

Unfortunately, fistula is but one of many debilitating, even life-threatening, disabilities that typify the perils of pregnancy in less developed countries. While some of these problems are of an acute nature, affecting the mother during or immediately after childbirth, others may constitute chronic conditions, negatively impacting her health and quality of life for months or years afterward. Included among the most serious are (1) **postpartum hemorrhage**, the leading cause of maternal death; (2) **blood poisoning (sepsis)** resulting from unsanitary conditions during delivery or abortion, sometimes leading to pelvic inflammatory disease; (3) **anemia**, low levels of iron in the blood, which is a major contributor to postpartum maternal death or illness; (4) **pregnancy-induced hypertension**, a complex of symptoms which, if not detected and treated, can

result in seizures or convulsions leading to death of the mother or chronic disabilities; and (5) **obstructed labor**, a situation in which labor may be prolonged for days because the mother's pelvis is too narrow to permit easy passage of the fetus through the birth canal.

Preventing problems such as these can be achieved through greater efforts to ensure that Third World women have the same access to good nutrition, family planning, prenatal care, obstetric care, and postnatal care that women in more developed nations already enjoy. Given the human misery and suffering caused by such largely preventable complications of pregnancy and childbirth, providing such assistance should be a moral imperative for the international health community.

References

Ashford, Lori. 2002. *Hidden Suffering: Disabilities from Pregnancy and Childbirth in Less Developed Countries*. Population Reference Bureau, MEASURE Communication (Aug).

United Nations Population Fund. 2003. *Population Issues: Improving Reproductive Health: Campaign to End Fistula*. http://www.unfpa.org/fistula/about.htm. Accessed Nov. 19, 2003.

---

35 are more likely than younger women to bear a child with congenital disorders such as Down syndrome (however, a Canadian study of more than half a million births revealed no greater risk of nonchromosomal birth defects among babies born to older mothers than among infants whose mothers were younger). In addition to concerns regarding birth abnormalities, mothers in their 30s and 40s have reason to worry about the general health of their babies. Up to age 30, a pregnant woman has an 89% likelihood of delivering a healthy baby; this level of assurance diminishes by 3.5% for each additional year of maternal age (Baird, Sadovnick, and Yee, 1991; van Noord-Zaadstra, 1991).

Interval between Births

Short birth intervals have long been recognized as an important factor contributing to infant mortality. Studies conducted in rural India demonstrated that babies born less than two years after a previous birth were 50% more likely to die before their first birthday than were babies born after a birth interval of more than two years. Researchers working with the U.S. Agency for International Development in Bangladesh report that efforts to encourage women to space their pregnancies had a greater impact on reducing infant mortality than did childhood immunization campaigns or oral rehydration therapy.

For years public health workers assumed that short birth intervals were equally harmful to the health of the mother. A condition called "maternal depletion syndrome," characterized by premature aging, weakness, and anemia, is frequently

Table 3-1   Complications of Pregnancy and Childbirth: Estimates for Less Developed Countries

Complication	Incidence as a Percent of Live Births	Maternal Disabilities that May Result
Severe bleeding (hemorrhage)	11	• Severe anemia • Pituitary gland failure and other hormonal imbalances • Infertility
Infection during or after labor (sepsis)	10	• Pelvic inflammatory disease • Chronic pelvic pain • Damage to reproductive organs • Infertility
Obstructed or prolonged labor	6	• Incontinence • Fistula • General prolapse • Uterine rupture, vaginal tears • Nerve damage
Pregnancy-induced hypertension (preeclampsia and eclampsia)	6	• Chronic hypertension • Kidney failure • Nervous system disorders
Unsafe abortion	16	• Reproductive tract infection • Damage to uterus • Infertility • Pelvic inflammatory disease • Chronic pelvic pain

Source: C. Murray and A. Lopez, eds., *Health Dimensions of Sex and Reproduction*, vol. 3 (Boston: Harvard Univ. Press, 1998), as summarized in L. Ashford, *Hidden Suffering: Disabilities from Pregnancy and Childbirth in Less Developed Countries* (Washington, DC: Population Reference Bureau, 2002). Used with permission.

observed among undernourished women in poor societies, where teenage marriage is often followed by about 20 years of uninterrupted pregnancy. Anemic women may indeed be at heightened risk of dying during or soon after childbirth due to their lower tolerance for blood loss. If one pregnancy quickly follows another, the intervening period may be too short for an anemic woman to make up the blood loss experienced during the earlier birth, thus increasing her risk of death due to hemorrhage or childbed fever during the next delivery. However, a study conducted in Bangladesh could find no evidence to support general claims of a direct link between birth intervals of less than two years and enhanced risk of maternal mortality. Short birth intervals, without question, pose real concerns regarding survival prospects of the baby; however, contrary to popular belief, it cannot be demonstrated that having several babies close together increases a woman's own likelihood of dying during pregnancy or childbirth (Ronsmans and Campbell, 1998).

Total Number of Births

Contrary to the popular notion that mothers with large numbers of children give birth "as easy as rolling off a log," statistics reveal that such women are especially prone to problem pregnancies and death during childbirth. Indeed, the total number of babies born to a woman during her lifetime can have a significant impact on her general state of health.

Generally speaking, a woman's second and third births are the safest; the first birth carries slightly greater risk statistically because it will reveal any physical or genetic abnormalities in the parents that could cause problems. With the fourth pregnancy, risk of maternal death, stillbirth, and infant death begins to rise, increasing sharply with the birth of the fifth and every succeeding child. Health workers in Bangladesh report triple the number of deaths among women giving birth to their eighth child as among those bearing their third. Degree of risk depends to a considerable extent on the socioeconomic status of the mother, the greatest hazards being faced by women from the lowest income groups. However, even among well-nourished, affluent women, every birth after the fourth involves an increased degree of danger for both mother and child.

Significantly higher rates of infant and child mortality among higher-order births in poor families seem to be due primarily to poor nutrition, as the limited amount of food available must be divided among many mouths. Unlike their older siblings, the latest born children must survive on reduced average portions during those early years when they are most susceptible to the effects of nutritional deficiency (Eckholm and Newland, 1977).

Thus a family-planning program that provides contraceptive protection for teenage women, women over 35, mothers who have already borne three or more children, and women who have recently given birth can make a very positive contribution to improving public health.

Contraceptive Safety

In assessing the health impact of family planning, one must of course take into account possible risks posed by contraceptive use. Questions have been raised regarding the safety of the birth control pill and the intrauterine device (IUD), prompting public concerns and causing potential contraceptors to turn to less reliable methods or to abandon attempts at birth control altogether. What indeed are the risks and benefits of the most commonly used contraceptives? A brief summary of the most popular methods used in the United States indicates that although various adverse side effects may accompany the use of contraceptives for some women, all common means of contraception entail fewer risks than do pregnancy and childbirth.

Hormonal Contraceptives

Such contraceptives are made of synthetic substances similar to the hormones that occur naturally in women's bodies. They prevent pregnancy by inhibiting ovulation.

Birth control pill.   Among American women aged 15–44 currently practicing contraception, approximately 15.6% use "the Pill," making this the second-most popular method of birth control in the U.S., behind female sterilization (PRB, 2002). Available either as a combination pill (containing both estrogen and a progestin) or as a "mini-pill" containing progestin only, oral contraceptives, when used correctly, are 97–99% effective in preventing pregnancy. Since the early 1960s when the birth control pill first became available, safety concerns centered around a possible increased risk of cardiovascular disorders such as blood clots, which could lead to a stroke or heart attack. For this reason medical authorities feel that a decision to use oral contraceptives should be made only after consultation with a health professional, and currently in all Western nations a doctor's prescription is required for the purchase of birth control pills. Nevertheless, the results of extensive epidemiological research on oral contraceptive safety over nearly four decades of pill use indicate that women over

Figure 3-1   Contraceptive Use among Married Women, Late 1990s

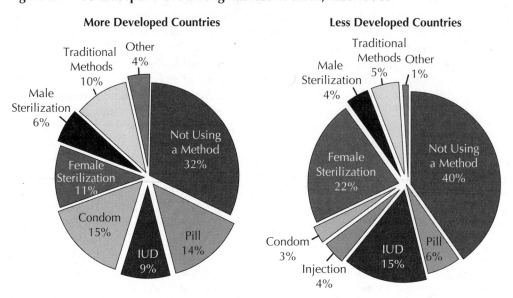

Source: Population Reference Bureau analysis of Demographic and Health Surveys and other contraceptive surveys.

40 are the only group for whom pill use poses a greater health threat than does child-bearing; among this group an increase in cardiovascular problems suggests the advisability of discontinuing pill use in favor of other contraceptive methods. However, for younger women, with the exception of those who smoke or have certain medical conditions (e.g., a history of blood clots, heart problems, cancer of the breast or female organs), medical evidence supports the view that the Pill is quite safe. Moreover, during the period they are taking contraceptive pills, users experience certain health benefits, including significant long-term protection against ovarian cancer (Riman, 2002), as well as reduced risk for ovarian cysts, endometrial cancer, pelvic inflammatory disease, iron-deficiency anemia, and fibrocystic breast disease. Persistent fears that women who use contraceptive pills might be at greater risk of developing cancer later in life were laid to rest in 1999 with the publication of results from a 25-year investigation of British women who had used oral contraceptives. The study convincingly demonstrated that ten years after they stopped taking contraceptive pills, the women experienced no higher risk of dying of cancer or stroke than did women who had never used oral contraceptives—good news for the 300 million women worldwide who have used the Pill at one time or another (Beral et al., 1999).

Depo-Provera.   After more than 20 years of use in over 90 countries worldwide, Depo-Provera won FDA approval in 1992 and is now the most popular non-oral hormonal contraceptive in the United States. Administered as an injection in the arm or buttocks every three months, Depo-Provera fills a need for women who want the reliability of hormonal contraceptives without having to worry about forgetting to take a daily pill. Depo-Provera is a synthetic form of progesterone that works by inhibiting ovulation, and it is 99% effective in preventing pregnancy. Worldwide, more than 30 million women have taken the drug since it was first introduced in 1969 and its overall safety record is good. Common side effects for women receiving a Depo-Provera injection include cessation of the menstrual period or irregular menstruation and modest weight gain.

Contraceptive patch, vaginal ring.   Two relatively new non-oral hormonal contraceptives, both the patch and the vaginal ring deliver hormones through the skin of the user. Both are self-administered, precluding regular visits to a clinic or health care provider and thus enhancing their appeal for women with busy lives. The Ortho-Evra™ patch, containing the same estrogen and progestin compounds found in birth control pills, is applied once a week for three consecutive weeks, then removed for the fourth week, at which time menstruation begins. The patch can be worn on the abdomen, the outside of the upper arm, the buttocks, or anywhere on the upper torso except for the breasts. Available only by prescription, the patch is 99% effective at preventing pregnancy when used correctly.

Unlike the patch, which must be changed weekly, the vaginal ring is inserted by the user once a month; after 21 days she removes it for the last 7 days of her cycle and then inserts a new ring. The NuvaRing™ delivers a lower dose of estrogen than do other hormonal contraceptives, but, like them, is 99% effective in preventing conception (Dieben, Roumen, and Apter, 2002).

Sterilization

The most widely adopted method of family limitation in the United States, sterilization is a logical alternative for those who have already attained their desired family size. Currently, sterilization is the contraceptive method of choice for almost 37% of contracepting couples, with nearly 13.2% opting for sterilization of the male partner, 23.8% for the female procedure (PRB, 2002). Vasectomy, or male sterilization, is a simple operation involving an incision in the scrotum to cut or block the vas deferens (tubes that carry semen from the testes to the penis). Vasectomy most often is performed under local anesthesia in a doctor's office, the entire procedure generally taking less than 30 minutes. In 2003 an alternative approach to male birth control was approved by the FDA. Vasclip™, a tiny clamp attached to each vas deferens to block the flow of sperm, has several advantages over a typical vasectomy. Vasclip™ is cheaper, less painful, and quicker (about 10 minutes) than the standard surgical procedure; the company that manufactures Vasclip™ is hopeful that future studies will demonstrate greater potential for reversibility as well, since it doesn't involve cutting or cauterizing the vas deferens (Good, 2003). In rare cases, minor postoperative infections may develop, but in general male sterilization is among the safest of all birth control methods. Female sterilization, or tubal ligation, entails a slightly higher degree of risk since it involves sealing off the fallopian tubes—an operating room procedure done under general anesthesia. Although major complications are rare, they occur in an estimated 1.7% of cases. A new incision-free form of female sterilization, Essure™, now provides an alternative to tubal ligation. This method, which can be performed in a doctor's office using only a local anesthetic, involves inserting a small metal coil into each fallopian tube, accessed through the cervix using a narrow catheter. Over a period of three months following insertion, the coils stimulate the formation of enough scar tissue to hold the coils in place and completely block the passage of eggs through the fallopian tubes (Minkin and Hanlon, 2003). Sterilization, both male and female, is more than 99% effective in preventing pregnancy and ends any further expense, fuss, or bother related to contraceptive use. However, sterilization is a permanent method of birth control and such a decision should not be made lightly. Efforts to date at reopening the vas deferens or fallopian tubes have met with minimal success, so sterilization should be regarded as irreversible.

Intra-uterine Device (IUD)

Once among the most popular forms of contraception in the United States and still widely relied upon by women in other countries (particularly in China and Russia where it is the most common method of birth control), the IUD today is the method of choice for less than 1% of contracepting American women. Indeed, by the mid-1980s IUDs had nearly disappeared from the marketplace, withdrawn by manufacturers fearing legal liability for alleged harmful side effects of the device (a situation brought about by thousands of lawsuits against the A. H. Robins pharmaceutical firm, charging that the company's Dalkon Shield had caused numerous cases of bleeding, pelvic infections, and resultant infertility among users). Nevertheless, physicians and manufacturers consider most IUDs both safe and reliable. Currently three types of IUD are being marketed in the U.S.—the Paragard™ T 380A, effective for 8–10 years; Progestasert™, a hormone-releasing IUD that must be replaced yearly; and Mirena™, another hormonal IUD intended to last 5 years. Among malnourished, anemic women IUD use has sometimes been correlated with increased blood loss during menstruation. For healthy, well-nourished women, however, IUDs are as safe as the Pill and nearly as dependable. The major problem associated with IUD use is an increased risk of pelvic inflammatory disease (PID) which, if severe, can result in permanent infertility. IUDs are not recommended for women who have never been pregnant and in general are considered most suitable for young women in mutually monogamous relationships (PID incidence is highest among women with several sex partners) who want no more children but are not yet ready for an irreversible surgical sterilization.

Spermicides

Spermicidal foams, creams, suppositories, or gels must be inserted into the vagina within an hour before intercourse and must be replenished if intercourse is repeated. They act to form both a physical and chemical barrier to sperm and are available without a prescription. While few problems are associated with spermicides (those who experience a burning sensation or irritation should avoid them), their effectiveness when used alone is only 70–80%.

Barrier Methods

Barrier methods employ some device that prevents the egg and sperm from uniting, thus preventing fertilization.

Vaginal contraceptives. Diaphragms, cervical caps, sponges, and the female condom all work by keeping egg and sperm apart. (The polyurethane female condom is also intended to provide some protection against sexually transmitted disease, but medical authorities caution that for best protection, male latex condoms are preferable.) When used with spermicides, vaginal contraceptives have few, if any, adverse effects and are moderately effective at preventing pregnancy. Both the sponge and the female condom have an estimated failure rate of about 1 in 4; the cervical cap and diaphragm are somewhat more trustworthy, with failure rates ranging from 6% for a diaphragm used with spermicide to 18% for the cervical cap.

Condoms. Like the vaginal contraceptives, condoms cause no adverse health effects other than an occasional allergic reaction to rubber among some individuals. Used alone, their reliability is significantly less than pills or IUDs, but in combination with vaginal contraceptives and in situations where legal, early abortion is available, they offer the safest means, other than sterilization, of totally effective fertility control. The third most commonly used contraceptive method in the United States and Canada, the condom is being actively promoted by health agencies in many countries not only for birth control reasons but also as an effective prophylactic against the spread of AIDS and other sexually transmitted diseases (STDs). As a case in point, efforts to promote condom use in Thailand have reduced the incidence of new HIV infections in that country's sex industry by 85% within the last few years, according to the director of the United Nation's AIDS program. A comprehensive report by the National Institutes of Health on the efficacy of male condoms for preventing such infections concluded that they are indeed effective in preventing transmission of HIV, gonorrhea, and chlamydia, so long as they are used correctly and consistently. The report emphasized the need for public health agencies to reinforce the message that condoms *do* work in preventing STDs and pregnancies and that the overwhelming issue affecting condom failure is non-use (NIAID, 2001).

Periodic Abstinence

Frequently referred to as the "rhythm method," this approach to birth control carries no health risk but has a consistently high failure rate. To utilize this method, a woman attempts to determine when she is ovulating by charting daily bodily functions such as basal temperature (i.e., temperature when the body is at its lowest level of metabolic activity, usually measured before getting out of bed in the morning) and by examining her cervical mucus. The problem is that many women experience monthly variations in their menstrual cycle, making accurate calculation of the fertile period problematic. In addition, the abstinence from sexual activity during fertile periods which must be rigorously observed by couples using natural family planning requires a high degree of motivation and cooperation between partners and can significantly limit the number of days each month when couples can have intercourse free from fear of unwanted pregnancy.

The success of the family-planning movement in the United States is evident from surveys which reveal that among sexually active women at risk of an unwanted pregnancy, fully 95% are using some method of birth control. In an age when sexual activity seems to be as popular a pastime as it ever was, an even more convincing indicator of contraceptive usage is the fact that the average number of children per U.S. couple is now just two, one of the lowest figures in our history. Apparently most Americans now agree with the family-planning sloganeers who affirm that "a small family is a happy family" (Piccinino and Mosher, 1998).

Family Planning in the Third World

Whereas the birth control movement in the United States and Europe grew out of the conviction that health and social considerations demanded that women receive help in regulating their fertility, the impetus for family planning in most Third World countries grew directly out of concerns over the high rates of post-World War II population growth and the awareness that this "population explosion" would impede their rate of economic development. Only after family-planning programs had been launched did Third World governments attempt to justify their support for such efforts on the basis of protecting maternal and child health and of guaranteeing couples the means for regulating the spacing and number of their children. This superficial shift in emphasis constituted a publicly acceptable rationale for reconciling the interests of the nation with those of individuals.

In most cases, the initial promoters of family planning in the Third World were private organizations such as International Planned Parenthood Federation, the Ford and Rockefeller Foundations, and the Population Council. By the 1960s, however, even earlier in some countries, national governments were becoming increasingly active in establishing their own family-planning programs, usually in conjunction with their ministries of health. Generally they were assisted by the private organizations mentioned and, in later years, by the U.S. Agency for International Development and such United Nations agencies as the World Bank and the UN Fund for Population Activities (UNFPA). Funds, both governmental and private, allocated for family-planning work increased sharply after the mid-1960s, but even today constitute a very small percentage of most national budgets. Today the vast majority of developing countries have some sort of family-planning program in operation. How effective those programs are in reducing national birth rates will in large part determine the success of such countries in raising living standards and ensuring a bright future for their people.

Spreading the Word

Since the main impetus for implementing family planning came from central governments or outside agencies rather than reflecting grassroots interest, as was the case in North America and Europe, success required intensive efforts to reach all elements of society, the majority of whom lived at subsistence level in rural areas, often isolated from adequate medical care and frequently illiterate. Such people had to be made aware of the existence of fertility-regulating methods, provided with regular access to the same, and convinced that it was in their own best interest to use them.

In pursuing this goal, family-planning workers in Third World countries adopted methods radically different from those used in Western nations. Mobile units in the form of specially equipped vans or buses have been essential in carrying health workers and equipment into villages far from any hospital. Trained field workers actively attempt to recruit contraceptive acceptors, meeting with women's groups, farmers, and so on, to persuade them of the advantages inherent in limiting family size. Considerable reliance has been placed on mass media communications. Advertisements in newspapers, on radio, and in cinemas regularly stress the benefits of small families while roadside billboards or posters on buses, in train stations—even painted on the hides of farm

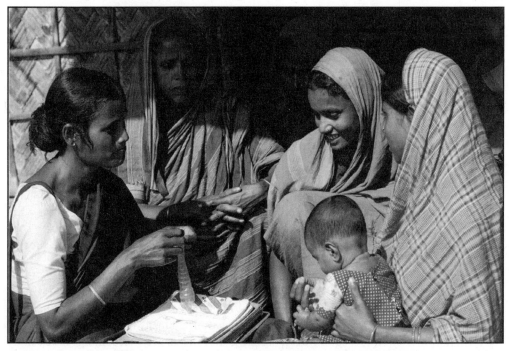

A community health worker in Bangladesh demonstrates condom use to local women. Such workers also provide child nutrition and family-planning advice. [*Mark Edwards/Still Pictures*]

animals—proclaim such messages as "Two or Three—Enough!" Some governments have attracted participation by offering gifts to contraceptive acceptors. In India thousands of men agreed to vasectomies in order to receive a free transistor radio; in Thailand the government has sponsored free distribution of condoms at sporting events or all-expense paid tours of Bangkok's temples for rural men agreeing to sterilization!

Most Third World programs, like those in the West, offer a choice of birth control methods and generally include information on spacing births, nutrition, and child care along with contraceptive services. Some also enlist the services of midwives, teachers, or other respected community leaders to act as distributors of contraceptives, particularly pills and condoms, thereby giving these influential individuals a vested interest in the success of such programs.

Motivation—The Key to Success

Efforts to reduce birth rates in developing nations have met with mixed results, though general trends have been encouraging. With the exception of the countries of sub-Saharan Africa, where fertility remains at traditionally high levels (a current average of 6 children per mother), birth rates have declined significantly in recent decades. Today in the developing nations as a whole, average family size is 3–4 children and nearly 50% of all married couples employ some form of contraception. A number of surveys conducted over the past 25 years have shown that the vast majority of women in the developing world are aware of the existence of at least one modern method of contraception. Nevertheless, a sizable proportion of these women—including many who told interviewers they wanted no more children—were, for one reason or

Wall paintings and billboards throughout India carry the family-planning message. This sign with the symbolic family of four bears the slogan, "Two are enough!" [*Agency for International Development*]

another, not practicing contraception. As a result, in almost every country surveyed, women were having more babies than they said they wanted. To some extent, failure to use contraceptives is related to easy access; not surprisingly, contraceptive use was higher in communities where a family-planning clinic or other source of contraceptive supplies was close by—a particularly important factor among people using either pills or condoms. Cost can also be a major deterrent to poor women; even when they have access to contraceptives, many cannot afford to buy them. A British physician visiting Sri Lanka reported meeting women desperate to control their fertility but too poor to buy more than 5 contraceptive pills at a time, rather than a full month's supply of 21 (Potts, 2000).

A far more important determinant of contraceptive practice, however, is motivation—the desire of couples to limit family size. In many parts of the developing world economic and social factors interact to perpetuate traditional attitudes toward childbearing. For very practical reasons, many Third World couples have concluded that although two or three children per family might be in the best interest of society, they want and feel they need a significantly larger number themselves. In the absence of coercion, when individual and societal needs conflict, personal desires generally prevail. Factors contributing to this continued preference for large families among many Third World couples include high infant mortality rates, the view of children as "social security," the desire for sons, and the low educational and economic status of women.

High infant mortality rates.   Although the drop in infant and child death rates in large part fueled the explosive growth of Third World populations, such rates are still substantially above the levels prevailing in developed countries. In many parts of Africa, for example, infant death rates are over 100, compared to 6.7 in the United States, 5.2 in Canada, and 3.0 in Japan (PRB, 2003). At the personal level, surveys have found that wherever childhood deaths are common, it is extremely difficult to convince parents to limit themselves to two births. For this reason, sharply lowering infant and child mortality rates is regarded as one of the key components in any population control program.

Children as "social security."   In most developing countries, lack of extensive social welfare programs means that most parents are dependent on their grown children for financial support in their post-retirement years. In such cultures, responsibility for elderly parents falls primarily on the sons; thus a couple may feel the need to produce at least two or three boys to ensure their being adequately provided for in old age. In addition, even young children may be regarded as financial assets, since their labor is needed on the farm or around the home. In such situations an additional baby is not viewed as another mouth to feed but rather as an additional pair of hands to gather wood, tend livestock, haul water, and so forth (Dasgupta, 1995).

Desire for sons.   Many family-planning program administrators fear that the preference for sons rather than daughters will keep fertility rates high in many developing countries. Son preference is apparent in surveys of American couples but is even more pronounced among parents in most Third World nations. In such cultures, doubt about whether they will have enough boys concerns parents who are asked to produce no more than two or three offspring. A woman's status, even the stability of her marriage, is dependent on her having sons. To some extent, such preferences are based on economic concerns: sons can support parents in old age while daughters are a financial liability, often requiring an expensive dowry at time of marriage. A fertility preference study conducted in Nepal found that although more than 80% of the

Box 3-3   Missing Girls

The latest census results from the world's two most populous nations, China and India, reveal a worrisome trend—a steady decline in the proportion of baby girls to baby boys. For human societies everywhere, the normal sex ratio at birth is 105–106 boys for every 100 girls (or, viewed in reverse, 94–95 girls for every 100 boys). Since the mortality rate for males is slightly higher than that for females in every age group, this gender imbalance at birth seems to be Nature's way of ensuring approximately equal numbers of young men and women during the prime reproductive years. However, the gender discrepancy revealed by Chinese census reports in 2000 showed 117 boys for every 100 girls, indicating a deficit of at least 980,000 girls. Similarly, in India, the 2001 census showed that for every 1,000 boys born, the corresponding number for girls was 927.

This recent unnatural widening of the gender gap suggests that something out of the ordinary is going on in countries where parental preference for sons has always been a fact of life. Both India and China are highly patriarchal societies, where sons are valued as a means of support for parents in their old age and for perpetuating the family line. A daughter, by contrast, leaves home to join her husband's family when she marries (in rural China a married daughter is no longer considered a member of her birth family) and thus represents more of a financial burden than an asset to her parents. This burden is particularly onerous today in India, where the custom of providing daughters with a huge cash dowry at the time of marriage imposes a crushing debt on many families. Dowry concerns don't trouble Chinese parents, but constraints imposed by China's strict family-planning laws do. In most parts of that country, severe penalties are imposed on couples having more than one, or at most two, children (in some counties parents are permitted to have a second child only if the first one is a girl); more than two, regardless of sex, is prohibited. These new legal realities impose added pressure to ensure that the one child is a son.

For centuries strong son preference in Chinese and Indian society occasionally manifested itself in the form of female infanticide. Even today, among poor families in some rural areas of India, the killing of girl babies immediately after birth remains far too common. One young mother, interviewed during a UN-sponsored study conducted in northwestern India, was unrepentant about killing her first two baby girls and said she would kill any others she might bear because she had hardly any money to give them at the time of their wedding. In China, the age-old practice of killing or abandoning unwanted baby girls was stamped out by the Communist government during the early decades of that regime, but following the 1979 introduction of China's "one-child policy," numerous cases were reported of newborn girls being murdered by parents who hoped that a second try would produce a boy.

More recently, the advent of modern medical technology and the legalization of abortion in both countries have given Indian and Chinese parents an effective new approach for ensuring they have a son. Amniocentesis was introduced decades ago as a means of prenatal determination of a wide variety of genetic disorders. However, the chromosomal analysis also revealed the unborn child's sex and as early as the 1970s was being used by some couples specifically for sex-selection purposes; if amniocentesis showed the fetus to be female, the mother frequently chose to terminate her pregnancy. One survey conducted in Bombay hospitals revealed that of 8,000 abortions performed, all but one were of female fetuses.

However, the fact that amniocentesis must be performed in a modern medical setting and is relatively expensive limited its use to urban areas and more affluent patients. Only with the introduction of ultrasound technology in the mid-1980s did the possibility of sex-selection become a reality for the masses—and the birth ratio of girls to boys began its steady downward slide. Ultrasound imaging for gender detection has several distinct advantages over amniocentesis: it presents no risk to the fetus or mother; can be performed earlier in the pregnancy (13–14 weeks vs. 18–20 weeks), costs half as much, and is widely available. By the 1990s, ultrasound technology had spread from urban areas into the countryside. At public hospitals and proliferating for-profit maternity clinics, demand for sex-determination services has continued to grow. Providing gender information has proven to be quite profitable for doctors, clinic operators, and the manufacturers of ultrasound scanners—a fact that helps to explain the spread of sex-determination services to the remotest corners of both countries, despite laws prohibiting the use of ultrasound for such purposes. Although medical practitioners in India are legally proscribed from telling expectant mothers what ultrasonography revealed about the sex of the fetus, the law is almost never enforced.

In China the likelihood that an abortion will follow determination that the fetus is a girl varies depending on the order of the pregnancy and the sex of previous children. Surveys in a rural area of that country suggest that if a couple has one daughter already and finds that a second pregnancy would result in another girl, chances are overwhelming that the mother will opt for abortion. Since the Chinese don't regard the fetus as a person, believing that human life begins at birth, the act of abortion itself raises no moral qualms. However, if the first child is a son, odds of an abortion to prevent the birth of a little sister are considerably less. By contrast, research in India reveals numerous first-pregnancy abortions of female fetuses, as well as among women who already had one living son.

The issue of sex-selective abortions has become increasingly controversial in both India and China, as concerns grow about the widening gender gap. Emotionally conflicted feminist groups in India deplore the situation as yet another example of the victimization of women in that male-dominated society, yet they strongly defend a woman's right to abortion as a matter of free choice and control over her own reproduction. Some commentators in India defend the practice on the grounds that it is preferable for a woman to abort unwanted daughters rather than produce six or seven children in order to have one or two boys. Others justify the practice on the grounds that the girls who *are* born will suffer less discrimination, while some predict that over the long term, a declining sex ratio will improve women's status in society as they become an increasingly scarce commodity. Unfortunately, the latter conjecture is contradicted by the reality in certain rural areas of China today where the paucity of young women in relation to young men has caused severe disruptions in the "marriage market." Rather than being accorded greater respect and better treatment, young women in that region are now at heightened danger of being kidnapped by criminal gangs and sold to village men desperate for wives.

The widespread practice of sex-selective abortion has prompted soul-searching discussion among Indian and Chinese policymakers and academicians about what, if anything, can be done to end this perverse use of medical technology. Imposing legal prohibitions obviously is not the answer; although India and China both have strict laws regulating the use of ultrasound scanners, the devices are now so widespread, corruption so rampant, the profit motive among service providers so strong, and the desire for sons so overwhelming that curbing the abuse of medical technology through legislation is likely to prove impossible. Given these realities, there is general agreement that the only lasting solution to the problem is a fundamental shift in societal attitudes toward women and the wide scale implementation of economic, social, and legal measures to promote gender equity. Until the status of women is improved to the point that the birth of a baby girl is welcomed as joyously as the birth of a boy, millions more girls are fated to "go missing."

References

Chu, Junhong. 2001. "Prenatal Sex Determination and Sex-Selective Abortion in Rural Central China." *Population and Development Review* 27, no. 2 (June): 259–281.

Oomman, Nandini, and Bela R. Ganatra. 2002. "Sex Selection: The Systematic Elimination of Girls." *Reproductive Health Matters* 10, no. 19:184.

United Nations Population Fund. 2003. *Missing . . . Mapping the Adverse Child Sex Ratio in India* (June).

couples surveyed named two to three children as the ideal family size, a substantial majority of both husbands and wives would opt for one extra child in order to achieve their preferred number of sons; almost half of the husbands and a third of the wives indicated their willingness to have more than twice the number of children they really wanted in order to attain the desired number of sons (two was the most commonly designated number of boys wanted). While over two-thirds of the couples questioned said they'd like to have one daughter, none had any desire to go beyond their stated ideal family size if the first two children were boys (Mahler, 1997).

Low educational and economic status of women. Birth rates today are highest in those parts of the world where women have little schooling and where opportunities for paid employment outside the home are few. In such societies, a woman's worth is measured in terms of her childbearing abilities. Such women, striving to maintain favor with their husbands and in-laws, are unlikely to respond favorably to the idea of family limitation. In addition, illiterate women or women with only an elementary education are less likely than better educated women to have heard about modern contraceptive techniques or to know how to use them. Surveys indicate that providing women with at least a secondary school education is one of the most effective ways of reducing the birth rate in developing countries. In general, fertility drops noticeably as the level of female education increases, primarily because educated women tend to marry later, have greater opportunity for employment outside the home, are more aware of the advantages of smaller family size, and understand how to practice contraception more effectively. The mother's education level is even more strongly correlated with improved childhood health and nutritional status. Women who have primary schooling or higher are much less likely to see their children die than are women who never attended school; children whose mothers completed high

Providing young women with at least a secondary school education is one of the most effective ways of reducing birth rates in developing countries. [*Jorgen Schytte/Still Pictures*]

school or college are much less likely to be underweight or short for their age in comparison with children whose mothers are less educated (Riley, 1997).

Such factors support the contention of many demographers that broad-based social and economic changes must precede or accompany population programs in developing nations if population growth is ever to be stabilized; simply making contraceptives more widely available will not be enough to overcome traditional biases that favor large families.

Population Policy: Moving Beyond Birth Control

Since the inception of both private and government-sponsored family-planning programs in the 1950s and 1960s, efforts have focused on increasing the availability of contraceptives while simultaneously trying to encourage their use. Numerous surveys conducted in many countries during these years demonstrated that many women were continuing to have more children than they desired, often because of misperceptions about the health effects of certain contraceptives, excessive cost of obtaining supplies, insufficient choice of contraceptive methods, or other problems related to access. Building new clinics and expanding social outreach programs seemed like the most straightforward approach to dealing with a problem that government leaders were beginning to view as increasingly urgent. By the 1980s, public opinion in many developing countries was supportive toward stabilizing growth rates and many Third World governments had begun implementing vigorous efforts to increase the percentage of couples practicing contraception. A declaration by delegates to the United Nations-sponsored International Conference on Population, held in Mexico City in 1984, for governments to make family-planning services "universally available" was hailed as a significant achievement by population control advocates.

During those same years, however, feminists and others concerned about women's health issues and civil rights were growing increasingly critical of the single-minded focus on distributing contraceptives, often with no follow-up and apparently with little concern for the welfare of the women they were recruiting as contraceptive acceptors. Particularly in Asian countries (India and China being notable examples), family-planning programs were target-driven, with administrators' job security based on how many IUDs their staffs inserted within a month or how many sterilizations they performed. Such quota systems inevitably lead to violations of patients' rights—sometimes to outright coercion—and critics charged that the emphasis on numerical goals diminished the quality of services provided.

In 1994 when the United Nations convened its third decennial international population conference in Cairo, Egypt, a grassroots insistence that contraceptives alone are not the answer to the world's population dilemma persuaded planners of the need for a radical change in focus. Reflecting the new emphasis, the name of the event itself was changed to the International Conference on Population and Development (ICPD), highlighting the conviction of those attending that fertility rates could be further reduced only in conjunction with broad-based development initiatives to improve health, reduce poverty, and improve the status of women. Attracting delegates from 180 different countries, as well as representatives of 1,200 nongovernmental organizations, many of them women's advocacy groups, the Cairo conference was the most comprehensive international meeting ever held on the population issue. While agreeing that both family planning *and* economic development are essential for reducing population growth rates, delegates for the first time acknowledged that empowerment of women will be a crucial factor in stabilizing world population size. Moving away

from the past emphasis on people-coun
Action coming out of Cairo was base?
should focus on individual needs, not o
of the 180 national delegations partici'
goals to be achieved by 2015. Among

1. To provide universal access t
   methods and related reprodui

2. To reduce infant mortality ra
   mortality rates (i.e., deaths of c

3. To achieve a maternal mortality

4. To increase life expectancy at bii
   in the countries currently experiei

5. To achieve universal access to and cc.
   the widest and earliest possible access by gii.
   higher levels of education.

To carry out this ambitious program will require a sustained ᵕ
national governments, as well as many billions of dollars to implement the ᵕ
reproductive health programs. Achievement of the designated goals is also incumbe..
on wrenching changes in lifestyle and cultural norms in societies reluctant to alter age-
old traditions regarding gender roles (Ashford, 1995). Whether the promise of Cairo
(and subsequent reaffirmation of these goals at the 2004 ICPD conference in France)
will be realized in an era of dwindling development dollars, when women's opportunities remain severely constrained in many countries and at a time when the developing
world is beset by pressing economic problems, remains to be seen.

References

Ashford, Lori S. 1995. "New Perspectives on Population: Lessons from Cairo." *Population Bulle-tin* 50, no. 1 (March).

Baird, P. A., A. D. Sadovnick, and I. M. L. Yee. 1991. "Maternal Age and Birth Defects: A Population Study." *Lancet* 337:527.

Beral, Valerie, Carol Hermon, Clifford Kay, Philip Hannaford, Sarah Darby, and Gillian Reeves. 1999. "Mortality Associated with Oral Contraceptive Use: 25-Year Follow up of Cohort of 46,000 Women from Royal College of General Practitioners' Oral Contraceptive Study." *British Medical Journal* 318, no. 7176 (Jan. 9): 96–100.

Dasgupta, Partha S. 1995. "Population, Poverty, and the Local Environment." *Scientific American* 272, no. 2 (Feb): 40–45.

Dieben, Tom, F. J. M. E. Roumen, and D. Apter. 2002. "Efficacy Cycle Control and User Acceptability of a Novel Combined Contraceptive Vaginal Ring." *Obstetrics and Gynecology* 100(3):585–593.

Dulitzki, M., D. Soriano, E. Schiff, A. Chetrit, S. Mashiach, and D. S. Seidman. 1998. "Effect of Very Advanced Maternal Age on Pregnancy Outcome and Rate of Cesarean Delivery." *Obstetrics and Gynecology* 92, no. 6 (Dec): 935–939.

Eckholm, Erik, and Kathleen Newland. 1977. "Health: The Family Planning Factor." *Worldwatch Paper* 10, Worldwatch Institute.

Good, Brian. 2003. "A Better Vasectomy Option." *Men's Health* 18, no. 7 (Sept): 34.

Kleinman, R. L., and P. Senanayake. 1984. *Breastfeeding, Fertility, and Contraception.* IPPF Medical Publications.

League of Women Voters Education Fund. 1982. *Public Policy on Reproductive Choice.* No. 286 (July).

Mahler, K. 1997. "Strong Son Preference among Nepalese Couples May Outweigh Their Desire for Smaller Families." *International Family Planning Perspectives* 23, no. 1 (March).

McLaren, Angus A. 1990. *A History of Contraception.* Oxford, England: Basil Blackwell, Ltd.

Toby Hanlon. 2003. "New: Permanent Birth Control." *Prevention* 55,

Allergy and Infectious Disease (NIAID). 2001. *Workshop Summary: Scien-*
Condom Effectiveness for Sexually Transmitted Disease (STD) Prevention, July 20.
J., and William D. Mosher. 1998. "Trends in Contraceptive Use in the United
2–1995." *Family Planning Perspectives* 30, no. 1 (Jan/Feb): 4–10.
., J. D. Blume, and S. M. DeMonner. 2002. "Young Maternal Age Associated with
sed Risk of Neonatal Death." *Obstetrics and Gynecology* 100(3):481–486.
n Reference Bureau (PRB). 2002. *Family Planning Worldwide: 2002 Data Sheet.*
. 2003. *2003 World Population Data Sheet.*
, Malcolm. 2000. "The Unmet Need for Family Planning." *Scientific American* 282, no. 1
(Jan): 88–93.
iddle, John M. 1992. *Contraception and Abortion from the Ancient World to the Renaissance.* Cambridge, MA: Harvard Univ. Press.
Riley, Nancy E. 1997. "Gender, Power, and Population Change." *Population Bulletin* 52, no. 1 (May).
Riman, T. et al. 2002. "Risk Factors for Invasive Ovarian Cancer: Results from a Swedish Case-
control Study." *American Journal of Epidemiology* 156 (4):363–373.
Ronsmans, Carine, and Oona Campbell. 1998. "Short Birth Intervals Don't Kill Women: Evi-
dence from Matlab, Bangladesh." *Studies in Family Planning* 29, no. 3 (Sept): 282–290.
Stokes, Bruce. 1980. "Men and Family Planning." *Worldwatch Paper* 41. Worldwatch Institute.
Van Noord-Zaadstra, B. M. et al. 1991. "Delaying Childbearing: Effect of Age on Fecundity
and Outcome of Pregnancy." *British Medical Journal* 302:1361.
Weiss, Peter. 1993. "The Contraceptive Potential of Breastfeeding in Bangladesh." *Studies in*
Family Planning 24, no. 2 (March/April).

4

THE PEOPLE-FOOD PREDICAMEN

Famine seems to be the last, the most dreadful resource of nature. The power of population is so superior to the power in the earth to produce subsistence for man, that premature death must in some shape or other visit the human race.
—Thomas Malthus, "An Essay on the Principal of Population" (1798)

The fierce debate sparked by Malthus' gloomy pronouncements over two centuries ago continues to reverberate today as policymakers and scientists argue about the planet's ability to meet the nutritional needs of additional billions of people in the decades ahead. Viewpoints vary widely, with many experts expressing cautious optimism that improvements in agricultural technology, coupled with declining birth rates, guarantee that future generations will be adequately fed. Other less sanguine observers insist that current trends are already seriously undermining the long-term sustainability of world agriculture and fisheries while simultaneously increasing the number of mouths to be fed.

The wide divergence in outlook stems from personal assumptions regarding future trends in human fertility, world economic growth, environmental degradation, and agricultural productivity—assumptions that may ultimately prove correct or radically off base. Until relatively recently, remarkable gains in agricultural productivity worldwide provided ample grounds for optimism that one day in the not-too-distant future, no child would go to bed hungry nor any family worry about the next day's meal. From 1950 until 1984 the world's farmers were successful in producing increased quantities of food more rapidly than the world's parents were producing babies. During this period world grain consumption per person increased by 38% in spite of spiraling population figures, resulting in impressive nutritional gains in many formerly food-short regions of the world. Global trends were somewhat misleading, however, since the world food production averages to a large extent reflected an enormous and disproportionate increase in North American crop yields during those years. These figures masked grimmer statistics showing that in many of the rapidly growing developing nations, per capita increase in food production had halted by the late 1950s due to high rates of population increase. Until the mid-1980s, global averages continued to convey the impression that all was rosy on the food front. Throughout this period, world grain harvests increased by almost 3% annually (compared with a world population growth rate at this time of about 2%). During the 1970s the resource-intensive technologies of the Green Revolution resulted in a major boost in Third World agricultural production; by the early 1980s news of huge crop surpluses dominated the farm pages of newspapers and laments of a worldwide "grain glut" were heard from Chicago to Melbourne. Even western Europe, reliant on food imports for the past 200 years, became a grain exporter during those golden years.

By the mid-1980s, however, some worrisome trends were becoming evident. After nearly 40 years of steady growth in world food output, a significant slowdown became apparent in many of the world's most populous countries. In India, grain production has been stagnant since 1983—at a time when India's population continues to increase by over 20 million yearly; in China, agricultural output has dropped since 1984's peak harvest; Indonesia and Mexico have witnessed a leveling off of their production, while in Japan, Taiwan, and South Korea grain output has been declining for years. In contrast to the 3% annual increases in grain harvests that characterized the period between 1950 and 1984, during the 1990s world grain output grew by just 1% a year—while world population figures continued to climb at a 1.4% annual rate. This gap between grain production and people production meant that food availability *per capita* had actually declined during the 1990s. By 2002, per capita global grain production had fallen to 294 kilograms per person, the lowest level since 1970, a year when the total harvest was slightly over half that of 2002. As a result, in 2003 grain reserves were at their lowest level in a generation (Halweil, 2003; Brown, 2003).

Of course, livestock production and fisheries also contribute significantly to human diets. Mirroring the per capita increase in grain harvests, production of beef and mutton tripled between 1950 and 1990; since then, a lowering of rangeland productivity due to overgrazing has resulted in a leveling off in production, with future increases unlikely unless more feed grains are diverted to livestock. Meat production overall has continued to grow by about 2% annually, thanks largely to big increases in poultry production, as well as to a continued expansion in the market for pork, the world's most popular red meat. While meat currently comprises a much larger proportion of the daily diet in rich countries than in the Third World, meat consumption is rising more rapidly in developing nations. China has now become the leading producer and consumer of pork, accounting for half the world's supply. Two-thirds of the world increase in meat consumption in 2002 occurred in developing nations, where rising incomes, urbanization, and food imports are prompting a major shift in dietary habits (Nierenberg, 2003). Growth in world fisheries, which witnessed a near-quintupling of the annual catch between the early 1950s and the early 1990s, now appears to be at or near its maximum sustainable yield; many stocks of preferred table fish species have already been fished to commercial extinction and marine biologists fear we may have already exceeded the carrying capacity of the world's oceans (Watson and Pauly, 2001).

While many national leaders tend to blame adverse weather conditions for food shortfalls, the true causes are more complex: loss of good cropland to erosion and nonfarm uses, inefficient agrarian structures, lack of investment in agriculture by city-oriented government officials, cutbacks in agricultural research, and *too many people.*

Factors Influencing Food Demand

While it is obvious that the total yield of the world's croplands, pasturelands, and fisheries constitutes the world's food *supply,* assessing food *demand* is slightly more complicated. **Population growth,** not surprisingly, is the single largest factor in determining food demand. Since 97% of the world's population increase is occurring in the countries of Asia, Africa, and Latin America, food supply problems currently are most acute in these regions. An additional factor must be considered in assessing food demand, however. **Rising personal incomes** that have characterized the economic development of most industrialized countries since the Second World War have greatly added to world food demand. This is not because the typical American, Swede, or Japanese eats tremendously greater quantities than the average Peruvian, Pakistani, or Sudanese, but because higher incomes generally translate into an increased demand for high-quality foods, particularly meat and dairy products. As you will recall from our discussion of trophic levels and energy transfer (chapter 1), it requires several times as much grain to produce a pound of human flesh from meat as it would if that same grain were eaten directly, due to inescapable inefficiencies of

Figure 4-1

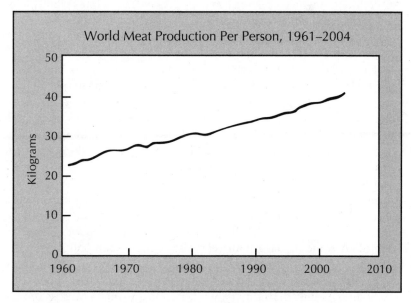

Source: Based on data from the Food and Agriculture Organization of the United Nations.

energy conversion. (Some animals are more efficient converters than others, however. The grain demand imposed by eating poultry is far less than that of eating beef, for example, since producing a pound of chicken requires just three pounds of feed grain, while it takes seven to ten pounds of grain to produce a pound of beef.) Currently nearly 40% of world grain production is utilized for livestock feed; with analysts predicting that world meat consumption is likely to increase at a 1.8% annual rate for the next twenty years, pressure on grain supplies will correspondingly increase (Pinstrup-Andersen, Pandya-Lorch, and Rosegrant, 1997).

Perhaps nowhere does the pent-up consumer craving for animal protein have more explosive potential than in China, where rapid economic growth is bringing hitherto undreamed-of prosperity to the world's most populous nation. Meat-eating has now become a status symbol in China, a way for Chinese to demonstrate their embrace of a modern lifestyle and a repudiation of past poverty that imposed a largely vegetarian diet (Gardner and Halweil, 2000). The rapid rise in personal incomes in East Asia and in many developing nations during the past decade is having a profound impact on both the type and amount of food people in those countries eat. As the people of China—and elsewhere—shift from primarily vegetarian to more heavily meat-based diets, world grain demand will grow even faster than mere population figures would suggest.

Extent of Hunger

Determining the number of hungry people in the world today is a rather tricky business. Certainly there is a quantum difference between the teenager coming home from school complaining, "When's dinner, Mom? I'm starving!" and a Somali child with sticklike limbs and protruding abdomen, dying of acute malnutrition. In an attempt to establish some basis for comparison, the Food and Agriculture Organization (FAO) of the United Nations has devised a concept called the **basal metabolic rate** (BMR). The BMR is defined as the minimum amount of energy required to power human body maintenance, not including energy required for activity. On this basis, the FAO considers anyone receiving less than 1.2 BMR food intake daily to be undernourished. Using this rather conservative figure (some authorities feel the cut-off point should be raised to 1.5 BMR), the FAO estimates that 840 million people in the world are undernourished, receiving insufficient food to develop their full physical and mental potential. Hunger, of course, is not equally shared among nations or even within nations. The vast majority of the world's hungry people inhabit the South Asian countries of India, Pakistan, and Bangladesh, parts of Southeast Asia, Africa south of the Sahara, and the Andean region of South America—all regions where rates of population growth continue to be high. Nevertheless, pockets of hunger can be found even within many affluent societies. In the United States malnutrition is distressingly common among the poor, the elderly, migrant farm workers, and Native Americans.

In developing nations as a group, as many as one-third of all children under 5 years old are malnourished, a figure that rises as high as two-thirds in India and Bangladesh. The World Health Organization (WHO) estimates that every day 19,000 children (over 6 million a year) die as a result of malnutrition and related ailments; malnutrition is the direct or indirect cause of more than half the deaths of children under age 5 in Third World countries (WHO, 1997). Women, too, are at disproportionate risk of malnutrition. This situation exists because within households in many cultures men, being the primary workers and providers, are served the best food before the rest of the family eats. Children and women, including both pregnant and

Figure 4-2   Countries Facing Food Emergencies

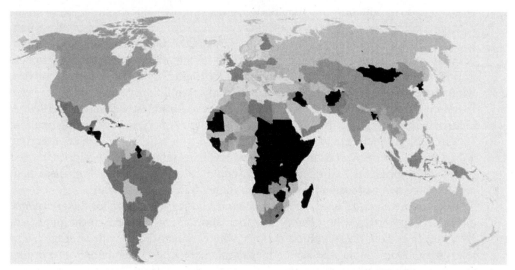

Africa: Angola, Burundi, Chad, Central African Rep., Dem. Rep. of Congo, Rep. of Congo, Cote d'Ivoire, Eritrea, Ethiopia, Guinea, Kenya, Lesotho, Liberia, Madagascar, Mauritania, Malawi, Sierra Leone, Somalia, Sudan, Swaziland, Tanzania, Uganda, Zimbabwe. **Asia/Near East:** Afghanistan, Bangladesh, Iraq, Korea, Maldives, Mongolia, Sri Lanka. **Latin America:** Guatemala, Guyana, Haiti, Honduras, Nicaragua. **Europe:** Russian Federation (Chechnya).

Source: "Foodcrops and Shortages," Issue no. 1 (Feb. 2005), Food and Agriculture Organization of the United Nations (www.fao.org/giews). Used with permission.

nursing mothers, whose nutritional needs in proportion to their size exceed those of men, subsist on whatever remains. In such situations, girl children frequently receive less than boys, since males are more highly regarded (Riley, 1997).

The hunger issue most frequently impinges on the public consciousness during periods of severe famine, generally caused by prolonged droughts, floods, or wartime upheavals. During recent years, media coverage of starving children and anguished parents in North Korea, Zimbabwe, Congo, and Ethiopia have kept us grimly aware of human suffering during times of calamity elsewhere in the world. Such periodic episodes of famine, tragic though they are, do not represent the world's major hunger problem, however. Rather, a "covert famine"—the chronic, undramatic, day-after-day undernutrition of those who know that, good harvest or poor, their bellies will never be full—constitutes today's most serious food supply dilemma.

Causes of Hunger

The existence of more than 800 million severely malnourished people seems paradoxical when one considers that the world's farmers, ranchers, and fishers produce enough food to supply every human on the planet with 3,800 calories per day—more than enough for good health (Bender and Smith, 1997). Most commentators conclude that resources exist to meet the food demands of the projected world population well into the 21st century and even to reduce existing levels of malnutrition. If this is so, why are so many people today suffering from inadequate diets? The current situation is caused largely by two factors: **uneven distribution** of food and **poverty**.

Although global averages suggest that there should be enough food for everyone, many of the areas where hunger is endemic are regions where there is a widening gap between food production and population growth; only imports from food-surplus areas prevent the problem from worsening further. However, as human numbers continue to climb, more equitable distribution of existing resources may not suffice—particularly if a high-quality diet rather than caloric content alone is the goal. Researchers at Brown University calculate that an even apportioning of the current world harvest, without any diversion of grain for livestock fodder, would provide an adequate vegetarian diet to a world population of 6 billion people—a milestone passed in 1999. A diet comparable to that currently consumed by South Americans, consisting of about 15% animal products, could be evenly distributed to 4 billion. To provide everyone with a typical North American or European-style diet (about 30% of calories derived from animal products), world population could barely exceed 2 billion—less than one-third the number currently dwelling on Planet Earth (Chen, 1990).

On a more practical level, however, the most basic explanation for the prevalence of hunger is poverty. Even in chronically food-short countries, the rich eat quite well. By contrast, even in the wealthiest nations, where markets bulge with a veritable cornucopia of foods, people who lack money to purchase groceries go hungry. According to World Bank estimates, over one billion people live in absolute poverty, earning less than the equivalent of $1 per day. These "poorest of the poor" include farmers whose land holdings are too small to be economically viable, rural landless laborers, and urban residents of the rapidly growing squatter settlements ringing many Third World cities. For these hungry people, and for 2 billion more who are only marginally better off, an increase in world food production will mean little unless corresponding social and economic improvements increase their ability to purchase food for their families.

Poverty's role as a determinant of hunger was clearly evident during the 1967 drought in Bihar, a state in eastern India threatened with severe famine due to near-total crop failure. Food aid rushed into the area by the United States and other donors was credited with averting large-scale loss of life, and interviews with villagers after the crisis was over revealed that many of them ate better during this period of natural disaster than at any other time in their lives. Why? Because the donated wheat was distributed to the needy free of charge and all received a share. During normal times the poorer segments of society lacked money to buy sufficient food in the marketplace and so went hungry. As George Verghese, editor of the *Hindustan Times* and information advisor to Prime Minister Gandhi during the famine eloquently described:

> For the poorest sections of the society, 1967, the Year of the Famine, will long be remembered as a bonus year when millions of people, especially the children, probably for the first time were assured of a decent meal a day . . . in a "normal year," these people hover on the bread line. They are beyond the pale, nobody's concern, they starve. In a famine year, they eat. Their health is better and the children are gaining weight. For them this is a year of great blessing. This is the deep irony, the grim tragedy of the situation.

Most observers are confident that until 2025 at least there will be adequate food to meet the demand of those who can afford to pay for it. For those who cannot, the outlook is dismal. In a number of the poorest countries, food production is falling farther and farther behind increasing food demand as their populations continue to grow. If their economies are unable to generate the foreign exchange necessary to purchase food from abroad, nutritional levels are likely to suffer. Free food aid and other forms of development assistance from the wealthy industrialized countries have declined substantially in recent years, further increasing the vulnerability of the world's poorest people. Food insecurity is expected to increase significantly in sub-Saharan Africa and South Asia during the first decade of the 21st century, with large proportions of the population in those regions too poor to purchase food at prevailing prices. Political instability, regional conflicts, greater variability in agricultural production due to climate change—all could have an impact on food price fluctuations that will determine who eats and who goes hungry (Pinstrup-Andersen, Pandya-Lorch, and Rosegrant, 1997).

Health Impact of Hunger

The most serious energy crisis in the world is the depletion of human energy—a depletion that comes about because the brain receives too few calories or too few proteins to think, and the body too few to act.

—Richard J. Barnet, *New Yorker*, March 31, 1980

Malnutrition

Hunger is more than a state of physical discomfort and a cause of political unrest. Even in the absence of acute famine, inadequate food intake has a profound impact on human health. Among the poor in developing countries, **protein-energy malnutrition** (PEM) is a leading cause of death and disease; numerous studies over the past decade have shown that protein-energy malnutrition is responsible, directly or indirectly, for 50–60% of all childhood deaths in developing countries. Such deaths are seldom due to outright starvation, but rather to a chronic deficit of calories and essential nutrients that leave a child underweight, weak, and vulnerable to infection (FAO,

---

Box 4-1   Supersized America: The Other Face of Malnutrition

Americans like to think of their country in superlative terms—the biggest and best of everything! A recently attained new world record is nothing to brag about, however: by the 1990s, Americans had indisputably become the fattest people on earth. Clinically, a person's body mass index (BMI), defined as one's weight in kilograms divided by the square of one's height in meters, determines whether that person is categorized as "overweight." A BMI over 25 is defined as overweight, while a BMI over 30 is considered obese. According to the Centers for Disease Control and Prevention (CDC), by 2004 65% of adult Americans were overweight or obese; of these, 5 million are regarded as "morbidly obese," more than 100 pounds overweight. Of even greater concern are figures showing that fully one-quarter of all American children under 19 are now either overweight or obese. These numbers are *double* those of 30 years ago and have prompted U.S. Surgeon General David Satcher to declare obesity a "national epidemic."

Bulging American tourists have become the butt of jokes and sniggering comments abroad, but expanding U.S. waistlines may be a harbinger of things to come elsewhere in the world as obesity becomes—according to an official World Health Organization pronouncement—"one of the greatest neglected public health problems of our time." For the first time in human history, there are now as many people overweight as underweight—1.2 billion of each (both conditions are regarded as a form of malnutrition; the overweight obviously are consuming more than enough calories, but their diets frequently lack sufficient vitamins and minerals). In the United Kingdom, for example, there are now three times as many obese Britons as there were 20 years ago. Even in developing countries where large segments of the population remain undernourished, those who can afford to eat heartily are getting fat; today an estimated 23% of Chinese city dwellers are overweight. Nevertheless, Americans remain pacesetters in the international march toward obesity, raising the inevitable question, "Why?"

At its most basic level, the answer is simple: too much calorie-dense food vs. too little exercise. Since the trends first became noticeable almost a half-century ago, nutritionists and government health agencies have been urging Americans to eat less and exercise more—admonitions that largely fell on deaf ears because of trends in American (and, increasingly, world) society that encourage excessive eating and sedentary lifestyles. Add to this humans' innate love of sweet and fatty foods (a hold-over from our old hunter-gatherer days when there was survival value in occasional gorging to store up energy for the lean times to come) and the propensity to lounge about when action isn't necessary, and the inevitable result is extra pounds.

A number of changes in the American food supply and in U.S. eating habits have converged to make this country what some nutritionists call a "toxic environment" when it comes to food. Some of the changes since the early 1980s that foster weight gain include the "supersizing" of food portions at restaurants and fast-food establishments; the extra ingredients (largely high-starch or high-fructose items) cost little and the customer's perception of "better value" sells. And, research has shown, when presented with bigger servings, consumers eat more whether or not they're hungry. Moreover, a single fast-food meal frequently exceeds the recommended daily intake of fat, sugar, cholesterol, and sodium. Emphasizing the "empty calories" represented by fast food—and the nutritional ignorance of the American public—questionnaire results on the food habits of typical Americans revealed that 20% of "vegetables" consumed by the group surveyed consisted of french fries and potato chips! School cafeterias, once a reliable source of at least one well-balanced meal a day, in recent years have increasingly succumbed to offers by fast-food companies and soft drink purveyors to take over the lunchtime feeding of America's schoolchildren in return for corporate financial contributions to school programs.

Another adverse influence, nutritionally speaking, is the fact that in today's hectic world, one out of every three meals is eaten outside the home and snacking (or "grazing"!) has become nearly continuous. Eating in public, considered extremely rude by previous generations, has now become omnipresent; the office coffeepot is now surrounded by doughnuts and other high-calorie treats. Sports TV-watching has become synonymous with snacking, as has movie-going. Virtually all these extra calories eaten outside the home consist of less nutritious fare than the home-cooked food of yesteryear; one depressing trend is that, even when home, Americans cook less than ever. By 1998, only 38% of American meals were truly homemade—cooked from basic ingredients. The majority were take-in, prepackaged, or convenience foods, quickly warmed in a microwave. Some observers suggest that the day is not far off when scarcely any Americans will have ever prepared—or tasted—a home-cooked meal. This is profoundly worrisome, not only in terms of lost cultural values. Fast foods and convenience foods contain higher concentrations of energy-dense fats and sugars than do the basic ingredients of home cooking; in other words, they're less healthy and more fattening—and we're eating more and more of them.

The impact of these consumption trends is most pronounced among the least-affluent segments of the population. The cost once associated with a high-fat diet has now declined precipitously as cheap corn syrup sweeteners and palm oil saturated fats replaced higher priced ingredients. As a result, millions of low-income people worldwide can now afford to indulge in richer foods than previous generations could ever have dreamed of doing. Consequently, obesity today disproportionately plagues the poor, especially those who are African American and Latino; rates of obesity in both groups are well above the already-too-high national average.

The flip side of the coin, of course, is insufficient exercise to burn up all those extra calories. Ever since the advent of the automobile, Americans have been walking less and sitting more. TV and video games have largely supplanted outdoor activities and have turned us into a nation of couch potatoes. Even in public schools, P.E. class is falling victim to school budget cuts and time constraints, as required sports are dropped in favor of state-mandated academic subjects. Children who ride buses to school and stay indoors watching television after school are thus increasingly deprived of their only remaining opportunity to get some badly needed physical activity. Middle-class and affluent children may compensate by joining health and fitness clubs or by attending summer camp; for the poor this generally isn't an option. Additionally, because they often live in neighborhoods lacking public parks and playgrounds—or considered by their parents as too dangerous for unsupervised play—poor children are even more likely than their wealthier classmates to spend out-of-school hours indoors in front of the TV, eating high-calorie snacks and gaining weight.

In the past, being overweight was a topic of public jokes and private humiliation; today it has become a national health issue as important as cigarette smoking in terms of its impact on physical well-being, longevity, and health care costs. Among the long list of diseases caused by or associated with being overweight or obese are cardiovascular disease, high blood pressure, several kinds of cancer (breast cancer in postmenopausal women, plus cancer of the endometrium, ovaries, colon, prostate, and gall bladder), and type 2 diabetes. The latter, a chronic, potentially crippling lifelong disease, is an ailment once confined almost exclusively to adults. In recent years, however, it has been documented with alarming frequency among obese children even before the age of puberty. From a national economic perspective, diabetes is imposing an enormous financial burden on the United States; the care and treatment of diabetes in this country now costs in the range of $100 billion a year, with the majority of new cases presenting as a direct result of excess weight.

Other health consequences of obesity include orthopedic problems such as arthritic joints and slipped hips; various forms of respiratory distress, such as obstructive sleep apnea, allergic asthma, and a condition called "Pickwickian syndrome," where large amounts of abdominal fat cause the patient to breathe in a rapid, shallow fashion, with increasing intervals of breathlessness. Excessive weight in pregnant women can significantly elevate the risk of stillbirth, death of the baby soon after birth, or a range of congenital birth disorders.

With so many serious health consequences inherent in America's current obesity epidemic, many nutritionists and other health experts are clamoring for effective action. It's obvious that simply exhorting the public to eat less and exercise more is not effective. Among the wide range of options that have been proposed, many based on the results of behavioral research, the following offer the most promise: (1) change the lunch menus in school cafeterias, eliminating or reducing fast-food and snack items, increasing fruit and vegetable offerings, and removing vending machines that sell soda pop and candy; (2) remove high-calorie snack foods from the home; (3) prohibit advertisements for candy, snacks, and soft drinks on TV shows commonly watched by children under age 10; (4) drastically limit the number of meals eaten outside the home; (5) serve from the kitchen rather than placing serving dishes on the table in order to make it more of an effort to get additional portions; (6) limit hours children are permitted to watch TV or play video games; (7) reinstate daily physical education classes in schools where these have been discontinued; (8) increase opportunities for people to be physically active by encouraging local governments to provide hiking/jogging trails, bike paths, swimming pools, tennis courts, ball fields; (9) levy a small tax on "junk foods," soft drinks, and new television sets to raise money for the public recreation programs cited above. These initiatives would require widespread cooperation among various levels of government, schools, health care providers, parents—indeed, from all levels of society. The task is daunting and past efforts have yielded discouraging results. Nevertheless, the consequences to the nation's health and wealth are too serious to ignore.

References

Critser, Greg. 2003. *Fat Land: How Americans Became the Fattest People in the World.* Boston: Houghton Mifflin.

Gardner, Gary, and Brian Halweil. 2000. "Underfed and Overfed: The Global Epidemic of Malnutrition." *Worldwatch Paper* 150 (March).

Nestle, Marion, and Michael F. Jacobson. 2000. "Halting the Obesity Epidemic: A Public Health Policy Approach." *Public Health Reports* 115 (Jan/Feb).

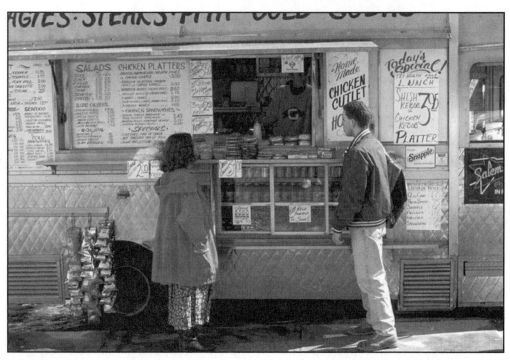

In the U.S., diets high in sweet and fatty foods have contributed to an epidemic of obesity. Most overweight Americans are considered malnourished because their diets lack sufficient vitamins and minerals. [© *Lee Snider/The Image Works*]

The propensity for physical activity that comes so naturally to young children diminishes significantly in adolescence, contributing to increased numbers of American children under age 19 being classified as overweight or obese. [© *Royalty-Free/Corbis*]

2002a). If children receive less than 70% of the daily standard food requirement, their growth and activity fall below normal levels; if food deprivation is prolonged, stunted physical development becomes irreversible and adult size is correspondingly reduced. The World Health Organization estimates that PEM affects one out of every four children worldwide to some extent, with 150 million underweight and 182 million exhibiting stunted growth.

Even more ominous than the link between malnutrition and decreased physical development, however, is the finding that severe malnutrition in children, especially very young infants, results in a permanent stunting of brain development, characterized by a decrease in the number of brain cells and an alteration of brain chemistry. Studies have shown that if a nutritional deficiency occurs just before or immediately after birth, the baby will suffer a 15–25% reduction in number of brain cells. If malnutrition afflicts the developing fetus and continues to persist in the postnatal period, the child's complement of brain cells will be lowered by 50–60%.

Two clinical manifestations of PEM, occurring most commonly among children in famine-stricken areas or under conditions of limited food supply, are **kwashiorkor** and **marasmus**. The former is a protein deficiency disease that affects millions of children in tropical areas, particularly in Africa. Although usually associated with food supply emergencies (drought, floods, or violent conflict), kwashiorkor can develop in babies who are weaned early and given only starchy, low-protein foods such as rice, cassava, or bananas to eat—common baby foods in many tropical regions. Symptoms of mild kwashiorkor include discoloration of the hair (in dark-haired children, hair may assume a reddish cast), white patches on the skin, retardation of physical growth, development of a protruding abdomen due to accumulation of fluids, and a loss of appetite. In more severe cases the hair may fall out painlessly in tufts, digestive problems arise, fluid collects in the legs and feet, muscle wastage and enlargement of the liver may occur, and the child becomes listless and apathetic. Once this stage of the disease is reached, shock and coma leading to death are likely unless the child receives medical attention. Victims who recover from severe cases of kwashiorkor never attain their full height and growth potential. In its milder forms, however, the effects of kwashiorkor are reversible and generally disappear as the child becomes older and is given a more varied diet.

Marasmus, the second of the two most commonly observed deficiency diseases among children, is an indication of overall protein-calorie deprivation—in essence, the child is starving. Most frequently striking babies under one year of age, especially those no longer being breast-fed, marasmus often occurs after the child has been suffering from diarrhea or some other disease. Victims of marasmus can be distinguished by their thin, wasted appearance, with skin hanging in loose wrinkles around wrists and legs and eyes appearing unusually large and bright because of the shrunken aspect of the rest of the body.

In addition to its direct impact on growth and mental development, malnutrition also greatly increases a child's susceptibility to infectious disease by reducing bodily defenses. Even mild levels of malnutrition can increase a child's risk of dying from common childhood ailments such as diarrhea, measles, or acute respiratory infections. As the severity of malnutrition (measured in terms of a child's weight-to-age ratio) increases, so does the risk of death due to infectious disease, from 2.5 times higher for mildly malnourished children to 4.6 times for those moderately underfed to 8.4 times excess risk for severely malnourished youngsters (FAO, 2002a).

Malnutrition takes its toll among older children and adults as well. Undernourished people lose weight and become less able to combat infections or environmental stress. They thereby become less economically productive and less able to care for

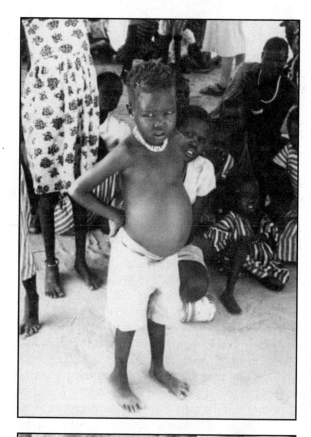

This child exhibits the protruding abdomen characteristic of kwashiorkor sufferers. [*R. Bafalis/U.S. Agency for International Development*]

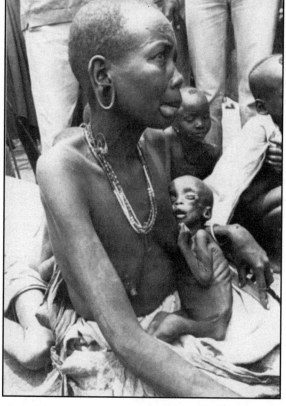

Victims of marasmus, an overall protein-calorie deprivation, can be identified by their thin, wasted appearance. [*World Vision*]

their families. Surveys in developing countries have shown that nutritionally deprived adults who are smaller and slighter than normal earn lower wages than their better-fed colleagues when employed in jobs requiring physical labor—proof that while poverty may be a cause of hunger, hunger can also cause poverty (FAO, 2002a). However, while adults suffering temporarily from severe food deprivation may become listless and apathetic, unable to engage in strenuous physical labor, they seldom experience the permanent damage characteristic of childhood malnutrition. At greatest risk, of course, are pregnant and lactating women. Such women, if malnourished, run a significantly higher risk of miscarriage or premature delivery than do adequately fed mothers. If they manage to carry their babies full-term, the child is likely to suffer from low birth weight (one of the most frequent causes of infant mortality) or to be stillborn. The old myth that nursing mothers draw on their own nutritional reserves to provide top-quality food for their infants is untrue—the milk of undernourished mothers is lower than normal in vitamins, fat, and protein content.

Micronutrient Deficiencies

A large portion of the world's undernourished population suffers as well from an inadequate intake of essential vitamins and minerals. This situation is largely a reflection of the lack of variety in the diet of the poor, who may subsist on little but rice, tortillas, or chappatis. However, micronutrient deficiencies are not limited to chronically hungry populations; many people receiving an adequate, even excess, daily intake of calories may still be malnourished in terms of vitamin or mineral deficiencies if their diets are heavily skewed toward starchy, low-nutrient foods. The WHO estimates that some 2.0–3.5 billion people worldwide are currently affected by micronutrient deficiencies that make them more susceptible to disease, stunt their mental and physical development, and sap their energy. Of particular concern because the condition is so widespread is insufficient intake of vitamin A, iron, and iodine.

Vitamin A deficiency (VAD). A public health problem among the poor in over 100 countries, VAD is the single most important cause of childhood blindness in low-income countries. VAD, seldom a concern among those whose diet includes eggs, dairy products, and green leafy vegetables, can result in a drying of the eye membranes or a softening of the cornea. Such conditions lead first to night-blindness and, if not treated, to total blindness of its victims. In areas such as South and Southeast Asia, Africa, Central America, Haiti, and northeastern Brazil, an estimated 100–140 million children suffer from VAD and 250,000–500,000 go blind as a result. Scientists have confirmed that VAD not only can lead to blindness, but also is an important determinant of child mortality due to its deleterious effect on the immune system. Vitamin A stimulates maturation of white blood cells, which aid the body in fighting disease; its deficiency provokes changes in the mucous membranes lining the respiratory, gastrointestinal, and urinary tracts, rendering them less effective in protecting the body against invading pathogens.

Efforts by the World Health Organization to combat VAD focus on several complimentary approaches. Promoting breast-feeding of infants is regarded as the best way to protect babies against VAD, since breast milk is a natural source of vitamin A. For children already suffering from VAD, administering mega-doses of vitamin A in capsule form twice a year has proven to be an easy-to-implement, cost-effective approach to reducing child mortality rates. However, because the effects of the capsules last only 4–6 months and because breast-feeding is time-limited as well, neither can be considered a long-term solution. Yet another approach involves fortifying some common dietary constituent such as sugar with vitamin A, a strategy that has been moderately successful in Guatemala. Educating parents to provide their children with foods rich in vitamin A seems to offer the best solution to the problem; such an approach can include promotion of home gardening to grow vitamin A-rich foods in regions where they aren't locally available in the marketplace or are too expensive. In the long run, however, eliminating VAD depends on reducing levels of poverty and raising living standards so that all families can enjoy an adequate and nutritious diet (Potter, 1997).

Iron deficiency. Iron deficiency anemia, the most common of all nutritional deficiency diseases, afflicts more people worldwide than any other single condition and may well be regarded as a public health epidemic. The WHO estimates that between 4–5 billion people (66–80% of the world's population) currently suffer from iron deficiency. Of these, 2 billion are anemic, primarily due to inadequate dietary intake of iron, especially among those subsisting on vegetarian diets, but also exacerbated in many tropical countries by malaria and parasitic worm infections. Anemia is surprisingly common in the United States as well, though for different reasons. Over-consumption of calorie-rich "junk foods" instead of nutritionally superior fare has contributed to a situation where almost 20% of premenopausal American women are iron-deficient—a figure that rises to 42% of pregnant African-American women living in poverty (Gardner and Halweil, 2000).

Anemia is characterized by lack of energy and low levels of productive activity. It is especially dangerous—and especially common—in pregnant women, where it increases the likelihood of maternal death, premature delivery, or stillbirth. Repeated pregnancies rapidly drain a woman's reserve supplies of iron; in India, where the problem is more severe than anywhere else in the world, 88% of pregnant women are anemic. Iron deficiency anemia is held responsible, at least in part, for the high female mortality rate in that country. While women need three times as much iron as men to replace losses during menstruation and pregnancy, their food intake is generally lower than that of their husbands, sons, and brothers. While increasing the consumption of red meat (the best source of easily assimilated iron) among poor women in developing nations may not be a practical option due to religious prohibitions or lack of purchasing power, the frequency of iron deficiency anemia could be significantly reduced by supplying ferrous salt tablets to pregnant and lactating women, as well as to children, living in areas with a high prevalence of this deficiency disease (WHO, 1997).

Iodine deficiency. Iodine deficiency disorders (IDD) currently affect over 740 million people—13% of the world's population—and threaten another 30%. IDD constitutes a serious public health problem in 130 developing countries, where it is particularly prevalent among pregnant women, preschool children, and the poor. Associated in the public mind with a condition called **goiter** (a disfiguring enlargement of the thyroid gland on the neck), IDD has far more serious health implications than goiter alone. Regarded by public health agencies as the world's single most important cause of preventable brain damage and mental retardation, IDD can reduce a victim's IQ by 15 points. The World Health Organization estimates that almost 50 million people currently suffer from some degree of IDD-related brain damage. If a pregnant woman is iodine-deficient, her fetus can incur irreversible brain damage, resulting in the baby being born dwarfed and mentally retarded, a condition referred to as cretinism. Serious iodine deficiency during pregnancy can also result in miscarriage or stillbirth. For those less severely afflicted, IDD's impairment of mental ability lowers the intellectual capacity of millions of people, with a corresponding impact on the economic productivity of regions most affected.

Fortunately, prospects for eradicating IDD worldwide now appear bright. In 1993 the World Health Organization launched its Universal Salt Iodization campaign, providing technical tools and guidance to countries wishing to create their own salt iodization programs. Because salt is widely available, eaten in consistent amounts year-round, and cheap to iodize (about 5 cents per person per year), it provides an ideal vehicle for international efforts at fortification, just as it did in the United States decades earlier. Progress in reducing IDD since initiation of the WHO effort has been dramatic. The number of countries with salt iodization programs has soared to 93, and the prevalence of IDD has been cut in half since the mid-1990s. As a result, global rates of goiter, mental retardation, and cretinism are falling rapidly, offering hope that one day in the not-too-distant future, iodine deficiency disorders will be regarded as ancient history, much like scurvy, beriberi, and pellagra.

Prospects for Reducing World Hunger

When confronted with stark pictures of starving babies or cold statistics on the growing prevalence of malnutrition, the typical reaction among most Americans is to say, "Let's do something about it!" Send a donation to CARE or OXFAM, eat a vegetarian meal once a week, write a letter to a congressional representative urging a "yes" vote on the next food aid bill. Certainly there has been no shortage of suggestions as to what might be done to ease the population-food crunch. Some of the approaches being tried have real merit, as well as limitations, while others are merely wishful thinking. It's important that people have some understanding of the key elements in the ongoing debate as to how best to eradicate hunger, since this issue is certain to assume even greater urgency in the years ahead. Some of the most frequently mentioned ways of increasing the world food supply are discussed in the following sections.

Expanding the Amount of Land Under Cultivation

From the beginning of the Agricultural Revolution right up to the early 1950s, increasing acreage put to the plow was the major, often the only, way of increasing food supply. Expanding the amount of cultivated land was accomplished by clearing forests, terracing mountainsides, or building irrigation systems—all of which permitted hitherto unproductive lands to be farmed. During the 1950s the Soviet Union vastly increased its agricultural acreage by opening up the "virgin lands" of Kazakhstan; at the same time the Chinese completed some major irrigation networks, substantially expanding their cultivated acreage and making it possible to raise two to three crops per year on the same land. Since that time, significant increases in highly productive farmland have been quite limited. Worldwide, total acreage devoted to agriculture expanded by just 8% since the mid-1960s, with almost all of this increase in developing countries. The hard truth is that the world's prime farmland is in finite supply, and after approximately 10,000 years of agricultural expansion most good land is already being cultivated. Since the 1950s most of the additional land cleared for farming has been so-called "marginal land"—land that is incapable of sustaining moderately good yields over any extended period of time due to its poor soil, erodability, or steep slope. Farmers who today are moving onto marginal lands, desperately trying to eke out a living for their families, do so only because the better lands are already overcrowded. The additional food that such lands will contribute to world harvests is negligible and the long-term ecological damage caused by removing the natural vegetative cover from such lands may eventually have an adverse impact on better lands elsewhere.

Some optimists look hopefully to regions of South America and Africa where nearly half of the yet-undeveloped land suitable for agriculture is located. However, such lands are far from current markets and lack the transportation infrastructure necessary for viable agricultural development. The huge amount of capital investment that would be required appears at present to be far beyond the financial capabilities of the nations involved. Moreover, increasing cultivated acreage in a few land-abundant regions is unlikely to provide additional food or benefits for land-scarce countries. In the world's two most populous nations, China and India, opportunities to expand farmland acreage are virtually nonexistent (Bender and Smith, 1997).

When assessing the contribution that additional farm acres could make to the total world harvest, commentators frequently overlook the other side of the coin; that is, the substantial amounts of good cropland that are currently being lost every year to erosion, desertification, salinization and water-logging of irrigated fields, and urban development. It is now recognized that the increase in world food production witnessed during the 1970s and early 1980s was achieved in part by plowing marginal lands unsuitable for sustained cultivation and by over-irrigating, which has resulted in drastic drawing-down of groundwater reserves in many areas. Today in many of the major grain-producing areas of the world, the cropland base is beginning to shrink as highly erodible lands are abandoned. The World Resources Institute reports that approximately two-thirds of the world's crop and pasturelands have suffered some degree of degradation over the past half century, with 40% of agricultural lands rated as strongly or very strongly degraded. The situation is sufficiently severe and widespread to reduce productivity on 16% of farmlands, particularly in Africa and Central America. While crop yields on a worldwide basis are expected to increase over the next few decades, the results of soil degradation surveys suggest that the long-term productivity of more than half the world's agricultural lands is being undermined by erosion and nutrient depletion (WRI, 2000). The following chapter will examine these trends in more detail, but it is important to bear in mind that while most of the lands currently being added to our agricultural base are marginal acres, those being lost are, for the most part, prime croplands that will never be returned to production.

Increasing World Fish Catch

When one considers that 71% of the earth's surface is water, it's understandable that many people look to the oceans as the source of apparently limitless high-quality animal protein. Such optimism seemed justified during the years between 1950–1989, when total world fish catch soared from about 22 million tons annually to 89 million tons—a four-fold increase that, even at a time of unprecedented population growth, resulted in a doubling in the per capita availability of seafood. Since fish provide approximately one-sixth of all the animal protein consumed by humans on a worldwide basis and constitute the primary protein source for one billion people, this bounty from the sea raised hopes for substantial progress in combating malnutrition.

Official statistics during the 1990s indicated that the annual world fish catch continued to rise slowly, fluctuating slightly up and down throughout the decade. However, a reexamination of the existing data by two Canadian researchers revealed that the global fish harvest statistics had been badly skewed by gross overreporting of the annual catch in China. Driven by politically inspired "productivity increases," the Chinese had been reporting catches nearly double the true amount. When the global fisheries data were readjusted, the researchers found that the annual world fish catch has been gradually declining, by about 700,000 metric tons a year, since the late 1980s (Watson and Pauly, 2001). Even more ominous than the slight drop in total fish harvest is the precipitous decline in large predator fish, once the mainstay of ocean fisheries. Overexploitation by industrial fishing fleets has reduced stocks of these species to a mere 10% of their former levels (Myers and Worm, 2003). As a result, stocks of species regarded as desirable table-grade fish—swordfish, haddock, hake, toothfish (a.k.a. Chilean sea bass), orange roughy—are now in sharp decline. For some the situation is even more dire; the International Union for Conservation of Nature and Natural Resources (IUCN) *Red List* now includes such overfished species as the Atlantic cod, Atlantic halibut, yellowtail flounder, and five species of tuna as headed toward extinction, at least over large expanses of their original range (WRI, 2000).

The fact that the total annual catch hasn't dropped precipitously is due to what some researchers refer to as "fishing down the food web" (Pauly et al., 1998), maintaining tonnage by hauling in many lower-trophic level species, such as anchovetas, herring, and mackerel, formerly regarded as "trash fish." Since the 1980s, low-value fish species have accounted for almost three-quarters of the overall increase in world fish catch. The FAO reports that approximately 47% of the major marine fish stocks are now fully exploited, yielding catches at or close to their maximum sustainable limits and therefore offering little hope for increased future harvests. Another 18% of stocks are already overexploited, making it likely that in the years ahead catches of these species will be further reduced unless remedial action is taken soon to lessen the pressures of overfishing. Ten percent of stocks are already significantly depleted or recovering from depletion and are far less productive than they once were. Fish stocks that are still underexploited or only moderately exploited, the group representing the greatest potential for increasing world marine fish catch, comprise just 25% of the major fish stocks for which information is available (FAO, 2002b).

Ocean fisheries, of course, don't account for the world's entire fish catch. Inland capture fisheries—those taking wild fish by line, net, or trap—supply about 12% of all fish consumed by people. Like their marine counterpart, however, inland fisheries are now being exploited at nonsustainable levels. Only through restocking and by introducing more productive fish species (a practice restricted to a few countries such as China) has it been possible to maintain some growth in inland fisheries (WRI, 2000). The declining capacity of the world's coastal and marine ecosystems to meet the growing demand for seafood will inevitably lead to higher prices. Already a major share of the world's marine fish harvest is exported to affluent consumers in Japan, the U.S., and other industrialized nations. In the years ahead, rising prices sparked by rising demand will further boost fish exports from developing nations, leaving fewer fish for local consumers and making fish protein less and less affordable for low-income families.

While the main factor affecting sustainability of capture fisheries is overexploitation, pollution is having an impact as well. It has not yet been possible to demonstrate a decline in the abundance of entire species in the open sea due solely to pollution, but experiments have shown that toxic contaminants such as hydrocarbons, heavy metals, and synthetic organic compounds—all common water pollutants—can kill or injure aquatic organisms. In the coastal waters that constitute some of the world's most productive fishing grounds, nutrients, primarily nitrates and phosphates from sewage discharges or farmland runoff, constitute the most extensive and serious pollution problem. A large area of sea bottom in the Gulf of Mexico offshore from New Orleans is now a virtual "dead zone," thanks largely to agricultural runoff from Midwest farmlands. The decline of Chesapeake Bay's crab and oyster harvest, once among the world's richest, can be traced to contamination from runoff as well. Shellfish are particularly susceptible to pollution of near-shore areas; if not directly killed by toxic contaminants, they are often declared unmarketable because of the health threat they pose to human consumers.

Development activities that destroy coastal habitats, particularly coastal marshes, mangroves, and sea grasses, also play a role in reducing populations of ocean fish because many commercially important species depend on coastal or estuarine waters for survival during some phase of their life cycle. Burgeoning urban populations along most of the world's coastlines are rapidly increasing development pressures in these areas, yet few countries are managing such growth in a manner that will protect the ocean's biotic resources.

Aquaculture

In contrast to the rather gloomy outlook for the capture fisheries, fish harvests from **aquaculture** (fish farming) have been growing rapidly. Production from fish farms exceeded 45 million metric tons in 2000; four times the amount harvested in 1985. At present, one out of every three fish eaten worldwide is farm-raised. Growth

---

Box 4-2 The Cost of Farmed Salmon

Atlantic salmon is a popular menu choice among diners looking for a tasty, "heart-healthy" meal—low in saturated fats and high in the omega-3 fatty acids that reduce risk of cardiovascular disease. That salmon has now become so widely available and affordable is largely due to the rapid growth of a salmon aquaculture industry that has experienced a five-fold increase in production since the late 1980s. By the early 1990s, farm-raised fish accounted for the majority of world trade in salmon. With once-abundant wild salmon stocks decimated by overfishing, dam-building, and habitat loss in both North America and Europe, farming salmon offered hope for reducing pressure on remaining wild fish while providing a healthy food product to consumers at a price most could afford. An item that had, for decades, been a luxury food now became, as an industry newsletter put it, "possibly the cheapest protein there is." The proliferation of salmon farming in a number of countries possessing extensive protected coastlines and cold ocean water— Norway, Canada, Chile, the U.K. (Scotland), and, to a lesser extent, the U.S.—has brought thousands of jobs to communities in economic decline and has made salmon an abundant year-round market commodity.

So why is the meteoric rise of salmon aquaculture not unqualified good news? Primarily because of the industry's negative impact on coastal ecosystems in the vicinity of salmon farms. In contrast to the majority of aquaculture operations that raise herbivorous fish in freshwater ponds—a practice that has minimal environmental impact— farming salmon, a carnivorous species, involves resource-intensive methods with significant and far-ranging impacts.

Although reared from eggs in on-shore hatcheries, the immature salmon, or smolts, are soon transferred to offshore net pens where they are then raised to maturity. Sea water flows freely through the mesh of the suspended pens, but the fish must be regularly fed and the wastes they generate removed. And this is where the problems begin.

The pelleted feed eaten by farmed salmon is made primarily of fish meal and fish oil, produced by grinding up enormous numbers of so-called "industrial fish," mainly small, oily deep-sea species such as sardines, anchovies, and herring, harvested from the already overexploited fisheries off the coast of Chile and Peru or the North Atlantic. Since it requires approximately three pounds of feed to produce a pound of salmon, it's obvious that eating farmed salmon does nothing to ease pressures on endangered marine fisheries. Not all of the pelleted feed tossed into the netpens is eaten, of course, so the excess, along with prodigious amounts of salmon feces, drift downward from the pens to the ocean floor. As they decompose, they release nutrients (primarily nitrogen and phosphorus) that can stimulate algal blooms, while the metabolic activities of the decomposer organisms themselves may severely deplete levels of dissolved oxygen in the surrounding waters. As a result, the sea bottom below salmon aquaculture operations frequently becomes a virtual dead zone, with biodiversity reduced to a few worm species throughout an area extending perhaps 100–500 feet in diameter beyond the aquaculture operations.

Unfortunately, fish food is not the only necessary input to a salmon-farming operation. Because the pens are so tightly stocked with salmon to maximize production, infectious diseases and parasitic infestations that seldom trouble wild salmon populations are rife in the aquaculture setting. In an attempt to control these and prevent wide-scale losses, farm managers make heavy use of vaccines, antibiotics, and parasiticides. These, is turn, subsequently enter the environment, posing a threat to marine life near the pens. Rampant disease within salmon farms presents a risk to the health of nearby wild salmon populations. One of the most serious problems of farmed salmon in northern waters is sea lice, tiny parasitic crustaceans that kill salmon by eating their flesh. Sea lice are seldom a threat to wild salmon, but because aquaculture operations are often located adjacent to wild salmon migration routes, infestations of sea lice in netpen areas frequently spread to wild stocks as well. Severe outbreaks of sea lice among wild salmon in Norway, Scotland, and British Columbia, resulting in a near-total loss of affected stocks, were attributed to lice infestations among nearby farmed salmon.

To some biologists wary of the rapid spread of salmon aquaculture, escaping fish themselves present the most serious ecological concern. Such escapes are a regular occurrence, both as massive outbreaks during storms and at chronic levels on a daily basis. Although farmed salmon are considered less fit for survival in the outside world, the fear is that the sheer number of escapees will adversely impact wild stocks by spreading disease and by competing for food and habitat. Contamination of the wild gene pool via interbreeding is another concern, though farmed Atlantic salmon don't seem capable of breeding with Pacific salmon. In areas where salmon farming is long established, it's probably too late to worry about escapees—in parts of Europe the process has been ongoing for so many years that today farmed fish comprise up to 90% of the salmon in some Norwegian rivers.

The economic clout of the large multinational companies now dominating the salmon aquaculture industry has limited governmental regulatory efforts to deal with these problems. Existing regulations, imposed by various federal, state, or provincial agencies, cover such issues as siting of operations; waste management; chemical use; protection of endangered species and marine mammals; health safety standards; and the prevention, reporting, and recovery of escaping farmed fish. Unfortunately, most of the regulations were not tailored specifically for the aquaculture industry and are relatively weak. They also are frequently ignored. Fines, when imposed, are far too low to pose a significant deterrent to noncompliance. On the other hand, industry has recently begun making tentative efforts to clean up its environmental act. Some farms in British Columbia and Washington State are trying to reduce fish escapes by strengthening netpen infrastructure and improving maintenance and monitoring of the pens. Farms in Norway and Iceland have abandoned pesticides in favor of millions of "cleaner fish" to pick sea lice off salmon. Motivated by rising feed costs, many salmon farms now use underwater cameras to monitor the amount of feed being dispensed into the pens, thereby reducing the amount of waste. However, such actions, while commendable, are local, piecemeal approaches to a problem of industry-wide proportions. Many environmental groups are convinced that the only way to protect coastal waters from pollution, disease, and fish escape problems is to require that facilities be moved onto land, with fish contained in large cement or fiberglass tanks. Doing this, however, would greatly increase the cost of raising salmon and, given the current low market price for the now overly abundant fish, the economic viability of what appears to be a technologically sound solution is rather doubtful. As salmon farming continues to expand (in British Columbia, the provincial government is striving to quadruple salmon aquaculture production in that Canadian province), demands for more effective regulatory controls are being expressed with increasing urgency by affected communities and grassroots activists. Absent such action, the environmental cost of providing salmon for the masses will be substantially higher than the supermarket tab indicates.

References

Naylor, Rosamund L., Josh Eagle, and Whitney L. Smith. 2003. "Salmon Aquaculture in the Pacific Northwest: A Global Industry with Local Impacts." *Environment* 45, no. 8 (Oct).

Ryan, John C., 2003. "Feedlots of the Sea." *World•Watch* 16, no. 5 (Sept/Oct).

of aquaculture has been particularly rapid in China, the source of almost half the total value of global aquaculture production. Today China, Japan, India, Thailand, South Korea, Indonesia, and the Philippines all obtain a substantial portion of their fish from aquaculture. While fish farming in the United States still accounts for less than 2% of world production, it already supplies most of the catfish, crayfish, and salmon sold in American supermarkets. Currently over 210 aquatic animals and plants are being raised in various freshwater or marine aquaculture operations around the world, with various species of finfish representing more than half of total production (FAO,

Aquaculture (fish farming) provides one-third of the total world fish harvest. Species that can be successfully raised include catfish, crayfish, salmon, trout, and tilapia. [*Archer Daniels Midland*]

2002b). While as much as a third of the wild fish catch is used to make fish meal and fish oil, farmed fish go directly to human consumers. It is anticipated that any future increases in fish consumption will have to come from aquaculture, since there is little hope of further increasing ocean fish catch. Unlike capture fisheries, however, aquaculture demands

Table 4-1   Top Ten Countries in Aquaculture Production

Producer	2002 (thousand tones)
China	27,767.3
India	2,191.7
Indonesia	914.1
Japan	828.4
Bangladesh	786.6
Thailand	644.9
Norway	553.9
Chile	545.7
Vietnam	518.5
United States	497.3

Source: Adapted from "The State of World Fisheries and Aquaculture 2004," Table 4. Food and Agriculture Organization of the United Nations. Used with permission.

significant resource inputs. Freshwater fish farms require considerable amounts of land and water, both of which must be diverted from other types of agricultural production. Concerns over cropland loss to fish production have already prompted Chinese authorities to restrict future farmland conversion to aquaculture. Additionally, farmed fish, unlike those caught on the open seas, must be fed by those who raise them. Fortunately, fish are among the most efficient energy converters, requiring just 2–3 pounds of feed to gain one pound of flesh. Ironically, the growth of fish farming has intensified pressures on ocean fish stocks because 10–15% of all fishmeal obtained from capture fisheries is fed to farmed fish. Like every other enterprise, aquaculture has its economic and environmental costs (see box 4-2).

Reducing Post-Harvest Food Losses

Implementation of better methods of handling and protecting food between the time it is harvested and the time it appears on the consumer's plate may not sound particularly exciting—rat-proof grain bins are not the stuff of which poetry is made—but, in the short-run at least, such simple, well-understood measures could help increase the availability of food in the marketplace. Each year enormous amounts of harvested foods are lost to pests and spoilage, particularly in tropical countries. Rats, birds, insects, and molds all consume or render unfit for human use large amounts of stored foods that would otherwise have been available for people. Cultural practices are partially responsible for such losses. In many countries grains are stored in the open or in easily penetrated sacks or bins. Lack of adequate refrigeration promotes spoilage, while poor transport facilities delay rapid movement of food from fields to consumers, thereby increasing chances of loss or spoilage.

In wealthier countries, consumers' insistence that food be cosmetically perfect results in substantial wastage of harvested crops, particularly fruits and vegetables. Tiny blemishes that in no way affect a food's taste or nutritional value frequently result in its being discarded because it doesn't meet market standards of aesthetic acceptability. Retailing, food service, and personal consumption habits also result in considerable wastage of food. Just these three stages of the marketing process account for the loss of almost 95 billion pounds of food annually in the United States—27% of all food available for consumption (Kantor, 1997). Of course there is no guarantee that less food wastage in rich countries would result in greater food availability for the poor, but some analysts suggest that if food losses could be reduced to 23% worldwide, an amount equivalent to 13% of global consumption would be saved, thereby reducing per capita food demand (Bender and Smith, 1997).

Eating Lower on the Food Chain

Humanitarians are frequently troubled by the apparent inefficiency of converting a substantial portion of the world grain harvest into meat or poultry to satisfy consumers' carnivorous cravings. The same amount of corn, wheat, or oats, they argue, could satisfy the caloric needs of millions of additional people dining on vegetarian fare. (To be consistent, they might also target the 10% of the U.S. corn crop diverted to the manufacture of corn syrup, much of which is used for sweetening soft drinks; that same amount of corn could make a lot of tortillas!)

The impact of diverting feed to food, even if fully implemented, might not be as great as proponents suggest, however. It has been estimated that abandoning the use of grain for feed entirely would increase market supplies of food by 20–30% at most (Ehrlich, Ehrlich, and Daily, 1993). If world population continues to grow as projections indicate, the one-time gains achieved by going vegetarian would soon be erased by the food demands generated by more and more people.

Regardless of whether promoting meatless diets would be an advisable or effective approach to increasing food availability, it is not a realistic option. While health concerns are prompting some individuals to reduce their consumption of high-fat animal products, no society in modern times has voluntarily reduced meat-eating by any significant amount. Indeed, as we have seen, trends in newly affluent areas of the world are in exactly the opposite direction as their citizens enthusiastically begin to ascend the "protein ladder." In fact, meat production in developing countries now exceeds that in the industrialized nations (Nierenberg, 2003). While consumers might simplify their diets in response to scarcity-induced higher prices, an appeal to altruism—asking diners to forego their steaks and sauerbraten so that strangers far away could enjoy a temporary increase in food supplies—is unlikely to meet with a positive response.

Improving Yields per Acre

Since mid-century the largest gains in world food supply have been obtained not by expanding our cropland base but by dramatically increasing per acre or per hectare (metric unit for land measurement, equivalent to 2.47 acres) yields on existing farmlands. In the United States, corn yields, which had remained stable for almost 70 years, more than quadrupled from 1940 to 1985. Impressive increases were also achieved for wheat, rice, barley, rye, peanuts, and sorghum. In Great Britain, where wheat yields are the world's highest, per hectare wheat production tripled from 1940 to 1984. These enormous gains were accomplished through the application of research and technological improvements gradually developed and perfected since the late 1800s, the major elements of which included new hybrid crop varieties, better farm machinery, tremendous expansion in the use of chemical fertilizers and pesticides, and increased use of irrigation.

The developed nations were not alone in realizing major gains in agricultural productivity during the past several decades. In the late 1960s, twenty years of plant breeding experiments to improve grain yields in tropical and semi-tropical regions resulted in the development of several strains of so-called "miracle wheat" and "miracle rice" which heralded the advent of what commentators have dubbed "The Green Revolution." Within a few years of its introduction, the new hybrid wheat was giving farmers from Mexico to India yields two to three times greater than the best formerly obtained from traditional strains. Since the introduction of the first miracle wheat in India in 1966, that country has more than doubled its wheat production. Pakistan,

Turkey, and Mexico were among more than 30 other countries whose farmers eagerly adopted the new technology and witnessed a corresponding surge in their wheat production statistics. Similarly, the miracle rice varieties developed at the International Rice Research Institute in the Philippines have approximately doubled the yields of this grain in situations where the hybrid seeds, along with proper fertilization and adequate irrigation, were employed.

The spectacular gains of the Green Revolution led many political leaders during the early 1970s to relax on the population issue, assuming that continued dramatic increases in food production had erased the Malthusian image of starving millions. Agricultural experts, however, were less sanguine regarding the food-population

Figure 4-3

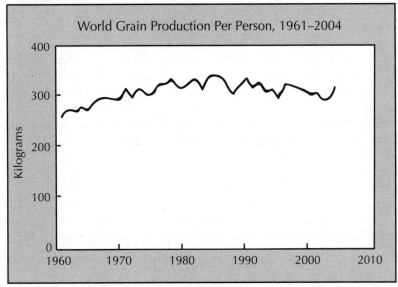

Source: Based on data from the Food and Agriculture Organization of the United Nations and the Census Bureau.

crunch and warned that it would be a fatal mistake to assume that plant scientists would be able to achieve another quantum leap in crop yields in the foreseeable future. Agronomist Norman Borlaug, "Father of the Green Revolution" and recipient of the 1970 Nobel Peace Prize for his key role in developing miracle wheat, cautioned dignitaries assembled for the awards ceremony in Oslo that his contribution would, at best, buy humankind about 30 years of food security—years during which they must tame the population monster, he warned. Unfortunately, Borlaug's gift of time has largely been squandered; in developed and developing nations alike the gains of the Green Revolution are losing momentum even as population figures continue to climb. The fact that many of the world's farmers are already fully exploiting the technologies that enabled them to double, triple, or even quadruple yields in the years prior to 1984 means that future gains will come in ever-smaller increments and will be increasingly difficult to achieve. Throughout the 1990s, increases in per acre grain yields averaged barely 1% annually, with analysts lamenting the "yield plateau" that now seems to characterize cereal production in most of the world's major grain-growing areas.

Some observers predict that in the not-too-distant future we are likely to encounter an absolute yield ceiling imposed by plants' photosynthetic efficiency. The plant breeders who developed the miracle strains of wheat and rice created these high-yielding genetic cultivars by boosting the proportion of sugars produced by photosynthesis that are diverted to seed production. While traditional varieties converted roughly 20% of these sugars into seeds, Green Revolution cultivars are able to convert over 50%. Scientists estimate that the absolute upper limit of sugar production that could go into seed formation without depriving the plant of energy needed for other vital functions is about 60%. Therefore, the opportunity for further yield gains through conventional breeding programs is extremely limited (Brown, Flavin, and French, 1999).

Similar limits are becoming apparent regarding fertilizer applications. Use of nitrogen fertilizers grew more than nine-fold between 1950–1998 and, along with hybrid seeds, receives much of the credit for the crop yield increases of the past 50 years. However, there are now signs that the Law of Diminishing Returns has set in and crops that have been receiving higher and higher levels of fertilizer applications for many years are approaching the limits of their physiological capacity to utilize nutrients. As an example of this, take the case of fertilizer use in America's "Corn Belt." During the 1950s and 1960s, for every extra pound of nitrogen applied a farmer could expect a yield increase of 15–20 extra bushels of corn. By the late 1970s, that increment was 5–7 bushels and falling. By the 1990s, growth in fertilizer use, both in the U.S. and Europe, had virtually halted, partly due to more efficient application methods but also in response to farmers' recognition that additional fertilizer inputs were not economically justified by the minimal boosts in yields per acre. In developing regions such as the Indian subcontinent where reliance on nitrogen fertilizer is more recent and less intensive, potential for increasing yields through additional fertilizer application still exists. In the longer term, however, the same laws of nature will impose an upper ceiling on production there as well. Unless plant scientists can develop new cultivars of wheat, rice, and corn that are even more responsive to heavy fertilization than those currently being grown, it is unlikely that the slowdown in annual growth of world harvests witnessed during the past decade will be reversed.

Other components critical to the success of Green Revolution technologies—irrigation and chemical pesticides—also may be approaching practical limits. High-yielding varieties can only achieve their maximum potential when supplied with abundant water. Today 40% of all crops harvested come from the 17% of world cropland under irrigation (WRI, 2000). For a number of reasons, the rapid expansion in irrigated acreage that occurred annually from 1950 to 1978 has tapered off since that time to less than 1% a year (Brown, Renner, and Flavin, 1998). In the absence of irrigation, miracle grains perform less well than lower-yielding traditional varieties—another reason why the recent slowdown in grain production is likely to continue. Chemical pesticide use is another factor critical in optimizing yields from new crop strains since they are highly susceptible to insects and fungal pathogens, but it is proving less effective than it was several decades ago. Overuse of these products has promoted development of resistant pest populations that are once again having an adverse impact on agricultural production.

Many people optimistically assume that biotechnology will soon present us with a new generation of super-high-yielding crop plants. Indeed, genetic engineers in both the United States and Japan are now hard at work to develop transgenic plants that have a more efficient photosynthetic apparatus. If successful, such plants could significantly boost crop yields. Scientists caution, however, that their work is progressing very slowly and any practical applications for such research lie years in the future (Mann, 1999). In the short term, biotechnology's main contribution to world agriculture is likely to be the introduction of disease- and insect-resistant crop varieties, as well as crops more tolerant of drought or salt. Such cultivars may boost current yields somewhat, but do not represent the quantum leap in production represented by the Green Revolution's miracle grains.

For all these reasons, experts seriously doubt that a doubling or tripling of world harvests can be repeated. In most of the world's major agricultural areas farmers have already reaped the full potential offered by miracle crops; in regions not yet touched by the Green Revolution, natural conditions such as lack of water resources or inadequate technology transfer may preclude them from ever enjoying its fruits. Even within countries where the new technologies have boosted food self-sufficiency, large areas remain mired in poverty and backwardness—northwest China, the Andean Mountain area, the highlands of Mexico, and large areas of central India are all notable examples. The outlook for improvement is perhaps most clouded in the semiarid regions of sub-Saharan Africa where yields of maize, the most important cereal crop, have remained stagnant at about one ton per hectare since 1961. A few countries in west and central Africa, however, have recently experienced some productivity increases, thanks to the introduction of new maize varieties (Pinstrup-Andersen et al., 1997). Food production in these chronically food-deficit areas could improve, despite maximum *genetic* yield barriers, if the use of existing production technology is further expanded. More on-site research to develop seed varieties adapted to local growing conditions, more attention to efficient water use and proper planting dates, greater emphasis on educational outreach programs to transfer the latest agricultural develop-

Table 4-2 Sample of Genetically Modified Organisms

GMO species	Genetic modification	Purpose of genetic modification	Primary beneficiaries
Maize	Insect resistance	Reduced insect damage	Farmers
Soybean	Herbicide tolerance	Greater weed control	Farmers
Cotton	Insect resistance	Reduced insect damage	Farmers
Carnation	Alteration of color	Production of different flower varieties	Retailers and consumers
Rice	Pro-Vitamin A	Increase Vit A supply	Consumers

Source: Adapted from "Biotechnology and Food Security," Food and Agriculture Organization of the United Nations. www.fao.org.

Box 4-3   GMOs: A "Second Green Revolution" or "Frankenfoods"?

As the quantum leaps in world grain production witnessed in the late 1960s tapered off and Third World population figures continued to soar, agricultural scientists began to ask "What's next?" in terms of a magic bullet for increasing global food supplies. By the mid-1970s remarkable progress was being made in DNA sequencing, making it possible to consciously design new forms of life; that is, to insert a gene from one organism (most commonly a virus or bacterium) into another species, thereby producing a GMO—a so-called "genetically modified organism." With the 1980 Supreme Court ruling (*Diamond vs. Chakrabarty*) confirming patent rights for living organisms, what some commentators have dubbed the "Second Green Revolution" was off and running.

This landmark Court decision made the resource-intensive laboratory work profitable and during the 1980s the new field of biotechnology grew by leaps and bounds. Giant corporations, most notably St. Louis-based Monsanto, poured millions of investment dollars into the race to market the first genetically engineered crop varieties. Competition was fierce, with seed companies and chemical manufacturers on both sides of the Atlantic scrambling to secure patents and get their products commercialized before their rivals beat them to the marketplace.

By the mid-1990s a host of genetically modified crops went commercial, generating headlines around the world. Rather than better taste or higher nutritional value—qualities of importance to consumers—the new transgenic crops featured herbicide and pest resistance, features that offered growers savings in labor and chemical costs but little of apparent benefit to the general public. By 1996–1997, vast acreages across the Midwest and South were planted in Roundup-Ready soybeans, cotton, corn, and canola, offering farmers an easy way to control troublesome weeds: just spray the Roundup-Ready crop with Monsanto's nonselective herbicide Roundup (glyphosate) to kill the vulnerable weeds while sparing the now genetically resistant crop plants. Soon Roundup-Ready GMOs were joined by a host of other crops genetically engineered to defend themselves against plant-devouring caterpillars. A gene from the bacterium *Bacillus thuringiensis (Bt)*, an organism that secretes a toxin lethal to larvae of many lepidopterous insects (i.e. moths and butterflies), was introduced into corn and cotton to protect those crops from pests such as the European corn borer and the tobacco budworm (a major pest of cotton) while simultaneously reducing use of environmentally damaging chemical insecticides. Today Roundup-Ready soybeans, *Bt* corn, and genetically improved cotton comprise fully 85% of all the transgenic crops grown worldwide.

In retrospect, it's probably unfortunate for the public image of transgenic crops that the first widely planted GMOs were ones whose benefits accrue almost exclusively to a small number of huge, private corporations that jealously guard their patent rights and act aggressively to control any products they commercialize. Throughout the industrialized world, gene power became bound to corporate power and many advocates for the poor fear that developing countries lacking the scientific and technical infrastructure to carry out their own research programs may find themselves growing ever more dependent on imported agricultural commodities and technologies they can ill afford—what some refer to as a growing "molecular divide" between rich and poor nations.

For many people, the problem goes far beyond resentment toward greedy capitalistic corporations exploiting powerless farmers and expropriating the earth's biological heritage for profit. Since the mid-1980s, anti-GMO activists have been warning that tinkering with plants' genetic material amounts to "playing God" by regarding life forms as mere commodities to be altered at will. They warn that insufficient research has been conducted on the possible harmful impacts of wide-scale release of GMOs into the general environment, suggesting that cross-breeding between Roundup-Ready crops and their wild relatives could produce new strains of "superweeds" or that the prevalence of *Bt* crop varieties will eventually lead to insects resistant to the *Bt* toxin, the primary weapon now used by organic farmers to protect their crops. GMO critics point out that almost all the safety testing for transgenic organisms has been done by the companies themselves and urge governments to require independent testing of the products' safety and environmental impact. They raise fears about the potential for allergens from one species to be introduced unintentionally into another, jeopardizing the health of consumers of genetically modified foods (to date there is no evidence that this has happened in any commercialized transgenic product). In general, the response among American consumers has been rather "ho-hum," with most expressing confidence that such food is safe and only a small minority perceiving GMOs as a serious food risk. Indeed, the fact that transgenic products have been present since the late 1990s in many of the foods Americans eat on a daily basis suggests that there is little to worry about so far as human health is concerned.

The public reaction in Europe and elsewhere has been far different, however. By chance misfortune, the European Commission had voted to accept Roundup-Ready soybeans in March 1996, just five days before the British Prime Minister announced that at least 10 people had died from a human variant of "mad cow disease." Reassurances to a skeptical public that the government could be relied upon to guarantee food safety carried little weight at that point and Greenpeace activists enthusiastically entered the fray to halt a threatened GMO invasion of Europe. By and large, the European media, especially in the U.K., supported those campaigning against so-called "Frankenfoods," conjuring up vivid images of monsters created by scientists run amok. The scientific communities in Europe and the U.S. were unable to convince European consumers that they should welcome genetically altered foods into their kitchens.

So how valid are concerns that "Frankenfoods" pose genuine long-term health and environmental risks? Most scientists are convinced that the danger is minimal—certainly no greater than threats posed by conventional foods, many of which contain natural toxins that seldom worry many consumers. Similarly, fears raised about pollen from transgenic crops contaminating conventional fields or harming wildlife seem exaggerated; the impact to date appears negligible—certainly far less than the impact traditional agricultural operations have had on wildlife, soil, and water quality. By reducing the quantities of chemical insecticides needed to control crop pests, GMOs may leave, on balance, a slightly positive environmental footprint.

From the standpoint of global food security, however, the promise of transgenic foods as a solution to world hunger has largely been squandered. Since poor Third World farmers offer few profit opportunities for the multinational companies that now control the biotech industry, virtually no work has been done on crops grown for local consumption in developing countries. Important Third World food crops such as cassava, lentils, chickpeas, sorghum, millet, and peanuts have been ignored by corporate scientists, as have desirable crop-improving traits such as drought resistance or enhanced nutritional value. While some work is underway on several transgenic temperate forest tree species to boost lumber production, genetic enhancement of tropical fruit trees has been almost totally neglected. Recent success in decoding the rice genome by independent teams in China and Switzerland offers promise for creating new, improved rice cultivars, but enthusiastic claims by GMO boosters that genetic engineering is humanity's "last, best hope" for ending world hunger sound rather hollow in light of negligible progress toward that goal thus far. Many observers fear that the food security needs of the poor will go unmet unless the industry giants now holding exclusive licenses on the technology relax their grip and allow researchers in developing countries to use these tools to work on improved versions of local crops.

GMOs are clearly here to stay, but the distrust and antagonism they arouse in many quarters show few signs of dissipating any time soon. Greater efforts on the part of the biotechnology industry to develop crops that meet real consumer needs and a willingness to share their expertise with poor nations could go a long way to redeeming the now-dubious promise of genetic engineering as a force for good in the world.

References

Charles, Daniel. 2003. *Lords of the Harvest: Biotech, Big Money, and the Future of Food*. Cambridge, MA: Perseus Publishing.

Fresco, Louise O. 2003. *A New Social Contract on Biotechnology*. Agriculture Department, Food and Agriculture Organization of the United Nations.

ments to cultivators in the field, adoption of government financial and economic policies that make it profitable for farmers to adopt new technologies—all offer potential for boosting currently modest yields in some Third World areas. However, population growth rates in those same areas demand that the governments of those nations give priority to modernizing their agricultural sectors in order to realize this potential. In addition, bountiful harvests alone will not eradicate hunger among those too poor to buy food for their families.

In the first decade of the 21st century, humanity is confronted by demographic projections indicating that global population will continue to climb by about 77 million each year—at a time when growth in per capita food supply has leveled off or even declined in some key areas of the world. While optimists continue to insist that human inventiveness will somehow find the means for feeding future billions, there are no new technologies on the horizon offering the quantum leaps in food production witnessed during the recent past. With a shrinking cropland base, falling water tables, diminishing impact of chemical fertilizers, and the long-term specter of adverse climatic change in some of the world's most productive agricultural regions (see chapter 11), farmers will be hard-pressed to meet future food demands at prices hungry people can afford. More vigorous efforts at stabilizing population size and reversing land degradation are urgently needed if we are to prove Malthus wrong.

References

Bender, William, and Margaret Smith. 1997. "Population, Food, and Nutrition." *Population Bulletin* 51, no. 4 (Feb).

Brown, Lester R. 2003. *Plan B: Rescuing a Planet under Stress and a Civilization in Trouble.* Earth Policy Institute. New York: W.W. Norton.

Brown, Lester R., Christopher Flavin, and Hilary F. French. 1999. *State of the World 1999.* New York: Worldwatch Institute/W.W. Norton.

Brown, Lester R., Michael Renner, and Christopher Flavin. 1998. *Vital Signs 1998.* New York: Worldwatch Institute/W.W. Norton.

Chen, R., ed. 1990. *The Hunger Report: 1990.* The Alan Shawn Feinstein World Hunger Program, Brown University.

Ehrlich, Paul R., Anne H. Ehrlich, and Gretchen C. Daily. 1993. "Food Security, Population, and Environment." *Population and Development Review* 19, no. 1 (March).

Food and Agriculture Organization of the United Nations (FAO). 2002a. *The State of Food Insecurity in the World 2002.*

———. 2002b. *State of World Fisheries 2002.*

Gardner, Gary, and Brian Halweil. 2000. "Underfed and Overfed: The Global Epidemic of Malnutrition." *Worldwatch Paper* 150, Worldwatch Institute (March).

Halweil, Brian. 2003. "Grain Production Drops." *Vital Signs 2003: The Trends That Are Shaping Our Future.* Worldwatch Institute.

Kantor, Linda S., et al. 1997. "Estimating and Addressing America's Food Losses." *Food Review* 20, no. 1.

Mann, Charles C. 1999. "Genetic Engineers Aim to Soup Up Crop Photosynthesis." *Science* 283, no. 5400 (Jan. 15): 314–316.

Myers, Ransom A., and Boris Worm. 2003. "Rapid Worldwide Depletion of Predatory Fish Communities." *Nature* 423 (May 15): 280–283.

Nierenberg, Danielle. 2003. "Meat Production and Consumption Grow." *Vital Signs 2003: The Trends That Are Shaping Our Future.* Worldwatch Institute.

Pauly, D., V. Christensen, J. Dalsgaard, R. Froese, and F. Torres Jr. 1998. "Fishing Down Marine Food Webs." *Science* 279:860–863.

Pinstrup-Andersen, Per, Rajul Pandya-Lorch, and Mark W. Rosegrant. 1997. *The World Food Situation: Recent Developments, Emerging Issues, and Long-Term Prospects* (Dec). Washington, DC: International Food Policy Research Institute.

Potter, Andrew R. 1997. "Reducing Vitamin A Deficiency Could Save the Eyesight and Lives of Countless Children." *British Medical Journal* 314, no. 7077 (Feb. 1): 317–318.

Riley, Nancy E. 1997. "Gender, Power, and Population Change." *Population Bulletin* 52, no. 1 (May).

Watson, Reg, and Daniel Pauly. 2001. "Systematic Distortion in World Fisheries Catch Trends." *Nature* 414 (Nov. 29): 534–536.

World Health Organization (WHO). 1997. *The World Health Report—1997.*

World Resources Institute (WRI). 2000. *World Resources 2000–2001: People and Ecosystems: The Fraying Web of Life.*

IMPACTS OF GROWTH ON ECOSYSTEMS

> To sustain an environment suitable for man, we must fight on a thousand battle-grounds. Despite all of our wealth and knowledge, we cannot create a redwood forest, a wild river, or a gleaming seashore.
> —President Lyndon B. Johnson (1966)

Certainly the issue of how to feed additional multitudes in the years ahead, when close to a billion of the earth's current inhabitants are malnourished, looms as a monumental task for future world leaders. However, population growth exerts many other socioeconomic and environmental impacts that may be less publicized than famine, yet have a profound influence on human well-being and on the sustainability of planetary life-support systems. In many parts of the world today evidence is mounting that large and still-growing human and livestock populations have already exceeded the carrying capacity of the land itself. In effect, at a time when we are trying to produce more and more from a given land area to sustain increasing numbers of people, the activities of those people are damaging natural ecosystems to the extent that they are becoming incapable of supporting their present population, much less future billions.

Giving evidence of the fact that population growth and ecological degradation are inextricably interrelated are the swelling numbers of **"environmental refugees"**—people seeking refuge abroad due to environmental problems at home. Oxford University ecologist Norman Myers estimates that 25 million people have been forced to leave their place of birth due to water scarcity, depleted soils, deforestation, desertification, or other environmental calamities. Regions most affected by this phenomenon include Central America, India, China, the Horn of Africa, and the Sahel. More ominously, Myers predicts that this number could double by 2010 as population growth in many of the world's poorest countries puts even more pressure on already-stressed local environments. Such vast movements of environmentally displaced persons could become one of the major political and national security issues in the years immediately ahead.

Degradation of Land Resources

> We abuse land because we regard it as a commodity belonging to us. When we see land as a community to which we belong, we may begin to use it with love and respect.
> —Aldo Leopold, *A Sand County Almanac*

The disruption of natural cycles resulting from human pressures on land resources is undermining the sustainability of ecosystems in many parts of the world today. A survey of soil degradation conducted by the International Soil Reference and Information Center estimates that 10% of the earth's vegetated surface is at least moderately degraded, while 9 million hectares (about 22 million acres) are so severely degraded that their original biotic functions have been completely destroyed (WRI, 1996). Although much of this land is still being cultivated, some of its natural productivity has been lost and could be restored only through implementation of expensive national programs to provide farmers with technical assistance and financial incentives. In the absence of such efforts, the condition of these lands will only deteriorate further. On those lands classified as "severely degraded," restoration, for all practical purposes, is impossible. The factors responsible for land degradation include overgrazing of livestock herds, faulty agricultural practices, and deforestation. While the environmental damage provoked by such activities theoretically could occur anywhere, certain natural areas are more vulnerable to long-lasting destruction than others. Tundra, desert, tropical rain forest, and arid grasslands are more easily impaired and take much longer to recover from disruption than does, for example, temperate deciduous forest. Because several of these areas today encompass the homelands of many millions of people whose well-being, and indeed survival, depends on the continued productivity of their land, it is important for us to take a closer look at some specific ways in which humans, consciously or not, are radically undermining the stability of natural ecosystems.

Overgrazing

Of the various activities contributing to soil degradation, none is more significant than overgrazing. According to Lester Brown, president of the Earth Policy Institute, approximately 20% of the world's rangelands have been degraded by the pressure of too many livestock. Since 1950, the world's cattle herd has more than doubled in size, from 720 million to 1.5 billion in 2001; similarly, flocks of sheep and goats have expanded in number from 1.04 billion to 1.75 billion during those same years (Brown, 2003). In India, more than half the land now regarded as "wasteland" was reduced to that status by goats, allowed by their owners to forage freely prior to slaughter. Municipal authorities in India's capital, New Delhi, have spent millions of rupees to replant shrubs and grass on hillsides near the city, but in the absence of efforts to control goat populations, such expenditures have been largely wasted (Tobias, 1998). Under natural conditions, grassland communities are well-adapted to a moderate level of grazing; herds of bison, antelope, wild horses, and so forth, have for millennia been the dominant animals in the grassland biome, evolving and adapting in conjunction with the native plants on which they are dependent. However, when livestock managers increase the number of livestock beyond a certain size or when they introduce types of grazing animals foreign to a particular plant community, the resulting pressure on that community often leads to an unraveling of the ecosystem.

The effects of overgrazing are first seen in the declining populations of those plant species least able to tolerate the increased cropping. As these plants disappear, species more tolerant of heavy grazing are then relieved of competition and expand to fill the niche vacated by the more vulnerable types. The loss of the latter, however, results in an overall reduction in the height, biomass, and total coverage of the grassland. If overgrazing persists, even the more resistant native plants will be unable to withstand the pressure and give way to invader weed species that were not members of the original community. Such plants are generally much inferior to the native plants in nutritive qualities and, as a result, the vitality of the herd is adversely affected. Eventually the weeds themselves may be trampled to such an extent that they, too, are reduced in coverage.

The soil, thus exposed to the forces of wind and water, may be worn away, leaving a barren mud flat or rocky hillside, devoid of any plant community (Whittaker, 1975).

While land degradation due to overgrazing is most pronounced in Australia (80%) and in Africa (49%), severe problems of overgrazing are all too evident in the Middle East, northern India, Central Asia, Mongolia, and much of northern China. Extensive areas of rangeland in the American West are severely affected as well. Of the approximately 270 million acres of publicly owned rangeland in 16 western states, over 60% are considered to be in unsatisfactory condition, degraded by years of overgrazing and mismanagement. The many native species of fish and wildlife inhabiting these rangelands have been severely affected by the deteriorating ecological conditions; close to 90 animal species on federal lands are now listed as endangered or threatened because of environmental damage provoked by overgrazing. Rangeland riparian habitats—the narrow bands of lush vegetation bordering streams and lakes—have been particularly hard-hit. When oversized herds of cattle or sheep congregate in or along the edge of waterways, they trample and eat vegetation, pollute the water, and damage streambank stability. The resulting soil erosion and sedimentation may result in streambeds becoming shallower, warmer, and more turbid, negatively affecting aquatic life. Overgrazing is now regarded as the leading culprit blamed for the decline of native trout populations in western states.

Soil Erosion

Throughout much of the world, including the rich farmlands of the American Midwest, the fertile topsoil that is the basis of agricultural productivity is thinning at an alarming rate. Around the globe, experts estimate that one-third or more of the world's agricultural land is losing soil faster than it is being replenished (Brown, 2003). Given the fact that under normal agricultural conditions it takes from 200 to 1,000 years to form an inch of topsoil, such losses could well undermine the productive capacity of farmlands if effective conservation strategies are not implemented. The Food and Agriculture Organization of the United Nations has warned that unless Third World countries give much higher priority to soil erosion control efforts, they could witness a 30% reduction in harvests by the end of the 21st century—at which time their populations will have increased by as much as sixfold over current levels.

Some degree of soil loss is, of course, a natural process and occurs even in the absence of human intervention. Poor agricultural practices, however, greatly increase the rate of erosion, and when the amount of topsoil lost exceeds that of new soil formed through the gradual decomposition of organic matter (an amount referred to in agricultural circles as **T-value** or, more simply, **"T"**), then the layer of topsoil becomes thinner and thinner until it disappears completely, leaving only the unproductive subsoil or, in extreme cases, bare rock. Topsoil loss has a direct negative impact on cropland productivity, though in recent decades the relationship between soil erosion and diminishing yields has been largely masked by the greatly expanded use of chemical fertilizers. We have, in a sense, been substituting chemical nitrogen and potash for topsoil in order to maintain good harvests. However, while chemicals can replace nutrients lost through erosion, they can't substitute for the lost organic material necessary for maintaining a porous, healthy soil structure. Some studies suggest that heavy fertilizer use can actually damage the soil by disrupting natural nutrient cycles and predict that future per-acre yields, even on lands receiving chemical inputs, will begin to drop if erosion trends aren't reversed (Smil, 1991).

Serious erosion control efforts in the United States grew out of the disastrous Dust Bowl years of the mid-1930s, when millions of tons of rich Great Plains topsoil were literally "gone with the wind" as a result of drought and unwise cultivation practices.

In 1935 the Soil Conservation Service (SCS) was created and Congress funded a major research effort to learn more about the processes of erosion and effective methods of control (in 1994 the name of this agency was changed to Natural Resources Conservation Service, or NRCS). By the 1940s and 1950s soil loss on U.S. farmlands was declining noticeably as American farmers followed the advice of Cooperative Extension

Sheet erosion after heavy rain robs farmland of valuable topsoil and causes water pollution and sedimentation problems in nearby streams and ditches. [*Gary Fak, Soil Conservation Service*]

An effective erosion-control method is the construction of grass ridge terraces such as the one pictured here. A terrace reduces soil runoff by shortening the length of the slope and diverting water in a horizontal direction. When planted in perennial grasses, the approximately 10–foot-wide area has the additional benefit of providing valuable wildlife habitat. [*Gary Fak, Soil Conservation Service*]

"Dust Bowl" years: an Oklahoma family runs for shelter during one of the numerous sky-blackening storms that afflicted the Great Plains states during the 1930s. [*U.S. Department of Agriculture*]

advisors (county agents) or SCS personnel to install terraces, plant windbreaks, contour strip-crop, build grass waterways—whatever method or combination of methods was most suitable to reduce erosion rates on the lands they were cultivating.

By the 1970s, however, soil loss due to farmland erosion once again began to accelerate, reversing the gains of the previous two decades. High commodity prices and the demand for agricultural exports to feed growing populations overseas combined to boost farm production—and promoted record levels of erosion. Citing the link between farm exports and land degradation, an official at the Illinois Department of Agriculture remarked at the time that " . . . for every bushel of corn we ship overseas, we send 1½ bushels of topsoil down the Mississippi River." In the push for expanded production, the traditional practice of crop rotation was abandoned in favor of continuous cropping of corn or soybeans, a practice that greatly increases erosion rates since this leaves the soil surface without any plant cover during a considerable portion of the year. Strong export demand prompted farmers to plow "from fencepost-to-fencepost" to reap the maximum possible profit. By doing so, however, they brought into production much highly erodible land that would have been better left in pasture—and it promptly began to wash away. In the Midwest, fall plowing came into vogue and contributed to substantial amounts of erosion by both wind and water during winter and early spring when fields are bare.

By the late 1970s it was evident that soil loss was once again becoming a serious national problem. In 1981 the USDA estimated that the inherent productivity of fully one-third of American farmlands was declining because of high rates of erosion. Efforts were launched at both the state and federal level to reduce soil loss to tolerable levels (i.e., to T-value). The main strategy for achieving this goal was the promotion of **conservation tillage,** a cultivation practice that involves leaving 30% or more of the soil surface covered with the previous year's crop residue. Variants on conservation tillage include **no-till,** in which crops are planted in the undisturbed residue of an old

No-till farming: young soybean plants emerge from a field whose surface is protected from erosion by a cushioning layer of corn stubble. [*U.S. Department of Agriculture*]

crop; **mulch-till,** a situation where crops are planted in a field where the entire surface has been disturbed, but at least the minimum amount of residue remains after planting; and **strip-till**, a variant of no-till, in which narrow (10"–12"), raised (3"–4") strips are plowed the length of the field, leaving the soil on either side of the strips untouched. Seeds are planted in the center of these strip rows and fertilizer applications are efficiently targeted to these areas. Strip-till cultivation is rapidly winning adherents in the midwestern Corn Belt, since the removal of a narrow band of crop residue in the seed bed promotes warming and drying of the soil during cool, wet spring weather, thus making it possible for farmers to plant earlier than they could under a conventional no-till system. These crop residues perform a number of protective functions: cushioning the impact of falling raindrops, decreasing wind access to bare soil, serving as mini-dams to restrict overland runoff from fields, and improving soil characteristics that resist erosive forces. Alone or in combination with such soil conservation measures as terracing or construction of grass waterways, conservation tillage can substantially reduce erosion rates while maintaining or even increasing crop yields. While conservation tillage is not appropriate for all crops, the practice has expanded rapidly during the past two decades, particularly in corn-and soybean-producing areas of the Midwest.

Erosion control efforts in the United States were given a major boost when Congress passed the **Food Security Act of 1985,** creating the **Conservation Reserve Program (CRP).** Under this landmark program, excessive production and soil loss are being curbed by offering farmers financial incentives to take highly erodible or environmentally sensitive land out of production for 10 to 15 years, converting them to pastures or woodlands. Surveys by the NRCS indicate a 19-ton per acre reduction in soil loss from lands under CRP contract. Modifications to the CRP since its inception in 1985 have broadened the focus of conservation activities. Though CRP's original goal of controlling soil erosion remains a top priority, improving wildlife habitat and water quality are now important components of the program. Landowners are encouraged to sign up for high-priority conservation projects such as developing filter strips (areas of grass or other vegetation at the low end of fields that can filter out soil particles or other pollutants suspended in farmland runoff) or windbreaks. The magnitude and far-reaching scope of the Conservation Reserve Program makes it the federal government's single largest environmental improvement program and represents a major success story in reversing soil loss on U.S. agricultural lands (USDA, 1997).

Similar efforts to reduce excessive soil erosion are desperately needed in many developing countries where the situation is even more serious. Indian agronomists estimate their country is losing 5 billion tons of topsoil annually, almost double the soil loss in the United States where the cropland area is about the same (Brown, 1988). In Ethiopia, erosion is depriving that nation's hard-pressed farmers of 1.5 to 2 billion cubic meters of topsoil every year; as a result, 4 million hectares (about 10 million acres) of Ethiopian highlands are now termed "irreversibly degraded." At the foothills of the Himalayas, in eastern Nepal, 38% of the land area consists of barren fields, abandoned because their topsoil has been lost to erosion (Stutz, 1993). In the lush farmlands of central Chile, the current prosperity may be short-lived because excessive rates of soil loss are undermining agricultural productivity even on the best lands; on the marginal lands where over half the country's peasant farmers live, erosion is seriously depressing crop yields and threatening farmers with large financial losses if current trends are not reversed (Faeth, 1994). In China, soil erosion is endangering increases in crop production desperately needed to feed a still-growing population. In China's northwestern Gansu Province, half or more of all arable land has already been lost to erosion and encroaching deserts.

Although soil erosion is the most obvious form of land degradation, other processes may play a role as well. Improper methods of mechanical tillage may cause compaction or crusting of soils. Repeatedly growing crops on the same land without sufficient fallow periods depletes soil nutrients, though this can be mitigated through the use of manure, cover crops, or appropriate amounts of chemical fertilizers. Extensive land degradation in arid regions of the world has been caused by poor water management on irrigated fields. Failure to drain such areas adequately can result in the salinization or waterlogging of soils. The former process occurs when salts naturally present in certain soils are dissolved by rising water tables under poorly drained irrigated fields and eventually accumulate at the soil surface, poisoning crop roots. Currently between 10–15% of all irrigated lands are plagued by waterlogging or salinization. In the case of salt-affected lands, restoration efforts may take generations, with some lands never recovering. In Australia, 10% of the land area is now suffering from salinization and experts there worry that the percentage could grow to 40% within the next 50 years. Other regions threatened by salinization include irrigated areas of Iraq, Turkey, Pakistan, northern India, China, and the American Southwest.

Deforestation

For the last ten thousand years humans have been cutting and burning woodlands at an ever-increasing pace in their quest for additional farmland, fuel, and building material. Forests still cover slightly over one-fourth of the world's land area (excluding Greenland and Antarctica), but recent decades have witnessed a significant decline in both the area covered by forests and in the quality of remaining woodlands. In spite of increased forest protection efforts in many parts of the world, during the 1990s the world's forests suffered a net loss of 96 million hectares (approximately 240 million acres), the greatest reduction in forested area of any 10-year period thus far (FAO, 2001). At the dawn of the 21st century, only 40% of lands categorized as "forested"

Figure 5-1 Loss of Original Forest Cover by Region as of 1999

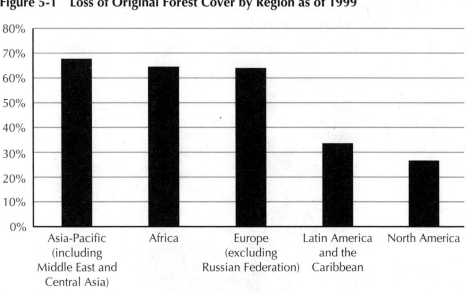

Source: Gardner-Outlaw, Tom, and Robert Engelman. 1999. "Loss of Original Forest Cover by Region."
Forest Futures: Population, Consumption, and Wood Resources. Washington, DC: Population Action
International. Used with permission.

are high-quality **frontier forests**—relatively undisturbed, extensive areas that remain
ecologically intact. The remaining 60% consist of secondary forests, tree plantations,
open woodlands, and brushlands. Frontier forests today are largely limited to the
northern boreal forests of Russia, Canada, and Alaska and to the tropical forests of
the northwestern Amazon basin and the Guyana Shield along South America's northern coast. These remaining frontier forests cover scarcely one-third the areas they
occupied before human activities set in motion the processes of deforestation that
have markedly accelerated within recent decades. As the rate of forest loss accelerates,
so do pressures on ecosystems in the form of species loss, soil erosion, and even climate change.

Deforestation, defined as the permanent decline in crown cover of trees to less
than 10% of its original extent, is particularly worrisome in regard to tropical forests,
where most of the deforestation of the past 30–45 years has occurred. Unfortunately,
rates of loss continue to accelerate. Between 1960–1990, one-fifth of tropical forests
were destroyed, including over 30% of those in Asia and approximately 18% in Latin
America and Africa (Abramovitz, 1998). FAO statistics suggest that the *rate* of tropical deforestation began to slow somewhat during the 1990s, but the UN agency
admits that its estimates are questionable, since reliable direct measurements are
scarce. Indeed, more recent studies suggest that forest loss in Brazil and Indonesia is
more extensive than FAO estimates indicate (WRI, 2000).

Elsewhere, in the semiarid regions of Asia, Africa, and Latin America where forests have always been scanty, existing forests have almost entirely vanished. Only in
Europe and, quite recently, in North America are forests being managed on a sus-
tained-yield basis. In the United States, wooded areas have expanded significantly
over the past 50 years, as once-cleared marginal farmlands revert to forest. The FAO
estimates that forested areas in the industrialized countries as a whole expanded by
2.7% between 1980–1995 (FAO, 2001). However, this overall increase in forest bio-

Box 5-1 Eco-Certification of Coffee: A New Approach to Saving Tropical Forests

Want to help save Latin America's tropical forests? If so, insist that your next cup of coffee bear the **Rainforest Alliance Certified** (formerly "ECO-O.K.") stamp of approval!

Throughout the highlands of Central America, Colombia, and the Caribbean, coffee cultivation has been a mainstay of the economy for almost 200 years. Introduced to New World settlements by European colonial powers (who had themselves been introduced to the stimulating brew several centuries earlier by Arab traders), coffee was well-suited to growing conditions in the mountainous terrain stretching from southern Mexico to Colombia. A shade-loving, small evergreen tree, coffee thrives on steeply sloping hillsides where temperatures are consistently mild, rainfall abundant, and the rich volcanic soil well-drained. As coffee farms proliferated throughout the region during the 19th and 20th centuries, extensive areas of primary forest were cut to make room for coffee plants. However, in contrast to the devastating ecological impact of clearing forests for cattle ranching or banana plantations, the traditional method of coffee cultivation was relatively benign in terms of its environmental "footprint." Individual coffee farms tended to be relatively small, with coffee trees spaced at intervals among dozens of other tree species—some indigenous to the original forest, others planted to provide the grower with supplemental income from fruit, fuelwood, or fiber. This method of production was beneficial both to the crop plant, providing essential shade and protection from the wind, and to the environment. The overarching canopy of diverse tree species and the leaf litter below provided abundant habitat for a wide variety of tropical birds, mammals, insects, and other

[Courtesy of Rainforest Alliance, www. rainforest-alliance.org]

wildlife. Traditional coffee farms, in fact, function ecologically in much the same way as the forests they replaced and are considered the least disruptive form of agriculture currently practiced.

Unfortunately, in recent years market forces and technological advances have been changing the way coffee is grown, undermining the ecological balance of coffee-producing regions. Seeking to maximize production and boost earnings, commercial coffee growers have been planting more sun-tolerant coffee tree varieties, adopting high-density methods of cultivation in which plants are closely spaced in hedgerows in vast open fields. This technique has increased yields by approximately 50%, but at a severe cost to the environment. Converting to sun-grown coffee plantations, growers have bulldozed millions of acres of traditional coffee farms, transforming them into what some observers call "biological deserts." The new coffee monocultures, unlike traditional shade-grown farms, are heavily dependent on chemical inputs to maintain high levels of productivity and to ward off insects, weeds, and fungal diseases. The proliferation of sun-grown coffee farms has been devastating to local biodiversity, with the number of species plummeting as a once richly varied habitat is rapidly simplified to broad expanses of nothing but coffee.

In 1987, concerns about worldwide tropical forest loss prompted formation of the Rainforest Alliance, an international nonprofit organization whose mission centers on developing and promoting economically sound and socially responsible alternatives to tropical deforestation. In 1991 this group created an eco-labeling program that focuses specifically on agricultural crops whose production has had a major negative impact on tropical ecosystems, with sun-grown coffee a prime target (bananas and oranges have also been subjects for Rainforest Alliance production standards). The concept of eco-labeling is a well-established method for encouraging "green" purchasing decisions by providing consumers with the assurance that the item in question has been produced in an environmentally sustainable manner. To ensure that such eco-labels represent more than just a promotional gimmick, certification programs have been established to evaluate the accuracy of environmental claims. The Rainforest Alliance's sustainable coffee-labeling program has developed a list of stringent standards that must be met by every farm they certify. A team of conservationists, scientists, representatives of relevant government agencies, and coffee farmers work together to develop certification criteria. Among the basic principles with which any certified farm must comply are agreements to: avoid any further deforestation; protect native plants and wildlife; prohibit hunting; protect streams and wetlands; maintain tree canopy cover; minimize applications of chemical fertilizers and pesticides; follow sound soil conservation practices; treat workers fairly and adhere to local labor laws; provide workers with safe and sanitary working conditions; and avoid racial discrimination. Farms desiring eco-certification must submit to a field evaluation by a team of Rainforest Alliance technicians who write a report specifying any changes that must be made in order to comply with certification criteria. A follow-up visit to confirm compliance will subsequently be made and a detailed report prepared for examination by a review board. If approved, coffee from the now-certified farm can be labeled with the Rainforest Alliance seal of approval, distinguishing it from other brands in the marketplace. To guarantee that a certified grower doesn't fail to uphold high standards, an annual audit is required to maintain certification.

What motivates growers to devote the effort it takes to earn certification? In part it is pride in their work and love of the land

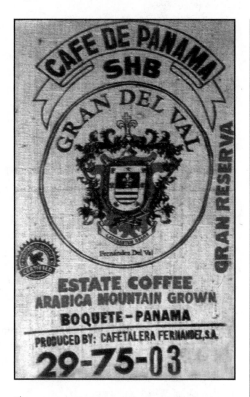

that many of them have cultivated for generations—coffee farmers, too, can be ardent conservationists. It can also be a sound business decision. At a time when world commodity prices for coffee are at record lows due to overproduction, shade-grown eco-certified brands occupy a unique market niche in the upscale gourmet coffee world. Known for superior flavor and carrying a cachet of social and environmental responsibility, shade-grown coffee bearing the Rainforest Alliance label guarantees growers a higher price than they could hope to earn from a higher-yielding but inferior quality sun-grown crop.

The ultimate success of this novel approach to saving forests depends, of course, on the willingness of coffee consumers to "vote with their pocketbooks" and opt for eco-certified brands. These are sold through an increasing number of online and retail outlets, an updated listing of which can be found on the Internet at Rainforest Marketplace, http://www.rainforestalliance.org/marketplace/index.html.

mass obscures the fact that large areas of temperate old-growth forest have been replaced by tree plantations, often comprising but a single species that is grown and harvested within a relatively short time period. Such plantations can be ecologically beneficial for reducing erosion, regenerating degraded soils (e.g., pulpwood plantations in the U.S. Southeast now thriving on abandoned cotton acreage), or providing fuelwood for local consumption. Nevertheless, they are much less biologically diverse than the primary forest ecosystems that once flourished in those regions.

The largest single cause of deforestation, particularly in Africa, is the **clearing of land for agriculture.** The population pressures behind this trend and the ecological damage caused by exploitation of marginal lands not suited for sustained cultivation have already been described. The Cote d'Ivoire (Ivory Coast) provides a classic example of such pressures. With an annual population growth rate averaging between 3–4% until quite recently, slash-and-burn farmers have destroyed fully 95% of the forest cover in that West African nation (Tobias, 1998).

Contributing to the degradation of forests in many poor countries is the **gathering of wood for fuel.** The FAO estimates that approximately half of all wood cut in the world today is used for firewood or for making charcoal. For approximately 90% of the people in the world's less-developed nations, today's true energy crisis is the scarcity of firewood. In most tropical countries wood is used largely for cooking, but in colder climates and mountainous regions it's used for heating as well. While nearly two-thirds of fuelwood is being gleaned from trees along roadsides, small woodlots, or from wood industries, the remainder comes from forest resources (WRI, 2000). The problem is particularly acute in semiarid regions where removal of vegetation leaves land at the mercy of wind and water. In once heavily forested lands such as Nepal, whole mountainsides are being stripped by villagers who now spend most of the day searching for a supply of firewood that a few decades ago could have been gathered in an hour. The investment in time and physical energy required just to obtain enough fuel to cook the family meal has thus increased tremendously in just one generation. Of greater concern to Nepali officials, however, and to their counterparts in the vast Indian subcontinent to the south is the fact that the progressive denudation of the Himalayan slopes is resulting in a massive increase in soil erosion in this ecologically fragile mountain region. As a result, not only is the productive capacity of the land rapidly decreasing, but also much more frequent and severe flooding is occurring downstream in the river valleys of northern India, Pakistan, and Bangladesh due to greatly increased amounts of runoff in the headwaters area of the Ganges, Indus, and Brahmaputra rivers. The devastating floods that regularly leave millions homeless and kill thousands during the subcontinent's monsoon season represent an "unnatural disaster" caused by increased runoff from the denuded Himalayan watershed upstream and increased rates of siltation in lowland deltas that diminish their water-holding capacity. While severe flooding used to occur perhaps twice in a century, "50-year floods" have become regular events, thanks to progressive deforestation in the Himalayas.

As the supply of fuelwood continues to diminish, prices rise accordingly, imposing additional burdens on already impoverished populations. Where people can't afford the high cost of wood, women and children spend much of their time scrounging the countryside for anything burnable—dry grass, fallen leaves, animal dung, garbage—a practice that in the long run further degrades the soil by robbing it of these natural fertilizers. In the industrialized nations, which until about 100 years ago had been just as dependent on wood for fuel as the developing countries are today, the substitution of coal, petroleum products, and natural gas for wood forestalled a growing pressure on their forests. In the developing world, increasing use of kerosene or bottled gas stoves has slightly eased the burdens on those nations' timber resources.

Unfortunately, for millions of the world's poorest people such wood substitutes remain priced out of reach.

In Southeast Asia, Central Africa, and tropical South America, **commercial lumbering** has become a major cause of deforestation, decimating valuable tropical hardwood reserves in order to supply the increased demands of industrial nations for furniture, plywood, and paper pulp. In Indonesia alone, lumbering operations—80% of them illegal—are converting 4 million acres of lush forest to barren wasteland every year; observers predict that by 2010 most of that country's lowland forests will be gone (Bonner, 2002). Until relatively recently, tropical forests largely escaped the logging pressures that earlier had decimated the virgin forests of Europe and North America, primarily because they were sparsely populated and not easily accessible. In addition, in tropical forests commercially valuable tree species are widely dispersed over a broad geographic area, interspersed with many less-desired species, a fact that made their large-scale exploitation economically unfeasible. This situation changed dramatically in the 1960s when mechanization of the timber industry and the arrival of giant multinational lumber companies made possible the ever-more-rapid felling of tropical forests. The methods employed by these companies have been particularly destructive and wasteful; in a typical operation only 10–20% of the trees are cut and removed (i.e., those species with commercial value), but 30–50% of nontarget trees are destroyed in the process. On many tracts, trees are felled by utilizing giant tractors, working in tandem, to drag huge link chains across the forest floor, pulling down everything in their path. This process causes such extensive soil damage that the land may never fully recover. During the 1990s, the use of fire to clear vast tracts of land became the principle means of deforestation in the Amazon and was widely employed in Indonesia as well. In late 1997, fires set to clear new land for rice cultivation and tree plantations burned out of control, spreading through at least 2 million hectares of forest and igniting underground deposits of peat. The fires cast a pall of smoke across much of Southeast Asia for several months, creating serious air quality problems as far away as Malaysia, Singapore, the Philippines, and Thailand (Abramovitz, 1998).

While commercial lumbering in the tropics has taken its greatest toll thus far in Southeast Asia, the near-exhaustion of primary forests in that region has prompted timber barons to shift their attention to South America, particularly to Bolivia, where logging concessions have been granted for more than half that nation's forest lands; to Guyana, where more than 80% of government-owned forests have been leased to wealthy Korean and Malaysian timber companies on terms extremely generous to the Asian firms; and to Chile, where the world's largest remaining expanse of still-pristine temperate rain forest is being felled at an alarming rate to meet the insatiable demands of Japanese paper producers for wood chips. Environmentalists fully expect to see the same well-documented pattern of land degradation and abuse that has accompanied logging operations in Africa, Malaysia, Indonesia, and Papua New Guinea repeated in South America. In countries where politicians control the distribution of timber concessions, bribery and corruption ensure the overexploitation of forest resources with minimal regulation of environmental damage. Careless logging practices frequently result in permanent ecological degradation and those charged with enforcing sound forest management practices are either bought off or become totally frustrated by their inability to prosecute loggers whose political connections insulate them from any enforcement actions. Land rights of indigenous forest peoples, 50 million of whom still make their home within the tropical rain forest, are another casualty of commercial logging operations in the tropics. Preexisting tribal claims are seldom considered when timber concessions are granted; a case in point was the Bolivian government's give-away of logging rights within Guarayo and Chiquitano de Monte

Verde indigenous territories in the late 1990s. Native peoples frequently suffer total impoverishment after logging destroys the forest resources that sustained these groups for millennia (Ayres, 2004; Colchester, 1994).

In Latin America, **cattle ranching** has imposed additional pressures on threatened forests. In such Central American nations as Costa Rica and Panama, cattle ranching has destroyed more hectares of tropical forest than any other activity—70% of the land formerly covered by trees in both countries is now utilized as pastureland (Coffin, 1993). During the 1980s much of this destruction was driven by the demand for cheap beef to supply fast-food chains in the United States. In Brazil, cattle ranching is a major cause of deforestation in the Amazon basin, the largest continuous tract of tropical forest in the world. Since the 1970s, ranchers have cleared more than 10 million hectares of rain forest for pastureland, a practice originally encouraged by generous tax breaks and subsidies from a Brazilian government eager to develop the vast interior of that nation while providing an abundant supply of inexpensive meat for working-class consumers in the country's large coastal cities. In recent years subsidy programs have been terminated, but ranchers continue to clear new pasture as a form of land speculation—a means of obtaining legal title to such lands at a time of rapidly rising property values. Unfortunately, as in the case of agricultural exploitation in Amazonia, grazing pressures on these deforested tracts can be sustained profitably for only a few years. When the fragile tropical soils wear out, their content of phosphorus and other nutrients depleted, ranchers simply move on, burn or cut down more trees, and thus perpetuate the destructive cycle.

Within the past few years commercial **soybean production** has emerged as yet another key factor fueling deforestation in Amazonia. To meet escalating global demand for soy, large areas of previously untouched jungle are being cleared for cultivation of Brazil's newest cash crop. In 2002, soybean fields were responsible for a 40% jump in the rate of Amazonian deforestation. Blairo Maggi, governor of the state of Mato Grosso (which translates as "dense jungle") is calling for a three-fold increase in soybean acreage within a decade and shrugged off the ecological implications of doing so with the remark, "To me, a 40% increase in deforestation doesn't mean anything at all, and I don't feel the slightest guilt over what we are doing here" (Rohter, 2003).

That destruction of the earth's forest cover will have a serious and adverse impact on terrestrial ecosystems—and on their human inhabitants as well—is undisputed. Past history should have taught us that heedless deforestation can lead to excessive erosion rates, decrease the soil's water-absorbing capacity, increase the amount of runoff and flooding, and lead to the transformation of once-productive environments into desertlike conditions. Today we have growing evidence to indicate that loss of forest cover also can lead to local climatic changes, with an increase in temperature and drop in annual rainfall when large expanses of woodland are cleared. More ominous is the possibility that deforestation will hasten the onset of global warming, due to the pivotal role forests play as a "carbon sink," absorbing CO_2 and thereby counteracting the so-called "Greenhouse Effect."

One might suppose that since the consequences of deforestation are well understood, a serious attempt to reverse current trends would be well underway. Unfortunately, in many of the countries most seriously affected reforestation efforts are negligible. Even where the political will exists and funds are available, large-scale tree-planting programs encounter serious difficulties that are inextricably related to the cultural, political, and economic facts of life in rural societies. In many areas saplings planted with high hopes are promptly devoured by overabundant and freely roaming goats, sheep, and cattle. In some places nomads passing through an area may deci-

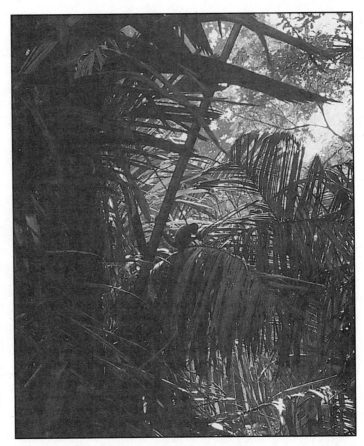

The tropical rain forest remains intact within Costa Rica's Tortuguero National Park.
[*Mathew Nadakavukaren*]

Cattle ranches now dominate the Costa Rican landscape in what was formerly lush tropical forest.
[*Mathew Nadakavukaren*]

The "slash and burn" methods used by Brazilian ranchers to create more pastureland has turned millions of acres of Amazonian tropical forest into "tree cemeteries." [© *Joao Luiz Bulcao/Corbis*]

mate a village's efforts at reforestation, while in still other areas villagers themselves may uproot young trees because they simply have no other source of fuel. Successful reforestation efforts require extensive administrative efforts to protect the plants for years—efforts that may be politically unrewarding to officials trying to win voters' approval for next year's election rather than a "job well done" 20 years in the future. There have been some reforestation success stories, most notably in India where approximately four hectares of trees are being planted for every one that is deforested. Although these tree plantations, which consist primarily of fast-growing eucalyptus or pine, lack the diversity of the native forest cover, they nevertheless provide soil and watershed protection while serving as windbreaks and a renewable source of fuel for local residents.

Ultimately the most serious obstacle to curbing forest loss is the continued rapid growth of human populations in the countries most affected. As a Costa Rican squatter on a partially forested ranch poignantly stated, "By subsisting today I know I can destroy the future of the forest and the people. But I have to eat today" (Hamilton, 1989).

Desertification

That humans can create desertlike conditions on once-productive land has been known, though largely ignored, since the time 2300 years ago when Plato bewailed the ecological fate of his native Attica, writing that "our land, compared with what it was, is like the skeleton of a body wasted by disease. The soft, plump parts have vanished and all that remains is the bare carcass." This sorry situation was brought about by the cutting of forests and overgrazing of livestock, which in that semiarid climate inevitably resulted in topsoil erosion and springs that dried up because they were no longer being recharged (due to rainwater runoff). The formation of cultural waste-lands, which occurred in ancient Greece and the lands around the eastern Mediterranean, is a process that so increased in extent during the 20th century that it was graced with the somewhat unwieldy, though descriptive, term **desertification.** Defined by delegates at the 1992 United Nations Conference on Environment and Development (UNCED) as "land degradation in arid, semiarid, and dry sub-humid areas resulting from various factors including climatic variations and human activities," desertification today is adversely affecting the lives and economic well-being of an estimated 900 million people in over 100 countries.

Contrary to the prevailing image of sand dunes relentlessly sweeping down over green fields and pastures, desertification seldom involves the steady influx of sands along a uniform front. Most often the process is set in motion when climatic fluctuations and abusive land-use practices interact to extend desertlike conditions irregularly over susceptible land. Spots of extreme degradation are especially likely to form around water holes when nearby pastures are heavily grazed and trampled and around towns when people denude adjacent lands in their search for fuelwood. Since desertification first captured world attention in the 1960s and 1970s, it has generally been assumed that population pressures have been the primary cause. More recently, however, data obtained from a decade's worth of satellite photos indicate that climatic variations exert a much more pronounced influence on the expansion of desertlike conditions than do human pressures. In the world's arid grasslands and semi-desert regions, year-to-year fluctuations of rainfall can be moderately destructive to biotic communities even under natural conditions, but in the long run natural processes can correct the imbalance and quickly reestablish pre-drought vegetational patterns. However, when environmental stresses due to normal climatic variation are coupled with such activities as overgrazing, gathering fuelwood, and poor cultivation practices, problems of land degradation are seriously aggravated. If such human pressures persist and intensify, they can sharply limit the regenerative capabilities of the land, hindering its recovery even after climatic conditions improve (Hulme and Kelly, 1993).

Whatever its cause, desertification is a process occurring today on an unprecedented scale. The human tragedy embodied in the great dust storms that blackened the skies in the American prairie states during the 1930s is being repeated today in sub-Saharan Africa, where nomadic herdsmen and their oversized flocks seem to have pushed the carrying capacity of the land beyond the point of no return; in northwest India, the world's most densely populated arid zone and, thanks to the large herds of cattle, camels, goats, etc., also perhaps the world's dustiest area; in North Africa, where soil erosion is accelerating the pace of desertification on lands that were once the granary of the Roman Empire; and in northwestern China, where once-productive rangelands are now blowing away and turning to desert due to overgrazing. Although the Chinese government is urging herders in the area to reduce their flocks by 40% in a desperate effort to combat desertification, China's Gobi Desert continues to expand eastward, forcing villagers to flee their homes to escape the encroaching sands. Huge dust storms in late winter or early spring occur with increasing frequency, producing "brown rain" as far afield as Korea and Japan and creating fears that northern China is turning into a "Dust Bowl" (Brown, 2003). Many of these areas still have the potential to reestablish their former grassland ecosystems if the constant pressure of overgrazing and overplowing could be lifted, but some have been irreversibly degraded by complete loss of topsoil. If human pressures continue to mount, degradation of arid lands will result in the permanent destabilization of existing ecosystems and a continuing impoverishment of both ecological and cultural conditions. Ecosystems, like civilizations, can decline and fall if pushed too far.

Wetlands Loss

Swamps, bogs, fens, tidal marshlands, pocosins, estuaries, ponds, river bottoms, flood plains, and prairie potholes all fall under the designation of **wetlands,** ecosystems characterized by soils that are inundated or water-saturated for at least a portion of the year and by the presence of certain water-loving plants ("hydrophytes"). In the not-too-distant past, most people viewed wetlands as a nuisance, useful only to frogs and mosquitoes, and thus prime candidates for draining or filling to convert them into more "profitable" areas for farming, mining, or urban development. As a result, over half the wetlands that existed in the contiguous 48 states at the time European settlers first arrived (estimated at about 247 million acres in AD 1600) have now disappeared. Fortunately, the rate of loss has declined in recent years, thanks to federal legislation protecting wetlands. In 1997 the U.S. Fish and Wildlife Service released its decennial estimate on wetlands status and trends, reporting that the average annual net loss of wetlands has dropped by about 60% since 1985, from 290,000 acres per year to a mid-1990s level of 117,000 acres lost annually. Today, wetlands cover just 5% (104 million acres) of the land surface in the lower 48 states. Alaska has another 160 million acres, with wetlands extending across half the North Star State. Outside Alaska, Florida and Louisiana have the largest remaining expanses of wetlands, though they are also among the states with the highest rates of wetlands loss in recent years. California has lost a greater percentage of its original wetlands than any other state (91%), but Florida has lost the largest number of acres (EPA, 1988; WRI, 1992). In recent years the significance of this loss has finally begun to be realized, and belated efforts to control wetlands conversion are now underway at both the federal and state level. Wetlands have been disappearing elsewhere in the world as well; globally the loss is estimated at about 50%, but in France and Germany wetlands destruction totals 80% (Hinrichsen, 2003).

Today the importance of wetlands in both ecological and economic terms is unquestioned. Their ability to retain large amounts of water makes them extremely valuable as nature's own method of preventing devastating floods. Not surprisingly, as wetlands along the Mississippi River Valley have been destroyed, the severity and frequency of floods in that region has escalated—a fact made tragically clear during the disastrous flooding along the upper Mississippi River Valley in the summer of 1993. Wetlands provide the major recharge areas for groundwater reserves and also serve as "living filters" for purifying contaminated surface waters as these percolate into the ground. Indeed, taking advantage of wetlands' capacity to act as "nature's kidneys," some communities are now utilizing constructed marshes to treat stormwater or secondary wastewater effluent by directing the flow through **engineered wetlands**, where living organisms remove pollutants efficiently and inexpensively. The sustained productivity of commercial fisheries is also heavily dependent on the existence of wetlands. Between 60–90% of fish caught along the Atlantic and Gulf coasts spend at least some portion of their life cycle, usually the vulnerable early stages, in coastal marshes or estuaries. Further inland in the Midwest, the system of lakes, marshes, and prairie potholes extending from the Gulf of Mexico north into Canada provides the major life-support system for millions of migratory waterfowl (half of all ducklings in North America are hatched in the prairie potholes of the Dakotas and Canada). A $1 billion recreational hunting industry, attracting 2.5 million duck hunters each year, is thus totally dependent on preservation of these vital wetlands breeding areas. Wetlands provide a habitat not only for ducks and geese but also for many other bird and mammal species—whooping cranes, river otters, black bears, and so on.

Although some wetlands are lost due to natural causes such as erosion, land subsidence, storms, or saltwater intrusion, human activities account for by far the greatest

Box 5-2   Everglades: Test Case for Wetlands Restoration

The Everglades, Florida's legendary "River of Grass" and the world's largest freshwater marsh, is today one of the most threatened ecosystems in the United States. Under incremental attack for more than a century by humans who have dredged, drained, and diked this once-vast swampland, the Everglades has shrunk to little more than half of its original 8 million acres, stretching from Lake Okeechobee in central Florida more than 100 miles south to Florida Bay. In 1948, following six months of torrential rains and devastating floods in the Miami area, Congress authorized the U.S. Army Corps of Engineers to launch the **Central and South Florida (C&SF) Project.** This mammoth, multi-purpose water management effort was intended to provide flood control, ensure a dependable water supply for urban and agricultural consumers, prevent saltwater intrusion into aquifers, and to preserve conditions beneficial to wildlife, navigation, and outdoor recreation. While the Corps continues to insist that the C&SF Project performed its functions well, making it possible for over 5 million people to live and work in the 18,000 square mile area, many view the Project's ultimate consequences as an ecological disaster.

The insatiable water demands of irrigated agriculture and of cities lining the Sunshine State's "Gold Coast," along with flood control projects and natural droughts, have disrupted the natural sheet flow of water that for millennia sustained the natural rhythms of life throughout the Everglades. The ecological damage caused by this disruption has been further compounded by serious degradation of water quality due to fertilizer-laden drainage from adjacent sugarcane fields. Phosphate pollution in particular has precipitated massive fish kills and algal blooms, as well as the explosive growth of cattails. Along South Florida's Atlantic coast, where polluted runoff from the Everglades discharges into the sea, periodic die-backs in the seagrass beds of Florida Bay, along with massive algal blooms, jeopardize the economic health of sports and commercial fisheries.

Another major threat to ecosystem stability in the Everglades has been the melaleuca tree, an exotic Australian species introduced in 1906 to help drain the swamp; it did its job only too well and, in the absence of natural enemies, has displaced many of South Florida's native plant and animal species. As a result of this triple onslaught (i.e., drainage projects, pollution, and melaleuca), wildlife populations in the Everglades have plummeted in recent decades—breeding pairs of waterbirds are down 90% from former levels and 33 species of indigenous animals are listed as either threatened or endangered. In the long run, degradation of the Everglades threatens not only flamingoes and alligators but Floridians as well, since the groundwater supplies on which the southern part of the state depends, naturally replenished through hydrologic contact with the Everglades, are not being recharged as rapidly as in the past. Soil resources also are threatened as drainage projects and intensive agricultural production have exposed the rich topsoil to oxidation and erosion. Some of the agricultural areas within the Everglades have lost more than 6 feet of topsoil—about half its original depth—due to the drying and oxidation of the peaty soils.

The slow ecological decline of this invaluable wetland resource has not gone unnoticed; since the early 1900s, activists have loudly protested the activities which, they warned, would destroy the very features that attracted people to South Florida in the first place. In 1947 proponents of preservation convinced Congress to set aside the southern portion of the giant marshland as Everglades National Park. More recently, the Everglades Coalition, now an assemblage of 45 national and local environmental groups, began pressing toward a far more ambitious goal—reengineering, and in some places undoing, the elaborate plumbing system that makes the Everglades the most intensively managed region on earth. The ultimate objective, as proclaimed in 1983 by then-Governor Bob Graham, was to make ". . . the Everglades look and function by the year 2000 more as it did at the turn of the century."

Restoration of the Everglades moved a giant step closer to reality in the fall of 1992 when Congress authorized a comprehensive review of the C&SF Project and the following year established the South Florida Ecosystem Restoration Task Force. The state of Florida remained an active partner in these efforts, passing the 1994 Everglades Forever Act that established a multifaceted program to restore large portions of the Everglades. Under the joint direction of the U.S. Army Corps of Engineers and the South Florida Water Management District, the review study focused on how the Everglades and Florida Bay ecosystems could be restored while still providing for the water needs of South Florida's agricultural producers and urban residents. In 1998 the Corps of Engineers released a far-reaching plan to restore a more natural water cycle to southern Florida, and in 2000 the U.S. Congress enacted legislation creating a $7.8 billion **Comprehensive Everglades Restoration Plan (CERP)**, described as the world's largest ecosystem restoration effort. Encompassing a 30+ year time span, including more than 60 major components, and covering 16 South Florida counties, CERP's primary goals are to restore the area's natural water flow patterns to the greatest degree possible, to improve wildlife habitat in order to protect and enhance biodiversity, and to reduce human pressure on ecosystems by restraining urban sprawl.

Of these goals, none are more fundamental to the project's ultimate success than increasing the capacity for storing water within the Everglades watershed. Plans for achieving this include the construction of channels and reservoirs that will capture much of the freshwater currently being discharged to the ocean during the rainy season, storing it in large surface impoundments, engineered marshes, and in underground aquifers. A portion of this water will be released during the dry season to flow in a sheetlike manner through the Everglades to Florida Bay, while the remainder of the stored water will be used for irrigation and to meet urban water demands. In an effort to remove existing barriers to the sheetflow of water through the area, approximately 500 miles of canals and levees are targeted for removal. Work has already begun on restoring the channelized Kissimmee River to a more natural state, helping to improve wildlife habitat in that section of the Everglades.

Engineering projects alone, however, won't be enough to restore the Everglades to good health. The water quality problems caused by fertilizer runoff from cane fields and vegetable farms present a politically charged dilemma. State law requires farmers to reduce the amount of phosphorus they release in their drainage water and to pay one-third of the cost of building phosphorus-scrubbing wetlands through which agricultural wastewaters must pass before draining into the Everglades. However, phosphate concentrations in agricultural runoff following wetlands treatment is still higher than the mandated 10 parts per billion limit, meaning that farmers will have to take additional steps to meet the effluent requirements. In 2003, environmentalists were outraged when narrow political interests beholden to "Big Sugar" convinced the Florida legislature to postpone the deadline date for compliance with the phosphorus regulations by 10 years, from the originally mandated 2006 to 2016.

Curbing urban development in rapidly growing South Florida is another essential element in protecting and restoring the Everglades ecosystem. By 2010 planners anticipate a population of 8 million in the Miami area, up from 6 million in 2000. In the absence of wise-growth policies, urban sprawl and the water demands of additional millions will severely jeopardize Everglades restoration efforts. Currently a regional program called "Eastward Ho!" is striving to redirect new growth toward vacant land in already-developed areas and to alter building and zoning codes to require higher-density housing in new suburban developments.

Whether or not such efforts will be successful remains to be seen; the Everglades Coalition has already voiced concern at what they see as betrayal of congressional intent by Corps of Engineers regulations which, they say, fail to give priority to restoration, catering instead to pressure from commercial interests. As examples, they cite Corps' approval of deep-pit limestone mining within the Everglades (the Corps justifies its action by saying that once the pits are mined out, some will be used as water storage reservoirs) and continued Corps-permitted ditching, draining, and development of natural areas in the western Everglades on the outskirts of Naples and Fort Meyers. Environmental activists vow to keep the pressure on Congress to ensure that the Corps makes restoration, not development, its top priority, as mandated by CERP, and to lobby vigorously to secure congressional funding for Everglades restoration projects.

The Everglades restoration effort now underway will be immensely challenging, representing the most ambitious and far-reaching environmental restoration effort ever attempted anywhere. Achieving the goals set will be difficult and expensive, but the cost of allowing continued ecosystem degradation would be even higher. Years ago, author Marjorie Douglas, a tireless crusader for preservation of Florida's wetlands, aptly described the task ahead, and its potential rewards, in a stirring call to action.

"The Everglades is a test," she proclaimed. "If we pass, we get to keep the planet."

References

Derr, Mark. 1993. "Redeeming the Everglades." *Audubon* (Sept/Oct).

Fauth, Laura. 2002. "Mining, Lack of Independent Review Threaten Everglades Restoration." *The Planet Newsletter*, Sierra Club (Nov/Dec).

World Resources Institute. 2000. "Replumbing the Everglades: Large-scale Wetlands Restoration in South Florida." *World Resources 2000–2001: People and Ecosystems.*

The Everglades, one of America's greatest natural treasures and the world's largest freshwater marsh, has been reduced to half its original size by agriculture, urban sprawl, and unwise water management. In 2000, the federal government launched a massive restoration project to restore the area's natural water flow pattern to the greatest extent possible. [*Pat Lynch, SFWMD*]

amount of loss. Draining swamps or bottomlands for agricultural purposes is the leading cause of wetlands destruction. The Fish and Wildlife Service estimates that in spite of federal incentive programs for farmers to preserve wetlands, fully 79% of current wetlands loss can be traced to drainage for agricultural use. Coastal development also has taken a heavy toll of wetlands, particularly along estuaries that provide vital habitat and breeding grounds for many commercially valuable fish and shellfish species. Dredging for canals and port construction, flood control projects, and road building have all had a negative impact on wetlands, as has urban sprawl. In the southeastern states, deep-soil swamps were cleared and drained for conversion to pine plantations, resulting in extensive wetlands loss until the EPA banned such activities in 1994. While there are no federal laws expressly prohibiting the draining, filling, or converting of most wetlands, Congress took a small step toward protecting our remaining wetlands when it included a section in the 1985 farm bill referred to as the "Swampbuster Provision," aimed at discouraging draining of wetlands for agriculture by stating that farmers who do so will lose their farm program benefits. The Conservation Reserve Program, enacted under that same legislation, provided farmers with financial incentives to protect lands taken out of cultivation and thereby fostered the restoration of critical wetlands habitat. In 1989 federal legislation created one of the most significant conservation programs in U.S. history. The North American Wetlands Conservation Act (NAWCA) provides matching grants for wetlands conservation programs throughout North America and since 1989 has helped finance over 960 projects in all 50 states, Canada, and Mexico. With private groups such as Ducks Unlimited and the Nature Conservancy matching federal money dollar for dollar, almost 9 million acres of wetlands have been restored and protected, thanks to NAWCA.

Since almost three-fourths of all wetlands acreage in the United States is privately owned, the ultimate success of wetlands preservation attempts hinge on efforts by both government and environmental organizations to educate landowners on the intrinsic value of wetlands, to encourage wetlands conservation and restoration, and to provide the technical assistance and financial incentives that will persuade property owners to protect this precious resource.

Loss of Biodiversity

Extinction of a species, like the death of an individual, is a natural process. As fossil evidence clearly indicates, many groups of plants and animals that dominated life on earth in past millennia have died out, only to be replaced by newly evolving organisms. The rise and fall of species throughout the course of earth's history was determined largely by a population's ability to adapt to changing environmental conditions or to become increasingly specialized for life in a particular ecological niche. As evolution proceeded, the number of plant and animal species proliferated as populations dispersed into far-flung geographic regions and adapted to life in a seemingly endless variety of ecological niches. Today biologists have described 1.75 million species (Heywood and Watson, 1995), but estimate that the actual number currently in existence, many yet undiscovered, ranges from 3 to 30 million, the largest number being small creatures living in tropical forests and in the deep oceans. Unfortunately, it is widely feared that many of these species will vanish before their existence is ever noted or recorded.

The sad truth of the present situation is that human actions have greatly accelerated the rate at which species are becoming extinct; indeed, for the first time since the last great die-off at the end of the Cretaceous Period 65 million years ago, species are vanishing more rapidly than new ones are evolving, resulting in a diminishing diversity of life forms. The first recorded animal extinction—that of the European lion—was documented in AD 80; more than half of the animal species that have disappeared since that time have become extinct since 1900. Just as human populations have been increasing at an ever-faster pace in recent centuries, so has the rate of species loss. While estimates indicate that over the vast span of geologic time one mammalian species suffers extinction every 400 years and one bird species every 200, the record for the past 400 years shows a dramatic acceleration in the rate of extinction: 58 mammalian species and 128 bird species. Even these numbers don't accurately rep-

Table 5-1 Number of Threatened Species by Major Groups of Organisms (1996–2004)

	Number of described species	Number of threatened species in 2004	Number threatened in 2004, as % of species described
Vertebrates			
Mammals	5,416	1,101	20%
Birds	9,917	1,213	12%
Reptiles	8,163	304	4%
Amphibians	5,743	1,770	31%
Fishes	28,500	800	3%
Subtotal	**57,739**	**5,188**	**9%**
Invertebrates			
Insects	950,000	559	0.06%
Molluscs	70,000	974	1%
Crustaceans	40,000	429	1%
Others	130,200	30	0.02%
Subtotal	**1,190,200**	**1,992**	**0.17%**
Plants			
Mosses	15,000	80	0.50%
Ferns and allies	13,025	140	1%
Gymnosperms	980	305	31%
Dicotyledons	199,350	7,025	4%
Monocotyledons	59,300	771	1%
Subtotal	**287,655**	**8,321**	**2.89%**
Others			
Lichens	10,000	2	0.02%
Subtotal	**10,000**	**2**	**0.02%**
TOTAL	**1,545,594**	**15,503**	**1%**

Source: Adapted from *2004 IUCN Red List of Threatened Species.* www.iucnredlist.org

resent the true toll, especially for recent decades, since, by international agreement, a species isn't classified as extinct until 50 years after its last sighting. In addition, with millions of species still undiscovered and unnamed, it is quite likely that large numbers are quietly disappearing, unnoticed and unmourned (Wilcove, McMillan, and Winston, 1993). In 2003 the World Conservation Union (IUCN) listed 25% of mammalian species and 11% of bird species worldwide as threatened with extinction. When *all* types of organisms are considered—not just the feathered or furry creatures that appeal to human emotions, but the myriads of insects, mollusks, fish, fungi, plants, and other organisms that greatly enrich the diversity of life—then current rates of extinction are even more alarming. Harvard biologist E. O. Wilson estimates that in tropical forest areas alone, home to a conservatively estimated 10 million species, the world is currently losing 3 species every hour, 74 per day, 27,000 each year. If present trends of rain forest destruction are not reversed, 10–20% of all rain forest species will be extinct within 30 years—a number equivalent to at least 5–10% of all species on earth (Wilson, 1992).

The magnitude of such a loss is staggering. Species diversity is generally considered a prime determinant of ecological stability; extinction of key species, particularly plant species, may lead to the collapse of whole ecosystems. Less spectacular but equally distressing from a human viewpoint is the prospect of many potentially useful plant species being lost before their food or medicinal value is discovered. Even today, one-fourth of all pharmaceutical products bought by Americans contain active ingredients derived from plant products. The discovery of taxol, a potent anticancer drug derived from the bark of the Pacific yew (formerly regarded as a weed tree in old-growth forests of the Pacific Northwest) is but one of the more recent additions to a long list of valuable medicinal products extracted from forest plants. From a philosophical viewpoint also, the implications of the wholesale destruction of nonhuman life is profoundly disturbing. Over a century ago Thoreau proclaimed that "In wildness is the preservation of the world." Much ethical discussion in recent years has centered around the question of whether humans have the moral right to exterminate another form of life, to abruptly terminate the product of millions of years of evolution. Undeniably, "extinction is forever."

Although the causes of accelerating species loss are by now fairly well understood, reversing these trends will be extremely difficult, particularly in regions where rapidly growing human populations are in direct competition with wildlife. Human pressures on other species can assume a variety of forms, as detailed below.

Direct Killing or Collecting of Wildlife for Food, Pleasure, or Profit

From the Paleolithic hunters who decimated the wooly mammoths and mastodons with primitive weapons to the modern Russian and Japanese fishing fleets that have brought several species of whale to the brink of extinction, predatory humans have totally eliminated a number of bird and mammalian species. Of all the animal extinctions known to have occurred within the past 400 years, the World Conservation Union estimates that nearly one-fourth (23%) were caused by overhunting. Collectors who dynamite reefs to obtain chunks of coral or capture rare tropical fish for sale to aquarium hobbyists; cactus "rustlers" who steal plants from nature preserves to satisfy the growing demand for rare houseplants; African poachers who shoot the endangered rhinoceros for the high profits its horn will bring in the markets of the Orient (powdered rhinoceros horn has long been considered an aphrodisiac in China and the Far East)—all contribute to the demise of species, as do the consumers who provide the incentive for such actions.

In an effort to remove the financial incentives for exploitation of wildlife, conservation groups mustered enough support to secure passage of the 1973 **Convention on International Trade in Endangered Species of Flora and Fauna (CITES).** Meeting twice a year, CITES' governing body regulates international trade in specified animal and plant products and flatly prohibits trade in products from endangered species. CITES has received much credit for stemming the slaughter of African elephants after issuing a ban in 1989 on ivory trading. A partial lifting of this ban in 1999 allowed Namibia, Botswana, and Zimbabwe to begin selling limited amounts of ivory to Japan; funds generated by this trade are supposed to be reinvested into wildlife conservation programs and may thus benefit elephant populations in those countries, so long as monitoring of the trade is rigorous enough to exclude illegally harvested tusks.

CITES has been less effective in curbing the illicit trade in tiger parts, which has resulted in such a precipitous decline in populations of the big cats that many wildlife biologists hold out little hope for the survival of tigers outside of zoos. In countries such as China and Taiwan, virtually every part of the animal's body brings premium prices due to their supposed medicinal benefits: tiger bones for potions to cure rheumatism, tiger whiskers to provide strength, tiger eyes to calm convulsions, and tiger penis, simmered in a soup, to rekindle male sexual prowess among senior citizens (only *wealthy* senior citizens need apply, however—a bowl of tiger penis soup may cost over $300!). The apparent lack of effort on the part of government officials to stem illegal commerce in tiger and rhino products brought strong CITES criticism of both

Box 5-3   Slaughter in the Jungle: Bushmeat's Tragic Toll

Bushmeat, a common term for the flesh of wildlife living in the jungles and shrub-land ("bush") of Africa, has always been a dietary staple for people inhabiting the vast forests of that continent. From time immemorial, subsistence hunters armed with bows and arrows, nets, and other traditional weapons have stalked, killed, and eaten a wide array of the native animals and birds whose habitat they shared. So long as human populations were relatively small and weapons primitive, when the hunters' goal was simply to secure enough meat to feed their own families or village, such predation had only a localized impact and was sustainable in terms of preserving stable wildlife populations.

That situation has now changed dramatically with the commercialization of hunting throughout the forests of western and central Africa. Horrified conservationists are now raising the alarm, warning that nothing—not even habitat loss—poses a greater threat to biodiversity throughout this vast region than does the relentless slaughter of wildlife for human consumption.

Each year the 30 million people living in the countries of the Congo River basin eat an estimated 5 million metric tons of forest antelopes, bush pigs, monkeys, gorillas, chimpanzees, elephants, monitor lizards, guinea fowl, and cane rats—among others. The demand for bushmeat is enormous and growing. Central Africans eat as much or more meat on a daily basis per person as do Americans or Europeans, but most of the meat they consume—about 80%—comes from wildlife rather than domestic animals. The lack of available grasslands for cattle grazing, the density of forests, and the prevalence of tropical diseases and insects lethal to temperate-zone livestock have made beef, mutton, and poultry rare items on Central African dinner tables; it's always been much easier and cheaper to look to the forest for the daily supply of meat. Rapidly growing urban populations in the region are increasing the demand for bushmeat; unlike the situation in rural areas where bushmeat is the cheapest source of animal protein, in the cities it is more expensive than shipped-in domestic meats. Many affluent Africans, however, are happy to pay premium prices for gorilla, chimpanzee, or other bushmeat,

regarding it as a status symbol and a way to maintain cultural ties and ethnic identity with their rural roots.

It is economics, however, that is driving the bushmeat business. Throughout central Africa, collapsing commodity prices for cash crops such as cocoa and coffee have caused widespread unemployment; to men desperate to support their families, the burgeoning bushmeat trade offers lucrative opportunities. As long as the supply of wildlife is abundant, hunters can earn from $400–1,100 per year, a sum higher than the average yearly income in the region (and greater than the salary paid to guards hired to prevent hunting). Resources needed to become a hunter are few and relatively inexpensive; a rifle, often borrowed, some cartridges, and perhaps some wire snares. Add to this the fact that few Africans see anything wrong with killing wildlife and it's not surprising that economic incentive coupled with cultural values gives the bushmeat trade widespread public acceptance.

Commercial hunting has been greatly facilitated and the demand for bushmeat substantially boosted by industrial logging operations in the Congo basin. Dozens of foreign timber companies have been granted logging concessions to extract timber from vast expanses of pristine tropical forests. The forest fragmentation caused by such operations and the network of access roads built to transport the logs to market have made native wildlife easy prey for hunters. By affording easy access to formerly impenetrable jungle and by allowing hunters to hitch rides on logging trucks, timber companies have, intentionally or not, greatly increased the supply of bushmeat and the profitability of the trade. Logging operations have also boosted demand; with thousands of itinerant loggers and their families moving into once sparsely settled areas, a market for bushmeat has arrived at the source of supply. Needing meat for their workers, some logging companies hire professional hunters directly or may provide them with guns and wire snares in return for a portion of the kill. Even without direct subsidies, bushmeat hunters ply a profitable trade among loggers who have money to spend, big appetites, and no other readily available source of meat. Elsewhere in the region, notably in the eastern section of the Democratic Republic of the Congo, wildlife has been decimated by the bushmeat demands of thousands of peasant farmers-turned coltan miners (coltan, a tantalum-containing ore, is a key component for circuitry in cell phones, video games, laptop computers, and other electronic devices). In the late 1990s, coltan prospectors began digging in Kahuzi-Biega National Park, supposedly a protected World Heritage Site. The hunters who arrived to supply them with food successively killed off the elephants, gorillas, chimpanzees, buffaloes, and antelopes. As the larger species were wiped out, hunters moved on to smaller prey; within a few years there was little left to shoot other than some small antelopes, birds, monkeys, and tortoises.

The scope of the ongoing massacre is immense. In some areas observers now refer to the "Empty Forest Syndrome"—regions where the jungle is relatively intact but devoid of all large animals. While the loss of any species is tragic, the plight of the region's great apes—gorillas, chimpanzees, and bonobos—is of special concern. Although these large primates comprise but a small percentage of bushmeat in the marketplace, perhaps just 1%, they are likely to be the first species hunted to extinction for their tasty flesh. Already rare, apes are exceptionally vulnerable to hunting pressures because of very low fertility rates. The fact that they are large, noisy, and gregarious makes it very easy for hunters to locate and shoot them and cultural values place a high premium on their meat, especially gorilla hands, which are considered a delicacy and fetch a high price. Since all great apes are classified as "endangered" or "highly endangered," it is illegal in every African country to kill them or to sell their flesh. Such laws are largely ignored, however, and seldom enforced. Recently, public health authorities have been raising an additional concern related to the bushmeat trade in chimpanzee and gorilla flesh, citing the potential for disease transmission. Evidence has been emerging of a possible link between exposure to dead apes and human outbreaks of HIV, Ebola, and Marburg virus. It is well-known that disease organisms can spread from one species to another and health officials fear that butchering and eating bushmeat places humans at increased risk of contracting deadly animal-borne diseases.

Unfortunately, prospects for any substantial curtailing of the bushmeat trade appear grim. With regional economies in a free-fall and government officials easy to bribe, the will and ability to monitor hunting and logging practices is largely nonexistent. Since the late 1990s international conservation groups have entered into cooperative agreements with some of the large logging companies, trying to enlist the industry's support for curbing the worst abuses of bushmeat trafficking while conceding that the timber industry has an important role to play in African development. Critics charge such associations give "green cover" to loggers who have been among the worst offenders in sanctioning the bushmeat business, adding that the agreements signed leave most of the costs for ameliorating problems with the "feel-good" environmental groups rather than with the highly profitable exploitive industries.

Barring a total moratorium on commercial hunting of bushmeat, extinction within the foreseeable future is a likely prognosis for many species in the Congo basin. With Central African populations doubling in size roughly every 25 years, bushmeat consumption is expected to increase by about 3% a year. With the current annual take already at an unsustainably high level, human demographic trends leave little room for optimism about Africa's large animals. While some might argue that well-fed Westerners have little right to criticize Africans' exploitation of their own natural resources—especially when so many of them are poor and have no other source of affordable protein—the fact remains that once the animals are eaten to extinction they are gone forever. African cooking pots will be empty and all of humankind will be the poorer for the demise of magnificent species, among them several of our closest relatives. How do we explain *that* to future generations?

References

Bushmeat Crisis Task Force (BCTF). 2003. *Bushmeat: A Wildlife Crisis in West and Central Africa and Around the World.* Silver Spring, MD: BCTF (accessed at www.bushmeat.org, Jan. 2004).

Peterson, Dale. 2003. *Eating Apes.* Berkeley: Univ. of California Press.

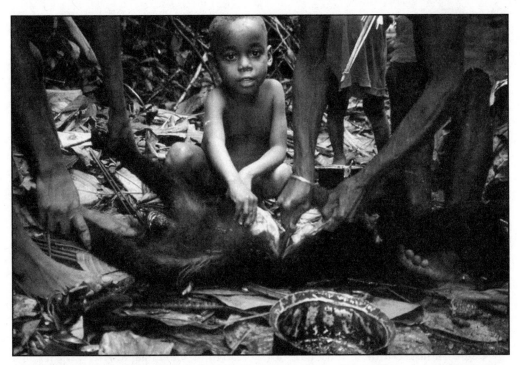

The indiscriminate hunting of "bushmeat" for both local consumption and large commercial markets has become the most immediate threat to the future of wildlife in the Congo Basin. [*Heidi Verhoef, courtesy of the Bushmeat Crisis Task Force*]

Taiwan and China. Since CITES has no enforcement powers of its own against treaty violators, the U.S., citing authority under the Pelly Amendment, in 1994 imposed trade sanctions on Taiwan. This action marked the first time any government had ever employed trade restrictions against another country specifically to protect endangered wildlife. Stung by the ban on export of their fish and wildlife products to the U.S., Taiwanese officials improved enforcement of their country's wildlife conservation laws and launched a public education effort to inform Taiwanese citizens about the endangered status of animals whose products were being used for medicinal purposes. As a result, Taiwanese trade in illegal wildlife parts fell sharply and in 1996 the situation had improved enough for U.S. sanctions to be lifted.

Unfortunately, trade sanctions imposed by individual countries to protect wildlife may conflict with international agreements to promote free trade, since the World Trade Organization (WTO) regards such unilateral actions as illegal. In 1998 the WTO ruled against a controversial U.S. ban on shrimp imports from certain Asian nations whose fishers refused to install turtle-excluder devices on their nets to reduce the accidental by-catch of several species of endangered sea turtles (Tuxill, 1998).

Introduction of Invasive Species

The deliberate or accidental introduction of nonnative plants, animals, or microbes into new environments has, until relatively recently, been the single most important factor accounting for species loss. Though now outranked by habitat destruction as the most critical threat to biodiversity, the growing number of "bioinvasions" has assumed such alarming proportions that in 1997 the United Nations established its Global Invasive Species Programme to focus international attention on the problem. In 1999, President Bill Clinton issued an executive order creating the

National Invasive Species Council which, two years later, released a management plan to enhance the United States' ability to minimize the impact of bioinvasions and to prevent their spread. The concern is economic as well as environmental; Dr. David Pimentel, an ecologist at Cornell University, estimates that in the U.S. alone, damages caused by invasive species and expenditures for their control add up to $137 billion annually. Biologists estimate that more than 6,000 exotic plant and animal species have now become permanent residents of the United States. While not all bioinvaders cause problems, many are now numbered among our most troublesome pests. Proliferating uncontrollably, threatening native ecosystems, or causing economic damage, these unwelcome newcomers are termed **invasive alien species**. Lacking natural enemies to curb their rampant spread, these aggressive invaders have overwhelmed and decimated many indigenous species—eating them, out-competing them for available resources, spreading disease, or in various ways altering ecosystems to the detriment of native flora and fauna.

Examples are legion: European starlings, forty pairs of which were deliberately released by a bird-lover in New York's Central Park in 1890, within 50 years had spread coast-to-coast, driving many less-aggressive songbirds from their original range; Eurasian cheatgrass, introduced when weed-infested seed grain carried by westward-bound immigrants fell alongside late 19th century wagon trails, subsequently spread over millions of acres of rangeland and even today greatly enhances the frequency of wildfires on the western plains; zebra mussels, first observed in Lake St. Clair near Detroit in 1988, have now spread throughout inland waterways in much of the eastern and central U.S., causing billions of dollars in damage to water intake pipes and overwhelming native mussel species. A notorious recent newcomer is the Asian longhorned beetle, native to China, Korea, and Japan. Discovered in 1996 on Long Island, in 1998 in Chicago, in 2002 in northeastern New Jersey, and in 2003 near Toronto, the large, shiny black-and-white beetle poses a serious threat to many species of hardwood trees, especially maples, into which it tunnels and feeds. Aggressive eradication efforts were launched in the localized areas where infestations have been identified and regulations have been imposed requiring that wooden shipping crates from China be heated and chemically treated to kill any beetles they might be harboring. Such precautions, unfortunately, didn't prevent the arrival of yet another uninvited guest from northeast Asia. In the summer of 2002, the emerald ash borer—a small, tree-infesting insect—was discovered in both Michigan and Ontario. Since then it has been identified in several nearby states and entomologists gloomily predict it will eventually spread throughout North America, killing untold millions of ash trees and causing enormous economic losses. In addition to such accidental arrivals, numerous fish-stocking programs since the 1950s have quite intentionally introduced nonnative brown and rainbow trout, as well as other game fish, into waterways where they previously didn't exist, pleasing sports fishermen but decimating populations of indigenous fish and amphibians. It's estimated that half the fish now on the "endangered" list are thus imperiled because of introduced exotics (Baskin, 2002).

The impact of nonnative species can be seen most dramatically in island ecosystems such as Hawaii, site of fully three-fourths of all known bird and plant extinctions in the United States. The goats, pigs, sheep, rats, and mongooses that came ashore with European settlers in the years after Captain Cook's voyage to the islands in 1778 are the most notorious of approximately 3,900 plant and animal species arriving in Hawaii over the past two centuries. Today, of the remaining native Hawaiian plants, one-fifth are endangered; for native bird species, nearly half are at risk, primarily due to the impact of exotic newcomers. On the Pacific island of Guam, the brown tree snake has virtually wiped out native bird populations since it was first introduced in

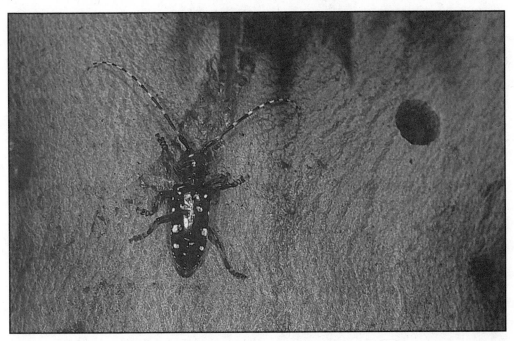

The Asian longhorned beetle threatens many species of hardwood trees, into which they tunnel large holes and then feed. Native to China, Korea, and Japan, the large beetle was discovered in Long Island in 1996, Chicago in 1998, and in northeastern New Jersey in 2002. In the U.S., only New York, New Jersey, and Illinois have seen outbreaks. [*Philip L. Nixon, Illinois Cooperative Extension Service*]

the mid-1940s. Nowhere, however, has the impact of alien species been more devastating than in Africa's Lake Victoria, a waterway once renowned for its amazing diversity of cichlid fishes—more than 300 species found nowhere else in the world. In 1959 Nile perch, a type of carnivorous fish growing up to six feet in length, were introduced into the lake by British settlers who thought they would enhance sports-fishing opportunities. Within 25 years the invaders had gobbled up so many of the native cichlids that several species disappeared completely; it is expected that eventually over half the native species will become extinct. The demise of the plant-eating cichlids has had far-reaching effects on the Lake Victoria ecosystem, leading to algal blooms, oxygen depletion, and the decline of many other lake species. While the decision to introduce the perch had no malicious intent, the catastrophic results of this act led a team of biologists to observe: "Never before has man in a single ill-advised step placed so many vertebrate species simultaneously at risk of extinction and also, in doing so, threatened a food resource and traditional way of life of riparian dwellers" (Wilson, 1992).

Problems due to invasive species are nothing new; for millennia as human populations moved about the globe they carried other species with them into new territories. What's different today is the quantum increase in numbers of species on the move, facilitated by more rapid transportation (permitting stowaways to survive long journeys), globalization of trade, and record numbers of people traveling to distant lands for business or pleasure. While some of the species introductions in recent years have been a deliberate result of commercial transactions, most are accidental consequences of the global distribution networks that facilitate international commerce. Exotic species frequently invade new territory attached to the hulls of ships; as stowaways in wooden crates or packing materials; hidden inside unprocessed logs, fruits, or seeds; as unticketed passengers on aircraft; or, most common of all, swimming in the ballast water discharged by ships entering ports (the zebra mussel's presumed route of entry). The impact of exotics has been particularly severe on coastal ecosystems. In San Francisco Bay alone, according to a spokeswoman at the Center of Marine Conservation, a new species is discovered entering the bay, on average, every 14 days.

At the level of international policymaking, stemming bioinvasions is more difficult and complex than curbing trade in endangered species. With the exception of various protocols that categorically exclude exotic organisms from Antarctica, there are no treaties specifically enacted to prevent bioinvasions. The 1992 Convention of Biological Diversity, which emerged from the UN-sponsored Earth Summit that year, requires signatory nations to prevent the introduction of alien species that pose a threat to ecosystem stability but to do so "as far as possible and appropriate"—a qualifying phrase that makes the treaty little more than a weak statement of noble intentions. For the foreseeable future, efforts at mitigating the impact of exotic species will likely remain a combination of port-of-entry inspections, prohibitions or controls of listed problematic species or items (e.g. potentially insect-infested logs from Siberia, nontreated wooden crates from China), and eradication or control programs targeting already established exotic pests. The task is daunting, but biologists are convinced that over the long term controlling exotic species will be just as important for protecting biodiversity as are efforts to save those that are threatened and endangered; indeed, the two activities may be but opposite sides of the same coin (Bright, 1998).

Pollution of Air and Water with Toxic Chemicals

The death of entire aquatic ecosystems due to acid rainfall is a recent example of the effect toxic pollutants are having on other forms of life. Particularly since the introduction of the synthetic organic pesticides after World War II, numerous wildlife species, especially carnivorous birds, have suffered sharp population declines. Contamination of rivers, lakes, and estuaries with industrial effluents threaten the sustained productivity of those ecosystems. The problem is even more acute in the developing nations, where environmental laws regulating toxic discharges are either weak or nonexistent and where many of the hazardous pesticides now banned in most industrialized countries are still widely and indiscriminately used (Tuxill, 1998).

The impact of pollution on wildlife was a major topic of international discussion in the summer of 1988 when beaches along Europe's North Sea and the U.S. East Coast were littered with the bodies of dead and dying seals and porpoises. Though the cause of the marine mammals' demise was ultimately determined to be a type of pneumonia, it was theorized that swimming in highly polluted coastal waters weakened the animals' resistance to disease and thereby contributed to their death. More recent casualties have been the beluga whales inhabiting the St. Lawrence River. Once numbering in the thousands, the belugas have dwindled to an estimated population of 700 animals, large numbers of which are afflicted with various types of tumors, ulcers, lesions, cysts, pneumonia, and reproductive problems. Scientists attribute the whales' plight to chemical contamination of the river with mercury, lead, PCBs, and various organochlorine pesticides. Analyses of tissue samples from dead belugas show concentrations of all these chemicals at levels far above those in whales from Arctic waters. While marine mammals and fish are particularly hard hit because of the toxic soup that constantly surrounds them in many waterways, polluted air also is taking its toll on sensitive species. In western Europe fungi appear to be dying off *en masse,* with a 40–50% loss of species in certain areas of Germany, Austria, and the Netherlands. Among those adversely affected are the mycorrhizal fungi that live in symbiotic association with plant roots, promoting the uptake of dissolved nutrients. The fact that these inconspicuous organisms play an important role in the normal functioning of many plant species gives their demise far-reaching significance (Wilson, 1992). Efforts to safeguard human health by curbing pollutant emissions will have a beneficial impact on the health of ecosystems as well.

Habitat Destruction

By far the greatest threat to biodiversity today—and the most difficult to control—is the destruction of those natural areas that wildlife require for breeding, feeding, or migrating. As the pressures of expanding populations and economies increase, forests are chopped down, swamps are drained, prairies are put to the plow, rivers are dammed. Some wildlife species can thrive in close proximity to humans; most cannot and perish when their natural habitat is destroyed or reduced in size below a critical minimum.

While there is little disagreement that preservation of biodiversity is a lost cause without a significantly greater commitment to conserving natural habitats, the question of how to maintain the integrity of dwindling expanses of forest, savannah, and grasslands at a time of exponentially increasing human needs is a vexing one for policymakers everywhere. Since 1872 when Yellowstone was established as the world's first national park, the conventional approach to preserving wild areas of great beauty or biological richness has been to set aside **protected areas** as wildlife refuges, national parks, or wilderness areas. Extending this concept to the ocean environment, some fisheries experts are now advocating marine reserves as the only effective way to save endangered fish stocks. Currently a few small, widely scattered "no-take zones" exist and have been very effective in boosting catches in nearby waters, but these collectively encompass only 0.01% of the ocean surface. Some biologists are calling for 20% of the oceans to be set aside as protected zones, though many concede that it would be virtually impossible to police such vast areas (Pauly and Watson, 2003). Today 4% of the earth's total land surface has been set aside in approximately 8,000 protected areas worldwide, their natural wealth safeguarded by limiting human access to such areas. A modification of this approach is now being proposed by a number of prominent biologists who fear the number of endangered species far outstrips current resources to protect them. They advocate a scheme to prioritize preservation efforts by identifying **biodiversity "hotspots"**—areas characterized by exceptionally high numbers of native species facing likely extinction due to extensive loss of habitat. By focusing available financial resources on these critical areas, society could reap the most benefit in terms of protecting species. These scientists have identified 25 such "hotspots" they deem worthy of special conservation efforts and are trying to attract funding to implement their proposals (Myers et al., 2000).

While the protected areas approach has been relatively successful, particularly in regions such as North America where population pressures are modest, trends suggest that in the years ahead preservation of critical habitat through reliance on government-established exclusion zones cannot adequately protect biodiversity and is ultimately doomed to failure. This is true for a number of reasons: (1) in most cases, the protected areas are too scattered, small, and fragmented to sustain the long-term stability of their biotic communities; ecologists have amply documented the adverse impact of crowding species into isolated "islands" of woodland or tropical forest, surrounded by a "sea" of farmlands or urban development. The "edge effect" experienced around the periphery of these fragmented habitats (i.e., increased exposure to wind, sunlight, decreased humidity, vulnerability to new predators) may result in the loss of many species highly adapted to life within a narrow range of environmental conditions; (2) many so-called protected areas, particularly those in developing countries, are protected in name only, since governments frequently lack the financial resources, the technical expertise, or the will to enforce their borders. The wide-scale poaching of endangered rhinos in East Africa or of tigers in India—both legally protected animals—is indicative of the difficulty many poor countries face in trying to safeguard their natural heritage; (3) finally, and perhaps most importantly, the protected area strategy doesn't take into account the fact that humans are an integral part of ecosystems also. Most of the areas set aside for wildlife once sustained the needs of local people who are now forbidden to hunt, fish, or grow crops on lands they once considered theirs to use. As growing human populations press against park boundaries, it will be impossible and, indeed, unjust, to forbid them the use of their own surroundings without providing viable alternatives for survival.

Accordingly, within the past two decades a radically different approach to conservation of habitat has slowly gained adherents, an approach that attempts to make local communities both the *beneficiaries* and the *custodians* of efforts to safeguard biodiversity. Referred to as **community-based conservation,** this new concept recognizes that the exclusionary policies of the past, as embodied in the wildlife reserves, cannot be sustained in the face of mounting human poverty and hostility to programs that seem to place greater value on elephants or pandas than on people. Community-based conservation relies on positive grassroots participation, relinquishing the traditional top-down planning by central government officials in favor of involving local people in the planning, design, and implementation of conservation efforts which will benefit them directly and give them a personal stake in the successful outcome of such ventures. Community-based conservation efforts are quietly underway in a number of areas around the world and involve situations as diverse as the "extractive reserves" in Brazilian Amazonia, subsistence farming combined with ecotourism in Papua New Guinea, forest management by community councils in India, or incentive payments to private landowners for fostering biodiversity in England (Wright, 1993).

Another interesting approach to involve local people in wildlife conservation efforts is that of **biodiversity prospecting**—enlisting residents of species-rich tropical countries to assist in the search for plants or animals of potential medicinal, pesticidal, or agricultural value. Several bioprospecting agreements have been signed since the early 1990s between drug companies and national governments or institutes in the developing world (the U.S. National Parks Service has also indicated an interest in similar arrangements involving bioprospecting in such unique ecosystems as the hot springs at Yellowstone National Park). Merck & Co., Inc., the world's largest pharmaceutical corporation, now pays a private nonprofit organization in Costa Rica to send the company a steady supply of plant, animal, and microbial specimens to be analyzed for possible medicinal properties. Merck has agreed to pay royalties to its Costa Rican partner, the Instituto Nacional de Biodiversidad (INBIO), for any commercial products developed from Costa Rican specimens. It is assumed that once the biochemically active ingredient of a newly discovered species is identified, it will be possible to mass-produce an identical synthetic compound, thereby avoiding further exploitation of the species in its native habitat. By intimately involving local people in cataloging their country's biodiversity, INBIO gives Costa Ricans an in-depth understanding of their natural heritage and a personal stake in protecting it. Similar arrangements involving other pharmaceutical firms are now in effect in Ghana, Nigeria, and Surinam (Tuxill, 1998).

The shift in focus from preserving wildlife to acknowledging the need to factor human needs into the equation may be the only practical approach to saving as much biodiversity as possible, particularly at a time when human-modified landscapes are relentlessly expanding. Convincing local people that their own well-being can best be ensured by conserving and sustainably using the biological wealth of their surroundings may ultimately be the key to species preservation.

Climate Change

Is the Costa Rican golden toad the world's first species doomed to extinction by global warming? Some researchers working in the Monte Verde Cloud Forest think this may be the case (Pounds, Fogden, and Campbell, 1999). Although habitat loss is currently the greatest threat to biodiversity, climate change may become an equally important cause of species loss in future decades. An international group of researchers based in the United Kingdom warns that anticipated increases in average global temperatures caused by human-generated greenhouse gas emissions may become a significant cause of species extinctions by the mid-21st century. As temperatures rise, provoking habitat change, many species living in those areas will either die out or move elsewhere. However, fragmentation of habitat could make such migration impossible and even if species succeed in reaching a new area of suitable climate, inappropriate soils or lack of food resources may prevent establishment of a viable population. For those species remaining in the original climate-altered habitat, the encroachment of invasive species moving in from disturbed ecosystems elsewhere may be the "straw that breaks the camel's back," precipitating their descent to oblivion. Estimates of the number of species "committed to extinction" vary in direct proportion to the amount of warming realized, with higher temperatures producing the greatest impact on species loss. Accordingly, concerned scientists are urging governments to implement policies for reducing greenhouse gas emissions as rapidly as possible in order to minimize the ultimate extent of climate change and thereby save a substantial percentage of species from extinction (Thomas et al., 2004).

Protecting Biodiversity: The Endangered Species Act

Since its enactment in 1973, the **Endangered Species Act (ESA)** has constituted the nation's most effective weapon for ensuring the survival of native plants and animals. Probably the toughest wildlife protection law anywhere in the world, the ESA prohibits the killing, collecting, harassment, or capture of any species listed by the U.S. Fish and Wildlife Service (FWS) as "endangered" or "threatened." It also provides strict protection for the critical habitat of endangered species and requires FWS to develop recovery programs for each species listed. By 2004, FWS had officially designated 1,260 species as endangered or threatened (516 animals and 744 plants), up from just 78 in 1967 when the original endangered species list was compiled. Thirty-one additional species (27 animals and 4 plants) were proposed for listing in the near future.

While environmentalists hail the ESA for noticeably slowing the pace of wildlife extinction in the United States, citing as evidence the fact that 60 endangered species have increased their numbers or expanded their range over the past quarter-century, opponents are working hard to weaken the law when it comes up for reauthorization. Charging that the Act has excessive power to supersede individual property rights, hinder economic progress, and threaten jobs, such disparate constituencies as land developers, Gulf Coast shrimpers, and loggers in the Pacific Northwest would like to see the Act significantly weakened. These groups raise the question of how much biological diversity can or should be preserved, especially when the species in question isn't particularly cute or fuzzy. Some people find it hard to get emotional about the Colorado squawfish or the scrub plum!

ESA defenders point out that, for the vast majority of protected species, recovery plans seldom provoke conflict. Perhaps one explanation for increasing antagonism toward ESA is the fact that in recent years the Act has begun to affect entire regions rather than just isolated projects, as was generally the case in the past. For example, in the early 1990s attempts to save the northern spotted owl by declaring large areas of the Northwest's old-growth forest off-limits for timber harvesting prompted vociferous complaints that the ESA favors wildlife over people.

In fact, contrary to detractors' claims, the Act *does* make an effort to accommodate societal concerns. Economic considerations are taken into account to some degree when designations of critical habitat are made; in situations where proposed projects threaten endangered species, the Act requires that an effort be made to find alternative means of carrying out the activity without endangering survival of the species in question. In those rare cases where the conflict is irreconcilable, an official panel (the "God Squad") can give the green light to projects deemed of sufficient importance, even if this action constitutes a death sentence for an endangered species.

Even supporters admit, however, that implementation of ESA is in need of improvement. To some extent, problems center around insufficient money and personnel to carry out the intent of the Act. Even more problematic is the cumbersome process of officially listing rare species as threatened or endangered. Frequently the official designation comes so late that populations of the species in question may already be too low to halt the slide into oblivion. In other cases, only costly rescue missions such as captive breeding programs can guarantee long-term survival, when earlier action could have achieved success through less extreme measures. Although studies suggest that a minimum population in the low thousands is a prerequisite for viable vertebrate populations, the average number of individuals remaining in vertebrate groups listed as endangered was just 1,075; for invertebrates it was even lower— 999. For plants, the average number of remaining specimens in at-risk populations at the time of official listing is a mere 120, making recovery of such species extremely difficult. Biologists suggest that the minuscule number of species that have rebounded and been removed from the endangered list can be explained by the fact that official designation often comes too late to implement effective recovery plans.

In spite of its limitations, the Endangered Species Act can claim its share of notable success stories. Although over the past 25 years only 15 species have been reclassified as "recovered," a number of others have made a remarkable comeback from near-extinction. These include the bald eagle, the American alligator, the whooping crane, peregrine falcon, California sea otter, grizzly bear, black-footed ferret, and the red wolf. All now have a new lease on life, thanks to the Endangered Species Act.

While ESA historically has focused on protecting individual species on a case-by-case basis, a 1982 amendment to the Act established an alternative approach to preserving biodiversity in the form of **habitat conservation planning (HCP).** Devised as a way of striking a balance between pressures for economic growth and habitat preservation, HCP allows landowners to develop property occupied by endangered species if they agree to minimize the loss of critical habitat or offset that loss by providing additional land nearby. While this approach implicitly permits the loss of some members of the endangered species in question, it guarantees that enough critical habitat will be preserved to sustain the remainder of that population indefinitely. Drawing up an acceptable plan may involve years of negotiations among developers, environmentalists, local governments, and Fish and Wildlife Service personnel who supervise the process and must ultimately approve the plan. Nevertheless, both environmentalists and property rights advocates are supportive of the HCP concept, the former seeing it as a way of winning concessions from landowners who might otherwise ignore the law, the latter preferring negotiated plans rather than blanket restrictions on land use.

By 2004, 437 habitat conservation plans had been approved, protecting more than 526 species. The HCP process has been particularly important in southern California, where intense development pressures on biologically rich natural areas have pitted preservationists against developers for years. In 1993 Interior Secretary Bruce Babbitt worked out an agreement between environmentalists and developers who had been at loggerheads for years over the fate of a diminutive songbird, the California gnat-catcher. Since fewer than 3,000 nesting pairs remained in the 250,000 acres of sage scrub stretching along the Pacific Coast from Los Angeles to San Diego, environmentalists had been demanding the Fish and Wildlife Service list the gnatcatcher as endangered; developers were adamant that such action, automatically triggering prohibitions on the use of valuable real estate, would impose serious economic hardships. Under the HCP brokered by Babbitt, the gnatcatcher was listed as merely "threatened" rather than "endangered," thus permitting a more flexible recovery plan; in return, development interests agreed to protect critical habitat by setting aside up to 12 reserves, an act that benefited not only the gnatcatcher, but as many as 40 other species as well. Habitat conservation planning has continued to win proponents throughout southern California, particularly in the San Diego area where what has been billed as a model HCP was approved by the city council in 1997. Under the agreed-upon arrangement, specified natural areas adjacent to the city will be acquired and permanently set aside for habitat preservation while other still-open lands will be available for unrestricted development.

While experience with habitat conservation planning is not yet extensive enough to render a verdict on its ability to save species, hopes are high that it provides a means for avoiding bitter confrontations and halting the decline of species long before their situation deteriorates beyond redemption.

References

Abramovitz, Janet N. 1998. "Taking a Stand: Cultivating a New Relationship with the World's Forests." *Worldwatch Paper* 140 (April).

Ayres, Ed. 2004. "The Hidden Shame of the Global Industrial Economy." *World•Watch* 17, no. 1 (Jan/Feb).

Baskin, Yvonne. 2002. *A Plague of Rats and Rubbervines: The Growing Threat of Species Invasions.* Washington, DC: Island Press/Shearwater Books.

Bonner, Raymond. 2002. "Indonesia's Forests Go Under the Ax for Flooring." *New York Times,* Sept 13.

Bright, Chris. 1998. *Life Out of Bounds: Bioinvasion in a Borderless World.* New York: W.W. Norton.

Brown, Lester. 2003. *Plan B: Rescuing a Planet under Stress and a Civilization in Trouble.* Earth Policy Institute. New York: W.W. Norton.

———. 1988. "The Changing World Food Prospect: The Nineties and Beyond." *Worldwatch Paper* 85 (Oct).

Coffin, Tristam, ed. 1993. "The Damage Done by Cattle-Raising." *The Washington Spectator* 19, no. 2 (Jan. 15).

Colchester, Marcus. 1994. "The New Sultans." *The Ecologist* 24, no. 2 (March/April).

Environmental Protection Agency (EPA). 1988. *America's Wetlands: Our Vital Link Between Land and Water.* OPA-87–016 (Feb).

Faeth, Paul. 1994. "Building the Case for Sustainable Agriculture: Policy Lessons from India, Chile, and the Philippines." *Environment* 36, no. 1 (Jan/Feb).

Food and Agriculture Organization of the United Nations (FAO). 2001. *State of the World's Forests 2001,* pp. 58–59.

Hamilton, John Maxwell. 1989. "Rescuing the Bounty of Rain Forests." *The Christian Science Monitor,* Jan. 26.

Heywood, V. H., and R. T. Watson, eds. 1995. *Global Biodiversity Assessment.* New York: Cambridge Univ. Press.

Hinrichsen, Don. 2003. "A Human Thirst." *World Watch* 16, no. 1 (Jan/Feb).

Hulme, Mike, and Mick Kelly. 1993. "Exploring the Links Between Desertification and Climate Change." *Environment* 35, no. 6 (July/Aug).

Myers, Norman, Russell A. Mittermeier, Cristina G. Mittermeier, Gustavo A. B. daFonseca, and Jennifer Kent. 2000. "Biodiversity Hotspots for Conservation Priorities." *Nature* 403 (Feb. 24):853–858.

Pauly, Daniel, and Reg Watson. 2003. "Counting the Last Fish." *Scientific American* 289, no. 1 (July).

Pounds, J. Alan, Michael P. L. Fogden, and John H. Campbell. 1999. "Biological Response to Climate Change." *Nature* 398 (April 15):611–615.

Rohter, Larry. 2003. "Relentless Foe of the Amazon Jungle: Soybeans." *New York Times*, Sept. 17.

Smil, V. 1991. "Population Growth and Nitrogen: An Exploration of a Critical Existential Link." *Population and Development Review* 17, no. 4.

Stutz, Bruce. 1993. "The Landscape of Hunger." *Audubon* 95, no. 2 (March/April).

Thomas, Chris D., et al. 2004. "Extinction Risk from Climate Change." *Nature* 427 (Jan. 8):145–148.

Tobias, Michael. 1998. *World War III: Population and the Biosphere at the End of the Millennium.* New York: Continuum Press.

Tuxill, John. 1998. "Losing Strands in the Web of Life: Vertebrate Declines and the Conservation of Biological Diversity." *Worldwatch Paper* 141 (May).

U.S. Department of Agriculture (USDA). 1997. *The Conservation Reserve Program.* Farm Services Agency, PA-1603 (May).

Whittaker, Robert H. 1975. *Communities and Ecosystems.* New York: Macmillan.

Wilcove, David S., Margaret McMillan, and Keith C. Winston. 1993. "What Exactly Is an Endangered Species? An Analysis of the U. S. Endangered Species List, 1985–91." *Conservation Biology* 7, no. 1.

Wilson, Edward O. 1992. *The Diversity of Life.* Cambridge, MA: Harvard Univ. Press.

World Resources Institute (WRI). 2000. *World Resources 2000–2001: People and Ecosystems: The Fraying Web of Life.* World Resources Institute.

———. 1996. *World Resources 1996–97: The Urban Environment.* New York: Oxford Univ. Press.

———. 1992. *World Resources 1992–1993.* New York: Oxford Univ. Press.

Wright, Michal, ed. 1993. *The View from Airlie: Community-Based Conservation in Perspective.* Liz Claiborne and Art Ortenberg Foundation, narrative sampling of discussions during workshop held at Airlie, Virginia, week of Oct. 17.

PART 2

OUR TOXIC ENVIRONMENT
DOES EVERYTHING CAUSE CANCER?

Unsanitary conditions prevailing in 19th-century urban areas.

We have met the enemy, and it is us.

—Walt Kelly, POGO (1972)

Newspaper headlines screaming "Ozone Alert!"; a $1 million damage settlement to an asbestos worker's widow; public protests over a leaking hazardous waste dump; migrant workers hospitalized for pesticide poisoning; accidental sewage discharge forcing closure of public beaches—such situations represent but a handful of the issues daily facing modern society in which some aspect of environmental quality has a direct impact on human health.

From primitive times up until the mid-19th century the idea that health and disease were determined, at least in part, by environmental factors was widely accepted (witness the belief that night air precipitated fever and chills). The middle 1800s, however, marked a period of rapid progress in research relating to disease causation. The discovery of the anthrax bacterium by the German microbiologist Robert Koch and his demonstration in 1877 that this organism was responsible for an important human disease revolutionized society's view of health. For the next 70 years virtually all human ailments were blamed on pathogenic organisms such as bacteria, viruses, and protozoans. It was widely assumed that the development of preventative vaccines or curative antibiotics should be our main focus in protecting public health.

More recently, however, recognition of the role that deprivation or stress can play in initiating serious health problems and the sharp increase, particularly in more affluent societies, of the so-called "degenerative diseases" (cardiovascular disease, cancer, hypertension) have led to the realization that good health depends on more than just the absence of disease-causing microorganisms. Some of today's most prevalent ills are increasingly blamed on toxic environmental contaminants—synthetic chemical wastes carelessly dumped in waterways or landfills, products of combustion spewed into the air, pesticide residues in the food we eat. Other illnesses are associated with personal habits that in the broad sense can be considered aspects of environmental quality—smoking, drinking, high-fat diets, lack of regular exercise. Perception of the threat that such factors pose to human well-being provided the main thrust behind the modern environmental movement. Preservation—or restoration—of environmental quality means far more than protecting bald eagles or ensuring that the last coastal redwood isn't converted into a picnic table; the prime emphasis among environmental advocates has always been the protection of human health, with the implicit recognition that human well-being is inextricably intertwined with the health and stability of the natural ecosystems of which we form an integral part.

While not a perfect standard, the health status of societies is often measured in terms of life expectancy—the number of years an average individual in that society can expect to live. In terms of longevity, health conditions in the Western world have improved markedly in recent centuries. Whereas in the days of Roman emperors the average life expectancy at birth was about 30 years, today in most industrialized countries it has reached 75 years, up from 50 years at the turn of the century (Japanese are currently the world's longest-lived people, with an average life expectancy of 82, compared to 77 in the United States and 79 in Canada). Among the developing nations average longevity is more variable, ranging from a low of 35 in Zambia (due largely to the AIDS epidemic) to the mid-40s in Afghanistan and some African countries to the mid-70s in parts of Latin America and the Caribbean. Many people, looking at such statistics, assume that the major factor accounting for increased longevity worldwide was the introduction of modern medicines and pesticides that provided the first really effective weapons against many of the infectious epidemic diseases. While medical science undoubtedly played a part in reducing mortality rates, many observers feel that a more fundamental factor was a general improvement in living conditions: better nutritional levels made possible by increased agricultural productivity; improved sanitary conditions as a result of sewer system construction; the provision of safe drinking water supplies; refuse collection; sewage treatment; the enforcement of housing codes, and so forth. Rising incomes, increasing levels of education, mass communications, and improved standards of personal hygiene also have been extremely important determinants in furthering the health advances observed in most parts of the world.

However, we seem to have now reached a longevity plateau and are no longer observing a continued rapid drop in death rates such as characterized the years between 1950–1960. Indeed, longevity is actually declining in Russia, where high levels of pollution, added to the ravages of alcoholism and substandard health care, have caused male life expectancy to fall to 58 years, the lowest for any industrialized country (female life expectancy has remained stable at 72 years). There appears to be general agreement that future gains will come, not so much through new medical discoveries, but when—and only when—essential preconditions of better health are everywhere available. These essential preconditions relate largely to environmental considerations: sufficient quantities of uncontaminated water, elimination of malnutrition, proper handling and disposal of human wastes, control of toxic pollutants, adoption of healthier personal lifestyles. The environmentally induced diseases currently plaguing much of humanity can best be controlled through a strategy of prevention, rather than cure, requiring not only application of technology but also social, political, and behavioral changes. Adopting such a strategy and enlisting the public support necessary to attain the goal of a healthful society require a thorough understanding of the issues and dilemmas involved. The following chapters will delineate the major concerns regarding our increasingly toxic environment and the health implications inherent in our present lifestyle; they also attempt to show that improving human health and enhancing environmental quality are but two sides of the same coin.

ENVIRONMENTAL DISEASE

Environmental illness is simply an incurable disease. There is no cure. It can only
be prevented.

—Barry Commoner, 1990

Polluted air and water, excessive levels of noise, sunshine, nuclear weapons fallout, overcrowded slums, toxic waste dumps, inadequate or overly adequate diet,
stress, food contaminants, medical X-rays, drugs, cigarettes, unsafe working conditions—these comprise but a partial listing of the many environmental factors which,
through their adverse impact on human health, can be regarded as causative agents of
environmental disease. In recent decades public concern about rising levels of pollution and environmental degradation has increasingly focused on the question of
whether such trends may be influencing disease rates, particularly ailments such as
heart disease, cancer, and stroke. If such a connection exists, as virtually all authorities
agree it does, then society's response should be clear: most environmentally induced
diseases, unlike those caused by bacteria or other pathogens, are difficult to cure but
theoretically simple to prevent; remove the adverse environmental influence and the
ailment will disappear. In other words, by preventing the discharge of poisons into our
air, water, and food, by avoiding exposure to radiation, by refusing to fill our lungs
with cigarette smoke or our stomachs with saturated fats, we can protect our health
far more effectively and cheaply than we can by desperately searching for a cure after
our bodies succumb to a malignancy or degeneration of vital organs or when our children are born deformed. The old adage, "Prevention is the best cure," has never been
more true than when applied to environmentally induced disease.

In spite of the fact that environmental factors can affect human health in many
ways, the focus of most environmental health concern today in this age of toxic pollutants is on those substances that, in ways not yet completely understood, act at the cellular level to initiate often irreversible changes that can kill or damage the cell in
question. Although health damage due to environmental pollutants may be manifested by outward symptoms, research has shown that the action of such contaminants in fact occurs at the level of an individual cell or cells. In spite of its small size,
the cell is an exceptionally complex structure—the end product of billions of years of
evolution and natural selection in response to existing environmental conditions.
Thus it should not be surprising to find that a sudden change in the environment (e.g.,
exposure to X-rays, synthetic organic chemicals, heavy metals, etc.) to which a cell
has become so finely adapted can kill or injure the cell. Cell death, in many respects, is
a lesser concern than cell injury because it has no further implications. Cell damage,

Box 6-1   Microbial Killers

Toxic chemical pollutants may be the current "hot button" issue among many environmentalists today, but historically the primary focus of environmental health practitioners has been reducing the incidence of infectious epidemic disease. Fostered by poor living conditions and spread through contaminated food and water, bacterial, viral, and parasitic pathogens have been responsible for the vast majority of human deaths from time immemorial until the early 20th century. Even today, throughout much of the developing world infectious killers such as tuberculosis, malaria, and diarrheal diseases remain leading causes of mortality.

In North America and Europe, however, deaths caused by infectious microbes began to decline noticeably about 100 years ago, thanks in large part to drinking water purification, sewage treatment, and vector control. In the United States, infectious disease mortality rates dropped by approximately 2.8% annually between 1900 and 1937 (with the exception of 1918 when a worldwide outbreak of "Spanish flu" sent death rates soaring everywhere). From 1937 until 1952, mortality rates due to infectious diseases dropped even more precipitously— 8.2% per year—as cases of pneumonia, influenza, and tuberculosis plummeted. These years witnessed the introduction of powerful new antibacterial drugs—sulfonamides, penicillin, streptomycin, isoniazid— but it's likely that a number of factors in addition to improved medications account for mortality declines. From the mid-1950s until 1980 infectious disease death rates continued to drop, albeit more slowly than during the preceding 15 years. By this time it had become an article of faith that humankind (or at least those fortunate enough to live in affluent, sanitized, well-fed nations) had forever left behind the "age of pestilence and famine"—characterized by high rates of infectious disease mortality, especially among children and young adults. We had transitioned, so it was believed, into the modern age of degenerative diseases where most deaths occur among the elderly and are due to chronic ills such as cardiovascular disease or cancer.

Dismissal of microbial threats as a thing of the past has proven premature, however.

In 1981 medical recognition of Acquired Immune Deficiency Syndrome (AIDS) reminded the world that pathogens still lurk among human populations. From 1981–1996 the U.S. witnessed a steady rise in mortality rates due to infectious diseases, primarily AIDS and tuberculosis. Unfortunately, AIDS was only the first of several frightening diseases to make headlines over the past several decades. Medical researchers now speak of "newly emerging pathogens" to describe outbreaks of previously unknown ailments such as Lassa fever, Legionnaires' Disease, toxic shock syndrome, Ebola virus, hantavirus, and E. coli 0157:H7 food poisoning. In addition, old microbial diseases are now showing up in new places, South America's cholera epidemic of the mid-1990s being a case in point.

Other killers of yesteryear are surfacing in new forms; in late 1997, "bird flu"—a strain of influenza previously documented only among avian species—broke out in Hong Kong, killing four of the 16 people infected. A new and even more ominous strain of avian influenza, H5N1, has recently surfaced in several southeast Asian countries. The causative virus, continually mutating to more dangerous forms, has already jumped from birds to people. Global health experts are extremely worried that if this highly lethal pathogen develops the ability to spread person-to-person, a global pandemic will result, ravaging populations worldwide, since no baseline immunity currently exists against this new disease.

AIDS may be the first large-scale modern epidemic of infectious disease, but almost certainly it won't be the last. The world today is more vulnerable than ever before to the global spread of infections. As evermore crowded human populations invade previously undisturbed ecosystems, especially in the tropics, opportunities for contact with animal pathogens proliferate. The rapid expansion of global commerce and tourism provide easy access for microbes on one continent to travel quickly to distant locations, either riding along with cargo, harbored by stowaway insects, or incubating in the bodies of travelers. Unfortunately, the Western world's single-minded preoccupation with finding a cure for cancer and other degenerative diseases has caused us largely to ignore the microbial pathogens that remain an ever-present threat. The nations of the world still lack an "early warning system" to ensure the quick detection of new diseases when they first appear or to identify old diseases when they show up in unexpected places or in clever disguises. Continued delay in confronting this challenge due to a misplaced faith in humanity's supposed conquest of infectious disease is a risky tactic. As Dr. Richard Krause of the U.S. National Institutes of Health commented more than 20 years ago, "Plagues are as certain as death and taxes."

References

Armstrong, G. L., et al. 1999. "Trends in Infectious Disease Mortality in the United States During the 20th Century." *Journal of the American Medical Association* 281, no. 1 (Jan. 6):61–66.

Garrett, Laurie. 1994. *The Coming Plague.* New York: Farrar, Straus, and Giroux.

on the other hand, has more ominous implications. The subject of extensive scientific and medical research for the past half century, cell damage can be manifested as mutations, birth defects, or cancer.

Mutation

Mutation, defined as any change in the genetic material, is perhaps the most worrisome type of cell damage because of its potential for harming not only the person or organism harboring the mutant cell but, if the mutation occurs in an egg or sperm, unborn generations as well. To understand the significance of mutation, it is necessary to examine the nature of the hereditary material itself.

The most conspicuous organelle in most cells is the nucleus, readily visible under an ordinary light microscope. The nucleus contains threadlike structures called **chromosomes;** each species of plant or animal has its own characteristic number of chromosomes per cell. In humans the normal chromosome number is 46. When cells undergo **mitosis** (cell division), each chromosome splits longitudinally into two daughter **chromatids,** one of which goes into each of the two newly forming cells. Thus the number of chromosomes per nucleus remains constant and the hereditary material contained within the chromosomes is equally shared.

Chemically, each chromosome consists of a single giant molecule of DNA (deoxyribonucleic acid) and associated histone and nonhistone proteins. The DNA molecule itself is composed of two antiparallel strands of alternating units of a five-carbon sugar and phosphate molecules, cross-linked by one of four different nitrogenous bases (adenine, guanine, thymine, and cytosine), and twisted into a helical configuration (see figure 6-1). The pairing of the nitrogenous bases is quite specific: adenine can pair only with thymine and guanine with cytosine. Along any one strand bases can occur in any sequence, but once the order on one strand is given, the sequence on the antiparallel strand is automatically determined. The adenine-thymine (A-T) or guanine-cytosine (G-C) combination making up each cross-connection is referred to as a **base pair.**

DNA is vitally important to cellular function and is often referred to as the "Master Molecule" because (1) it passes genetic information from one generation to the next and (2) it controls cellular metabolism by giving the instructions for protein synthesis. The hereditary characteristics are controlled by **genes** along the length of the chromosome. In essence, a gene is a section of chromosome consisting of thousands of base pairs. Genes are responsible for the production of proteins necessary for proper cell function. It is absolutely essential that the integrity of the DNA molecule

The complexity of cell structure can be seen in this electron micrograph of a plant cell showing such organelles as nucleus, chloroplasts, ribosomes, endoplasmic reticulum, mitochondria, and vacuoles. Environmental toxins act here at the cellular level within organisms.
[*Mathew Nadakavukaren*]

be maintained if the correct information for protein synthesis is to be passed from one generation to the next. Any change within the gene constitutes a mutation.

Types of Mutations

There are two basic types of mutations recognized.

"Point" mutation (single gene mutation). By far the most common type of mutation, point mutations involve a change at the molecular level within a gene. Such a change could consist of the deletion, addition, or substitution of a single base pair or could involve a small portion of a single gene (e.g., a so-called "jumping gene," more properly referred to as a **transposable element**). Any of these changes would result in the "misreading" of the genetic code (the sequence of bases along a DNA strand is all-important; any change can result in the wrong protein being formed). The severity of a point mutation depends on precisely where within a gene the change occurs; it can range from being lethal to causing an almost imperceptible loss of vigor. Point mutations are now known to be responsible for several serious human ailments, including sickle-cell anemia, hemophilia, diabetes, and achondroplastic dwarfism. Though such ailments are tragic for the victim (prior to modern forms of treatment, which are only partially effective, these diseases invariably resulted in death at a fairly early age), many geneticists are more concerned about the accumulation of sub-lethal mutations in populations. Such sub-lethal mutations don't kill their victims outright, but render them

Figure 6-1   DNA Double Helix

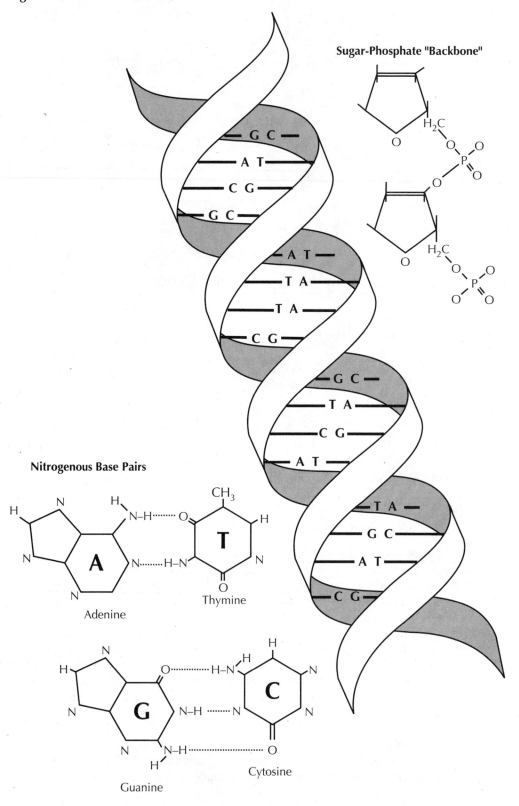

Sugar-Phosphate "Backbone"

Nitrogenous Base Pairs

Adenine

Thymine

Guanine

Cytosine

less fit than they would otherwise be. Examples of the types of impairment that could result from a sub-lethal mutation include reduced physical or mental vigor, shortened life span, increased susceptibility to disease, or varying degrees of malformation of some organ. Such changes, though possibly debilitating, nevertheless permit afflicted individuals to survive, reproduce, and pass altered genes on to succeeding generations.

Chromosome abnormalities. Chromosome abnormalities are thought to be the leading cause of fetal loss, responsible for half of all first trimester miscarriages and 20% of spontaneous abortions during the second trimester. They also are regarded as the primary cause of mental retardation. Chromosome abnormalities can include the loss or addition of sizeable pieces of a chromosome or the reversal of parts of the same chromosome—events that most commonly occur during a stage of meiosis (reduction division) when the homologous chromosomes are in synapsis and crossing-over takes place. Although some of these rearrangements seem to have little outward effect, others can have serious consequences. In humans, the reciprocal translocation of sections of chromosomes 9 and 22 represents a specific chromosomal abnormality (the "Philadelphia chromosome") that results in the development of chronic myelogenous leukemia, a form of cancer. Rearrangements of chromosomal material have now been observed in more than 40 different kinds of cancer (Jorde et al., 1999).

A second type of chromosome abnormality involves a change in the number of chromosomes within the nucleus of a cell. This situation occurs when paired homologous chromosomes fail to separate (nondisjunction) during meiosis, resulting in some cells with more than the normal chromosome number, others with less. In some cases, a change in chromosome number can be lethal. Having three copies (**trisomy**) of chromosome 16 is relatively common in the very early stages of human development; however, none of the fetuses characterized by this condition ever survives to birth. Trisomy of chromosomes 13 and 18 also is seen relatively often in fetuses miscarried during the first few months of pregnancy, but the condition is extremely rare among liveborn infants and almost all of them die soon after birth (Sack, 1999). The best known human ailment resulting from a change in chromosome number is Down syndrome. Afflicting about one baby out of every 800 live births, Down syndrome, in most cases, results in mental retardation (IQ seldom exceeds 70) as well as below-average physical and psychomotor skills. Victims often exhibit heart malformations and respiratory problems; few live beyond the age of 50. Down syndrome occurs due to the presence in the victim's cells of 47 chromosomes instead of the normal 46 (to be more precise, three copies of chromosome 21 rather than two). Interestingly, the likelihood of a woman's giving birth to a Down syndrome child increases as the mother gets older. While the likelihood of a 30-year-old woman giving birth to a Down syndrome child is one in 1,000, the risk at age 35 rises to one in 400; at age 40 it increases tenfold, to one in 100; at 45, it is still higher—one out of every 50 infants is likely to be a Down syndrome baby. Although the reason for the increased frequency of this birth defect among older mothers is not known with certainty, the prevailing theory is that the rate of nondisjunction is considerably higher among older women, possibly due to impairment of aging egg cells (since each female child is born with all the egg cells she will ever have, by the time the mother is 45 years old, her eggs are 45 years old also). Given the enhanced risk, it is now common practice for pregnant women 35 or older to undergo a prenatal diagnostic procedure such as **amniocentesis** or **chorionic villus sampling**. By removing and culturing fetal cells, medical personnel can determine whether the developing child has Down Syndrome or any of approximately 100 other genetic diseases. If test results are positive, the parents then have the option of terminating the pregnancy.

It is widely recognized that congenital abnormalities occur with greater frequency among babies of older mothers, but less commonly known that older fathers also have a greater chance of passing on defective genes to their offspring. Approximately 20 different genetic disorders have been correlated with increasing paternal age, including achondroplastic dwarfism, Apert syndrome (characterized by head, facial, and limb abnormalities) and schizophrenia. Since the number of mutations present in sperm cells increases as men grow older, some European countries now prohibit men from becoming sperm donors once they pass a certain age (Thacker, 2004).

Two other human abnormalities resulting from a change in chromosome number are Klinefelter's syndrome, found only in males, and Turner's syndrome, restricted to females. Whereas a normal man has an X and a Y sex chromosome, victims of Klinefelter's syndrome have an extra X, or 47 chromosomes altogether. This condition, one of the most common of all genetic abnormalities, can cause a variety of problems, ranging from learning disabilities, language difficulties, behavioral problems, infertility, and, in about one-third of cases, enlargement of the breasts following puberty. Many of these symptoms respond to therapy, enabling Klinefelter males to lead normal, productive lives even though they will never be able to father children (nevertheless, many marry and are sexually active). The frequency of Klinefelter's births is relatively high—about one out of every 1,000 male births—and is more prevalent among children of older mothers. Turner's syndrome, by contrast, occurs when one X chromosome is missing; i.e., the victim has only one sex chromosome, for a total of 45 instead of the normal 46. This malady is outwardly expressed by retarded sexual development (no breast development, failure to menstruate or ovulate), unusually short stature (generally under 5 feet), a webbed neck, and broad chest. Treatment methods developed within recent years have made it possible for an increasing number of Turner's syndrome women to live near-normal lives. Interestingly, the incidence of Turner's syndrome is far lower than that of Klinefelter's—about one in 3,000 female births. This discrepancy appears to be due to a very high rate of intrauterine deaths among fetuses with only one sex chromosome (Jorde et al., 1999).

Cause of Mutations

That mutations occur is not in question; their underlying cause is less well understood. A great many mutations occur spontaneously due to natural causes. Some of these spontaneous mutations have been attributed to radiation exposure from cosmic rays and radioactive minerals in the earth's crust. However, it is thought that such relatively low levels of background radiation are insufficient to account for the majority of spontaneous mutations, the cause of which remains a mystery.

Since the early 1900s, several substances identified as capable of inducing mutations have been introduced into the human environment and have raised serious concerns within the scientific community regarding their potential for increasing mutation rates. Such substances are known as **mutagens**. X-rays were the first mutagens to be recognized, their mutagenic effect on fruit flies being described in 1927 by the great geneticist H. J. Muller at Indiana University. Subsequently a number of chemical compounds have been found to possess mutagenic properties, among them formaldehyde, mustard gas, nitrous acid, colchicine, and vinyl chloride. Many other candidates are now under suspicion as being possible mutagens.

Mutation Rates

Although the probability of any given human gene in an egg or sperm cell undergoing a spontaneous mutation is difficult to estimate accurately, it is generally regarded as low. However, one must keep in mind that each person has about 20,000–25,000 genes (Human Genome Sequencing Consortium, 2004). The chances of a mutation occurring in at least one of those genes are thus quite large. In fact, the English geneticist Harry Harris asserts that, on the average, every newborn child may be "expected, as the result of a new mutation in either of its parents, to synthesize at least one structurally variant enzyme or protein." Since only those mutations that occur in an egg or sperm have the potential to be passed on to subsequent generations, studies of mutation frequency have focused on these so-called genetic mutations. Typically, mutations occurring in a person's sex cells have no effect upon him or her but present a risk to succeeding generations of offspring. On the other hand, a mutation occurring in any cell other than an egg or sperm (somatic mutation) can adversely affect the person who sustained the mutation, but such injury will not be inherited by his or her children and thus represents no threat to the human gene pool.

In this context, it is of interest to note that about a third of pregnancies spontaneously abort after implantation of the fertilized egg (it's unknown how many are lost prior to implantation). Geneticists estimate that at least 10–15% of conceptions exhibit some chromosome abnormality and that a significant portion of fetal loss can be attributed to these mutations (Jorde et al., 1999).

The great concern among geneticists today is that exposure of populations to the artificial mutagens so common in the modern environment could further increase mutation rates. Since most mutations are harmful to some degree, it is in humanity's long-term interest to keep mutation rates as low as possible.

Birth Defects

As we have seen in the previous section, mutations in parents' sex cells can result in their children being born with structural or functional abnormalities, but by no means are all birth defects due to mutations. The CDC (Centers for Disease Control and Prevention) estimates that approximately 120,000 infants in the United States are born with birth defects each year; mutations are believed to account for approximately 25% of the total. Since birth defects constitute the leading cause of infant mortality in the United States, responsible for the deaths of approximately 8,000 babies within a year after birth, efforts to understand why fetal malformation occurs and how to prevent such a tragic course of events assume added urgency.

Living things are far more sensitive to adverse environmental influences during their early stages of development than they are at any other time. Embryos that are perfectly normal genetically can be seriously or fatally damaged if exposed to extraneous hazards. Investigations over the past several decades have revealed the sad truth that the womb is not the safe haven it was once assumed to be.

The likelihood that all abnormal development is triggered by some aspect of the environment (even hereditary disorders were at some point initiated by a mutation) has given rise to the science of **teratology**—the study of abnormal formations in animals or plants—and to the search for **teratogens,** substances that cause birth defects.

Interest in birth abnormalities is undoubtedly as old as humanity itself, although prior to the 20th century most ideas regarding birth defects involved considerably more fantasy than fact. From ancient times until fairly recently, some societies believed that the emotional state and visual impressions of an expectant mother could influence the physical development of her child. For this reason women in ancient Greece were encouraged to gaze at statuary representing the ideal human form, while Norwegian mothers-to-be were cautioned against looking at rabbits, for fear their

Table 6-1   Some Known Human Teratogens

Teratogen	Effect
Ionizing Radiation	central nervous system disorders, microcephaly, eye
X-rays	problems, mental retardation
Nuclear fallout	
Pathogenic Infections	
German measles	congenital heart defect, deafness, cataracts
Syphilis and herpes simplex type 2	mental retardation, microcephaly
Cytomegalovirus	kidney and liver disorders, pneumonia, brain damage
Toxoplasmosis	fatal lesions in the central nervous system
Drugs and Chemicals	
Thalidomide	phocomelia
Methyl mercury	mental retardation, sensory and motor problems
DES	vaginal cancer in girls, genital abnormalities in boys
Dioxin	structural deformities, miscarriages
Anesthesia	miscarriages, structural deformities
Alcohol	mental retardation, growth deficiencies, microcephaly, facial irregularities
Cigarette smoke	low birth weight, miscarriage, stillbirth
Dilantin	heart malformations, cleft palate, harelip, mental retardation, microcephaly
Valproic acid	spina bifida
Accutane	cardiovascular abnormalities, deformation of the ear, hydrocephaly, microcephaly
Tegison	same effect as for Accutane

babies would be born with harelip! The Babylonians and Sumerians regarded certain types of malformations as portents of coming events; medieval Europeans regarded them as evidence that the mother had indulged in intercourse with Satan or other demons and occasionally used this event as an excuse to execute the unfortunate mother and child. The so-called "Theory of Divine Retribution," also prevalent in Europe during the Middle Ages, viewed the birth of a defective child as God's punishment on the parents for past sins. With the rebirth of scientific inquiry in the Western world following the Renaissance, less mythical interpretations of teratogenesis were sought. In the 17th century birth defects were attributed to such factors as the narrowness of the mother's uterus, poor posture of the pregnant woman, or to a fall or blow on the abdomen during pregnancy. Though inaccurate, these explanations at least were an attempt to find a rational explanation for what remained a mysterious phenomenon. Gregor Mendel's discovery of the laws of genetics, followed by an explosion of research into the mechanism of heredity, led in the early 20th century to acceptance of the idea that all developmental errors could be attributed to faulty genes. This view prevailed until the mid-20th century, but a series of significant discoveries and observations since that time has once again altered our perception regarding teratogenesis and has given new impetus and urgency to the field of teratology.

The first key discovery to contradict the prevailing view that heredity is all-important emerged from animal studies investigating the influence of maternal diet on the outcome of pregnancy. In 1940 a report was published showing that specific types of nutritional deficiencies in pregnant rats caused predictable types and percentages of malformations in their offspring (Warkany, 1972). This finding effectively shattered old ideas about the overriding importance of genes and the conviction that the fetus could parasitize the mother if necessary to ensure normal development. Continued research into the influence of maternal diet on fetal development has confirmed and broadened these original findings. It is now known that a wide range of nutrients, from proteins to trace minerals to specific amino acids, are essential for normal development. Conversely, an excess of some of these necessary substances (e.g., phenylalanine, vitamin A) can exert teratogenic effects. Among the birth abnormalities associated with a specific nutritional deficiency are neural tube defects such as spina bifida and anencephaly. Recognition that up to 75% of these devastating birth abnormalities could be prevented simply by increasing a pregnant woman's dietary intake of **folic acid**, one of the B vitamins, led the FDA to mandate the fortification of flour, corn meal, pasta, and rice with this micronutrient. The FDA action, which took effect on January 1, 1998, marks the first time the federal agency has required fortification of a food for the express purpose of preventing a birth defect.

In 1941 an unusually large number of babies in both the United States and Australia were born suffering from congenital cataracts, heart defects, or deafness. Epidemiological studies launched to try to determine the cause for such an outbreak found that the only common thread linking all the victims was the fact that during the first trimester of pregnancy, their mothers had contracted German measles *(Rubella),* which had reached epidemic proportions that year. The fact that a virus could cross the placental barrier and damage the fetus was thus established.

While these two developments demonstrated that mammalian embryos are vulnerable to such commonplace environmental influences as inadequate diet and infections, the most dramatic confirmation that certain environmental factors (in this case an artificially synthesized drug) must be regarded as a potential risk to the unborn came in the early 1960s with revelation of what has since become known as the "Thalidomide Tragedy."

Thalidomide was a drug first synthesized by a pharmaceutical company in Germany in 1953 and subsequently developed and widely marketed in western Europe as a mild sedative and as a treatment for morning sickness. Preliminary testing on laboratory animals indicated that thalidomide had little injurious effect even when taken in quantity (in fact, humans who attempted to commit suicide using the drug survived extremely large doses). With evidence of its safety regarding overdosing, but with virtually no testing for other side effects, the German manufacturer put thalidomide on the market as a nonprescription sleeping pill. Thanks to an aggressive advertising campaign stressing its safety, thalidomide (sold under the trade name *Cantergan*) became the most widely used sedative in Germany and was extensively sold in the United Kingdom; altogether, the drug was marketed in 48 countries during the early 1960s. Two American drug companies initially showed interest in acquiring thalidomide but concluded from their own tests that the drug was less effective than the brands they were already marketing. Somewhat later another American firm, impressed by the growing popularity of thalidomide in Europe, began another series of tests and released the drug for prescription use in Canada. In the United States, however, a doctor with the Food and Drug Administration had nagging doubts about some unexplained neurological results among long-term thalidomide users and restricted use of the drug in this country to a small clinical human trial. At about this time (1960) the European medical community was becoming increasingly puzzled by the sudden increase in what had formerly been an extremely rare type of birth abnormality. In near-epidemic proportions children were being born with a condition known as **phocomelia** (seal-limb), in which there is typically a hand or foot attached directly to the torso without an arm or leg. In some cases, however, even the hands and feet were absent, the babies being born with only a head and torso. The presence of large numbers of babies with such an obvious deformity couldn't be overlooked, but intense questioning of the parents regarding their hereditary background, blood type, radiation exposure, or chromosomal aberrations in other children failed to reveal a common link. Finally two alert physicians made the connection between thalidomide use early in pregnancy to the birth of limbless babies. Subsequent studies revealed that 40% of the women who had taken thalidomide during their first trimester of pregnancy delivered babies afflicted with phocomelia. As proof of thalidomide's teratogenic properties gained acceptance, use of the drug was gradually discontinued in country after country, but not before nearly 12,000 children had been permanently disabled.

Ironically, thalidomide's unsavory reputation may yet be redeemed. Research demonstrating that thalidomide acts by inhibiting blood vessel growth has suggested its potential for combating a number of serious human ailments, including brain cancer, AIDS, and lupus. The drug also offers hope for treating diabetic retinopathy and macular degeneration, the two leading causes of blindness in the United States. In July 1998, the FDA approved the use of thalidomide for treating a serious inflammatory skin condition in patients with leprosy (*erythema nodosum leprosum*), and by October of that year thalidomide became commercially available in the U.S. for the first time. Produced exclusively by Calgene Corporation under the trade name "Thalidomid," thalidomide is now being prescribed for hundreds of critically ill cancer patients as tests of its safety and efficacy are ongoing (Henderson, 1999; FDA, 1998).

In the early 1970s, not long after the heart-breaking photos of thalidomide babies had receded from media attention, another teratogenic chemical made headline news. Diethylstilbestrol, or **DES**, was first synthesized in 1938 and widely prescribed to pregnant women in the United States and Latin America for several decades thereaf-

This young girl is but one of the approximately 12,000 children born with missing arms or legs as a result of fetal exposure to thalidomide—a nonprescription sedative widely used in Europe during the early 1960s. [*March of Dimes Birth Defects Foundation*]

ter. Because its biological action resembles that of natural estrogen, doctors began administering it to women experiencing problem pregnancies in the mistaken belief that it would prevent miscarriages. In the late 1950s one drug company, touting the miraculous properties of DES, even urged that *all* pregnant women use the drug to produce "bigger and stronger babies!" Eventually it was demonstrated that DES had no beneficial health effects; in fact, when given in high doses before the 20th week of pregnancy, DES actually *increased* the risk of miscarriage. Gradually the popularity of the drug began to wane, but not before an estimated 5 million pregnant women had used it. Little more was heard about DES until the late 1960s when doctors at Massachusetts General Hospital in Boston made the connection between a rare form of vaginal cancer (clear-cell adenocarcinoma) in young female patients and the use of DES by their mothers during pregnancy. The fact that teratogenic effects could lie hidden for years, only to manifest themselves when the affected child became an adult hit the medical world like a bombshell—obviously birth defects don't have to be immediately visible to be important. Over the years that followed, several hundred cases of vaginal cancer were diagnosed among "DES daughters." While DES-related troubles initially focused on the daughters of women who had taken the drug, it gradually became apparent that girls were not the only victims nor was vaginal cancer the only problem. Many DES sons exhibit congenital deformities of the reproductive system and reduced fertility—problems experienced by DES daughters as well. DES daughters are at heightened risk of tubal pregnancies, miscarriages, and premature deliveries—if they are able to become pregnant in the first place. Perhaps most ominous of all are recent research results suggesting that DES exposure *in utero* causes genetic changes in a female embryo's egg cells that may pose a cancer threat to yet a third generation—the DES *granddaughters*. Unfortunately, hopes that the sad saga of DES would be confined to the generation exposed in the womb may prove too optimistic (Colborn, Dumanoski, and Myers, 1996; Newbold et al., 1998).

The thalidomide and DES episodes not only emphasized the importance of testing new drugs for their teratogenic effects, but also raised the profoundly disturbing question of what other drugs and medicines widely used by pregnant women might be doing to their unborn babies. That harmful effects could indeed result from medications used by pregnant women was confirmed again in the early 1980s when a French physician linked numerous cases of spina bifida to maternal use of valproic acid to control epileptic seizures (Harris and Wynne, 1994). A very beneficial medication for the mother's health problems, valproic acid proved devastating for unborn children exposed to the medication *in utero*. Valproic acid and thalidomide produced such distinctive types of abnormalities that they could scarcely go unnoticed. Conceivably, however, other teratogens that result in slight impairment of mental abilities, slight physical abnormalities, or diminished vigor might never be suspected as harmful.

These tragic episodes stimulated research, still ongoing, into what other substances present a threat to the unborn. Though much remains to be learned, investigations over the past several decades have implicated an increasing number of drugs and chemicals as proven or suspected teratogens. Among them, in addition to thalidomide and DES: dioxin, organic mercury, lead, cadmium, anesthetic gases, alcohol (see box 6-2), and cigarette smoke. While nonsmokers of any age can suffer health problems when exposed either to mainstream smoke exhaled by a smoker or from the sidestream smoke emanating from the end of a burning cigarette, infants in the womb are the most vulnerable. When a pregnant woman smokes—and nearly a quarter of expectant mothers in the U.S. *do* smoke—she is exposing her fetus to nicotine, carbon monoxide, radioactive polonium, and numerous other toxic chemicals. Carbon monoxide appears to be the most fetotoxic of these, causing a rise in carboxyhemoglobin

Box 6-2 A Totally Preventable Tragedy

Fetal Alcohol Syndrome (FAS) afflicts 1–3 of every 1,000 babies born in the world today and is the leading known cause of mental retardation. In the United States, an estimated 6–22 FAS-afflicted infants are born every day and the lifetime cost to care for each of them will exceed $1.5 million. Fetal Alcohol Syndrome is a lifelong, permanently disabling condition that cannot be reversed by providing prenatally damaged children with a high-quality, stable home environment after birth. Because it forever deprives its victims of a normal, productive life, FAS can justifiably be regarded as an extreme form of maternal child abuse.

As the name suggests, Fetal Alcohol Syndrome is a birth defect resulting from alcohol consumption during pregnancy. More toxic than any other abused drug, alcohol rapidly crosses the placental barrier from mother to fetus; within a few minutes after a pregnant woman drinks, blood alcohol levels in her fetus approximate her own.

Although surveys indicate most women are aware that drinking during pregnancy poses risks to a developing fetus, many choose to indulge regardless. Survey statistics published in 2004 revealed that each year approximately half a million pregnant women in the U.S.—about one in eight—report some degree of alcohol use, with 80,000 admitting to binge drinking.

Admittedly, not all babies born to heavily-drinking mothers have FAS—perhaps as few as 4 out of 100 have the full complement of symptoms. Why this is the case remains a subject of research, with individual genetic factors assumed to be the most likely explanation. However, the fact that all babies born with FAS have mothers who drank heavily during pregnancy supports a direct cause-and-effect relationship.

Fetal Alcohol Syndrome was first described in the early 1970s as a complex of physical and neurobehavioral defects resulting from prenatal alcohol exposure. Some of the more common physical features associated with FAS babies include smaller than average body size and weight—a characteristic that persists throughout childhood; facial abnormalities, the most apparent of which are small eye openings, skin webbing between the eyes and base of the nose, thin upper lip, indistinct or absent groove between the nose and upper lip, low nasal bridge, short nose, small jaw, and low-set ears. FAS children often exhibit congenital heart defects, cleft lip and palate, kidney and urinary tract defects, and/or malformed genitals. Skeletal defects such as a small head, deformed ribs and breastbone, hip dislocations, curved spine, and fused, webbed, or missing fingers or toes may also be manifest. Some of these physical characteristics become less obvious as the child grows older, but the same cannot be said of the neurobehavioral traits that are a result of alcohol's devastating effects on the central nervous system (CNS) and which frequently become even more noticeable after puberty. Because prenatal alcohol exposure damages the developing brain, FAS children often, though not always, experience some degree of mental retardation and low I.Q. Learning disabilities—particularly difficulty with arithmetic—are common, as is short attention span, hyperactivity, and poor body, hand, and finger coordination. As they get older, outbursts of aggression and lack of impulse control become an issue, schooling is frequently disrupted, and the children have difficulty maintaining friendships. As adults, FAS victims often experience mental health problems, find it difficult to hold a regular job, and not infrequently find themselves in trouble with the law. They typically exercise poor judgment in making decisions, have little understanding of danger, and find it difficult to use past experience in planning and organizing future actions. As a result, many are unable to care for themselves adequately, with homelessness often a result.

Combating FAS requires a thorough understanding of causation and although three decades of research have revealed a great deal of information, a number of questions remain unresolved. Confounding easy answers is the fact that, as a teratogen, alcohol produces a continuum of effects, making diagnosis problematic. While some children show the classic symptoms of FAS, less extreme cases may display only a few or no facial abnormalities, yet still exhibit the behavioral dysfunction characteristic of alcohol-induced CNS damage. These children are said to be suffering from Fetal Alcohol Effects (FAE), a condition almost twice as common as full-blown FAS—an estimated 3–5 cases out of every 1,000 live births worldwide. Whether prenatal alcohol exposure results in FAS or FAE appears to be dependent on dose; children whose mothers are confirmed alcoholics suffer more severe effects than those whose mothers drank only moderate amounts during pregnancy. However, the question of "how much is *too* much?" has proven difficult to answer. Until relatively recently, medical researchers believed that a pregnant woman could safely consume one drink per day (one drink is defined as 12 ounces of beer, 5 ounces of wine, or 1.5 ounces of hard liquor) without incurring any greater risk of harm to her baby than that of women who abstained completely. A study published in 2002, however, showed that mothers who had only 1½ drinks per week gave birth to babies who were shorter, weighed less, and had smaller heads than infants whose mothers never drank during pregnancy.

Regardless of the total amount of alcohol consumed, studies have conclusively shown that consuming a large number of drinks within a short time period (so-called binge drinking) is significantly more harmful to the fetus than drinking the same total quantity in smaller amounts over a period of several days. The stage of fetal development at the time of alcohol exposure is an important determinant of the specific type of damage inflicted on the fetus. During the first trimester, when the basic organs of the body are forming, maternal drinking results in the facial abnormalities typically associated with FAS; at this time exposure can also result in skeletal deformities and, if occurring during the 3rd–4th week of gestation, in malformation of the heart. During the second trimester, alcohol disrupts nerve formation in the brain, while in the third trimester it interferes with nervous system development. Both the second and third trimesters are critical periods for fetal growth, so alcohol exposure during these periods has a pronounced dose-dependent effect in terms of reduced body weight, length, and head size. As one might expect, the most severely damaged children are those whose mothers drank heavily throughout their pregnancy.

Health care professionals are now striving to develop effective ways of identifying and helping alcohol-dependent pregnant women. The need to reach and educate sexually active teenagers is considered especially urgent, since many become pregnant and continue using alcohol, often with little or no understanding of the risks or consequences of FAS/FAE. Doctors and staff at prenatal clinics could be effective educators by asking these young women about their drinking habits and encouraging them to cease using alcohol while pregnant. Altering behavior of chronically alcoholic women is much more difficult than dealing with binge-drinking teenagers, since even when they understand the risk, many are unable to break their addiction. Warning labels regarding the dangers of drinking while pregnant, now required on all alcoholic beverages, have raised awareness of the problem but have had minimal impact in changing the behavior of long-time heavy drinkers who tend to have numerous other problems, including drug abuse, smoking, and malnutrition.

For the majority of expectant mothers who are not alcohol-addicted but may be social drinkers, constant reminders by friends, relatives, and health care providers about the hazards of drinking while pregnant are appropriate. Since science has yet to identify a foolproof method for determining which infants are genetically predisposed to harm from even very low exposure to alcohol in the womb, it is only prudent for every pregnant woman to assume that her fetus is in this extra-vulnerable category and act accordingly. Although the global incidence of FAS/FAE continues to climb, the strategy for eliminating this cruel but completely avoidable birth defect is utterly straightforward: while pregnant, women should not drink any amount of alcohol—period. It's that simple.

References

Carroll, Linda. 2003. "Alcohol's Toll on Fetuses: Even Worse Than Thought." *New York Times*, Nov. 4, D1.

Eustace, Larry W., Duck-Hee Kang, and David Coombs. 2003. "Fetal Alcohol Syndrome: A Growing Concern for Health Care Professionals." *Journal of Obstetric, Gynecologic, and Neonatal Nursing* 32, no. 2 (March/April):215–221.

Floyd, R. L., and J. S. Sidhu. 2004. "Monitoring Prenatal Alcohol Exposure." *American Journal of Medical Genetics*, 127 C (1):3–9 (May 15).

Maternal consumption of alcohol during pregnancy is now recognized as a serious problem worldwide, its most dramatic consequences manifested here in the birth defect known as Fetal Alcohol Syndrome (FAS). FAS children generally suffer from low IQ, attention deficits, memory problems, and hyperactivity. The majority exhibit abnormalities of the upper lip, teeth problems, and an unusual shape of the head, face, ears, palms, and back/neck/spine. [*From "Fetal Alcohol Syndrome in Adolescents and Adults" by Ann Pytkowicz Streissguth, PhD., et al., JAMA, April 17, 1991 265. Courtesy of FAS Research Fund*]

in the blood of both mother and child and resulting in retarded fetal growth rates. Pregnant women who smoke 20 or more cigarettes daily are at heightened risk of bearing an infant with cleft lip and palate; maternal smoking during pregnancy also is associated with a significantly higher chance of giving birth to a mentally retarded child. Medical experts estimate that 20–40% of all low-weight births can be directly attributed to maternal smoking during pregnancy. Infants born to smoking mothers weigh on the average about 10% less at birth than do babies of nonsmokers. Since low birth weight is a major risk factor for infant mortality, it is not surprising that approximately 10% of all U.S. neonatal deaths each year are blamed on maternal smoking. Smoking during pregnancy also is blamed for an estimated 50,000 miscarriages annually and for 11–14% of all premature births, the risk of which rises the more heavily the mother smokes (Drews et al., 1996; Shaw et al., 1996). In spite of the gruesome lessons of past tragedies, pregnant women continue using various drugs (e.g., aspirin, antacids, barbiturates, tranquilizers, cough medicines), drinking, and smoking, even though it is generally accepted that excess use of any of the above substances carries some risk of fetal damage.

Self-administered drugs or medications are not the only source of teratogenic exposure, of course. Hundreds of thousands of American workers currently are employed in occupations that expose them to reproductive hazards—lead, anesthetic gases, ethylene oxide (used as a sterilant for many hospital supplies), and certain pesticides. While few well-documented associations between specific workplace chemicals and reproductive problems (i.e., miscarriage, reduced fertility, neonatal death, birth defects) exist at present, this doesn't mean such a linkage is nonexistent. Very few well-designed clinical or epidemiologic studies on the issue have been conducted, making it impossible to draw definitive conclusions. Nevertheless, a 1985 review of 2,800 chemicals evaluated for their ability to induce birth defects in animals indicated that more than a third exhibited some teratogenic potential (Chivian et al., 1993). Unfortunately, most workplace teratogens are identified only after significant numbers of employees experience personal tragedies. Among the more recent reproductive hazards to make headlines are two glycol ethers, widely used as solvents in the manufacture of computer chips. Studies conducted on female workers exposed to the chemicals during the chip-making process found that the women suffered miscarriages 40% more frequently than did nonexposed women in the industry and experienced 30% fewer pregnancies. As a result of these findings, several of the corporate giants in the semiconductor industry are allowing pregnant female employees to work outside the chip fabrication area of the plant and have announced their intention to phase the hazardous chemicals out of the production process altogether (Markoff, 1992; "Solvents Used," 1992). The widespread assumption that such workplace precautions need apply only to female workers is now being challenged by provocative, though inconclusive, evidence that a *father's* exposure to environmental hazards may also lead to defective offspring. It has long been observed that men working as painters, farmers, or mechanics—jobs involving exposure to certain solvents and pesticides—tend to be at higher risk of fathering children with birth defects than do men in other occupations. These observations have stimulated a new look at the impact that mutagenic or teratogenic substances might have on sperm production or on the chemical composition of semen, and thereby on the development of a fertilized egg (Stone, 1992).

While some progress in elucidating the mechanism of teratogenesis has been made in recent years, much more research is needed. Nevertheless, some broad generalizations about the causation of birth defects can be made. Perhaps most critical is the finding that fetal vulnerability to teratogens depends on the stage of development at the time of exposure. By far the most sensitive period is the time of tissue and organ formation (organogenesis), a period lasting from about the 18th day after conception to approximately the 60th day, with the peak of sensitivity around the 30th day. During this time, interference with development can result in gross structural defects. In the case of the thalidomide episode, it was found that virtually all of the thalidomide mothers had taken the drug precisely during those few days when the limb buds were forming. Those women who used thalidomide before or after this critical time gave birth to normal babies. Similarly, DES exposure after the 20th week of pregnancy did not result in reproductive tract deformities, while exposure before the tenth week increased the risk of cancer in DES daughters. During the first week after conception, when the embryo is a relatively undifferentiated mass of cells, any damage caused by teratogenic exposure will be lethal to the developing embryo. After the 8th week, though the fetus is barely an inch long, its organs are already basically formed. Exposure to teratogens after this time can cause such harm as mental retardation, blindness, or damage to the external sex organs, but the time for major structural deformation has passed. It must be recognized, however, that individual genetic differences in both mother and child will determine the extent of damage caused by teratogenic exposure. No teratogen causes birth defects in 100% of those exposed; if a group of women, all at the same stage of pregnancy, were exposed to equal concentrations of the same teratogen, some would give birth to babies with serious abnormalities, others with only moderate damage, and some would deliver infants who were perfectly normal (Harris and Wynne, 1994).

A second widely accepted generalization about teratogenesis is that as the dosage of a teratogen increases, the degree of damage increases. Basing their assumptions on the results of animal studies, teratologists thus presume the existence of a threshold below which no injury of any kind can be demonstrated. Determining exactly where that threshold is for any particular substance is, however, uncertain at best, and expectant mothers are well advised to limit their exposure to potential teratogens to the greatest extent possible.

Cancer

Few words arouse such emotions of sheer terror and hopelessness today as does the term "cancer." As the second leading cause of death in the United States (heart disease ranks first), and with over 1.3 million new cases diagnosed annually, cancer appears to have assumed epidemic proportions. Throughout the industrialized nations, cancer now accounts for 20–25% of all deaths each year; worldwide, according to the World Health Organization, cancer claims almost 6.5 million victims annually. In the United States, over 1,500 people die of cancer every day, with a yearly toll exceeding 560,000. Cancer is not an age-specific disease; although incidence rates are considerably higher among the elderly, cancer is the second-leading cause of death, after accidents, among children aged 1–14. In general, cancer death rates are considerably higher in developed countries than in the developing world, but the *types* of cancer that are most prevalent in various parts of the world differ sharply. Malignancies associated with cigarette smoking, asbestos exposure, or high-fat diets are far more common among populations in industrialized countries, while cancers linked to certain food preservatives, viral infections, or fungal toxins in food are more prevalent in the developing world.

In the United States, the *incidence* rate for all cancers as a group climbed steadily from 1973 to 1992, the peak year for new cancer cases, but has been gradually declining since then (cancer incidence for certain sites continues to increase however, most notably for breast cancer among women over the age of 50). The same trend holds true for cancer *mortality* rates. Since cancer record-keeping began in 1930, cancer death rates increased inexorably, year after year, reaching a peak in 1990. In 1991,

Figure 6-2 Leading Sites of New Cancer Cases and Deaths—2003 Estimates*

Estimated New Cases*		Estimated Deaths	
Male	**Female**	**Male**	**Female**
Prostate 220,900 (33%)	Breast 211,300 (32%)	Lung & bronchus 88,400 (31%)	Lung & bronchus 68,800 (25%)
Lung & bronchus 91,800 (14%)	Lung & bronchus 80,100 (12%)	Prostate 28,900 (10%)	Breast 39,800 (15%)
Colon & rectum 72,800 (11%)	Colon & rectum 74,700 (11%)	Colon & rectum 28,300 (10%)	Colon & rectum 28,800 (11%)
Urinary bladder 42,200 (6%)	Uterine corpus 40,100 (6%)	Pancreas 14,700 (5%)	Pancreas 15,300 (6%)
Melanoma of the skin 29,900 (4%)	Ovary 25,400 (4%)	Non-Hodgkin lymphoma 12,200 (4%)	Ovary 14,300 (5%)
Non-Hodgkin lymphoma 28,300 (4%)	Non-Hodgkin lymphoma 25,100 (4%)	Leukemia 12,100 (4%)	Non-Hodgkin lymphoma 11,200 (4%)
Kidney 19,500 (3%)	Melanoma of the skin 24,300 (3%)	Esophagus 9,900 (4%)	Leukemia 9,800 (4%)
Oral cavity 18,200 (3%)	Thyroid 16,300 (3%)	Liver 9,200 (3%)	Uterine corpus 6,800 (3%)
Leukemia 17,900 (3%)	Pancreas 15,800 (2%)	Urinary bladder 8,600 (3%)	Brain 5,800 (2%)
Pancreas 14,900 (2%)	Urinary bladder 15,200 (2%)	Kidney 7,400 (3%)	Multiple myeloma 5,500 (2%)
All sites 675,300 (100%)	All sites 658,800 (100%)	All sites 285,900 (100%)	All sites 270,600 (100%)

*Excludes basal and squamous cell skin cancers and in situ carcinoma except urinary bladder.
Percentages may not total 100% due to rounding.   ©2003, American Cancer Society, Inc., Surveillance Research

Source: American Cancer Society's Cancer Facts and Figures–2003. www.cancer.org. Reprinted by the permission of the American Cancer Society, Inc.

however, overall U.S. cancer mortality rates began a slow but steady decline that researchers are convinced will continue for at least 20 years. The welcome reversal is attributed to a variety of factors: decades of anti-smoking campaigns and other preventive efforts, earlier detection when malignancies are more likely to respond to treatment, and improvements in medical care (Cole and Rodu, 1996). For some types of cancer, the turnaround in mortality rates was achieved long before the 1990s. For over a half-century, deaths due to cancer of the uterus, cervix, and stomach have fallen by more than 70% in the United States. In the case of uterine and cervical cancers, credit for the decline in death rates is attributed to widespread use of the Pap smear test, which provides early diagnosis when the disease is still treatable. Experts estimate that a further 90% reduction in the current annual number of U.S. cervical cancer deaths could be achieved if all American women would take advantage of this simple procedure. Regarding stomach cancer mortality, which is lower today in the United States than anywhere else in the world (at present the East Asian countries and several of the former Soviet republics, including Russia, have the highest incidence of stomach cancer mortality), favorable trends are probably due to improved methods of transport and to refrigeration, which have made fresh produce available year-round. These advantages of modern life are significant in terms of cancer prevention because they have led to increased consumption of fresh fruits and vegetables (known to contain anticarcinogenic compounds), thereby lessening dependence on the salted, pickled, or smoke-preserved foods that are thought to pose a cancer risk.

More recently, colorectal cancers have also begun to decline in both North America and western Europe; liver cancer, bladder cancer, and childhood leukemia mortality rates exhibit similar downward trends. Most encouraging, however, is the long-awaited reversal in the lung cancer death rate. Although lung cancer remains by far the leading cancer killer among Americans of both sexes, death rates for this disease are finally beginning to drop for U.S. men. The only significant increases in cancer death rates since the early 1990s are for lung cancer among women and non-Hodgkin's lymphoma for both sexes.

Cancer, of course, is not a new disease; ancient societies were familiar with the ravages of cancer. Indeed, all multicellular organisms, plant and animal, are subject to the occasional development of malignancies. However, cancer's rapid rise to prominence as a leading cause of illness and death during the 20th century has imbued it with an aura of dread and fatalism. Until recently, progress achieved in the so-called war against cancer remained disappointingly limited after decades of intensive medical research and the expenditure of billions of dollars. Major gains *were* achieved in prolonging a cancer patient's survival time after the initial diagnosis, and notable successes were scored in reducing deaths from childhood leukemia and Hodgkin's lymphoma; nevertheless, the "magic bullet" that would provide a cure for cancer was nowhere in sight. Research and observation strongly suggested that a majority of cancers were associated with environmental causes (using the term "environment" in its broadest sense to include diet, smoking, sun exposure, chemical pollutants, and so forth), yet the mechanism for such interaction remained unknown. During the past two decades, however, several major breakthroughs in cancer research have revolutionized our understanding of carcinogenesis. While a great deal more remains to be learned, these findings have provided important information on how once-healthy cells become malignant and offer new hope for both prevention and treatment of this formidable killer.

What Causes Cancer?

"Cancer" is a collective term used to describe a number of diseases that differ in origin, prognosis, and treatment. It is essentially a condition in which the regulating forces that govern normal cell processes no longer function correctly, leading to uncontrolled cell proliferation. Cancerous cells, unlike normal ones, continue to divide and spread, invading other tissues where they interfere with vital bodily functions and eventually lead to death of the organism. The search for agents responsible for initiating this chain of events has been ongoing for years and has focused on a number of possibilities including pathogens, hereditary factors, oxidation damage within cells due to normal metabolic processes, and exposure to a wide range of environmental **carcinogens** (substances that can cause cancer) such as toxic chemicals and radiation.

Viruses have long been known to cause some forms of cancer in animals (e.g. viral leukemia in cats, Rous sarcoma in chickens). It is now recognized that at least seven viruses cause cancer in humans as well; among the most significant are the hepatitis B and C viruses that predispose infected individuals to liver cancer (about 70% of all liver cancers are a result of hepatitis infections) and the herpes papillomavirus associated with approximately 90% of all cervical cancers (Parkin et al., 1999). For decades it had been assumed that **bacteria** had no part to play in the cancer drama, but in the early 1990s researchers found that both gastric cancer and non-Hodgkin's lymphoma of the stomach are markedly higher among people infected with the bacterium *Helicobacter pylori*, the common microbe recognized as the leading cause of stomach ulcers. Interestingly, while non-Hodgkin's lymphoma of the stomach is extremely rare in the United States, it is relatively common in the Veneto region of Italy where 90% of the population is infected with *H. pylori* (Parsonnet et al., 1994; Isaacson, 1994). Together, viruses and bacteria are now viewed as causative agents for almost 15% of all human cancers—over a million new cases annually—with viruses responsible for the large majority of these (Parkin et al., 1999).

Since the rediscovery of Mendelian principles of genetics in the early 1900s, **heredity** has been a prime suspect for cancer causation, particularly because certain kinds of malignancies are more common in some families than in others. It is well established that a few types of cancer *are* hereditary; among the best known inherited cancers are retinoblastoma, a cancer of the eye, and familial polyposis, a rare type of colon cancer. For the most part, however, studies carried out decades ago discounted heredity as a significant factor in cancer causation. These studies compared the incidence of specific types of cancer among descendants of immigrants to the United States and members of the same ethnic group remaining in the homeland. For example, a 1944 study of the incidence of liver cancer showed that African-Americans have much lower rates of this disease than do native African populations; similarly, Japanese-Americans exhibit low rates of stomach cancer—comparable to those of the general American population—while stomach cancer remains very common in Japan. By contrast, these Japanese-Americans, like other U.S. residents, experience typically high rates of colon cancer, a disease quite rare in Japan. A subsequent study of immigrants to Australia and Canada found that a woman's risk of breast cancer shifted from the rate prevailing in her country of origin toward the rate observed among native-born women in the country to which she moved. Thus women who emigrated from England, where breast cancer rates are relatively high, experienced a lowering of risk in their new country of destination; conversely, female emigrants from Asian countries, where breast cancer rates are lower than those prevailing in Canada and Australia, were more likely to develop breast cancer in their adopted countries than were women in their homelands. Study results strongly suggest that risk of breast cancer has little to do with heredity, but rather is associated with as-yet unidentified environmental and lifestyle factors. Since most of the women emigrated as adults, it also suggests that one's risk of breast cancer can be altered later in life (Kliewer and Smith, 1995).

Although few types of cancers are directly associated with "cancer genes," a tidal wave of new discoveries during the past two decades has demonstrated the existence of an inherited *predisposition* to cancer that explains the prevalence of specific types of malignancies within certain families. These findings not only help to explain why some people exposed to known carcinogens remain hale and hearty while others sicken and die, but also offer promising therapeutic approaches for reducing cancer mortality among those likely to develop the disease. A classic example of genetic predisposition to cancer is that of hereditary non-polyposis colon cancer, a common type of colorectal malignancy. Victims of the disease carry an inherited defective gene which, in its normal state, produces a DNA repair protein that acts as a cellular "spell checker," correcting errors in the order of nucleotide base pairs during DNA replication. In mutated form, the gene is no longer able to produce its key protein, so mistakes occurring after replication rapidly accumulate throughout the genetic material, creating a situation that may eventually result in cancer (Leach et al., 1993; Fishel et al., 1993). For individuals with a predisposition for hereditary non-polyposis colon cancer (about 10% of all colon malignancies), the chances of eventually developing colon cancer range between 70–90%, with many victims developing tumors before the age of 50. The practical significance of these recent findings is therefore immense: if carriers could be identified through genetic screening programs, they could begin having regular colonoscopic examinations at an early age in order to detect precancerous polyps when they can be easily removed. Similarly, identified bearers of the defective gene could be strongly advised to adopt the low-fat, high-fiber diet that is known to reduce the risk of colorectal cancer (Weinberg, 1998; Papadopoulos et al., 1994; Bronner et al., 1994).

A great many **environmental agents** such as cigarette smoke, radon gas, sunlight, heavy metals, X-rays, chemical pesticides, some air pollutants, and high-fat diets are

---

Box 6-3   Lab Tests for Carcinogenicity—Are They Valid?

In 1977 a Canadian study documenting an excess incidence of bladder cancer among male rats fed a 5% diet of saccharin created a furor among an American public unconvinced that the food additive posed a real health threat and dismayed at the possible banning of the only noncaloric sweetener on the market at that time. Intelligent assessment of the implications of the saccharin research was not helped by the statement by a top FDA official that humans would have to drink 800 cans of diet soda daily to consume an amount of saccharin equivalent to that fed the experimental rats. The issue was widely aired in outraged letters to Congress and newspaper opinion pages, laughed about on late-night talk shows, and used as the butt of cartoonist's jokes. The public was given the impression that the tests were meaningless as far as human health was concerned, an attitude aptly expressed by Congressman Andrew Jacobs of Indiana who proposed passage of a bill requiring that products containing saccharin bear the label: "Warning: the

Canadians have determined that saccharin is dangerous to your rat's health."

Unfortunately, the Congressman's remarks, echoed by millions of his fellow Americans, revealed a profound lack of understanding regarding the methods routinely used for determining the safety of new chemicals. The objections raised to the Canadian saccharin tests—and to animal testing procedures in general—focus primarily on two points:

1. The question of dosage. Does *everything* cause cancer when present in excess? Contrary to popular belief, only carcinogens cause cancer. A test animal might be fed a mountain of sugar or salt and die of toxemia, but it will not develop a malignancy because neither substance is a carcinogen (some would qualify this statement by pointing out that because hyper-obesity is a risk factor for certain types of cancer, excessive consumption of chocolate fudge sundaes could lead to cancer; nevertheless, it would be difficult to argue that ice cream is an environmental carcinogen in the same sense that aflatoxins or nitrosamines are known to be). Feeding or exposing test animals to extremely high doses of a suspected chemical is a widely accepted procedure necessary for obtaining meaningful results within a reasonable period of time, given the constraints of such experiments. In a typical study, for reasons of expense and space considerations, only 50 to 100 experimental animals are used in each test group. Such animals have a relatively short life span in comparison with humans, so in order to compensate for the long latency period involved in cancer initiation and to increase the chances for a weak carcinogen to be revealed in the small study population, massive doses are used. This method simply facilitates the collection of data within a reasonable time and at considerably less expense than would be possible using larger test populations and lower dosages.

That such tests are valid and that administration of large doses, per se, does not lead to carcinogenesis are supported by the results of past experimentation. A researcher at the National Cancer Institute some years ago reported that of 3,500 suspected carcinogens tested in the routine manner, only 750 proved, in fact, to be carcinogenic—hardly support for the thesis that large doses in themselves are cancer-causing.

2. Animals aren't humans. Do the substances that cause cancer in mice, monkeys, or rats predict cancer causation in humans? The prevailing assumption among researchers is that the basic biological processes in all mammals are fundamentally the same. For ethical reasons it is impossible to prove the thesis that any chemical that causes cancer in animals also causes the disease in humans—to do so would require deliberately exposing humans to a known animal carcinogen and waiting to see if cancer develops! However, numerous tests have been successfully carried out to prove the reverse: every substance known to induce human cancer causes cancer in animals as well (with the sole exception of arsenic, a heavy metal that is a human carcinogen, is mutagenic to bacteria and to cells grown in tissue culture, yet has never been shown to have carcinogenic potential in animals). Thus it seems logical to assume that the opposite is true also and that animal testing

is a valid method for determining which chemicals are carcinogenic. What animal testing cannot tell us, however, is how strong or weak a given carcinogen will be in humans. This is because different species show varying degrees of sensitivity to the same substance, some developing cancer only at high levels of exposure while others are vulnerable to relatively low doses. Unfortunately, it is not possible to calculate the level of human risk based on the risk level in animals. We may be more or less vulnerable; the tests indicate only which substance can be expected to result in a given number of human cancer cases.

Animal models, of course, provide but one of several methods for studying the mechanism of carcinogenesis. Other approaches for advancing our understanding of cancer include: **mutagenesis studies using bacteria** which, due to their very large population size and short generation time, allow rapid screening of numerous potential carcinogens; **tissue culture research**, which permits examination of DNA damage and mutagenesis in eukaryotic cells (as opposed to prokaryotic bacterial cells); and **epidemiologic studies** of cancer incidence among human populations. Each of these lines of investigation has inherent limitations, and results yielded by one type of study may not always correspond with conclusions drawn from an alternative mode of inquiry. For example, nickel compounds are potent carcinogens in both humans and animals but are not mutagenic to bacteria. Conversely, organic mercury compounds damage DNA in bacterial cells and are mutagenic to cells in tissue culture, but have not been shown to induce cancer either in humans or animals. Cadmium and chromium, however, show carcinogenic potential in all four systems.

The disturbing lack of consistency in results among these various test models has led some observers to question the validity of current testing procedures and to challenge government regulations based on the results of carcinogenicity studies on animals. Most investigators would argue, however, that in an admittedly imperfect world, we must continue to use the only tools currently available, always bearing in mind their limitations and exercising due caution when interpreting data or extrapolating results from such experiments.

known to be carcinogenic. These environmental factors, acting in conjunction with an individual's inherited predisposition to cancer and with acquired susceptibility, are believed to be responsible for an estimated 80% of all human cancers. The exact mechanism by which such agents induce a malignancy is still not completely understood, but recent progress in unraveling cancer's mysteries has brought us tantalizingly closer to that goal (Perera, 1997).

How Does Cancer Develop?

The exact mechanism of carcinogenesis is still being unraveled, with various theories being proposed as new findings emerge from medical research. The currently prevailing hypothesis is that cancer develops as a multistep process that begins when a single cell undergoes a mutation. The mutant cell then slowly proliferates to form a small group of genetically identical precancerous cells. This first step, termed **initiation**, is possibly provoked by a brief interaction between the target cell and a carcinogenic agent. It has been demonstrated that many environmental carcinogens (e.g., ultraviolet light, aflatoxin, vinyl chloride, certain components of tobacco smoke, etc.) bond tightly with DNA to form DNA-carcinogen **adducts**, causing genetic damage that can eventually lead to cancer. Researchers can utilize the unique "biomarkers" left at characteristic locations along certain genes to identify the causative agent of a specific cancer (Semenza and Weasel, 1997).

Cells that have undergone initiation do not inevitably give rise to malignancies, however. Tumor progression is dependent on the **promotion** of initiated cells by long-term exposure to nonmutagenic agents that stimulate cell proliferation, thereby expanding the number of initiated cells and increasing the likelihood that additional mutations will occur within this population. Unlike initiation, which is an irreversible event, promotion can be reversed if the promoting agent is removed (Pitot, 2002). It has long been observed that onset of malignant disease almost always occurs many years after initial exposure to a cancer-causing agent. This characteristically long **latency period** can be explained by the fact that **progression** of cancer requires considerable time (10–30 years or more, depending on the type of cancer) for a precancerous tumor to accumulate the three to seven additional independent, random mutations generally needed to cause malignant growth—a fact which may explain why the chances of developing cancer increase exponentially after the age of 55 (Levine, 2002).

During the 1990s, a number of significant findings by cancer researchers further clarified the nature of the molecular changes within genes that lead to the outward manifestation of cancer. It is now known that two major types of genes are of fundamental importance in cancer causation: **proto-oncogenes** and **tumor-suppressor genes**, both of which play an essential role in regulating the cell cycle. Proto-oncogenes tell the cell when to begin dividing; in so doing, they orchestrate orderly fetal development, the routine replacement of worn-out cells, healing of wounds, and so forth. Mutant versions of these genes, called **oncogenes** (from the Greek word *onkos*, meaning "lump" or "mass"), cause cells to divide endlessly when they should not. By contrast, normal tumor-suppressor genes halt uncontrolled multiplication of cells, acting in a manner analogous to the brakes on an automobile. In mutant form, normal gene function is inactivated, resulting in runaway cell proliferation. Approximately 100 oncogenes and 25 tumor suppressor genes have now been identified as key contributors to the development of many cancers. The *ras* oncogene is known to occur in 50% of colon cancers and 90% of pancreatic cancers. Even more ubiquitous is the tumor-suppressor gene, *p53*, found in altered form in the tumors of more than half of all cancer patients, regardless of the type of cancer involved. Normal functioning of *p53* is especially important because, in addition to preventing uncontrolled cell division, the gene gives instructions for a cell to self-destruct when it detects irreparable damage to DNA during cell division. Because of its role in preventing the dangerous proliferation of mutant cells, *p53* is sometimes referred to as the "guardian of the genome."

Research has shown that the progression of a precancerous tumor to a full-blown malignancy requires a series of mutations that both activate specific oncogenes and inactivate specific tumor-suppressor genes. This sequence of events can be, and usually is, blocked by a number of different bodily defense mechanisms that limit the number of times a cell can divide before dying (cell mortality) or that cause defective cells to self-destruct (apoptosis). Only when all such obstacles are surmounted does cancerous growth commence (Weinberg, 1998).

Undoubtedly, the next few years will witness unprecedented expansion of our knowledge regarding cancer causation—knowledge that will provide an increasing number of weapons for fighting and eventually controlling this dreaded disease. In the meantime, however, society must continue ongoing efforts to prevent exposure to the myriad of environmental agents that are believed responsible for the majority of cancers. While new evidence of inherited predisposition to specific cancers explains why some people are more likely to develop cancer than others, it holds true nevertheless that with most cancers even susceptible individuals are unlikely to develop a malignancy in the absence of adverse environmental exposure. Conversely, even individuals who are not genetically predisposed can experience the DNA damage leading to carcinogenesis if exposure to cancer-causing agents is excessive. By eliminating contact with known carcinogens, one can drastically reduce the incidence of a malignancy—as in so many other realms of life, prevention is the best cure for cancer.

Environmental Carcinogens

The fact that an environmental agent can cause cancer was first reported more than two centuries ago when, in 1775, an English physician, Sir Percival Pott, recognized an association between cancer of the scrotum and exposure to soot. Every patient he examined with this relatively rare ailment had, as a child, worked as a chimney sweep, being lowered naked into chimneys to clean out the soot that accumulated there. In the process, the boys were covered with soot and grime themselves and with the low standards of personal hygiene that characterized those times, some of this soot remained in the folds of the scrotum for long periods, eventually resulting in the development of scrotal cancer years later (more recently the active ingredient in this soot was identified as benzopyrene, known as a very potent carcinogen). Not until the 20th century, however, was much research directed toward detecting environmental carcinogens. Work during the early 1900s revealed the cancer-causing properties of a number of coal tar products and of X-rays, but not until mid-century as age-adjusted cancer rates began to soar did the search for cancer causation acquire new urgency. Since that time the public has been bombarded with so many dire warnings that the average citizen may be excused for thinking that indeed *everything* causes cancer. This of course is untrue, but the very large number of new chemicals and products that are introduced each year, many without adequate testing for harmful side effects, justifies concern. Epidemiologic surveys carried out on the "geography of cancer" indicate that the incidence of certain types of cancer is elevated in heavily industrialized areas.

Researchers and environmentalists alike continue to debate the extent to which present cancer rates reflect exposure to chemical pollutants as opposed to personal habits such as smoking or diet. The outcome of this controversy is obviously of political and economic importance, since extensive regulation would be required to control the former, while education and persuasion represent the practical limits to modifying

Box 6-4 Synergism: 1 + 1 = 5

Virtually all laboratory tests to determine carcinogenicity of suspected substances are based on responses to single-source exposures. Results of such testing methods may significantly underestimate risks in the real world because it is now well known that certain substances in combination are far more hazardous than either one would be if acting independently. For example, people who smoke cigarettes are 10 times more likely to develop lung cancer than are nonsmokers; asbestos workers incur significantly higher risk of lung cancer than do people not exposed to asbestos. However, a person who both smokes cigarettes and works with asbestos is 60 times more likely to get lung cancer than is a person exposed neither to cigarette smoke nor to asbestos—far higher than the risk factor for either type of exposure separately. This phenomenon, where the interaction of two or more substances produces an impact greater than the sum of their independent effects, is known as **synergism** and can perhaps be most easily thought of as a situation where 1 + 1 = 5.

Synergistic effects are well documented in relation to interactions between various air pollutants, water pollutants, and so forth and will be mentioned again in the chapters dealing with those topics. Synergism has been most studied, however, in the context of cancer and smoking in an effort to demonstrate the degree of risk inherent in various types of smokers' lifestyles. In addition to the smoking-asbestos connection, other synergistic associations with smoking include:

1. Smoking and alcohol consumption—as much as a thirtyfold increase in the risk of mouth and throat cancer.

2. Smoking and living in areas of high air pollution—elevated risk of lung cancer.

3. Smoking and working with chemicals or in uranium mines—high lung cancer risk.

the latter. Several of the most prominent public concerns in relation to cancer causation include the following.

Smoking. Tobacco use, particularly cigarette smoking, is now recognized as far and away the leading contributor to cancer mortality. Rates of lung cancer are most reflective of the impact of smoking on health, and the drastic rise in this disease in the United States neatly parallels the increase in the smoking habit in American society. Today about one-third of all U.S. cancer deaths are due to lung cancer, and of the 170,000 new lung cancer victims diagnosed annually in recent years, 87% are cigarette smokers (most of the others are individuals industrially exposed to carcinogens such as asbestos fibers or those exposed to radon gas inside their homes). Death rates among lung cancer victims, as opposed to victims of some other types of cancer, are quite high largely because lung malignancies are seldom diagnosed before the mass has reached a size of about 1 cm in diameter. By that time it has been growing for about 10 years and has usually spread to other parts of the body.

Lung cancer rates began their steady rise in the mid-1930s, approximately 20 years or so after cigarette smoking became popular. Interestingly, until the mid-1950s it was widely assumed that women were resistant to the disease because the incidence of lung cancer among females was negligible compared to that among men. However, over the past 50 years, the incidence of lung cancer among women has soared by 600%, reflecting the growing social acceptance of women's smoking following the "female emancipation" of the 1920s and 1930s. In 1987 lung cancer surpassed breast cancer as the leading cause of cancer mortality among women, making it for the first time the number one cancer killer among both sexes. As the advertisement for Virginia Slims puts it, "You've come a long way, Baby"—all the way from virtually no lung cancer prior to the 1950s to the current situation where more than 80,000 American women are diagnosed with lung cancer each year (Patel, Bach, and Kris, 2004). Thanks to increasing public awareness of the many adverse health impacts of tobacco use following the 1964 Surgeon General's report, the incidence of cigarette smoking among adults in the United States steadily declined from a national average of 42% in 1965 to 21.6% in 2003, holding relatively steady for the last several years. The percentage varies widely among states, with a high of 32.6% in Kentucky and a low of 12.7% in Utah (the U.S. Virgin Islands does even better, with smokers constituting only 9.5% of the adult population). Smoking prevalence is higher for men (24.1%) than for women (19.2%) and is highest among Native Americans (39.7%) as compared with other ethnic groups. Smoking prevalence is inversely associated with educational level, reaching its peak among adults with a GED diploma (44.4%) and lowest (7.5%) among those people with master's, doctoral, or professional degrees (CDC, 2005; 2004a).

Since most smokers acquired their habit as teenagers, health officials have been closely watching trends in tobacco use among young people. They were heartened to note that between 2000–2002, cigarette smoking by high-school students dropped from 28% to 22.9%; it dropped even further by 2003, with 21.9% of teenage females and 21.8% of teenage males using cigarettes. The use of other tobacco products such as cigars, bidis, kretek, and smokeless tobacco declined as well. Unfortunately, there was not a corresponding drop in smoking among middle school students during the same period; 13.3% of children surveyed in grades 6–8 reported using some form of tobacco, most commonly (10.1%) cigarettes. Among both groups, girls were just as likely to smoke as boys, a disturbing fact considering the well-documented adverse impact of maternal smoking in relation to problem pregnancies and birth defects (CDC, 2004b; 2003b).

Elsewhere in the world, the toll of tobacco-related disease mirrors that in the United States. Smoking prevalence in other industrialized countries has equaled or exceeded that in the U.S. for many years and in recent decades many newly affluent developing nations also witnessed an explosive increase in cigarette sales and per-capita cigarette consumption. As a result, throughout the world lung cancer is the leading cause of cancer mortality. There are currently an estimated 1.1 billion smokers worldwide and the consequences of their addiction are evident in the 4.9 million deaths globally caused each year by smoking-related illnesses. The number of victims today is almost evenly divided between those living in developed vs. developing nations—evidence that tobacco is an equal-opportunity killer (Ezzati and Lopez, 2003).

Such trends cause dismay to those who realize that cigarette smoke contains more than 4,700 chemical compounds, of which at least 43 are known carcinogens, including benzo(a)pyrene, arsenic, cadmium, benzene, and radioactive polonium. Since these substances are inhaled, it is not surprising that the lungs are the tissue most directly affected. However, smoking also has been documented as a major cause of cancer of the mouth, esophagus, larynx, and pharynx, and contributes to the development of bladder, kidney, pancreatic, and colon cancer. Smoking also significantly increases the risk of breast cancer for women who began using tobacco at an early age. Research has shown that girls who start smoking within 5 years of their first menstrual period have sharply higher rates of breast cancer during middle age than do women who began smoking after a full-term pregnancy. The presumed explanation for this observed fact is that cells within the breasts of adolescent girls are not yet fully differentiated and are thus quite susceptible to the effects of environmental carcinogens like cigarette smoke; breast cells become fully differentiated only after a first pregnancy, after which they are much less sensitive to carcinogenic chemicals. Such findings make it especially important to intensify public health efforts aimed at discouraging cigarette smoking among young teenage girls. Interestingly, older women who have never been

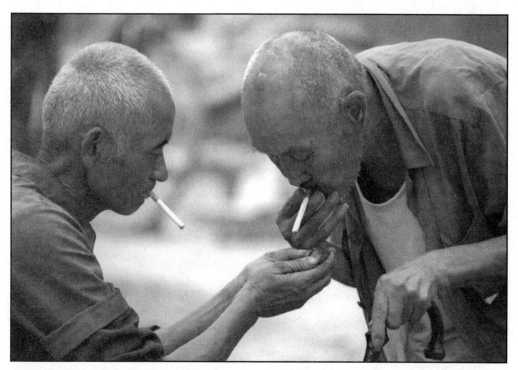

In China, 70% of adult males smoke, and the number of cigarettes smoked per day has been rising steadily, prompting health officials to brace for an epidemic of smoking-related diseases in the years ahead. [*Reuters / Corbis*]

pregnant and who have been heavy smokers (20 or more cigarettes daily) for at least twenty years are also at increased risk of developing breast cancer (Band et al., 2002).

Whatever their age, smokers who quit live longer than those who continue to smoke. However, they continue to have a higher risk for certain types of cancer than do people who never used tobacco. During the past few years, a growing number of smokers report cutting back on the frequency of smoking, using cigarettes some days but not on others. Whether this trend is due to higher taxes on tobacco products, to smoking restrictions, or to personal health concerns is not clear, but research has shown that individuals who reduce their tobacco use, even by 50%, as opposed to quitting entirely are just as likely to die of smoking-related diseases as those who are heavy smokers. Risk begins to decline only with complete cessation of smoking (CDC, 2003a).

Most troubling are research findings that smoking during childhood or adolescence, when lung tissue is particularly sensitive, confers a heightened lifelong risk of cancer even when the individual involved subsequently kicked the habit. Such results are especially disturbing in light of the growing numbers of very young smokers. As one cancer researcher remarked, "We have a generation of people who smoked as teenagers, quit, changed their lifestyles, and now are just walking time bombs for cancer to develop" (Wiencke et al., 1999).

Altogether, it is estimated that smoking is responsible for fully 30% of all cancer-related deaths. In light of these realities, those who look forward to a long and healthy life would do well to consider the categorical advice offered by a former U.S. Surgeon General:

> There is no single action an individual can take to reduce the risk of cancer more effectively than to stop smoking—particularly smoking cigarettes.

Box 6-5 International Initiative to Fight Tobacco: The Framework Convention on Tobacco Control

As the number of smokers in the United States, Canada, and many Western countries continues to fall, tobacco companies seeking to maintain sales and profits are looking to the nations of Asia, Africa, and eastern Europe, where millions of new smokers are taking up the habit. Of the estimated 1.3 billion smokers in the world today (47.5% of all men and 10.3% of women currently use tobacco, according to WHO statistics), 84% live in low or middle-income countries. The global tobacco epidemic, which began in North America and western Europe, is now taking a heavy toll in the developing nations where nearly half of the 4.9 million smoking-related annual deaths occur. Unless action is taken to reverse present trends, experts fear annual global mortality caused by tobacco could rise to 10 million by 2030, with smokers in poor and middle-income countries accounting for 70% of these fatalities. In China, where approximately 70% of males smoke, researchers warn that a million men per year are likely to die of tobacco-related diseases during the first few decades of the 21st century—a number predicted to rise to 3 million annually by 2050 (until quite recently, only 1% of Chinese women smoked, hence the restriction of tobacco-related mortality to men in that country). Russia and the eastern European nations constitute several of the most rapidly growing markets for tobacco sales; Russians now lead the world in per capita cigarette consumption, a fact with ominous implications for Russia's health statistics in the years ahead.

As tobacco-related deaths and disease continue to climb throughout the world, many governments—particularly those in developing countries whose health care budgets are already stretched thin trying to deal with infectious diseases—are beginning to implement antismoking initiatives similar to those already widespread in the United States and some European countries. The international community as a whole became actively involved in fighting the scourge of tobacco-related disease in 1999 when Gro Harlem Brundtland, then Director-General of the World Health Organization, decided to make global tobacco control a WHO priority. During the next four years, representa-tives from around the world negotiated the details of what was to become the **Framework Convention on Tobacco Control (FCTC)**, an international treaty unanimously approved by delegates from 192 countries in March 2003. Despite efforts by "Big Tobacco" to undermine FCTC and to exert pressure on governments to spurn the agreement, the treaty entered into force and became legally binding on Feb. 27, 2005, 90 days after ratification by the requisite 40 signatory nations (the U.S. signed the treaty in 2004 but has not yet ratified it). Stating that FCTC's goal is "to protect present and future generations from the devastating health, social, environmental, and economic consequences of tobacco consumption and exposure to tobacco smoke," framers of the Convention incorporated numerous provisions to achieve this objective, the most significant of which include:

- **Encouragement of higher cigarette taxes.** Experience in several countries has shown that increasing the cost of tobacco products via higher taxes is the most effective means of discouraging smoking, particularly among adolescents. At least 32 U.S. states have raised cigarette taxes during the past several years, in part to enhance state revenues but usually with the justification that doing so served as a deterrent to teenage smoking. In France, where over half of all 15–24 year-olds smoke, the government has recently imposed sharp hikes in the tobacco tax in an effort to reverse teen smoking trends. In the UK, where the cigarette tax in 2004 was $5.03/pack, a 70% increase in the cost of cigarettes over the past 20 years is credited, at least in part, for a 35% decrease in the number of cigarettes smoked. In Norway, the first nation to ratify the FCTC, the cigarette tax is a whopping $5.99/pack. Governments that ratify FCTC are urged to consider national health objectives when deciding how to tax tobacco products and are also encouraged to restrict or prohibit their duty-free sale.

- **A comprehensive ban on tobacco advertising and promotion** within 5 years of ratification. Sponsorship of sporting events by tobacco companies—a more recent tactic by tobacco companies to evade advertising bans—would also be prohibited, as would cross-border advertising (e.g., TV or Internet ads that could be seen by viewers in another country) originating within nations that ratified the treaty.

- **Requirement for prominent warning labels:** FCTC calls for health warning labels to cover at least 50% of the principle display area of the packet and stipulates that these warnings be printed in the language of the country where the product is sold. Within three years of ratification, parties to the agreement must also prohibit misleading terms.

- **Protection of nonsmokers.** Legislating smoke-free workplaces, public transport, and other indoor public spaces was a concept pioneered in the U.S. and constitutes another requirement of FCTC. Supported by scientific research proving that secondhand smoke can cause death and illness among exposed nonsmokers, mandatory smoking restrictions have been adopted by numerous U.S. cities and most states; more recently, other countries have followed suit, recognizing that only a complete ban on public smoking can effectively protect nonsmokers.

The trend toward smoke-free areas seems to be spreading and, in some countries, restrictions are even more comprehensive than the antismoking laws in the United States. By 2005, Ireland, Norway, and the Netherlands, despite considerable controversy, had imposed nationwide bans on smoking in restaurants and bars (immediately after Ireland's prohibition on smoking in pubs went into effect in March 2004, sales of outdoor heaters and awnings for installation outside pubs soared). Most far-reaching of all are the actions of the small Himalayan kingdom of Bhutan which, on the last day of 2004, banned cigarettes completely, making the sale of tobacco products illegal and imposing fines on anyone caught smoking in public.

Additional issues addressed by FCTC provisions include requirements to eliminate tobacco smuggling, to include in national health programs services to help smokers break the habit, to prohibit the sale of tobacco products to minors, and to

encourage litigation against tobacco interests as an antismoking strategy.

Even before the treaty became legally binding on the countries that had ratified it, FCTC motivated many governments to strengthen their own national antismoking programs. Examples include the United Kingdom's reassessment of its policies on exposure to secondhand smoke in public places; Thailand's crackdown on cigarette smuggling; Tanzania's prohibition on smoking in public places; and North Korea's doubling of cigarette prices. In Europe, where the percentage of adults who smoke remains considerably higher than in the U.S., large black-and-white warning labels bearing such blunt admonitions as "Smoking May Cause a Slow and Painful Death" are now mandatory under European Union law. By mid-2005, tobacco advertising on television, radio, and the print media had become illegal throughout the EU; tobacco sponsorship of sporting events has been banned as well, beginning in 2005.

Of course laws are one thing, enforcement another matter entirely. Antismoking advocates acknowledge that achieving a smoke-free environment, regardless of legal victories, will not be easy. Even in countries like France and Germany where laws already call for restaurants to provide nonsmoking sections, few establishments comply. In some countries, especially in southern Europe, it's commonplace to see smokers puffing away while leaning against a "NO SMOKING" sign!

Nevertheless, bit by bit, attitudes are beginning to change as public and policy-makers alike contemplate the devastating health and financial impact wrought by smoking-related disease and acknowledge the validity of the WHO's declaration that:

"A cigarette is the only legally available consumer product that kills through normal use."

References

Action on Smoking and Health (ASH). 2004. "International Tobacco Treaty Has Strong Provisions . . . But We Must First Get It Ratified." *ASH Smoking and Health Review* 34, no. 1 (Jan/Feb):4–5.

Ezzati, Majid, and Alan D. Lopez. 2003. "Estimates of Global Mortality Attributable to Smoking in 2000." *The Lancet* 362, no. 9387 (Sept. 13):847–852.

The European Union's (EU) Commissioner for Health and Consumer Protection recently unveiled a database of 42 new hard-hitting warning labels for cigarette packages as European policymakers intensify their antismoking efforts. [© *European Community, 2005*]

Dietary factors. Approximately one-third of all U.S. cancer deaths are believed to be due to dietary factors, but judging from media accounts, most of us misidentify the main culprits. Recent scares about everything from coffee to charcoal-broiled meat to peanut butter having the potential to cause cancer have prompted consumers to fear that many food additives and contaminants are potential carcinogens—a concern that is reflected in the growing popularity of so-called "natural" or "organic" foods. This topic will be discussed at greater length in chapter 9. Suffice it to say here that although some food additives—particularly the coal tar dyes used for artificial coloring and sodium nitrite in hot dogs—are known to be carcinogenic in tests on laboratory animals, no solid evidence yet exists to indicate that human cancer rates are rising because of these substances in food. However, bearing in mind the long latency period of many forms of cancer and the fact that many additives have been widely used for only a few decades, it may yet be too early to state categorically that such chemicals won't cause future problems.

Ironically, while many people worry, perhaps unjustifiably, about synthetic food additives, they pay little attention to findings regarding naturally occurring carcinogens in food. Substances called **aflatoxins,** potent carcinogens produced by the fungus *Aspergillus flavus*, cause liver cancer in both humans and animals and are suspected of contributing to the high rates of that disease observed in parts of Africa and Southeast Asia. Aflatoxins are known to act synergistically with the hepatitis B virus and with chronic alcohol consumption (National Research Council, 1996). The toxin-producing mold grows on peanuts, pistachios, corn, rice, and certain other grains and nuts when temperatures and humidity are high. If large quantities of aflatoxin are present in the food, liver damage and death may occur very quickly; in small amounts, consumed over a period of time, aflatoxins are among the strongest carcinogens known. Other natural carcinogens in food include safrole, an extract of sassafras long used to flavor root beer until banned by the FDA in 1960, and oil of calamus, used until 1968 to flavor vermouth. On a more cheerful note, it also has been demonstrated that many foods contain *anti*carcinogenic compounds whose regular inclusion in one's diet can be protective against many types of cancer. Most notable in this regard are members of the cabbage family—broccoli, cauliflower, cabbage, kale, and brussels sprouts—whose cells contain **sulforaphane**, one of the most potent anticarcinogens yet discovered. Cooked tomato products rich in **lycopene**—especially tomato sauce, tomato juice, and pizza—have long been associated with a reduced risk of prostate cancer. Other tasty sources of protection against cancer include yellow and green vegetables, citrus fruits, apricots, cantaloupe, brown rice, wheat germ, soy products, onions, and garlic (Giovanucci et al., 1995; Kliewer and Smith, 1995; Davis, 1990).

Perhaps most important of all in reference to food and cancer is the conviction among many researchers that there is a direct correlation between high fat intake and rates of colon and prostate cancer, as well as a relationship between stomach cancer and consumption of smoked, salt-pickled, and salt-cured foods. In addition, being excessively overweight seems to favor development of cancer of the endometrium and gall bladder (Doll, 1996; Willett, 1994). Women who are more than 50 pounds overweight are also at significantly enhanced risk of breast cancer, particularly after menopause (Rose, 1996). However, the widespread suspicion among health experts that breast cancer incidence is closely associated with high-fat diets was dispelled by results of a 14-year study of almost 89,000 women, which demonstrated that those who consume large amounts of fat have no higher risk of developing breast cancer than women whose diet is low in fat. Reducing dietary fat intake confers significant benefits in preventing heart disease, but apparently has no impact one way or the other in reducing breast cancer risk (Holmes et al., 1999). Although much remains to be learned concerning the relationship between dietary factors and cancer, current scientific evidence strongly suggests that a diet rich in a wide variety of fruits, vegetables, beans, and grain products and low in meat, dairy products, and other high-fat foods can significantly reduce overall cancer risk.

Air pollution. It has long been known that urban air contains a number of carcinogenic substances, benzo(a)pyrene among the most potent. Obtaining conclusive proof that breathing polluted air, by itself, induces cancer has been complicated by the fact that many cancer victims living in regions of poor air quality are also smokers. However, a number of well-designed epidemiologic studies, along with research utilizing techniques from molecular genetics, have yielded results demonstrating a clear association between polluted air and increased incidence of lung cancer. In southern California, a study of more than 6,000 nonsmoking Seventh-Day Adventists who had lived in areas with elevated levels of particulate matter, sulfur dioxide, and ozone found an excess rate of lung cancer among both men and women within this population (Beeson, Abbey, and Knutson, 1998). Halfway around the world, in a heavily industrialized region of Poland where coal combustion for industry and home heating has fouled the air for decades, studies have shown a close correlation between lung cancer incidence and residence in highly polluted neighborhoods. Scientists working in Krakow have demonstrated how air contaminants can damage the molecular structure of genes. Examining DNA from white blood cells of Polish central-city residents, researchers found that certain polycyclic aromatic hydrocarbons (PAHs) produced from burning coal bond to the DNA molecule to form PAH-DNA adducts. Since adducts at that location on the gene had previously been linked to elevated lung cancer risk, this finding provides additional evidence that certain air pollutants damage the genetic material and hence play a direct role in cancer causation (Whyatt et al., 1998).

Occupational exposure.   Since the days of Sir Percival Pott's observations on scrotal cancer among chimney sweeps, it has been recognized that certain occupations entail heightened risk of specific diseases. In recent decades the proliferation of new synthetic chemicals in industry, as well as the continued use of older substances only recently recognized as hazardous, has been reflected in cancer rates far higher among certain segments of the workforce than among the general public. Estimates of the number of American workers potentially exposed to chemicals considered by the National Institute of Occupational Safety and Health (NIOSH) to be proven or likely carcinogens range from 3–9 million; many others work with materials suspected to be carcinogens but on which the necessary testing has not yet been done. Although there has been considerable difference of opinion between industry and labor regarding the health impact of exposure to carcinogens in the workplace, researchers estimate that occupational exposure accounts for 4–38% of U.S. cancer incidence (Chivian et al., 1993). Until passage of the Toxic Substances Control Act in 1976, giving the federal government the power to require testing of potentially hazardous substances before they go on the market, hundreds of new chemicals with unknown side effects came into industrial use each year. Unfortunately, the carcinogenicity of many substances was recognized only after exposed workers, like human "guinea pigs," fell sick or died. Some of the most significant industrial carcinogens thus discovered include:

- **Asbestos,** one of the best-known occupational hazards, which is expected to cause the death of 30–40% of all asbestos workers
- **vinyl chloride,** a basic ingredient in the manufacture of plastics, found in 1974 to induce a rare form of liver cancer among exposed workers
- **anesthetic gases** used in operating rooms have been identified as the reason nurse anesthetists develop leukemia and lymphoma at three times the normal rate and also experience higher rates of miscarriage and birth defects among their children
- **benzene,** long known to be a powerful bone marrow poison capable of causing aplastic anemia, has now been shown to cause leukemia as well
- **coke oven emissions** have been linked with cancers of the lung, trachea, bronchus, and kidneys and are now regulated as hazardous air pollutants when vented to the outdoor air
- **benzidine, naphythylamine,** and several other chemicals associated with rubber and dye manufacturing pose an excess risk of bladder cancer to exposed workers in those industries
- **hardwood dust** inhaled by cabinet and furniture makers can lead to malignant nasal tumors
- **radioactive mine dusts** have been a particular problem in uranium mines, resulting in lung cancer rates among miners four times higher than the national average

Although pressure from labor unions and adoption of protective government legislation have resulted in some improvements in reducing occupational hazards, standards set for protecting workers are far less stringent than those set for protecting society at large. In addition, until relatively recently workers often lacked basic information about the nature of the materials with which they worked and were thus unable to take precautions even if they desired to do so. A major step forward in this regard was promulgation by the Occupational Safety and Health Administration (OSHA) in 1983 of its Hazard Communication Standard, intended to provide employees in manufacturing industries access to information concerning the hazards of chemicals that they encounter in the workplace. Essentially a federal "Employee Right-to-Know" law, this ruling requires that U.S. manufacturers inform their employees of any workplace hazards and how they can minimize risk of harm. Manufacturers must also ensure that all chemicals are properly labeled and that Material Safety Data Sheets for each chemical are available for any employee who requests them.

Reproductive/sexual behavior. The National Cancer Institute estimates that 7% of all cancer deaths can be linked with reproductive factors or sexual practices. For reasons thought to relate to hormone levels, breast cancer incidence is significantly higher among women who experienced early onset of menstruation, childless women or women who first gave birth at a late age, and women who were older than average at the time of menopause. Conversely, research suggests that mothers who breast-feed, especially *teenage mothers* who nurse their babies for at least six months, cut their risk of developing breast cancer before menopause nearly in half. For women in their 20s and 30s, prolonged breast-feeding reduces cancer risk by approximately 22%. Although such risk factors are largely beyond the control of the women involved, those who fall into one or more of these categories should be especially conscientious about having regular mammograms once they reach age 40.

Risk factors for cervical cancer are more subject to self-control: early age at the time of first intercourse and multiple sex partners predispose a woman to subsequent development of this type of cancer. Chances of contracting uterine cancer are enhanced by early onset of menstruation, late menopause, a failure to ovulate, a history of infertility, or by excessive obesity (Pitot, 2002).

Preventing Cancer

The preceding discussion should make it apparent that while we still have much to learn about the nature of carcinogenesis, we have already discovered enough to suggest a variety of personal actions that individuals can take to reduce substantially their own risk of developing cancer. Malignancies caused by tobacco use, responsible for more than 170,000 U.S. cancer deaths every year, could be prevented entirely. Eating generous amounts of fruits and green and yellow vegetables daily, while cutting down on meat and total calories could, along with regular exercise, significantly reduce the estimated one-third of fatal cancers attributed to dietary factors. Avoiding excessive sun exposure and using a high-SPF sunscreen when such exposure is unavoidable could have a major impact on reducing new cases of skin cancer, currently totaling over one million annually in the United States. More widespread use of vaccines and antibiotics to prevent or treat infections known to cause several major types of cancer could have a significant impact on lowering cancer incidence, particularly in developing countries where such infections are rampant. Although medical science continues its aggressive search for a cancer cure, even the most optimistic researchers affirm that *preventing* cancer from ever developing is the most effective way of combating this dreaded, but certainly not inevitable, disease.

References

Band, Pierre R., Nhu D. Le, Raymond Fang, and Michele Deschamps. 2002. "Carcinogenic and Endocrine Disrupting Effects of Cigarette Smoke and Risk of Breast Cancer." *The Lancet* 360, no. 9339 (Oct. 5):1044–1049.

Beeson, W. Lawrence, David E. Abbey, and S.F. Knutson. 1998. "Long-Term Concentrations of Ambient Air Pollutants and Incident Lung Cancer in California Adults: Results from the AHSMOG Study." *Environmental Health Perspectives* 106, no. 12 (Dec):813–828.

Bronner, Eric C., et al. 1994. "Mutation in the DNA Mismatch Repair Gene Homologue hMLH1 Is Associated with Hereditary Non-polyposis Colon Cancer." *Nature* 368 (March 17).

Centers for Disease Control and Prevention (CDC). 2005. "Cigarette Smoking Among Adults—United States, 2003." *Morbidity & Mortality Weekly Report (MMWR)* 54, no. 20 (May 27):509–513.

———. 2004a. "State Specific Prevalence of Current Cigarette Smoking Among Adults—United States, 2002." *Morbidity & Mortality Weekly Report* 52, no. 53 (Jan. 9):1277–1280.

———. 2004b. "Cigarette Use Among High School Students—United States, 1991–2003." *Morbidity & Mortality Weekly Report* 53, no. 23 (June 18):499–502.

———. 2003a. "Prevalence of Current Cigarette Smoking Among Adults and Changes in Prevalence of Current and Some Day Smoking—United States, 1996–2001." *Morbidity & Mortality Weekly Report* 52, no. 14 (April 11):303–307.

———. 2003b. "Tobacco Use Among Middle and High School Students—United States, 2002." *Morbidity & Mortality Weekly Report* 52, no. 45 (Nov. 14):1096–1098.

Chivian, Eric, M.D., et al., eds. 1993. *Critical Condition: Human Health and the Environment.* Physicians for Social Responsibility. Cambridge, MA: The M.I.T. Press.

Colborn, Theo, Dianne Dumanoski, and John P. Myers. 1996. *Our Stolen Future.* New York: Dutton, Penguin Books USA.

Cole, Philip, and Brad Rodu. 1996. "Declining Cancer Mortality in the United States." *Cancer* 78, no. 10 (Nov):2045–20248.

Davis, Debra Lee. 1990. "Natural Anticarcinogens: Can Diet Protect Against Cancer?" *Health & Environment Digest* 4, no. 1 (Feb).

Doll, Richard. 1996. "Nature and Nurture: Possibilities for Cancer Control." *Carcinogenesis* 17, no. 2 (Feb):177–184.

Drews, Carolyn D., Catherine C. Murphy, Marshalyn Yeargin-Allsopp, and Pierre Decouflé. 1996. "The Relationship Between Idiopathic Mental Retardation and Maternal Smoking during Pregnancy." *Pediatrics* 97, no. 4 (April):547–553.

Ezzati, Majid, and Alan D. Lopez. 2003. "Estimates of Global Mortality Attributable to Smoking in 2000." *The Lancet* 362, issue 9387 (Sept. 13):847–852.

Fishel, Richard, et al. 1993. "The Human Mutator Gene Homolog MSH2 and Its Association with Hereditary Nonpolyposis Colon Cancer." *Cell* 75 (Dec. 3).

Food and Drug Administration (FDA). 1998. "Once-Feared Drug Provides Relief for Leprosy Symptoms." *FDA Consumer* 32, no. 6 (Nov):2.

Giovanucci, E., A. Ascherio, E.G. Rimm, M. J. Stampfer, G. A. Colditz, and Walter Willett. 1995. "Intake of Carotenoids and Retinol in Relation to Risk of Prostate Cancer." *Journal of the National Cancer Institute* 87, no. 23 (Dec. 6):1767–1776.

Harris, John A., M.D., and Jackie W. Wynne. 1994. "Birth Defects Clusters: Evaluating Community Reports." *Health & Environment Digest* 7 (Feb).

Henderson, Charles W. 1999. "Thalidomide Making Comeback to Treat Cancer, AIDS." *Cancer Weekly Plus* (Jan. 25).

Holmes, Michelle D., David J. Hunter, Graham A. Colditz, Meir J. Stampfer, Susan E. Hankinson, Frank E. Speizer, Bernard Rosner, and Walter C. Willett. 1999. "Association of Dietary Intake of Fat and Fatty Acids with Risk of Breast Cancer." *Journal of the American Medical Association* 281, no. 10 (March 10):914–920.

Human Genome Sequencing Consortium. 2004. "Finishing the Euchromatic Sequence of the Human Genome." *Nature* 431 (Oct. 21):931–945.

Isaacson, Peter G., M.D. 1994. "Gastric Lymphoma and Helicobacter Pylori." *New England Journal of Medicine* 330, no. 18 (May 5).

Jorde, Lynn B., John C. Carey, Michael J. Bamshad, and Raymond L. White. 1999. *Medical Genetics.* St. Louis, MO: Mosby.

Kliewer, Erich, and Ken Smith. 1995. "Breast Cancer Mortality among Immigrants in Australia and Canada." *Journal of the National Cancer Institute* 87, no. 15 (Aug. 2):1154–1161.

Leach, F. S., et al. 1993. "Mutations of a mutS Homolog in Hereditary Nonpolyposis Colorectal Cancer." *Cell* 75, no. 6 (Dec. 17).

Levine, Arnold J. 2002. "The Origins of Cancer and the Human Genome." In *The Genomic Revolution: Unveiling the Unity of Life,* edited by Michael Yudell and Robert DeSalle. Washington, DC: Joseph Henry Press, with the American Museum of Natural History.

Markoff, John. 1992. "Danger of Miscarriage Found for Chip Workers." *New York Times,* Dec. 4.

National Research Council. 1996. *Carcinogens and Anti-Carcinogens in the Human Diet.* Washington, DC: National Academy Press.

Newbold, Retha R., Rita B. Hanson, Wendy N. Jefferson, Bill C. Bullock, Joseph Haseman, and John A. McLachlan. 1998. "Increased Tumors but Uncompromised Fertility in Female Descendents of Mice Exposed Developmentally to DES." *Carcinogenesis* 19, no. 9 (Sept):1655–1663.

Papadopoulos, Nickolas, Nicholas C. Nicolaides, et al. 1994. "Mutation of a mutL Homolog in Hereditary Colon Cancer." *Science* 263 (March 18).

Parkin, D. M., P. Pisani, N. Muñoz, and J. Ferlay. 1999. "The Global Health Burden of Infection Associated Cancers." *Cancer Survey* 33: *Infections and Human Cancer:* 5–33.

Parsonnet, Julie, M.D., et al. 1994. "Helicobacter Pylori Infection and Gastric Lymphoma." *New England Journal of Medicine* 330, no. 18 (May 5).

Patel, J. D., P. B. Bach, and M. G. Kris. 2004. "Lung Cancer in U.S. Women: A Contemporary Epidemic." *Journal of the American Medical Association* 291, no. 14 (April 14):1763–1768.

Perera, Frederica P. 1997. "Environment and Cancer: Who are Susceptible?" *Science* 278, no. 5340 (Nov. 7):1068–1073.

Pitot, Henry C. 2002. *Fundamentals of Oncology.* 4th ed. New York: Marcel Dekker, Inc.

Rose, P. G. 1996. "Endometrial Carcinoma." *New England Journal of Medicine* 335: 640–649.

Sack, George H. 1999. *Medical Genetics.* New York: McGraw-Hill.

Semenza, Jan C., and Lisa H. Weasel. 1997. "Molecular Epidemiology in Environmental Health: The Potential of Tumor Suppressor Gene *p53* as a Biomarker." *Environmental Health Perspectives* 105, suppl. 1 (Feb):155–162.

Shaw, Gary, Cathy R. Wasserman, Edward J. Lammer, Cynthia D. O'Malley, Jeffrey C. Murray, Ann M. Basart, and Marie M. Tolarova. 1996. "Orofacial Clefts, Parental Cigarette Smoking, and Transforming Growth Factor-Alpha Gene Variants." *American Journal of Human Genetics* 58, no. 3 (March):551–561.

"Solvents Used in Making Computer Chips Linked to Workers' Miscarriages at IBM." 1992. *Environmental Health Letter,* Sept. 16.

Stone, Richard. 1992. "Can a Father's Exposure Lead to Illness in his Children?" *Science* 258 (Oct. 2).

"Studies Yield Conflicting Findings on Environment's Link to Cancer." 1994. *Environmental Health Letter,* April 27.

Thacker, Paul D. 2004. "Biological Clock Ticks for Men, Too: Genetic Defects Linked to Sperm of Older Fathers." *Journal of the American Medical Association* 291, no. 14 (April 14):1683–1685.

Warkany, J. 1972. "Trends in Teratologic Research." In *Pathobiology of Development,* edited by E. Perrin and M. Finegold. Baltimore, MD: Williams and Wilkins.

Weinberg, Robert A. 1998. *One Renegade Cell: How Cancer Begins.* New York: Basic Books.

Whyatt, R. M., R. M. Santella, W. Jedrychowski, S. J. Garte, D. A. Bell, R. Ottman, A. Gladek Yarborough, G. Cosma, T. L. Young, T. B. Cooper, M. C. Randall, D. K. Manchester, and F. P. Perera. 1998. "Relationship Between Ambient Air Pollution and DNA Damage in Polish Mothers and Newborns." *Environmental Health Perspectives* 106, suppl. 3 (June):821–826.

Wiencke, John K., Sally W. Thurston, Karl T. Kelsey, Andrea Varkonyi, John C. Wain, Eugene J. Mark, and David C. Christiani. 1999. "Early Age at Smoking Initiation and Tobacco Carcinogen DNA Damage in the Lung." *Journal of the National Cancer Institute* 91, no. 7 (April 7):614–619.

Willett, Walter C. 1994. "Diet and Health: What Should We Eat." *Science* 264 (April 22).

TOXIC SUBSTANCES

> What is it that is not poison?
> All things are poison and nothing is without poison.
> It is the dose only that makes a thing not a poison.
>
> —Paracelsus (16th Century)

Human illness or death due to contact with toxic materials in the environment is certainly not unique to the modern age. Hippocrates described the symptoms of lead poisoning as early as 370 BC; mercury fumes in Roman mines in Spain made work there the equivalent of a death sentence to the unfortunate slaves receiving such an assignment; for centuries Turkish villagers in central Anatolia who live in homes built of asbestos-containing volcanic rock have been dying of lung disease. Yet for the most part, such examples of illness caused by direct contact with toxic substances have been confined to certain occupational groups or to people who, by chance, happened to be living in an area where there was an unnaturally high concentration of some toxic material. By and large, in the past large populations seldom, if ever, were exposed to significant amounts of toxicants on a sustained basis. Today, however, that situation is changing, thanks in part to the tremendous increase in industrial production since the early 20th century, as well as to the "chemical revolution" that has introduced thousands of new synthetic compounds into widespread use in recent decades. Some of these substances, several of which were briefly mentioned in the preceding chapter, are largely confined to an occupational setting and pose little threat to the general public. Others, however, are now virtually omnipresent throughout the human environment and are generating considerable controversy as to the degree of public health threat they present.

In this chapter we will describe the process by which chemicals are tested for toxicity and their health risks assessed. We will then take a closer look at several of these substances—some naturally occurring, others artificially produced—to which human exposure is nearly universal and which are known to cause serious health damage.

Testing for Toxicity

"Toxic" or "toxicant" are terms scientists use to describe a chemical that provokes an adverse systemic effect on living organisms. That is, **toxicants** have the ability to cause harm to organs or biochemical processes away from the site on the body where exposure occurred. In this sense they differ from other harmful chemicals such as corrosives or irritants, which damage only the tissues they contact. For example, spilling concentrated acid on one's hand will result in a painful chemical burn, followed by loss of skin, but damage is localized to that area. By contrast, ingesting small amounts of arsenic over an extended time period can result in cirrhosis of the liver, skin discoloration, and peripheral nerve damage, among other problems. "Poison," a word many people use as a synonym for toxic, actually has a much narrower meaning, referring to a chemical that can cause illness or death at a very low dose of exposure—approximately 3/4 of a teaspoon for an adult or 1/8 of a teaspoon for a toddler. Very few chemicals are capable of causing death in such low amounts, hence the list of true poisons is much shorter than commonly believed. Another term frequently equated with "toxic" is "hazardous," whose actual meaning is more complex. The hazardous nature of a substance is dependent both on its inherent capacity to do harm (e.g., its degree of toxicity, corrosiveness, flammability, etc.) and, equally important, on the likelihood of that substance coming into contact with people. Methyl parathion, one of the most toxic insecticides, presents an extreme hazard to migrant farm workers entering a just-sprayed field without protective clothing; the very same chemical presents virtually no hazard when stored in its original container inside a securely locked storeroom.

The study of toxic substances, or **toxicology**, in an informal sense is probably as old as the human species. Long before written records were kept, ancient peoples learned through trial and error which plants and animals should be avoided because of their toxic properties. Among classical civilizations, knowledge of mineral toxicants was well established and was extensively applied to the art of poisoning one's enemies! Modern toxicology is a relatively recent offshoot of pharmacological science, its origin as an independent field of inquiry prompted initially by the needs of occupational medicine. Toxicology has gained added importance in recent decades due to the rapid growth of the chemical industry and associated public concerns regarding health effects of toxic chemicals.

Whether a chemical provokes a toxic effect—or any effect at all—is dependent on a number of variables, the most important of which is the **dose-time** relationship, that is, the amount of the chemical in question (dose) and the duration of exposure (time). Depending on the nature of the dose-time relationship, toxicity can be categorized as either acute or chronic. A chemical's **acute toxicity** refers to its ability to cause harm as a result of one-time exposure to a relatively large amount of the substance. Most accidental childhood poisonings (e.g., drinking a liquid pesticide stored in a cola bottle) represent harm caused by acutely toxic chemicals. **Chronic toxicity**, by contrast, refers to a chemical's ability to impair health when repeated low-dose exposure to the chemical occurs over a long time period. Interestingly, the effects of acute vs. chronic toxicity for the same chemical are often quite different in terms of symptoms and bodily organs involved. As an example, with acute exposure lead poisoning manifests itself as severe abdominal pains, while chronic lead toxicity provokes anemia and nervous system damage. Not only is there no correlation between acute and chronic toxicity symptoms, there also is no connection between their relative potency. A chemical that is very toxic in acute exposure situations may be nontoxic chronically. Similarly, a chemical with minimal acute toxicity may present a greater danger when exposure is chronic.

Another parameter influencing toxicity is the chemical's route of exposure. Toxic substances can enter the body through the mouth when a person eats, drinks, or smokes (**oral**); through the skin (**dermal**); or via the lungs if the substance is inhaled (**respiratory**). Depending on the chemical in question, toxicity will vary, depending on the route of exposure—very few chemicals are equally toxic by all three routes.

Toxicity is also profoundly affected by species, a fact that troubles those questioning the validity of animal testing procedures. Chemicals that are very toxic to some animal species may be only slightly toxic or nontoxic to others, including humans. Close taxonomic relationship is no predictor of how a particular species will react in a toxicity test. For some chemicals, toxicity in both humans and monkeys is very similar, while for other substances humans may join cats and dogs in being highly sensitive while monkeys suffer no adverse effects. Just as genetic variability *among* species influences toxicity, so do genetic differences *within* a population. Individual susceptibility, based on each person's (or each guinea pig's) biochemical makeup, explains the range of effects among members of a group exposed to exactly the same dose of any substance.

Determining the acute, subchronic, and chronic toxicity of a chemical is necessary in order to establish protective regulations. Acute toxicity is generally described using the technical term LD_{50} (LD=lethal dose), which refers to the amount of the chemical, administered in one dose, that is required to kill 50% of a population of test animals within a 14-day period. LD_{50} is expressed as the number of milligrams of chemical per kilogram of body weight. Thus the lower the LD_{50}, the smaller the dose required to kill; in other words, the lower the LD_{50}, the more acutely toxic the chemical is (substances legally termed "poisons" are those with an LD_{50} of 50 or less). For obvious reasons, acute toxicity testing is restricted to populations of laboratory animals; thus when results are used to estimate lethal doses for humans, considerable judgment must be exercised, recognizing that humans may be more or less sensitive than the test species. For some chemicals, unfortunately, direct human results may supplement animal data. When known quantities of a toxicant are involved in accidental poisonings, suicides, murders, or industrial accidents, these quantities can be related to the severity and type of symptoms and then compared with animal test results. If such data indicate the chemical is more or less toxic to humans than to animals, the human results supersede the animal data.

Testing for subchronic and chronic toxicity is more difficult, time-consuming, and expensive than acute toxicity testing and considerably less is known about the long-term effects of a chemical than about its acute effects. Symptoms of chronic toxicity may take months or years to manifest themselves, and because such symptoms are often similar to other common health complaints they may be misdiagnosed.

Testing for subchronic and chronic toxicity involves animal-feeding experiments, most commonly using rats or dogs. After determining the daily dose of chemical the animals are likely to be able to tolerate for long periods (a determination based on the chemical's LD_{50}), the animals are divided into three or more test groups, plus a control group. Each group will have the same number of animals and a balanced male/female ratio. Beginning at the time the animals are weaned, each group of test animals is fed a specified level of the toxicant mixed with its feed. One group receives a dose expected to have significant sublethal chronic effects; one group receives an amount of the toxicant predicted to have no effect; the third group is fed a level of toxicant intermediate between the other two. The control group is treated in exactly the same manner as the other animals except that no toxicant is added to its food. Subchronic toxicity tests typically are run for 90 days, their main intent being to establish levels of exposure at which no adverse effects can be observed and to identify which organ or organs suffer damage after repeated exposure to the toxicant being tested. Daily records are kept detailing the animals' appearance and behavior. At the end of the three-month test period, the animals are killed and autopsied, being carefully examined for evidence of organ damage or other adverse changes. Tests for chronic toxicity are conducted in the same manner as described for subchronic testing, except that the duration of exposure to the chemical is considerably longer. Chronic toxicity tests are usually carried out for a time period equivalent to the average lifespan of the test animals (generally rats or mice). Since determination of a chemical's carcinogenicity is a prime goal of chronic toxicity tests, autopsies performed at the conclusion of the test period are focused specifically on the incidence and location of tumors.

The data collected from these studies are plotted on a **dose-response curve**, which has three parts. The first portion of the curve, on the far left, is horizontal—an indication that low doses of the toxicant produce no ill effects. The middle portion of the curve begins at a point called the **threshold**, where increasing dosage is beginning to provoke adverse symptoms. The curve continues to climb upward as the dose increases until, in its final portion, it again flattens out after reaching its maximum effect (i.e., death). The dose-response curve describes one of the most basic principles of toxicology—the greater the dose of a toxicant, the greater the effect. If all groups of test animals displayed the same symptoms of harm, or if the group fed the lowest level of toxicant suffered more adverse health effects than the group receiving the highest dose, it could be concluded that something other than the toxicant caused the observed problems. Demonstration of the existence of thresholds is also of great importance to an understanding of toxicity. Because the threshold of toxicity for a chemical varies among species, as well as within a population of the same species and even in the same individual, depending on age and health status, it will probably never be possible to determine precisely where the threshold of tolerance is for any particular person. Nevertheless, knowing that there *is* a safe level of exposure facilitates regulation by providing a basis for establishing **margins of safety**—a buffer zone between the highest level of a chemical that produces no adverse effect in an animal species and a level of exposure assumed to be safe for humans. In the United States, a hundredfold margin of safety has traditionally been employed for regulatory control of toxic substances. This number was arbitrarily chosen, based on the assumptions that (1) humans are 10 times more susceptible to the toxic effects of chemicals than are laboratory animals and (2) the more vulnerable members of the population—young children, the elderly, the immunocompromised—are 10 times more sensitive than the average healthy adult. In spite of the uncertainties inherent in such assumptions, the fact that legal exposure limits to toxicants are well below the no-effect level should lend comfort to citizens beset by the chemophobia so widespread in modern society (Ottoboni, 1991).

Figure 7-1   Dose-Response Curve

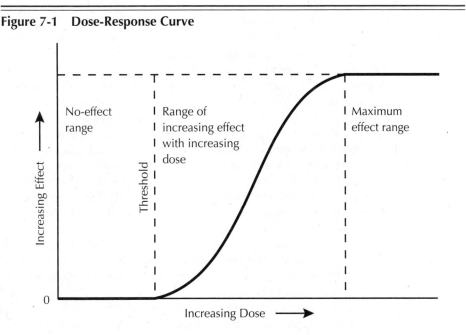

Assessing Health Risk

As fears of the potentially harmful health effects of chemical exposure have increased in recent decades, a concerned public has demanded that government act to manage such risks. Doing so effectively requires decision makers to determine whether a particular substance presents a greater danger than society is willing to accept, to examine the available options for controlling such hazards, and then to adopt policy measures (i.e., regulatory controls, product bans, market-based incentives, educational efforts) that reduce or eliminate unacceptable risk. **Risk management**, however, is dependent on accurate **risk assessment**—determining whether something suspected of presenting a human health threat is in fact dangerous, estimating how much injury or harm is likely to result from a given level of exposure, and determining if those consequences are serious enough to warrant action.

Health risk assessment began to receive serious professional attention early in the 20th century when adverse effects associated with certain types of occupational exposures were described. Investigations into the relationship between levels of exposure and the observed human health effects led to the identification of **no-observed-effect-levels (NOELs)** and the establishment of adequate margins of safety for exposure. By the early 1970s, creation of the U.S. Environmental Protection Agency and the Occupational Safety and Health Administration—agencies charged with writing regulations and implementing the provisions of a number of far-reaching new environmental, health, and safety laws—gave health risk assessment a major boost. By necessity, risk assessment became a prime component of the regulatory decision-making process, and modern quantitative methods of analysis emerged in response to this need. During the past 35 years, health risk assessments have been employed for a wide range of regulatory issues: food additives, pesticide residues, drinking water contaminants, indoor air pollutants, and so forth. Although hazardous substances can adversely affect human health in various ways—immune system dysfunction, reproductive or teratogenic effects, organ damage, nervous system impairment—the potential carcinogenicity of suspect chemicals has been the main focus of health risk assessments in recent years.

Health risk assessment constitutes a four-step process:

1. *Hazard identification.* Aimed at determining whether a particular substance or agent has an adverse effect on human health (e.g., is the substance carcinogenic?). Such a determination is typically made on the basis of animal testing, as described in box 6-3. If these tests indicate no harm from exposure, there is no need for further investigation; on the other hand, if exposure to the substance causes death or injury to some of the test animals, risk assessment proceeds to the next step.

2. *Dose-response assessment.* Since health effects of the same substance can be either harmful, beneficial, or neutral, depending on the amount of exposure received, determining the dose at or below which no effects are detected is important for establishing safety standards. For noncarcinogenic toxic substances this is a relatively straightforward process; empirical evidence has shown that biological effects of exposure to noncarcinogenic chemicals appear only after a threshold level has been exceeded. Exposing laboratory animals to varying doses of the agent in question permits identification of the lowest-observable-effect-level (LOEL), the no-observed-adverse-effect-level (NOAEL)—the dose at or below which no *harmful* effects are observed, and the no-observed-effect-level (NOEL). This dose-response information facilitates the determination of threshold levels of exposure.

For carcinogens, however, the situation is complicated by a working assumption, adopted by regulatory agencies on the premise it's better to be safe than sorry, that there is *no threshold* for cancer-causing substances—even one molecule of a carcinogen can initiate cancer. Evidence has been growing that this assumption is incorrect and that, for some carcinogens at least, a threshold does, in fact, exist. Nevertheless, the no-threshold approach to regulating carcinogens still applies. All parties to the controversy agree, however, that the risk of developing cancer is much greater when the exposure dose is high than when it is low.

3. *Exposure assessment.* Attempting to determine the numbers and types of people (age, sex, health status, etc.) who might be exposed to the substance in question, as well as estimating the duration, magnitude, and geographic extent of exposure, constitute the third step in the risk assessment process. In many real-life situations, some of the necessary information is unavailable—particularly actual exposure data—and those performing the analysis frequently must resort to computer modeling based on generalized assumptions about human behavior and how chemicals move in the environment. Generalizations on behavior include guesses on the kinds and quantities of food individuals in the target population eat each day; how much water they drink; how much time they spend indoors vs. outdoors. Assumptions regarding the environmental mobility of a chemical deal with its chemical stability, whether it dissolves in water or animal fat, how quickly it evaporates, or whether it binds to soil. The validity of assumptions about such parameters, in the absence of actual measurements, is questionable, making exposure assessment one of the weaker links in the information chain.

4. *Risk characterization.* Combining the information obtained from the first three steps of the risk assessment process, analysts produce a comprehensive picture of the types of adverse health effects likely to occur in exposed populations and the frequency with which such effects can be expected to occur. Risk is usually expressed in terms of quantitative probability; for example, one cancer death per 10,000 exposed population or 10^{-4} risk. For noncarcinogens, the risk characterization typically yields **Acceptable Daily Intakes (ADIs)** derived from dividing animal study NOELs by safety factors.

Information gathered through the risk assessment process is of great value to risk managers, but such data are incapable of answering many of the values-based questions with which decision makers wrestle: How safe is "safe enough"? What trade-offs between risks, benefits, and costs of control are justified? Will reducing an existing risk merely replace it with a newer, more dangerous one? Which among competing risks merits the greatest attention and resource allocation for abatement? Societal values and priorities must inevitably be taken into account in resolving these issues. Trade-offs among competing interests, political considerations, legal obligations, and scientific uncertainties are all factors that risk managers weigh as they decide how best to reduce hazards and protect public health. Risk assessment, while not perfect, provides a valuable tool for making appropriate decisions (American Chemical Society, 1998).

Polychlorinated Biphenyls (PCBs)

In 1964 Dr. Soren Jensen, a Swedish chemist at the University of Stockholm, began a project to determine DDT levels in human fat and wildlife samples; instead he discovered that the tissues he was examining contained large amounts of synthetic organic chemicals called PCBs. His findings, published in 1966, were greeted with widespread surprise and disbelief because PCBs, unlike DDT and other chlorinated hydrocarbon pesticides, were not being deliberately released into the environment but were restricted to use in industrial settings. Despite the initial skepticism, subsequent studies by researchers in many countries confirmed Dr. Jensen's findings. Virtually every tissue sample tested, from fish to birds to polar bears to animals living in deep sea trenches, contained detectable levels of PCBs. Extensive research during the decades that followed revealed that of all the chemical contaminants known, PCBs are the most widespread throughout the global environment.

How Could This Situation Come About?

Polychlorinated biphenyls were first synthesized in 1929, their production being taken over in 1930 by Monsanto, which sold the chemical under the trade name Arochlor. PCBs, which range in consistency from oily liquids to waxy solids, are extremely stable substances with a high boiling point, high solubility in fat but low solubility in water, low electrical conductivity, and high resistance to heat—all qualities that made them valuable for a wide variety of industrial uses. Primarily employed as cooling liquids in electrical transformers and capacitors, PCBs also have been used in hydraulic fluids, in carbonless carbon paper, insulating tapes, adhesives, paints, caulking compounds, sealants, and as road coverings to control dust.

The chemical stability that made PCBs so attractive to industry, however, is the very characteristic that has made them such an environmental and health hazard. Although designed for industrial use, there are many ways in which PCBs can inadvertently escape and contaminate the environment:

1. Discharge of PCB-laden wastes from factories into waterways have resulted in mammoth pollution problems, the most notorious episodes being Outboard Marine Corporation's dumping of PCBs into Waukegan Harbor (on Lake Michigan) and a similar situation in the Hudson River, traced to two General Electric plants.

2. Vaporization from paints or landfills or burning of PCB-containing material can result in the chemical becoming airborne and then reentering the ecosystem with precipitation. EPA estimates that approximately 89% of PCBs entering Lake Superior are deposited via airborne fallout (EPA, 1994). A classic example of fire causing extensive PCB contamination occurred early in 1981 in Binghamton, New York, where PCB-containing electrical equipment in the basement of the newly built State Office Building caught fire. Although the blaze was quickly extinguished, inspectors subsequently discovered that contaminated soot had been carried through the air conditioning system and deposited throughout the entire building. Air sampling indicated that this soot contained 10–20% PCBs, as well as lesser amounts of dioxin and dibenzofurans formed during the combustion process. The ensuing cleanup operation took seven years to complete and cost New York taxpayers $37 million (Fawcett, 1988).

3. Leaks in industrial equipment have resulted in numerous instances of PCB contamination, such as the case during the summer of 1979 when 200 gallons of PCBs leaked from an electrical transformer at a feed processing plant in Billings, Montana, contaminating about a million pounds of meal used in chicken feed. Subsequently, $2.7 million worth of chickens and eggs had to be destroyed because the birds had eaten the contaminated meal before the leak was discovered (Regenstein, 1982).

4. Accidental spills or illegal dumping are a source of concern because the high cost of legally disposing of PCB wastes has tempted some haulers to dump such materials along roadsides, in ditches, or other out-of-the-way places. In the summer of 1978 such "midnight dumpers" opened the discharge pipe of their truck while driving along 243 miles of back roads in 14 North Carolina coun-

ties, releasing 31,000 gallons of PCB-laden waste oil along the roadside where it remained until a major remediation effort, jointly funded by the EPA and the State of North Carolina, was launched to remove the contaminated soil and bury it in a hazardous waste landfill constructed for that purpose in 1983.

Whatever the route, once PCBs enter the environment they persist there for decades, resisting breakdown. Contamination of living organisms with PCBs generally occurs via the food chain, the concentration of the chemical increasing as it moves from lower to higher trophic levels ("biomagnification," see chapter 8). Within an individual organism, especially among higher-level consumers such as carnivorous birds, fish, and humans, PCBs accumulate in fatty tissues such as liver, kidneys, heart, lungs, brain, and breast milk. By 1976, after more than forty years of PCB production and use, 99% of all breast milk sampled in the United States contained PCBs. A quarter of the samples tested exceeded the legal level of contamination, which would have caused a commercial product to be banned from sale (Steingraber, 1997). With continuing exposure, PCB concentrations in the body increase over a period of time, a process known as **bioaccumulation**.

PCB Threat to Health

Widespread human exposure to PCBs has concerned health and regulatory officials because laboratory testing has shown the chemicals to be toxic to several animal species even at very low concentrations. In experiments with rodents, minks, and Rhesus monkeys, PCB exposure has resulted in the development of a number of adverse health effects: liver disorders, miscarriage, low birthweight, abnormal multiplication of cells, and (in rats only) liver cancer. Researchers presumed that chemicals that could produce such effects in some mammalian species were likely to have similar effects on humans, and the knowledge that virtually everyone on the planet has been exposed to at least trace amounts of PCBs was considered cause for alarm. Evidence that many foods, especially freshwater fish, were contaminated with PCBs prompted the U.S. government to take regulatory action. In 1973 the FDA established tolerance levels for PCBs in food; passage of the Toxic Substances Control Act in 1976 specifically banned the production, sale, distribution, and use of PCBs in open systems; and in 1977, Monsanto, the sole U.S. manufacturer of the chemicals, terminated PCB production.

In the meantime, research on the human health impact of PCBs continued and today a wealth of scientific data exists on the chemical's toxicological effects. Contrary to popular perception, the acute toxicity of PCBs is quite low. The most frequent complaint provoked by high levels of PCB exposure is the appearance of an acne-like skin disorder referred to as chloracne. Regarded as the most characteristic symptom of PCB poisoning (or poisoning with any of the related group of chemicals known as chlorinated hydrocarbons), chloracne was an occasional occupational health problem among workers during the early years of PCB production and use. Recognition of this hazard led to the establishment in 1942 of recommended maximum allowable concentrations in the workplace. Since then, with the exception of a few cases of chloracne and possibly diminished liver function, scarcely any adverse health effects attributable to PCB exposure have been documented, even among workers who were exposed to PCBs over a period of many years.

For humans, exposure to PCBs could occur via skin absorption if a person happens to touch PCB-containing lubricants or oils leaking from old equipment or if he/she were to swim in PCB-contaminated waters. Dermal exposure, however, poses far less of a health risk than does either inhalation or ingestion of PCBs. People living near hazardous waste sites or landfills where PCBs are present can be exposed to these chemicals by inhaling PCBs evaporating from the soil into the air or by drinking contaminated groundwater. The most common route of entry, affecting the largest number of people, is consumption of sports fish caught in PCB-contaminated lakes and rivers. Meat and dairy products may also constitute dietary sources of PCBs, though to a lesser degree than fish (ATSDR, 2000).

Concerns about PCBs in fish made news in 2004 with the publication of research indicating that farmed salmon, one of America's most popular fish, contains potentially dangerous levels of PCBs, as well as dioxin and several organochlorine pesticides. The presence of these contaminants in farmed salmon is blamed on the fact that these fish are raised on a concentrated feed made of various PCB-tainted fish oils and fish meals (a mixture that is already being modified in response to the adverse market reaction to this news). Interestingly, PCB levels in farmed salmon vary widely, depending on the area where they are raised; those from European salmon farms tested highest for contamination, while those from Chile were lowest, with North American salmon registering levels somewhere in between. The report's authors concluded that because of the high PCB levels, farmed salmon consumption should be limited to one meal per month in order to avoid increased risk of cancer. Such advice is hotly disputed by other scientists who point out that, although elevated, the PCB levels documented aren't high enough to pose serious danger and don't outweigh the undisputed nutritional benefits of farmed salmon, specifically the protection against heart attacks conferred by their omega-3 polyunsaturated fatty acids. Part of the dispute between scientists on both sides of the debate relates to the fact that the "safe" level set by the Food and Drug Administration (FDA) for PCBs in fish sold in supermarkets—a level based on nutritional benefits as well as safety considerations—is 40 times higher than EPA's standard for fish caught by sports fishers, for which health is the sole consideration. According to FDA standards, the PCB levels detected in farmed salmon are not excessive, while under EPA guidelines they are. As the experts wrangle over these questions, aquaculturists are hard at work, experimenting with new feed mixtures that will eliminate the PCB problem. One approach would substitute the fish oil component with a variety of transgenic canola oil containing a precursor to omega-3 fatty acids (Hites et al., 2004; Stokstad, 2004).

Since few members of the general public ever receive the relatively high levels of exposure experienced by workers in an occupational setting, the main concern about PCBs' possible health impact has focused on chronic toxicity, specifically their potential to cause cancer. Since animal studies indicate that PCBs are carcinogenic in rodents, it was feared that the same would be true in humans—one of the main reasons advanced to justify banning the chemical. However, after decades of research, no link between chronic PCB exposure and human cancer has been found. In 1999, the largest epidemiologic study to date found no increase in cancer deaths among more than 7,000 workers exposed to PCBs from 1946–1976 (Kimbrough, Doemland, and LeVois, 1999). The evidence thus appears convincing that even among those occupationally exposed to the chemical, PCBs do not cause cancer in humans. PCBs have not yet been acquitted of all charges of adverse human health effects, however. Their role as one of a group of so-called "endocrine disruptors" is now being actively investigated (see box 7-1) and may yet vindicate the legal action taken against them a quarter century ago.

Although PCB production in the United States halted in 1977, the chemicals remain very much a part of the American scene. During the years 1929–1977, 1.4 billion pounds of PCBs were produced in the United States. Decades later, millions of pounds remain in use, mainly in closed systems such as high-voltage capacitors (com-

Box 7-1   Hormonal Havoc

Until recently, PCBs, dioxins, and a host of other persistent organic pollutants were the focus of public fear and scientific scrutiny largely because of their presumed role as major contributors to rising cancer rates. Decades of intensive research have failed to support the widespread conviction that these chemicals are important environmental carcinogens, but a growing body of evidence now suggests they play a more insidious role as **endocrine disruptors.**

At least 50 different chemicals have now been identified as capable of interfering with the normal functioning of the endocrine system in both animals and humans. The culprits include lead and mercury—both naturally occurring heavy metals—but the majority are synthetic compounds, including many long-lasting chemicals that concentrate as they move up the food chain and tend to be dispersed widely throughout the environment. PCBs, dioxin, DDT, chlordane, atrazine, lindane, phthalates, and styrene are but a few of the synthetic organic chemicals known to act as endocrine disruptors. Although several of these compounds, including DDT and chlordane, are no longer being manufactured or used in most developed countries, they are still detectable in trace quantities throughout the environment and, unlike conventional toxicants, can wreak hormonal havoc even when present in extremely minute concentrations. Indeed, in terms of dose-response relationships, endocrine disruptors are unusual in that low levels of exposure tend to elicit a greater adverse response than do high doses.

Endocrine hormones play a pivotal role in regulating such vital processes as fetal development, sexual differentiation, reproduction, brain development, and immune system functioning; anything that prevents the correct chemical messages from being received is bound to cause trouble. Endocrine disruptors are believed to interfere with these processes by acting as "hormone mimics," replacing the natural hormones that bind to the hormone receptor molecules within cells, or as "hormone blockers," preventing natural hormones from attaching to a receptor. Embryonic development is particularly vulnerable to the effects of endocrine disruptors. Exposure that provokes only temporary effects in adults can produce permanent and far-reaching damage to an embryo or fetus if it occurs at a critical developmental stage.

Evidence demonstrating the harmful impact of endocrine-disrupting chemicals has come primarily from wildlife studies. As early as the 1950s and 1960s, researchers noted that animal populations as diverse as eagles in Florida, trout in Lake Ontario, and commercially raised mink in Michigan were experiencing reproductive failure, a problem eventually traced in part to their exposure to synthetic insecticides, dioxins, and PCBs, respectively. In the 1970s, biologists in California reported another strange phenomenon among western gull populations—females nesting with other females. Over the next 20 years, similar same-sex pairings were observed in waterfowl populations in the Great Lakes, Puget Sound, and off the coast of Massachusetts. In the late 1980s, wildlife biologists in Florida, searching the shores of Lake Apopka for alligator eggs, discovered to their dismay that only a small percentage of the eggs collected were viable, and half the baby alligators from the few eggs that did hatch died within ten days. Even more surprising was the fact that when male alligators were captured and examined closely, approximately 60% exhibited abnormally small penises. Alligator populations in other Florida lakes were flourishing, indicating some sort of localized problem. Researchers knew that almost a decade earlier, a spill from a nearby chemical factory had polluted Lake Apopka with the insecticide dicofol, but by the time biologists were scratching their heads over alligator reproductive failures, the lake appeared to be clean again. Whatever was causing the observed problems was obviously potent in very minute quantities.

Reports of abnormal sexual development and behavior, congenital abnormalities, and immune system dysfunction began appearing with increasing frequency in scientific journals during the late 1980s and early 1990s. More and more, researchers attributed the problems they were seeing to substances that acted like the sex hormones estrogen, progesterone, or testosterone to alter normal sexual development, or that interfered with thyroid metabolism, thereby adversely affecting development of the brain or reproductive organs. Knowing that differences between endocrine system functioning in humans and other animal species are negligible, scientists were concerned that the problems they were observing among wildlife populations might be occurring in humans as well.

Direct evidence for human health damage caused by endocrine disruptors is less compelling than that for wildlife effects, however. Demonstration of a link between fetal exposure to diethylstilbestrol and subsequent abnormalities of the reproductive system in DES-sons and daughters provides the most clear-cut association, but the fact that the exposure dose received by these individuals was much higher than the levels of endocrine disruptors in the general environment makes it problematic to extrapolate findings from long-term DES studies to the wider public. In the 1980s several European studies that documented a dramatic decline in human sperm counts over the past several decades attracted considerable attention and caused some observers to speculate that endocrine disruptors might be responsible. However, subsequent surveys in various parts of the world have yielded conflicting results, some corroborating the earlier research, others indicating no change in sperm counts or even an increased count in some groups studied. To date, investigators have been unable to reach a consensus on whether sperm counts are falling or not and on the extent to which endocrine disruptors are responsible for such a decline if it has, in fact, occurred.

Another source of evidence cited as suggestive of human health damage is a study that focused on the children of mothers consuming significant amounts of PCB-tainted Lake Michigan fish during pregnancy. Babies whose mothers had eaten the most fish tested highest for blood PCB levels and were smaller at birth than babies born to mothers who hadn't consumed Lake Michigan fish. Developmental testing of these children continued at intervals during their childhood years; researchers found that the children whose pregnant mothers had eaten the most fish were less cooperative in terms of behavior, had poorer memories, lower IQ, and had a shorter attention span than did the children of nonfish-eating mothers. These results are particularly worrisome because the PCB levels to which these children were exposed were not a great deal higher than concentrations prevailing among the general population.

Accurately assessing the human impact of endocrine disruptors is fraught with difficulties, not the least of which is the lack of a control population to compare the effects of exposure vs. nonexposure. Even in the most remote spots on the planet, people carry a measurable body burden of PCBs, DDT, and other persistent organic pollutants. Indeed, the Inuit people inhabiting islands in the Canadian Arctic, west of Greenland, exhibit some of the highest PCB levels ever detected in human populations. Another challenge is accounting for the additive or synergistic effects of exposure to the dozens of different chemicals to which humans are simultaneously exposed every day.

Despite these difficulties, intensive research efforts are currently underway to assess whether and to what extent endocrine disruptors are undermining our biological future as individuals and as a species. In the United States a number of federal agencies and institutes have launched close to 400 research projects dealing with the issue; many state environmental agencies are actively investigating the problem also, as is the chemical industry itself. Overseas, a number of national governments and international organizations, including the World Health Organization, are engaged in research efforts as well. It may be many years before these projects provide definitive answers, but in the meantime there are a number of actions individuals can take to reduce exposure to hormone mimics and hormone blockers: (1) avoid use of chemical pesticides to the greatest extent possible; don't permit children or pets to play on pesticide-treated lawns; (2) heed state-issued fish advisories; don't fish downstream from golf courses due to pesticide runoff from these heavily-treated grasses; (3) limit consumption of fatty meats and dairy products; (4) wash fruits and vegetables thoroughly to remove pesticide residues; better yet, grow your own chemical-free produce; and (5) when using a microwave oven, don't allow plastic wrap to touch food.

Reference

Colborn, T., Dumanoski, D., and Myers, J. P. 1996. *Our Stolen Future*. New York: Dutton.

mon on ordinary utility poles), electrical transformers, and fluorescent light ballasts. In addition, approximately 500 million pounds of PCBs have been dumped into land-fills and waterways where they continue to pose an environmental threat. As existing PCB-containing equipment becomes obsolete and is replaced, safe methods for dis-posing of this material must be found. Currently, high-temperature (2200° F or above) incineration is the EPA-approved method for destroying wastes containing high con-centrations of PCBs.

Many of the locations where PCB wastes were carelessly or illegally dumped years ago have now been targeted for remedial cleanup by state environmental agen-cies or, in the most serious cases, under the federal Superfund program (see chapter 16). Of the slightly more than 1,500 federal Superfund sites, approximately 500 involve PCB contamination. At present, one of the major projects scheduled for Superfund remediation is a 40-mile stretch of the Upper Hudson River where Gen-eral Electric dumped its toxic wastes decades ago. EPA is requiring GE to pay for dredging and removal of approximately 2.65 million cubic yards of PCB-contami-nated sediment.

Dioxin (TCDD)

In the wet spring of 1983 public apprehension about the dangers of dioxin soared when the U.S. Environmental Protection Agency announced that inhabitants of the tiny riverside community of Times Beach, Missouri, should abandon their homes and evac-uate the town. Soil analyses had revealed high levels of dioxin contamination due to oil-ing of roads for dust control in the early 1970s; the oil had been scavenged from a trichlorophenol factory by a waste hauler and was heavily laced with the toxic chemical.

Times Beach is but one of numerous places around the world where industrial accidents, deliberate dumping, or inadvertent use of dioxin-tainted pesticides have resulted in environmental contamination. Public concerns have been heightened by debatable statements by some researchers that "dioxin is the most toxic substance ever created by humans," and by allegations of a wide range of health problems and genetic disorders among American servicemen exposed to dioxin during their tour of duty in Vietnam. Widespread fears that serious human health damage can be caused by infini-tesimally small amounts of the chemical have led to such controversial regulatory actions as the evacuation of Times Beach and the suspension of the selective herbicides 2, 4, 5–T and silvex, yet the results of numerous follow-up studies on exposed popula-tions fail to show a single case where human death has resulted from dioxin exposure. What are the facts about this chemical whose very name seems to generate hysteria?

Chemically related to PCBs and other chlorinated hydrocarbons, dioxins form a large group of chemicals of widely varying levels of toxicity. The most dangerous dioxin is 2, 3, 7, 8–tetrachlorodibenzo-p-dioxin, generally referred to as TCDD or, simply, "dioxin." TCDD, unlike its chemical cousin PCB, has no industrial usefulness and has never been intentionally manufactured; it is formed as an unwanted by-prod-uct in the production of certain herbicides and the germ-killer hexachlorophene. Dioxin can escape into the atmosphere when it evaporates from TCDD-contaminated soil and water or when dioxin- or other chlorine-containing compounds are burned (EPA researchers say that municipal and medical waste incinerators currently consti-tute the leading source of dioxin emissions in the United States). Airborne dioxins can be carried long distances before they eventually are rained out or settle as dry deposits on soil, plant surfaces, or bodies of water. There they bind tightly to soil particles or sediment at the bottom of lakes and streams. Although TCDD undergoes rapid photolysis, if protected from light exposure dioxin breaks down very slowly—experimental evidence suggests that its half-life in soil may exceed 10 years. Thanks to regulatory controls on industrial emissions and the banning of 2,4,5–T, dioxin levels in the environment have fallen by about 50% since the late 1980s. Nevertheless, TCDD in minute quantities is still very widespread, present in soil, dust, chimneys of wood-burning stoves and furnaces, eggs, fish tissues, and animal fat. Most humans have accumulated small amounts of dioxin in their fatty tissues largely through consumption of meat, fish, and dairy products, with only 1% or less of the total body burden coming from such sources of exposure as contaminated air or water.

Statements asserting that dioxin is the "most toxic of all synthetic chemicals" are somewhat misleading because they are based on the observation that extremely low doses of TCDD are fatal to guinea pigs, by far the most sensitive species to the chemical's lethal effects. Hamsters, by contrast, can tolerate doses of dioxin up to 1,900 times the amount that would kill a guinea pig. For other test species, dioxin's lethality ranges somewhere between these extremes. However, dioxin is capable of producing many adverse effects other than death, and while any given species may exhibit a biological response at the far end of the range for a particular TCDD-induced problem, most species, humans included, respond similarly for most effects. For example, dioxin produces chloracne in rabbits, monkeys, mice, and humans at roughly equivalent levels of exposure. Interference with immune system function, fetal toxicity, and cancer are other adverse effects of dioxin exposure to which humans, rats, guinea pigs, and hamsters exhibit similar sensitivity. On the other hand, some of TCDD's effects are strikingly species-specific. Teratogenic effects of dioxin are apparent only in mice, which develop cleft palates at doses below the lethal level. Similarly, while dioxin acts as a liver toxin in a number of species, no signs of liver damage have yet been observed in highly exposed humans. By contrast, TCDD is carcinogenic in most species, producing malignant tumors at multiple sites—but only at high levels of exposure. Perhaps most significant among dioxin's long-term effects revealed by animal tests (presumed valid for humans as well) is the chemical's ability to disrupt the hormonal systems that control reproduction. Evidence from both wildlife and laboratory studies shows that exposure to dioxin (and to chlorinated organic chemicals in general) may result in reduced fertility, fetal loss, changes in sexual behavior, thyroid dysfunction, and suppression of the immune system. Indeed, some scientists conclude that these effects are far more significant than the carcinogenicity concerns that have been the focus of most toxicological research in relation to dioxin (Colborn, Dumanoski, and Myers, 1996; Birnbaum, 1994).

The implications of all this so far as human exposure is concerned remains somewhat problematic. Over the years thousands of people, particularly chemical industry workers, have had extensive exposure to the chemical at relatively high levels (e.g., a 1976 explosion at a trichlorophenol factory near Milan, Italy, released a toxic cloud that settled on the nearby suburb of Seveso, exposing 37,000 people of all ages to considerable amounts of dioxin). It is estimated that additional millions have been exposed to low concentrations (e.g., the farmers and ranchers using dioxin-contaminated herbicides, military personnel exposed to Agent Orange, residents of Times Beach and other communities where dioxin-laced waste oils were sprayed on dirt roads, consumers of TCDD-tainted fish, etc.). With the exception of a group of chemical industry workers whose dioxin exposure was 500 times greater than that experienced by the general public, the only confirmed human health problems associated with TCDD have been acute symptoms such as chloracne, muscle aches and pains, nervous system disorders, digestive upsets, and some psychiatric effects. TCDD's potential for causing such problems became international headline news in 2004,

Viktor Yuschenko is shown in photos from March 2002 (left) and December 2004 (right). The Ukrainian opposition leader (now president) was scarred by deliberate dioxin poisoning. [*AP photo/Viktor Pobedinsky/Efrem Lukatsky*]

when Ukrainian opposition leader and political candidate (subsequently elected president) Viktor Yuschenko was diagnosed with a severe case of dioxin-induced chloracne resulting from a bizarre assassination attempt.

Among the thousands of Seveso residents exposed to dioxin fallout from the 1976 industrial accident, the only health problems reported in the months following the explosion were about 200 cases of chloracne, almost all of them involving children, though over 200 animal deaths in the area were reported (Ottoboni, 1991). Nevertheless, a statistically significant increase in deaths due to soft tissue sarcoma (a type of cancer) and respiratory cancer has been confirmed among a group of men who were highly exposed while working for more than 20 years in chemical manufacturing plants. Among this group, workers who had been exposed to dioxin for the longest period of time had TCDD blood levels of 3600 ppt (parts per trillion). By comparison, for adults living in the industrialized world, the average blood level of dioxin is 6 ppt, while members of the U.S. military who handled dioxin-contaminated Agent Orange exhibited peak levels around 400 ppt (Fingerhut et al., 1991). In 1993, publication of a study carried out by a team of Italian researchers reviewing the medical records of thousands of Seveso residents documented an increase in soft tissue sarcomas, cancer of the gall bladder, and multiple myelomas among citizens exposed to the highest levels of dioxin ever recorded among civilian populations. However, the overall cancer rate for the region was lower than expected. Another study of U.S. chemical industry workers whose exposure to TCDD averaged less than one year revealed average blood concentrations of 640 ppt—a level 90 times higher than the national norm—yet the cancer death rate among these men 20 years after exposure was scarcely distinguishable from that of the general public (Dickson and Buzik, 1993). In 1997 the International Agency for Research on Cancer officially classified TCDD as a group 1 human carcinogen, basing its designation on studies showing an excess of all cancers among several groups of highly exposed workers. Results from a follow-up study of one of these groups, involving over 5,000 U.S. chemical workers, confirmed an increased cancer incidence due to dioxin exposure, but only among those who experienced doses 100–1,000 times higher than those encountered by the general public (Steenland et al., 1999). Such findings have led most researchers to the conclusion that while dioxin *does* cause cancer in humans at very high levels of exposure, it poses a minimal threat of malignancies at the low concentrations commonly encountered.

For those charged with protecting the public health and setting regulatory requirements regarding TCDD exposure, the dioxin issue presents some difficult decisions. Without question the chemical is acutely toxic to laboratory animals and produces serious chronic health problems in many animal species as well. However, in spite of extensive human exposure to TCDD, only a handful of transitory acute effects have been confirmed in people. It must be noted that one of the problems in determining the health effects of dioxin is the fact that TCDD virtually never occurs alone; rather, it is one of many chemicals in a mixture that may include PCBs, dibenzofurans, chlorophenols, and other dioxins. Since the identity of these other chemicals is frequently not known or not reported, it could be risky to attribute a given observed health effect to TCDD alone. While some investigators argue that dioxin presents less of a health threat to humans than to other animal species, others are convinced that the subtle effects observed in laboratory animals are having an impact on people as well. Citing animal data regarding TCDD's adverse impact on reproduction and on immune system function as justification for continued regulatory controls, such authorities are convinced of the necessity to limit human exposure to dioxin as much as possible (Colborn et al., 1996).

Asbestos

Probably no other hazardous substance has resulted in so many deaths and cases of disabling disease as has asbestos, the collective term for a group of six fibrous silicate minerals (amosite, chrysotile, tremolite, actinolite, anthophyllite, and crocidolite) found almost worldwide. The major asbestos producers currently are Canada, Russia, China, Brazil, Zimbabwe, and Kazakhstan.

Utilized by humans ever since Stone Age potters employed the substance to reinforce their clay, asbestos was woven into cloth during Greek and Roman times and was regarded as having magical properties because of its invulnerability to fire. In modern times asbestos has acquired great economic value as an essential component in over 3,000 commercial products. By the period of peak production in the late 1970s, over 5 million tons of asbestos were being produced each year worldwide. Production of asbestos has declined significantly since then, with somewhat over 2 million tons being mined annually at present. Over 70% of the world's current yearly production is used in Asia, Latin America, and eastern Europe. Although asbestos has been used in brake linings, insulation, textiles, roofing paper, ironing board covers, caulking compounds, floor tiles, and a host of other products, over 85% of all asbestos produced today is incorporated into asbestos-cement construction materials (LaDou, 2004).

Unfortunately, in addition to being very useful, asbestos is an occupational hazard of major proportions. Public health experts estimate that until asbestos exposure is eliminated, as many as 10 million people—the majority of them individuals occupationally exposed to asbestos fibers—may die of asbestos-related cancer. The number of workers exposed to asbestos far exceeds those involved in mining and processing the ore; an estimated 20–40% of adult men worldwide report some degree of occupational contact with asbestos, primarily through the replacement, repair, or maintenance of materials containing the fibers (Tossavainen, 2004). Exposure to asbestos is primarily through inhalation of tiny fibers suspended in the air. While airborne fibers may occur naturally in regions characterized by outcroppings of the mineral, they are more commonly associated with the deterioration of manufactured asbestos-containing materials or with the demolition or renovation of buildings containing asbestos. Fiber levels tend to be highest near asbestos mines or factories and are higher in cities than in rural areas, but virtually any air sample, regardless of where it is taken, will contain some asbestos fibers. Once inhaled, asbestos fibers are deposited in the air passages and cells within the lungs. Most of these are quickly carried away by the mucus that lines the respiratory tract, being transported up to the throat where they are swallowed, carried to the stomach, and eventually excreted with the feces. Some, however, remain trapped deep in the lungs and may never be removed.

Although inhalation represents the primary route by which asbestos enters the human body, people may also be exposed to the mineral in drinking water. Asbestos fibers can be released into water supplies when cement asbestos pipes corrode or when asbestos-containing wastes piled near mine sites are washed into lakes or rivers. Asbestos that is swallowed, fortunately, presents much less of a health hazard than that which is inhaled. Most fibers are simply carried through the stomach and intestines and are excreted within a few days. A small portion, however, may lodge in the cells lining the gastrointestinal tract, while a few may move through the intestinal lining and enter the blood stream. These may either become trapped in other tissues or be excreted in the urine.

Asbestos-Related Diseases

Several different types of asbestos-related diseases are known, the most significant being the following.

Asbestosis. A chronic disease characterized by a scarring of the lung tissue, asbestosis most commonly occurs among workers who have been exposed to very high levels of asbestos dust. It is an irreversible, excruciatingly painful, progressively worsening disease, the first symptom of which is shortness of breath following exertion. Lung function is adversely affected, the maximum volume of air a victim can inhale being reduced. In most cases, it takes 20 years or more of exposure to asbestos before symptoms of the disease appear; unfortunately, by this time asbestosis has usually reached an advanced state. The severity of asbestosis is influenced not only by the duration of exposure, but also by the type of asbestos fibers inhaled and by the synergistic effects of cigarette smoking. Until the 1940s, when concerns about workers' health led to regulations regarding dust levels in asbestos factories, asbestosis was the leading cause of death among asbestos workers. Since then, rates of asbestosis have been reduced, but even today cases continue to be diagnosed among individuals exposed to large quantities of asbestos fibers years ago.

Lung cancer. With the gradual reduction in dust levels in asbestos factories, deaths due to asbestosis have been decreasing, allowing workers to live long enough to develop today's leading cause of asbestos-related mortality, lung cancer. Approximately 5–7% of all lung cancer cases today can be attributed to occupational exposure to asbestos, with roughly 20,000 new victims diagnosed each year in developed nations with a long history of asbestos production and use (Tossavainen, 2004). It is estimated that as many as 20–25% of asbestos workers now succumb to this disease. The risk is especially great when exposure to asbestos fibers is accompanied by expo-

Box 7-2   Deadly Dust

No community in the United States is suffering more grievously from the ravages of asbestos-related disease than the small town of Libby, Montana, located in the scenic northwest corner of the state. Today Libby is the site of an extensive EPA hazardous waste cleanup effort under the federal Superfund program, a belated response to almost seven decades of massive contamination with tremolite asbestos fibers from a nearby vermiculite mine, an economic mainstay of the community from the 1930s until its closure in 1990. By 2001, shortly before remediation efforts got underway, over 200 residents of the area had died of asbestosis or asbestos-caused cancer and nearly 1,400 were being treated for asbestos disease. According to a 2000 report from the federal Agency for Toxic Substances and Disease Registry (ATSDR), the number of asbestos-related deaths in Libby is 60 times higher than the U.S. average and, given the long latency period associated with the onset of asbestos disease symptoms, the toll is likely to increase further in the years immediately ahead.

The events culminating in this tragic situation began with the discovery in 1919 of one of the world's largest deposits of vermiculite a few miles outside the town. The economic potential of Libby's immense vermiculite deposits prompted an entrepreneurial mining engineer to stake a claim in the early 1920s to approximately 1,200 acres of mineral-rich land and to open a mine which, by the 1930s, was shipping out ever-increasing quantities of a vermiculite product the company dubbed "Zonolite." By the early 1970s the Libby mine was producing over 200,000 tons of vermiculite each year—80% of the world's total.

Throughout these years, mine workers, grateful for well-paying jobs, seldom complained that the workplace environment subjected them to enormous quantities of airborne particulates as the ore was crushed and processed. Miners would return home covered with a thick layer of white dust on their clothes, skin, and hair, exposing family members to the material. To the workers, such conditions were simply an unavoidable part of their job—nothing to worry about, since company officials assured them it was nothing more than "nuisance dust," certainly not a health threat. Vermiculite itself is, indeed, harmless; but what the workers and townspeople were never told was that the vermiculite deposit at Libby was highly contaminated with asbestos, formed by the same geologic processes responsible for the presence of vermiculite. Although the dangers weren't recognized when the mine first opened, by 1956 asbestos had been officially listed as an ingredient in the Libby mine dust, with concentrations noted as ranging from 8–21% of the total (a subsequent analysis in 1982 revealed concentrations in the 21–26% range). State regulatory officials as well as mine owners were aware of the fact, yet workers were never told of the problem nor given protective equipment other than paper masks, which none of them wore; by 1959 chest X-rays showed that over one-third of the mine workers exhibited lung abnormalities. A few years later, laboratory analysis identified the type of asbestos fibers in the mine dust as tremolite, one of the most dangerous forms of asbestos.

The cover-up continued after W.R. Grace purchased the mine in 1963 and expanded production. Occasional inspections of the facility by state regulators revealed that miners were being exposed to levels of asbestos far higher than the so-called "safety limit" (in fact, there is *no safe* level of asbestos exposure), yet no government enforcement action was taken against the company. Although W.R. Grace installed a new ventilation system intended to eliminate indoor dust, smokestacks at the mill were emitting an estimated 5,000 tons of dust and fiber daily. At the same time, Grace was allowing waste vermiculite to be spread throughout Libby—in homes and gardens, on schoolyards, children's ballparks, and the high school running track. Grateful Libby residents admired Grace as a good corporate citizen, helping to improve community life; they never realized until it was too late that, as a result of the company's largesse, everyone in town was now in direct daily contact with one of the world's most pervasive environmental hazards.

By the 1960s overt signs of asbestos disease began to appear among individuals who had started working at the mine several decades earlier. As the years went by, more and more people became ill—not only miners, but wives and children as well. At first many attributed their poor health to "bronchial problems," but eventually those who traveled to Seattle or Spokane to seek medical advice were informed they had asbestosis, a disease many of them had never before heard of.

Elsewhere in the country, growing awareness of the extent of asbestos-related disease and of the massive industry cover-up of the problem (in legal terms, the "failure to warn") had resulted in a steady escalation in legal action against asbestos companies. Since the late 1970s, approximately 600,000 lawsuits have been filed in the U.S. and with irate juries awarding plaintiffs first hundreds of thousands and, later, millions of dollars in compensatory and punitive damages, even the wealthiest corporations began to buckle under the financial pressure. Eventually over fifty U.S. corporations, including W.R. Grace in 2001, sought protection under Chapter 11 bankruptcy proceedings. Demand for products containing asbestos underwent a steady decline in most developed nations and in 1990 W.R. Grace ceased operations at its plant in Libby.

By the 1990s, several Libby asbestos victims had filed suits against Grace, but all settled with the company out of court, agreeing to accept a monetary award in return for a promise not to talk about their case. It was only in 1998 that a claimant who had lost both parents to asbestosis and was determined to bring Grace to justice insisted on her lawsuit going to trial. During the proceedings some of the most influential testimony came from an asbestos expert from Brown University who told the court that among men who had worked at the mine for twenty years, 92% were diseased: "The highest reported rate of lung disease in any group of workers exposed to an asbestos form of mineral that I've seen." The woman won her case, becoming the first Libby resident to sue W.R. Grace successfully. To her disappointment, however, the world outside Libby continued to ignore what was happening there. Even among community leaders, concern about the town's image created pressure to downplay the severity of local health and environmental problems.

Although Grace had closed the mine and ceased its operations in Libby, the company had been ordered to remediate the site and had posted a cleanup bond, as required, to ensure that it would do so. In 1999 the local newspaper carried an article stating that Grace considered its work complete and was filing a request to recover the unused portion of its bond. The same resident who had successfully sued Grace the previous year spotted this story and decided to see for herself whether the cleanup had truly been finished. Driving to the site, she found few signs of reclamation; mine tailings were exposed to wind and rain, ensuring further dissemination of deadly asbestos fibers. Furious, she repeatedly contacted the appropriate Montana state regulatory agencies, insisting they come to Libby to view the mess for themselves. When they finally arrived several weeks later, they found conditions just as she had described them. At that point, the press was contacted and suddenly—finally—Libby's plight became national news. Shortly thereafter an EPA Emergency Response Team arrived from the Denver regional office and launched what turned out to be a two-year investigation. Federal agents were amazed at the community-wide extent of the contamination, in numerous cases affecting whole families. Almost 20% of the people who submitted to testing exhibited abnormal lung X-rays, a sure sign of asbestos-related disease. None of the investigators had ever before encountered such widespread poisoning, particularly among residents who had never themselves worked with asbestos. By the end of 2001, intervention by Montana's governor resulted in Libby being placed on the National Priority List for Superfund remedial action. Cleanup got underway in the summer of 2002, proceeding house-to-house in an effort to undo decades of contamination. It is unlikely that work will be finished before 2006 at the earliest, but Libby residents finally feel assured that an end is in sight to their decades-long nightmare of pollution and disease.

References

Bowker, Michael. 2003. *Fatal Deception: The Untold Story of Asbestos*. New York: Rodale.

sure to cigarette smoke. Studies have shown that while asbestos exposure alone increases an individual's risk of lung cancer death by a factor of seven, exposure to both asbestos and cigarette smoke entails a 60 times greater risk of lung cancer.

Mesothelioma. This previously rare cancer of the lung or stomach lining today kills more than 5% of all asbestos workers. Like many other forms of cancer, mesothelioma is characterized by a long latency period, onset of disease symptoms occurring 25–40 years after initial exposure. For this reason, peak levels of mortality from mesothelioma may not occur until 2010–2020, when workers exposed during the asbestos production boom of the late 1970s begin to sicken and die. Some health officials predict that western Europe alone will experience 250,000 mesothelioma deaths during the first three decades of the 21st century as a result of past asbestos exposure (LaDou, 2004). About half of all victims will be construction workers and men employed in shipyards, where for almost half a century asbestos materials were used on virtually every ship (Tossavainen, 2004). Even very low levels of asbestos can result in mesothelioma, as evidenced by cases among young adults whose only contact with the mineral involved childhood exposure to their fathers' asbestos-contaminated work clothes. Mesothelioma is of special interest to researchers because, unlike other forms of cancer, the only known causative agent for this disease is asbestos. Thus mesothelioma is considered a "marker disease" indicating asbestos exposure. Since no effective treatment exists, mesothelioma is an invariably fatal ailment, with death generally occurring within two years of diagnosis.

Although research has not yet been able to establish conclusively the degree of asbestos exposure necessary to initiate cancer, evidence suggests that some individuals who were exposed to high levels of asbestos for only one day developed cancer years later as a result. For this reason the current presumption is that there is *no safe level for asbestos exposure.* Some scientists have argued that the development of asbestos-related disease is dependent on the mineral type of asbestos to which an individual is exposed. However, most researchers believe that fiber *size* is a more important determinant of asbestos' cancer-causing potential than are its chemical or physical properties. Experimental data suggest that long fibers (those exceeding 1/5,000 of an inch in length) are more injurious than short fibers (less than 1/10,000 of an inch).

While *any* amount of asbestos exposure entails some degree of hazard, the extent of that risk is determined by a combination of several factors, among the most important of which are:

- level and duration of exposure
- time since exposure occurred
- age at which exposure occurred
- personal history of cigarette smoking
- type and size of asbestos fibers

While asbestos workers constitute by far the largest percentage of victims, others may be affected through indirect exposure. Mesothelioma has claimed casualties among people living in the vicinity of asbestos factories and among children of asbestos workers. When asbestos is brought into the home, it becomes a permanent part of the domestic environment, embedded in carpets and draperies and suspended in the air where it constitutes a 24-hour/day source of exposure not only to the less vulnerable healthy adults of the household but also to the very young, the sick, and the elderly who are the groups most susceptible to any type of environmental irritant. For this reason, asbestos workers today are cautioned to shower and change clothes at the workplace in order to avoid inadvertent contamination of their homes with asbestos fibers.

Asbestos Problems in Public Buildings

Until the mid-1970s most asbestos-related health concerns were focused on the millions of workers who had experienced significant levels of occupational exposure to the hazardous fibers. It thus came as an unwelcome surprise when the EPA warned that the general public has been receiving asbestos exposure for years simply by working or living in any of the estimated 700,000 commercial, governmental, or residential buildings that contain friable asbestos ("friable" refers to asbestos material which, when dry, can be crumbled to a powder by hand pressure).

Of greatest concern was the revelation that as many as 2–6 million schoolchildren and 300,000 teachers in 31,000 primary and secondary schools across the nation might be inhaling asbestos fibers on a daily basis. During the years 1946–1973, asbestos-containing fireproofing materials were extensively used in constructing or renovating schools throughout the country. By 1973 increasing documentation of the health threats posed by asbestos had caused the EPA to ban all spray applications of asbestos in insulating and fireproofing materials, and in 1977 new restrictions totally halted the spray application of asbestos. Such regulation had no effect, however, on existing asbestos-containing materials which, by this time, were beginning to deteriorate in many schools, releasing potentially dangerous fibers into the classroom environment. When asbestos-containing dust is swept up by janitors or disturbed by students' coming and going, it becomes resuspended and can remain in the air—at breathing level—for as long as 80 hours. The high levels of asbestos fibers measured in the indoor air of many schools prompted concerns for elevated rates of lung cancer and mesothelioma among today's schoolchildren 20–40 years hence. The initial EPA response to this perceived threat was to issue an advisory to school districts throughout the country, informing them of the situation and requiring that they inspect their buildings for the presence of asbestos-containing materials (ACM). If friable asbestos was found, the districts were to notify parents or the PTA of that fact. The federal authorities apparently assumed that if an asbestos hazard were identified, parental concerns about their children's safety would be sufficient to ensure prompt remediation of the problem. Such did not prove to be the case, however, as financially strapped school districts, in the absence of a firm federal mandate, postponed expensive remediation projects. By 1983, 66% of the nation's school districts had not yet even inspected for asbestos or had failed to report doing so to the EPA.

Consequently, in the fall of 1986, President Reagan signed into law the far-reaching Asbestos Hazard Emergency Response Act (AHERA), requiring that all primary and secondary schools be inspected for the presence of asbestos; if such materials were found, the school district was required to file and carry out an asbestos abatement plan. EPA was charged with promulgating rules detailing correct inspection procedures, establishing asbestos abatement standards, certification programs for contractors, and standards for the transportation and disposal of asbestos.

Asbestos Abatement

When an asbestos hazard is identified, those charged with remedying the situation have several options from which to choose:

1. *Encapsulation.* This is a technique in which exposed asbestos is heavily coated with a polymer sealant to prevent further release of fibers.

2. *Enclosure.* Feasible when the area affected is relatively small, this process involves building a nonpermeable barrier between the source of exposure and surrounding open areas.

3. *Removal.* A labor-intensive process whereby all asbestos containing materials are physically removed from the structure.

Asbestos insulation is exposed in the ceiling of a hallway in a New York City public school that ultimately was closed in 1978 due to pressure from parents. [© *Bettmann/Corbis*]

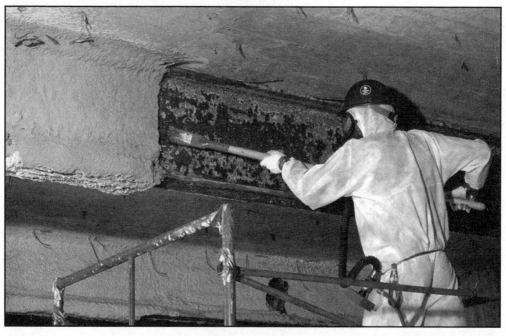

A heavily protected worker carries out asbestos abatement work in a public building in Chicago. [© *Donald C. Johnson/Corbis*]

Of the various abatement alternatives, complete removal is the most expensive and time consuming. It also entails the risk of worker exposure to asbestos fibers and, if carelessly done, could endanger the public as well. However, since removal absolves a building's owner of future liability and because encapsulated asbestos requires periodic reinspection, removal may, in the long run, be cheaper than encapsulation. In addition, federal laws require that any buildings that are going to be demolished or renovated, other than private homes or apartments with four or less dwelling units, must be inspected for the presence of asbestos-containing material. If any friable asbestos is found it must be removed before work can commence. Essentially this means that if a school district chose encapsulation as its asbestos abatement option and subsequently decided to tear down or substantially renovate that building, it would first have to hire a contractor to remove all encapsulated asbestos materials, thereby paying twice to have the job done. For these reasons, even though encapsulation is an acceptable method of reducing asbestos exposure, most asbestos abatement projects today involve complete removal.

Asbestos removal projects must adhere to strict federal and state regulations to protect both workers and the general public. Under the Clean Air Act provisions for hazardous air pollutants, EPA has set a standard of "no visible emissions" for any asbestos removal activities. Asbestos-containing materials must be wet down before work commences and must be kept damp throughout the course of the project, right up to final disposal. Damp asbestos wastes must be containerized in thick plastic bags or plastic lined containers, tagged with an appropriate warning label, and transported in a covered vehicle to an approved sanitary landfill. Since asbestos is not classified as a hazardous waste, the EPA-approved method of asbestos disposal is to bury the material in an area of the landfill separate from other household wastes, covering the containers with at least six inches of soil or with some other nonasbestos materials before compacting. Final cover of an additional 30 inches of nonasbestos material is required.

Legal Status of Asbestos

The mass of evidence documenting asbestos' adverse health impact has led to a total ban on the importation, manufacture, marketing, and use of asbestos throughout the countries of the European Union, effective in 2005. A number of other nations have also implemented complete or partial prohibitions of asbestos-containing products, and a vigorous "Ban Asbestos" movement has been working actively to persuade additional governments that the only solution to the worldwide epidemic of asbestos cancer is to discontinue all mining and use of the material (Harris and Kahwa, 2003). Among industrialized countries, the two major holdouts are Canada and the United States. As the largest exporter of asbestos, primarily to Third World nations, Canada continues to promote asbestos use and to oppose international efforts to outlaw the material (LaDou, 2004). In the United States, an EPA-mandated phase-out of all asbestos-containing products was announced in 1989 but was subsequently overturned on a legal technicality in 1991; as a result, a number of asbestos products continue to be marketed in the U.S. with little government regulation (Bowker, 2003).

Nevertheless, in the absence of a total ban, action against asbestos in the U.S. is proceeding on several fronts. Occupational exposure, which in the 1970s was lowered first to 5 and subsequently to 2 fibers/cm^3 of air, has now been reduced to 0.1 fibers/cm^3 over an eight-hour time-weighted average. Employers are required to sample at factory sites every six months and daily at construction sites unless employees are wearing respirators. In situations where fiber levels exceed standards, employers must install exhaust ventilation, dust-control systems, and air-vacuuming methods to reduce worker exposure to asbestos dust. Employers also must monitor workers' health, provide and launder protective clothing, maintain respirators, and provide showering and changing facilities. For the protection of the general public, the federal government has banned the use of asbestos in a number of consumer products: certain pipe coverings and patching compounds, artificial fireplace logs, sprayed-on decorations, and hair dryers. Since 1997, production of asbestos-containing materials for home construction and use has been banned. In spite of these prohibitions, however, consumers cannot always assume that products they buy are asbestos-free. Items imported from countries without legal restrictions on asbestos (Canada being a notable example) may still contain the mineral. Even in the United States, asbestos-containing products are not legally required to be labeled as such and therefore buyers wishing to know product content are advised to contact the manufacturer or the U.S. Consumer Product Safety Commission.

Lead

Lead poisoning is entirely preventable, yet it is the most common and societally devastating environmental disease of young children.
—Dr. Louis Sullivan,
former Secretary of Health and Human Services

Dr. Sullivan's remarks regarding the impact of lead on children's health were prompted by the recognition that 3–4 million American youngsters at that time had blood lead levels high enough to impair their brain function. This situation galvanized the public health community to redouble efforts to identify children affected by subclinical (i.e., lacking visible disease symptoms) lead toxicity and to remove sources of lead exposure. As a result of these initiatives, the number of children testing positive for elevated blood lead levels dropped steadily throughout the 1990s. By 1999–2000, a national survey of children aged 1–5 reported that an estimated 434,000 children—2.2% of those in that age group—exhibited blood lead levels above the threshold at which medical intervention is recommended; in 1978, the number so affected was estimated at 4.7 million. Obviously the situation is improving, but with nearly half a million children still lead-poisoned, the battle is far from over. Future medical historians may regard it as ironic that in the early years of the 21st century, a substance whose toxicity has been well established for millennia is regarded as the single most important environmental health problem affecting American children.

Human contact with lead, a mineral element naturally occurring throughout the environment, dates back to at least 4000 BC when it was first smelted as a by-product of silver processing. Because it is malleable and easy to work; doesn't rust, corrode, or dissolve in water; and binds readily with other metals, lead has been widely used since ancient times as an alloy; as an ingredient in paints, glazes, and cosmetics; and for gutters and piping. Indeed, the word "plumbing" is derived from the Latin word for lead, *plumbum*—hence lead's chemical symbol, Pb.

Among those who worked with the metal, it early became apparent that in addition to being commercially valuable, lead is a potent human poison. Over the centuries, evidence of the multifaceted aspects of lead's toxicity has continued to mount. More than two thousand years ago, Roman doctors were describing patients suffering with symptoms of gout, an ailment associated with chronic lead poisoning; modern commentators theorize such problems may have been caused by the Roman practice of lining wine casks, cooking pots, and aqueducts with lead. Lead poisoning may also have contributed to the low birth rate and high incidence of mental retardation among the Roman aristocracy. A major source of exposure to the metal among wealthy

Figure 7-2 Concentration of Lead in Blood of Children Ages 5 and Under

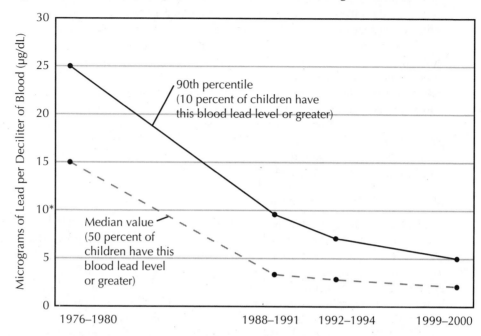

*10 µg/dL of blood lead has been identified by CDC as elevated, which indicates need for intervention. There is no demonstrated safe concentration of lead in blood. Adverse effects may occur at lower concentrations.

Source: U.S. Environmental Protection Agency, 2003. America's Children and the Environment: Measures of Contaminants, Body Burdens, and Illnesses. www.epa.gov/envirohealth/children, based on data from Centers for Disease Control and Prevention, National Center for Health Statistics, National Health and Nutrition Examination Survey.

Romans is thought to have been a grape juice syrup, *frumentum*, which was brewed in lead pots and subsequently used to sweeten foods and wine; even one teaspoonful of this syrup would have been more than enough to cause chronic lead poisoning. Unfortunately, later generations learned little from the Roman experience; during medieval times, Europeans in large numbers fell victim to "Saturnine poisoning," a result of using soluble lead acetate to sweeten sour wine, and even in the 16th century widespread outbreaks of lead poisoning occurred in France as a result of storing wine in lead-lined vessels.

Sources of Lead

Today, as in centuries past, lead is used in a wide range of industrial products. The single largest use of lead, over 70% of total U.S. consumption of the metal, is for lead storage batteries (virtually every car on the road contains 20 pounds of lead in its battery); other lead-containing products include ammunition, brass, coverings for power and communication cables, glass TV tubes, solder, and pigments. With world production estimated at more than 3 million tons annually, lead is produced in larger amounts than any other nonferrous metal. Not surprisingly, lead is now found throughout the environment—in soils, water, air, and food. Until the mid-1980s, automobile emissions constituted the major source of environmental lead. With the phase-out of leaded gasoline in the United States and a number of other countries, amounts of lead entering the atmosphere have declined sharply. Correspondingly, Americans' blood lead levels have fallen as well, down by more than 80% since the mid-1970s. In the approximately 100 countries where leaded gasoline is still used, however, environmental contamination from this source remains a serious problem. Researchers in India report that over half the children in six large metropolitan areas have elevated blood lead levels, a fact they blame on fallout of lead particles from automobile emissions (Sharma, 1999). In the United States today, airborne lead originates primarily from the burning of lead-contaminated used oil, from the smelting of ores and other industrial processes, and from the incineration of municipal refuse. Currently more lead is released into soil than into the air, primarily as the result of lead-containing solid wastes being dumped in landfills (aware of this hazard, a number of states have passed laws banning landfill disposal of lead batteries). Weathering of lead-based paints, particularly around the foundations of older structures, and fallout of airborne lead further contribute to the buildup of lead in soils.

Route of Entry into Body

In years past, ingestion of lead-tainted food and water constituted the main source of lead intake for most Americans. Canned foods and beverages represented a significant hazard because over 90% of such cans had lead-soldered seams. Leaching of the toxic metal from the solder into the cans' contents was commonplace, especially when the food items were acidic (e.g., tomato products, citrus, or carbonated drinks). Airborne fallout of lead from automobile emissions onto vegetables or fruits growing near busy highways was responsible for lead concentrations as high as 3,000 ppm on such crops. Drinking water, too, has been identified as a source of exposure for as many as 40 million Americans whom EPA estimates live in homes where tap water contains elevated levels of lead due to the presence of lead pipes or lead solder in household plumbing. Other sources of drinking water contamination include brass faucets on kitchen or bathroom sinks and brass pump fittings in private wells, all of which can leach dissolved lead into tap water (see chapter 15). Fortunately, Americans' exposure to lead from all these sources has been declining sharply since the phaseout of leaded gasoline (a process completed in the U.S. by 1995), the substitution of plastic (PVC) for metal piping in new and replacement home plumbing systems, and the 1991 prohibition on the manufacture of lead-soldered food or soft drink cans. However, imported foods continue to pose a hazard since few other countries restrict the use of lead solder.

Ironically, house paint remains the most important source of lead poisoning problems, even though the use of lead in paints was halted years ago. Lead was used in residential paint in the U.S. from 1884–1978; until 1953 the use of paint containing as much as 50% lead by weight was common in the United States. In that year a consensus was reached within the industry to reduce paint lead levels, resulting in a steady decline in the manufacture and use of interior lead-base paint (most European countries had recognized the problem decades earlier, signing a treaty in 1921 to prohibit the use of *interior* paints containing lead). Exterior lead-base paint continued to be widely available until the mid-1970s, although its lead content by then was considerably less than that of paint produced prior to the 1950s. In 1977 the Consumer Product Safety Commission banned all house paints, interior or exterior, as well as paints on toys or furniture, which contained more than 0.06% lead by weight. Lead-base paint can still be used, even today, for painting bridges, ships, and other steel structures and for a variety of industrial and military applications and sometimes this paint ends up being applied in homes by workers who have access to the material and fail to realize its hazardous nature ("Preventing Lead Poisoning," 1991).

Although the use of leaded paint has been illegal for more than 25 years, the U.S. Department of Housing and Urban Development (HUD) estimates that approximately 24 million dwellings nationwide are still lead contaminated, 4.4 million of them home to one or more children under the age of 6 (CDC, 2001). In such structures, deterioration or renovation activities may expose older layers of paint, providing access to toddlers who may inadvertently consume the poison chips or paint dust. While at one time it was believed that chewing on windowsills or eating flakes of the sweet-tasting paint was the major lead-poisoning hazard to children, researchers are now convinced that the prime culprit is ordinary household dust, contaminated by tiny particles of lead from the gradually deteriorating paint. Simply by playing in their own homes and doing what children normally do—putting dirty fingers in their mouths—youngsters can swallow enough lead to cause serious health problems. Recognizing the extent of lead contamination in the nation's housing supply, the federal government now requires anyone selling or renting a home or apartment to sign a form disclosing any knowledge of lead-based paint in the structure and to agree, if requested by the buyer or renter, to have the building tested for the presence of lead.

Lead presents a hazard outside as well as inside homes. Soil or dust adjacent to housing once painted with lead-base paints may contain lead levels high enough to pose a risk to small children playing in such locations; soil near busy streets or highways frequently has high lead levels also, thanks to airborne fallout of lead emissions from motor vehicles. Once deposited, lead may remain in soils as long as two thousand years. Researchers estimate that in the United States alone, more than 50 years of leaded gasoline use has left an environmental residue of 4–5 million metric tons of lead dust, the bulk of this amount being deposited along busy highways running through cities. This disproportionate concentration of lead in urban areas further increases the lead hazard for poor and minority children in inner-city areas, already at risk due to dilapidated housing conditions. Studies have shown that children living in neighborhoods where soil lead content is high often exhibit elevated blood lead levels (Mielke, 1999).

Interestingly, *ingested* lead poses a much greater hazard for young children than it does for adults. Whereas only 10% of lead swallowed by adults passes from the intestine into the bloodstream, 40% of the lead ingested by preschoolers remains within their bodies, making such youngsters the highest risk group for lead poisoning within our population. The fact that development of the blood-brain barrier isn't complete until a child reaches approximately three years of age means that lead can readily move into the central nervous system, further explaining why lead exposure is more hazardous for infants and toddlers than it is for other age groups. Particularly vulnerable are malnourished children; absorption of lead from the gastrointestinal tract occurs more readily among youngsters suffering from deficiencies of protein, calcium, zinc, or iron. Thus poor nutritional status is considered an additional risk factor for childhood lead poisoning (Chao and Kikano, 1993).

While young children constitute the primary victims of lead poisoning, people of any age are susceptible to the metal's toxic effects. The National Institute of Occupational Safety and Health (NIOSH) estimates that over 3 million Americans work in occupations involving potential lead exposure; of these, tens of thousands are estimated to suffer from lead poisoning each year, primarily through inhalation of airborne lead (30–40% of inhaled lead reaches the bloodstream and is deposited in the lower respiratory tract where it is almost completely absorbed). Occupational exposure to lead has been regulated since 1978 through specified **permissible exposure limits (PELs)** to airborne lead concentrations and by standards for allowable blood lead levels. Nevertheless, standards are not sufficiently enforced, with the result that significant worker exposure is an ongoing problem (Stauding and Roth, 1998). Those most at risk are construction workers who renovate or demolish bridges, approximately 90,000 of which in the United States are coated with lead-base paints. Such work is often performed without training or the use of personal protective equipment and may involve the use of acetylene torches or sandblasting, either of which can result in workers' inhalation of lead fumes or dust. After several weeks or months of such exposure, blood lead levels of workers can rise well above the point at which symptoms of acute lead poisoning are apparent.

In addition to bridge maintenance, other occupations that may involve excessive worker exposure to lead include battery manufacturing, shipbuilding, radiator repair, smelter and foundry operations, and certain crafts. Police or military personnel working at firing ranges have also reported symptoms of lead toxicity, a result of inhaling fumes released when lead-containing ammunition is fired (CDC, 1993; Franklin, 1991). Occasionally, some rather bizarre instances of lead poisoning illustrate the challenges facing those in the environmental health profession: over a period of seven months during 1991, eight individuals in Alabama were diagnosed with various symptoms of lead poisoning (e.g., anemia, abdominal pains, weakness in the arms, seizures, and nervous system damage) which developed as a result of drinking illegal "moonshine" distilled in an old automobile radiator containing lead-soldered components! Such a practice, which results in the leaching of lead from the solder into the home-brewed liquor, is a frequent source of lead poisoning in some rural Alabama counties and accounts for the fact that moonshine may contain up to 74 µg/L of lead (CDC, 1992).

Although lead concerns understandably focus on human health problems, it shouldn't be overlooked that environmental lead constitutes a hazard to other species as well. Especially vulnerable are waterfowl, large numbers of which have died after eating lead fishing sinkers lost by anglers. In the mid-1990s, EPA banned the manufacture and distribution of lead sinkers in order to alleviate this problem.

Regardless of whether the route of exposure is ingestion or inhalation, upon entering the body, lead first moves into the bloodstream where its half-life is estimated at 36 days. For this reason, measurements of blood lead levels, calculated as micrograms of lead per deciliter of blood (µg/dL), are considered to give the most accurate indication of short-term lead exposure. Some lead makes its way into soft tissues such as the brain and kidneys; approximately 50–60% of the lead that enters the body is excreted relatively quickly, mainly through the feces but also in urine. Over a period of time the remaining lead is slowly deposited and stored in the bones, particularly in the long arm and leg bones where it can remain for years (the estimated half-life of lead in bones is 27 years). Lead also accumulates in children's baby teeth, which have been used in research to indicate a child's lead burden. Lead in bones can act as a cumulative poison, becoming increasingly concentrated over an extended time period. Although once thought to be inert, it is now known that lead in bones can be suddenly released back into the bloodstream by a number of conditions such as high fever, osteoporosis, or pregnancy, resulting in cases of acute lead poisoning.

Biological Effects

A potent toxin that can adversely affect people in any age group, lead can damage human health in a number of ways. It interferes with blood cell formation, often resulting in anemia; lead can cause kidney damage, sterility, miscarriage, and birth defects. Because lead has a strong affinity for nerve tissue, injury to the central nervous system is perhaps the most serious manifestation of lead poisoning. Depending on the degree of exposure, lead poisoning can be reflected by hyperirritability, poor memory, or sluggishness at lower levels all the way to mental retardation, epileptic convulsions, coma, and death at high levels.

Lead is a poison that exhibits what health experts refer to as a **continuum of toxicity**; any amount of exposure, however small, carries with it some degree of harm. Not surprisingly, as levels of exposure increase, risk of adverse health effects rise correspondingly (as is the case with exposure to any hazardous substance, identical levels of lead may provoke a varying range of responses in different people). Until about the 1960s, it was widely believed that a diagnosis of "lead poisoning" was appropriate only when blood lead levels were high enough to cause such overt symptoms as anemia, kidney disease, brain damage, or death. Such conditions can be manifested when blood lead levels exceed 70 μg/dL (typically, brain damage only occurs at blood lead levels above 100 μg/dL). At that time, levels of blood lead below 60 μg/dL weren't regarded as dangerous enough to warrant monitoring or treatment. By the early 1970s, however, new evidence regarding lead's deleterious effects on biological systems prompted a reevaluation of the U.S. Public Health Service's level of "undue lead absorption"—the blood lead level at which medical intervention is recommended. In 1971 that level was lowered to 40 μg/dL, further lowered to 30 μg/dL in 1975, to 25 μg/dL in 1985, and, most recently, in 1991 was again reduced to 10 μg/dL (CDC, 2003; Florini, 1990). The justification for the steadily declining levels of blood lead that define a case of lead poisoning can be found in the results of numerous studies carried out over the last several decades, which have conclusively shown that even at levels previously considered safe, chronic low-level exposure to lead can inhibit the normal development of children's intellectual abilities. A landmark study launched in 1979 in the Boston suburbs of Somerville and Chelsea among second-grade students revealed that those whose baby teeth (which they had willingly withheld from the Tooth Fairy to contribute to science!) had a relatively higher lead level also exhibited a greater incidence of unruly classroom behavior, a lesser ability to follow instructions, and lower scores on I.Q. tests than did classmates with low lead levels in their teeth (Needleman et al., 1979). Yet none of the children would have been categorized as lead-poisoning victims based on the prevailing view at that time regarding "safe" levels of lead. Eleven years later, in 1990, a follow-up study was carried out to see whether the effects of low-level childhood lead poisoning persist into young adulthood. In light of the millions of children who have experienced some lead exposure, the results of this investigation were depressing: in comparison with classmates whose baby teeth had minimal levels of lead, the higher-lead students, by then 18-year-olds, exhibited a significantly greater school drop-out rate, higher incidence of reading disabilities, lower class rank, and higher absenteeism—all a legacy of childhood lead exposure (Needleman et al., 1990).

Lead Poisoning: Treatment and Prevention

Children with blood lead levels of 45 μg/dL or higher typically are treated through the use of chelation, a process that employs a drug that binds to lead, sequestering the metal and facilitating its excretion from the body. Most commonly, chelating agents are administered in a hospital setting where the patient must remain for a five-day period of treatment and testing (another type of chelating agent that can be given orally at home has been approved for use in less serious cases). Some forms of chelation therapy can be quite painful and the process, while essential in forestalling further impairment to the nervous system, cannot reverse damage that has already occurred. Nor is chelation a one-time solution to lead-poisoning problems. Since the chelating agent is generally unable to reach all of the lead stored in bones and teeth, blood lead levels frequently rebound following chelation therapy, the result of additional lead moving from bony tissues into the bloodstream. Many lead-poisoning victims are forced to suffer repeated bouts of hospitalization for years after the initial treatment. Children whose lead-poisoning symptoms are relieved by chelation therapy frequently require special education and therapy long after cessation of treatment and, in the all-too-common situation where they return to the same lead-contaminated environment responsible for the initial poisoning, their symptoms will promptly recur. For this reason, removal of the child from the source of exposure or, conversely, removal of lead from the child's environment, constitutes the prime strategy in restoring a lead-poisoned child to good health. Unfortunately, evidence suggests that mild brain damage persists in lead-poisoned children even after their blood lead levels were markedly reduced (Tong et al., 1998).

Preventing Childhood Lead Poisoning

Since the health impact of lead, even at very low levels, has been shown to be so devastating and because damage, once it occurs, may never be completely reversed, *prevention* of lead poisoning should be a high-priority societal goal. As mentioned previously, the near-total phase-out of the use of lead in gasoline, paint, food containers, and home plumbing has drastically reduced human exposure to this toxic metal in recent years. Nevertheless, over 400,000 U.S. preschoolers continue to exhibit elevated lead levels due to lead-contaminated paint and dust still present in millions of homes. Other household items may present a threat as well. Vinyl miniblinds, introduced to the U.S. in the late 1980s, include several brands containing lead. A study of childhood lead poisoning cases in North Carolina revealed that for 9% of the children surveyed, miniblinds were the main source of exposure. While no-lead blinds are now available, a product recall on the lead-containing versions has never been issued and the latter remain in widespread use (Norman, 1998). Food or juice served from improperly fired pottery or china coated with a lead-containing glaze has caused sporadic cases of lead poisoning, as has consumption of wine or other alcoholic beverages stored in lead-crystal decanters. Lead hazards continue to surface from unexpected sources; in 2003, health officials in both California and New Jersey issued health advisories targeted at "chapulines"—salty fried grasshopper snacks imported from Oaxaca that were popular among Mexican immigrants, unaware they were contaminated with high levels of lead. That same year public health workers in Rhode Island reported several cases of severe lead poisoning caused by a medicinal powder called "litargirio," widely used among immigrants from the Dominican Republic for purposes as varied as eliminating body odor and as a cure for sore feet (several of the Rhode Island victims were teenagers who had been using litargirio as a deodorant). One brand of litargirio tested by Rhode Island authorities contained 79% lead (Pérez-Peña, 2003; Urbina, 2003). Children may be inadvertently exposed when a family member engages in such hobbies as making pottery (lead glaze), stained glass, oil painting (some artists' paints contain lead), or furniture refinishing. Parents who work in occupational settings involving lead exposure may unintentionally carry lead dust home on work clothes, thereby exposing children to the toxic metal. A two-pronged national effort has been launched to combat childhood lead poisoning through environmental intervention to remove sources of lead exposure, and through screening programs to identify at-risk youngsters.

For the most part, environmental intervention entails removal of lead paint and lead dust from those structures where lead-poisoned children are living; prevention of future lead-poisoning cases would require removing lead paint from all homes, with special emphasis on residential units where such paint is deteriorating and presents an imminent and constant hazard (EPA, 1995). Since soils around homes with exterior lead-base paints commonly exhibit elevated concentrations of lead (in some cases as high as 11,000 ppm), a number of health authorities also recommend soil abatement programs for neighborhoods where childhood lead poisoning is prevalent. Such efforts would involve removing the top 6–7 inches of soil, replacing this with clean dirt, and then revegetating the area. However, recent epidemiologic studies have shown that in urban areas where children were experiencing low-level lead exposure, blood lead levels declined only slightly when soil abatement activities were carried out. Thus, although lead in soils *does* contribute to children's body burden of the metal (studies have shown that blood lead levels rise by 3–7 μg/dL for every 1000 ppm increase in soil or dust concentrations), the considerable expense of contaminated soil removal may not be cost-effective; significantly greater health benefits can be achieved by targeting available funds to interior paint abatement. In many situations where potential exposure to lead in soil is a concern, simply covering bare soil with sod, indoor-outdoor carpeting, or planting foundation shrubs along the base of the structure can eliminate or greatly reduce the opportunity for children to come into contact with contaminated soil—and at a much lower cost than removal activities would entail. However, in situations where soil lead levels are extremely high or where a child suffering from lead poisoning has a condition called pica—a tendency to eat nonfood items, including soil—then soil abatement could effect beneficial results (Mielke, 1999; Weitzman et al., 1993; Xintaras, 1992).

In the absence of a strong federal commitment to environmental lead remediation, the focus of prevention efforts on the part of government has shifted to blood lead screening to identify children at risk and to provide prompt treatment to those with elevated blood lead levels before damage becomes irreversible. Since many youngsters live in areas where the risk of lead poisoning is extremely low, screening efforts are being targeted at children living in older homes and children from low-income families. Although the prevalence of lead poisoning and its more severe manifestations have steadily declined since the 1970s, the fact that the disease still affects large numbers of young children means that society must persevere in efforts to eradicate humanity's most ancient toxic hazard.

Mercury

This liquid metal, the "quicksilver" of ancient times, has been used for a wide variety of purposes for at least 2,500 years—and has been contributing to illness and death among those exposed to it for an equal period of time. Although at very low levels of exposure mercury does not appear to be damaging, the margin of safety is small. Mercury is a valuable constituent of many industrial products and processes. It has been used as a catalyst in the manufacture of plastics, as a slime retardant in paper making, in fluorescent light bulbs, as a fungicide in paints, as an alloy in dental fillings, as an ingredient in many medicinal products (mercury's first medicinal use was for the treatment of syphilis when that disease reached epidemic proportions in 16th-century Europe), in the manufacture of scientific instruments, and for many other purposes.

Mercury has always been present in the environment in trace amounts, entering soil or water from vaporization and weathering of mercury compounds in the earth's crust or via volcanic activity. However, concentrations have increased three-fold in modern times due to coal combustion, mining and smelting of mercury-containing ores, and incineration of mercury wastes. Industrial processes such as electroplating, paper milling, mining and ore processing, chlorine and caustic soda production, textile manufacturing, and pharmaceutical production produce a mercury-laden effluent that is sometimes discharged into waterways. Evaporation of mercury from paints during the drying process can add significant quantities of this substance to the air;

Box 7-3   Mercury in Fish: The Regulatory Challenge

In the United States and around the world, human exposure to health-threatening levels of mercury is most likely to occur by eating mercury-tainted fish. How to deal with this situation and reduce the risks to their citizens—either by regulating sources of emissions or by educating consumers on food safety—constitute a challenge with which national governments and international organizations are currently grappling.

As evidence regarding mercury's adverse impact on neurological development of fetuses and young children accumulates, pressure has been mounting on governments to impose regulatory controls on the major industrial sources of mercury emissions. Attention first focused on municipal and medical waste incinerators, and between 1995–1997 those in the U.S. were required to reduce their mercury output by 90–94%. The results, while difficult to quantify, seem to be positive; a study conducted in the Everglades indicated that by late 2003, mercury levels had declined by as much as 75% in many of the fish and wading birds sampled.

Regulatory attention in the U.S. has now shifted to the approximately 1,100 coal-burning power plants that currently contribute about 40% of U.S. mercury emissions. Not affected by the restrictions imposed on waste incinerators in the mid-1990s, power plants were the target of regulations promulgated in March 2005 under EPA's Clean Air Mercury Rule. Although the agency had originally proposed that new and existing coal-fired utilities be required to curb mercury emissions using the "maximum achievable control technology" standard which would have sharply lowered emissions by 2007, the Bush Administration opted instead for a more industry-friendly approach that will reduce power plant emissions of the toxic metal by almost 70% from their 1999 level when the rule is fully implemented in 2018. To achieve this reduction, EPA has adopted the "cap-and-trade" system pioneered by the federal acid rain control program, making mercury emissions a tradable commodity. The agency asserts that a market-based system will motivate some utilities to make earlier-than-required reductions and should spur development of new, more effective mercury control technologies.

The determination of allowable mercury emission levels continues to be a subject of intense political controversy, both in the U.S. and internationally. Critics of strict new regulations argue that scientific studies have yet to establish a clear-cut quantitative relationship between the amount of mercury deposition and corresponding concentrations of the metal in fish. As a result, it is not yet possible to predict with certainty the extent to which emissions must be cut in order to reduce mercury in fish to a safe level. They also point out that the most widely consumed species of fish exhibiting high mercury concentrations are caught far offshore where the effects of reduced power plant emissions are likely to be negligible. Many policymakers also doubt the efficacy of emissions reductions imposed at the *national* level, since much of the mercury deposited within the boundaries of one country originated outside that nation's jurisdiction—a persuasive argument for international action. On the other hand, some researchers contend that up to 50% of airborne mercury is deposited locally, near the source facility. They argue that EPA's decision to allow less efficient utilities to buy pollution credits from facilities emitting less than the allowable level will expose communities near these "hotspots" to a continuous hazard even as other areas experience a decline in mercury fallout.

The impact of various deadline dates for achieving compliance with emission standards also generates controversy. Because soils and lake sediments in some regions have been accumulating mercury for over a century, researchers once assumed that cuts in current mercury emissions would have a minimal effect on levels of contamination in fish because the large environmental reserves of the metal would constitute a continuous source of exposure to aquatic organisms. However, evidence cited above from the Everglades, as well as preliminary results from the METAALICUS project in Ontario, Canada, indicate that emissions reductions might produce a much faster-than-expected decline in environmental mercury levels. In the Canadian study, researchers deliberately added mercury isotopes to the area around a small Ontario lake and found that they were converted to methyl mercury much more rapidly than was the case for mercury in lake sediment. Such results suggest that regulatory action to decrease mercury emissions could result in much faster cleanup of lake waters than previously imagined and argues in favor of a speedier timetable for compliance with stricter emissions standards.

The EPA and the Food and Drug Administration (FDA) have issued advisories to the public on fish species presenting the most serious mercury threat and have recommended limits on their consumption. Warnings are targeted primarily at pregnant women, since children continually exposed to mercury *in utero* are at increased risk of subtle developmental delays and learning disorders. The EPA estimates that as many as one out of every six babies born in the U.S. each year could be at risk for developmental disorders due to prenatal mercury exposure. Because mercury tends to concentrate in the umbilical cord, levels of the toxin there may be 1.7 times higher than in the mother's blood. Thus mercury levels in a newborn could exceed the safe concentration level, set by the EPA at 5.8 ppb, even when the mother's mercury level is well below that amount.

Since the health effects of mercury at the levels currently encountered in foods are so subtle, it's not surprising that some researchers argue that the hazards associated with dietary mercury may be exaggerated. In fact, several epidemiological studies aimed at quantifying the health risks came up with opposite conclusions. One study was conducted over a period of several years in the Faeroe Islands, a Danish island group in the North Atlantic. The diet of the Faeroe Islanders is based heavily on deep sea fish and pilot whale meat, all known to contain significant levels of methyl mercury. Results indicated that the children with the highest levels of prenatal mercury exposure performed worse on tests that measured such variables as attention span, memory, and language ability than did children whose exposure levels in the womb were lower. A similar research project carried out in New Zealand came up with similar findings. By contrast, a comprehensive study conducted in the Seychelles Islands in the Indian Ocean among another population group who relies on fish as the mainstay of its diet arrived at completely opposite results. Women in the Seychelles, who eat fish approximately 12 times per week, have body burdens of methyl mercury considerably higher than those found in most Americans, yet no resulting developmental damage can be found in their children. According to the National Research Council, neither of the studies cited above appears to have any serious flaws in the manner in which it was designed and carried out and as yet there is no explanation as to why the results are so contradictory.

In 2004, EPA and FDA issued a joint advisory, *"What You Need to Know About Mercury in Fish and Shellfish,"* aimed at pregnant women, women who might become pregnant, nursing mothers, and young children. The advisory emphasizes that although most fish and shellfish contain at least traces of mercury, for most people the nutritional benefits of eating fish far outweigh any health risk due to mercury. Several of the most popular fish species, in fact, exhibit low mercury levels and up to 12 ounces of these can safely be eaten each week: salmon, catfish, pollock, shrimp, and light tuna (by contrast, albacore, or "white" tuna, has higher levels and should be limited to one serving per week). The relatively short list of fish that shouldn't be eaten at all because of high mercury levels includes: shark, swordfish, king mackerel, and tilefish from the Gulf of Mexico. In some parts of the country, certain game fish may have high mercury concentrations, so those who enjoy recreational fishing should check local or state advisories regarding the safety of eating particular fish. If no information is available, the best advice is to eat no more than 6 ounces (one average-size meal) of locally caught fish per week and none from other sources. All of these advisories pertain to adult portions and amounts served to children should be reduced proportionately. While the situation regarding mercury in fish doesn't warrant public panic, prudence dictates a degree of caution in dining until the day that effective controls on mercury emissions succeed in substantially lowering environmental levels of this toxic metal.

References

Lutter, Randall, and Elisabeth Irwin. 2002. "Mercury in the Environment." *Environment* 44, no. 9 (Nov):24–40.

Stokstad, Erik. 2004. "Uncertain Science Underlies New Mercury Standards." *Science* 303, no. 5654 (Jan. 2):34.

studies have shown that mercury concentrations in indoor air may be one thousand times higher immediately after a room is painted than they were before painting. Several well-publicized cases of children developing symptoms of mercury poisoning after mercury-containing latex paints were applied to their homes led to an agreement among U.S. paint manufacturers to stop adding mercury to their products. Nevertheless, although the production of interior paints containing mercury halted in 1990, followed by similar action regarding exterior paint in 1991, the fact that many people keep partly used containers of paint for future use means that paint will remain a potential source of mercury exposure for years to come.

Mercury emissions to the environment are gradually declining in North America and Europe due to a decrease in demand for the metal, especially in the paint and chlor-alkali industries and for battery and wire manufacturing. Mercury recycling initiatives to divert mercury wastes from landfills and incinerators are helping to curb environmental releases, as are efforts to substitute mercury-free products for those containing the toxic metal (i.e., digital thermometers in place of mercury thermometers). However, emissions in Asia have been rapidly increasing and now constitute half of all mercury emissions worldwide (Selin, 2005).

Health Effects of Mercury Exposure

The action of mercury on the human system depends primarily on the form of mercury to which the victim is exposed, either inorganic metallic mercury or the far more toxic organic mercury.

Inorganic metallic mercury. This form of mercury frequently attacks the liver and kidneys; it also can diffuse through the alveolar membranes of the lungs and travel to the brain where it can cause such neurological problems as lack of coordination. Inorganic mercury can enter the system either by inhalation of mercury vapors or by absorption of mercury compounds through the skin after prolonged contact. Examples of human poisoning with inorganic mercury include a malady prevalent among hatmakers in 17th-century France called the "Mad Hatters' Disease" (immortalized by a character of the same name in Lewis Carroll's *Alice in Wonderland*). This neurological disorder, manifested as tremors and mental aberrations, resulted from the practice at that time of soaking animal hides in a solution of mercuric nitrate for purposes of softening the hairs. Since the hatmakers' bare arms and hands were in frequent contact with the solution as they manipulated the hides, skin absorption of mercury led to development of the disease symptoms.

Poisoning by inhalation is more common than skin absorption, however, and represents the most common form of occupational exposure to mercury. A survey conducted by NIOSH estimated that 70,000 American workers may be exposed to mercury vapors on the job. These include nurses, lab technicians, machine operators, miners, plumbers, dentists and dental hygienists, and many others. Even the families of potentially exposed workers may be at risk if mercury is carried home from the occupational setting on contaminated work clothing. Exposure to mercury vapors from dental fillings (standard amalgams are approximately 50% mercury by weight) has provoked concern about the potential for chronic poisonings, but there is no convincing evidence to support such worries. Most authorities feel the amount of mercury that dental fillings contribute to the average person's daily body burden of the metal is too small to pose any credible health risk.

Many people have become ill and some deaths have been reported among people exposed to mercury fumes when large quantities of mercury were accidentally spilled within confined, inadequately ventilated areas. If such an accident should occur, the mercury should be cleaned up as quickly as possible, regardless of how small an amount is involved, because vaporization of the metal over time could pose a serious health hazard to anyone in the vicinity, particularly small children and pregnant women. If the spill is on a smooth surface, such as a countertop or uncarpeted floor, a piece of paper can be used to roll the beads of mercury carefully onto another piece of paper and then placed in a zip-lock bag or glass jar with a tight-fitting lid. Never try to blot or wipe up mercury with a rag or paper towel—since the metal is not absorbent, doing so will simply disperse the mercury into smaller droplets and make it even more difficult to collect. If the spill occurs on carpeting, cleanup will be more difficult and usually requires seeking advice and assistance on decontamination from local health authorities. Because of the severe inhalation hazard posed by metallic mercury, a vacuum cleaner should *never* be used to clean up mercury droplets, since this will only exacerbate the problem by hastening vaporization and increasing air concentrations of the metal. People cleaning up spilled mercury need not worry about suffering acute inhalation poisoning, but they should either wear gloves or remove any rings, because mercury readily forms an amalgam with gold. Good ventilation with outside air during cleanup operations is important; windows should be opened and a fan used to direct air out of the room for at least an hour. Mercury collected should be kept in a tightly sealed container and disposed of in a manner recommended by local health or environmental officials (ATSDR, 1999).

In contrast to the serious dangers posed by *inhalation* of mercury, *swallowing* the metal—as could occur if a child bites down on an oral thermometer—poses no health threat. Metallic mercury is poorly absorbed by the gastrointestinal tract and is soon excreted in the feces.

Organic mercury.   Far more toxic than elemental mercury are the organic mercury compounds such as methyl mercury which, being extremely soluble, can readily penetrate living membranes. Organic mercury circulates in the bloodstream bound to red blood cells and gradually diffuses into the brain, destroying the cells that control coordination. Symptoms of organic mercury poisoning generally don't appear until a month or two after exposure, showing up initially as numbness in the lips, tongue, and fingertips. Gradually speech becomes slurred and difficulty in swallowing and walking becomes apparent. As mercury levels rise, deafness and vision problems may develop and the victim tends to lose contact with his or her surroundings. Before the nature of mercury poisoning was understood, such people were often thought to be neurotic or mentally ill and were occasionally placed in insane asylums.

Several tragic episodes involving methyl mercury poisoning have been documented in past decades. In 1972 more than 6,500 Iraqi villagers became seriously ill and 459 died after eating bread that had been made from seed wheat coated with an organic mercury fungicide. Contributing to this tragic accident was the fact that the brightly colored warning dye typically used to indicate treated seed had been washed off and the instructions on the bags were printed only in English (Bakir et al., 1973). A similar situation, fortunately on a much smaller scale, occurred in the United States three years earlier when several members of a family in Alamagordo, New Mexico, suffered permanent neurological impairment after they butchered and ate a hog that had been fed fungicide-treated seed corn. Undoubtedly the most infamous episode of mass poisoning with methyl mercury occurred during the years 1953–1961 in the coastal town of Minamata on the Japanese island of Kyushu. A plastics factory, Chisso Corporation, had for a number of years been discharging inorganic mercury wastes into the waters of Minamata Bay where many of the local residents earned their livelihood by fishing. In the anaerobic conditions among the sediments at the bottom of the bay, the inorganic mercury was converted into highly toxic methyl mercury by the bacterium *Methanobacterium amelanskis*. Readily soluble, the methyl mercury thus began moving through the aquatic food chain, being passively absorbed by microscopic algae which were subsequently eaten by zooplankton, which were eaten by small fish, etc., the methyl mercury becoming increasingly concentrated at each higher trophic level (mercury concentrations in predator fish at the top of aquatic food chains commonly reach levels 100,000 times higher than those present in the surrounding water).

Trouble first became apparent in Minamata when the town cats developed what residents first thought must be a strange viral disease, yowling continuously and sometimes leaping into the sea to drown. When the townspeople themselves started to complain of vague maladies such as extreme fatigue, headaches, numbness in their extremities, and difficulty in swallowing, it was first suspected that they were contracting some sort of illness from the sick cats. Eventually the true nature of their mutual problem was discovered—methyl mercury poisoning derived from a diet composed primarily of mercury-contaminated fish. By this time more than 100 people had been stricken with such symptoms as mental derangement, inability to walk or use chopsticks, visual disturbances, and convulsions. Forty-four of the Minamata victims died during this period and many others were permanently disabled. As this sad episode unfolded, the teratogenic properties of methyl mercury became apparent. Twenty-two brain-damaged babies were born during this period to mothers who themselves exhibited no outward signs of mercury poisoning, though several mentioned experiencing a slight numbness of the fingers during pregnancy and analysis showed a high level of mercury in their hair. Subsequent studies have revealed that methyl mercury has a special affinity for fetal tissue, easily crossing the placental barrier where it severely damages the developing child while leaving the mother unharmed. The ultimate human toll of Chisso's poisoning of Minamata Bay included 700 deaths and 9,000 individuals left with varying degrees of paralysis and brain damage. Estimates are that as many as 50,000 people living within 35 miles of the bay who consumed its fish have suffered at least mild symptoms of mercury poisoning (Weisskopf, 1987). After years of legal wrangling over compensation, several thousand plaintiffs reached a settlement with Chisso in 1996, agreeing to drop lawsuits in return for a $24,200 lump sum payment to each Minamata Disease victim, plus additional payments to five national victims' groups. A year later, in 1997, the regional government (Kumamoto Prefecture) declared that Minamata Bay is once again safe for fishing with mercury in the waterway's marine life having fallen below the level the government considers dangerous (Pollack, 1997).

Ironically, as Japan's tragic episode of methyl mercury poisoning draws to a close, Minamata Disease is now claiming new victims along the Amazon. Brazil is in the throes of a modern-day gold rush, with an estimated half-million prospectors roaming the Amazon basin, searching along riverbeds for traces of the precious metal. Employing methods that would have looked entirely familiar to California's "Forty-niners" a century and a half ago, prospectors utilize mercury to separate gold from the muck dredged from the river. In doing so they are releasing an estimated 250 tons of mercury into the Amazon watershed each year. Following the same sequence of events that transpired decades ago in Minamata, mercury has reached high concentrations in Amazonian fish. Villagers who eat the tainted fish are now showing signs of neurological disorders and have detectable body burdens of methyl mercury. A visiting epidemiologist from the Japanese Ministry of Health, surveying the scene, remarked on the suffering still endured by survivors in Minamata and observed, "It should not happen again" (Pearce, 1999).

Figure 7-3   Distribution of Concentrations of Mercury in Blood of Women of Childbearing Age, 1999–2000

Note: EPA's reference dose (RD) for methylmercury is 0.1 micrograms per kilogram body weight per day. This is approximately equivalent to a concentration of 5.8 parts per billion mercury in blood.

Source: U.S. Environmental Protection Agency, 2003. America's Children and the Environment: Measures of Contaminants, Body Burdens, and Illnesses. www.epa.gov/envirohealth/children, based on data from Centers for Disease Control and Prevention, National Center for Health Statistics, National Health and Nutrition Examination Survey.

In addition to the toxic materials discussed in this chapter, there are many other substances capable of causing health damage in humans when present in more than trace amounts or when exposure to even very low levels persists over an extended time period. Cadmium, fluorides, selenium, copper, nickel, chromium, and arsenic are but a few of the naturally occurring toxins that are known, under certain conditions, to affect human health adversely. Unfortunately, because the symptoms of exposure to toxic substances are often so vague or so similar to those of other more common ailments, they are frequently either ignored or misdiagnosed. Thus it would not be surprising to find that health damage due to such toxins is more prevalent than commonly assumed at present.

References

Agency for Toxic Substances and Disease Registry (ATSDR). 2000. *Public Health Statement for Polychlorinated Biphenyls (PCBs)* (Nov). http://atsdr1.atsdr.cdc.gov/ToxProfiles/phs8821.html, accessed March 24, 2004.

———. 1999. *Toxicological Profile for Mercury.* U.S. Dept. of Health and Human Services, Public Health Service.

American Chemical Society. 1998. *Understanding Risk Analysis.*

Bakir, R., S. F. Damluji, L. Amin-Zaki, M. Murtadha, A. Khalidi, N. Y. Al-Rawi, S. Tikriti, H. I. Dhahir, T. W. Clarkson, J. C. Smith, and R. A. Doherty. 1973. "Methylmercury Poisoning in Iraq." *Science* 181:230–241.

Birnbaum, Linda S. 1994. "The Mechanism of Dioxin Toxicity: Relationship to Risk Assessment." *Environmental Health Perspectives.*

Bowker, Michael. 2003. *Fatal Deception: The Untold Story of Asbestos—Why It Is Still Legal and Still Killing Us.* New York: Rodale.

Centers for Disease Control and Prevention (CDC). 2003. "Surveillance for Elevated Blood Lead Levels Among Children—United States; 1997–2001." *Morbidity & Mortality Weekly Report, Surveillance Summaries,* September 12, 2003/52 (SS10):1–21.

———. 2001. "Fatal Pediatric Lead Poisoning—New Hampshire, 2000." *Morbidity & Mortality Weekly Report* 50, no. 22 (June 8):457–459.

———. 1993. "Lead Poisoning in Bridge Demolition Workers—Georgia, 1992." *Morbidity & Mortality Weekly Report* 42, no. 20 (May 28).

———. 1992. "Elevated Blood Lead Levels Associated with Illicitly Distilled Alcohol-Alabama, 1990–1991." *Morbidity & Mortality Weekly Report* 41, no. 17 (May 1).

Chao, Jason, M.D., and George D. Kikano, M.D. 1993. "Lead Poisoning in Children." *American Family Physician* (Jan).

Colborn, Theo, Dianne Dumanoski, and John Peterson Myers. 1996. *Our Stolen Future.* New York: Dutton, Penguin Books USA.

Dickson, L. C., and S. C. Buzik. 1993. "Health Risks of Dioxins: A Review of Environmental and Toxicological Considerations." *Veterinary and Human Toxicology* 35, no. 1 (Feb).

Environmental Protection Agency (EPA). 1995. "Report on the National Survey of Lead-Based Paint in Housing: Base Report." EPA A747–R95–003.

———. 1994. "Deposition of Air Pollutants to the Great Waters." EPA-453A/R-93–055, May.

Fawcett, Howard H. 1988. *Hazardous and Toxic Materials: Safe Handling and Disposal.* New York: John Wiley & Sons.

Fingerhut, Marilyn A., et al. 1991. "Cancer Mortality in Workers Exposed to 2,3,7,8–Tetrachlorodibenzo-p-Dioxin." *The New England Journal of Medicine* 324, no. 4 (Jan. 24).

Florini, Karen L. 1990. *Legacy of Lead: America's Continuing Epidemic of Childhood Lead Poisoning.* Environmental Defense Fund.

Franklin, Deborah. 1991. "Lead: Still Poison After All These Years." *Health* 5, no. 5 (Sept-Oct).

Harris, Lilieth V., and Ishenkumba A. Kahwa. 2003. "Asbestos: Old Foe in 21st Century Developing Countries." *The Science of the Total Environment* 307, no. 1–3 (May 20):1–9.

Hites, Ronald A., Jeffery A. Foran, David O. Carpenter, M. Coren Hamilton, Barbara A. Knuth, Steven J. Schwager. 2004. "Global Assessment of Organic Contaminants in Farmed Salmon." *Science* 303, no. 5655 (Jan. 9):226–229.

Kimbrough, R. D., M. L. Doemland, and M. E. LeVois. 1999. "Mortality in Male and Female Capacitor Workers Exposed to Polychlorinated Biphenyls." *Journal of Occupational and Environmental Medicine* 41, no. 3 (March 10):161–171.

LaDou, Joseph. 2004. "The Asbestos Cancer Epidemic." *Environmental Health Perspectives* 112, no. 3 (March).

Mielke, Howard W. 1999. "Lead in the Inner Cities." *American Scientist* 86 (Jan–Feb):62.

Needleman, H. L., et al. 1990. "The Long-Term Effects of Exposure to Low Doses of Lead in Childhood." *The New England Journal of Medicine* 322:83–88.

———. 1979. "Deficits in Psychologic and Classroom Performance of Children with Elevated Dentine Lead Levels." *The New England Journal of Medicine* 300:689–95.

Norman, Edward H. 1998. "Childhood Lead Poisoning and Vinyl Miniblind Exposure." *Journal of the American Medical Association* 279, no. 5 (Feb. 4):342.

Ottoboni, M. Alice. 1991. *The Dose Makes the Poison.* New York: Van Nostrand Reinhold.

Pearce, Fred. 1999. "A Nightmare Revisited." *New Scientist* 161, no. 2172 (Feb. 6):4.

Pérez-Peña, Richard. 2003. "Powder Cure is Dangerous, Officials Say." *New York Times,* Nov. 6.

Pollack, Andrew. 1997. "Japan Calls Mercury-Tainted Bay Safe Now." *New York Times,* July 30.

Preventing Lead Poisoning in Young Children. 1991. U.S. Dept. of Health and Human Services, Centers for Disease Control.

Regenstein, Lewis. 1982. *The Poisoning of America.* Washington, DC: Acropolis Books.

Selin, Noelle Eckley. 2005. "Mercury Rising: Is Global Action Necessary to Protect Human Health and the Environment?" *Environment* 47, no. 1 (Jan/Feb).

Sharma, Dinesh C. 1999. "Alarming Amounts of Lead Found in Indian Children." *The Lancet* 352, no. 9153 (Feb. 20):647.

Stauding, Kevin C., and Victor S. Roth. 1998. "Occupational Lead Poisoning." *American Family Physician* 57, no. 4 (Feb. 15):719–728.

Steenland, Kyle, Laurie Piacitelli, James Deddens, Marilyn Fingerhut, and Lih Ing Chang. 1999. "Cancer, Heart Disease, and Diabetes in Workers Exposed to 2,3,7,8–Tetrachlorodibenzo-p-dioxin." *Journal of the National Cancer Institute* 91, no. 9 (May 5):779–786.

Steingraber, Sandra. 1997. *Living Downstream: An Ecologist Looks at Cancer and the Environment*. Addison-Wesley.

Stokstad, Erik. 2004. "Salmon Survey Stokes Debate About Farmed Fish." *Science* 303, no. 5655 (Jan. 9):154–155.

Tong, Shilu, Peter A. Baghurst, Michael G. Sawyer, Jane Burns, and Anthony J. McMichael. 1998. "Declining Blood Lead Levels and Changes in Cognitive Function During Childhood: The Port Pirie Cohort Study." *Journal of the American Medical Association* 280, no. 22 (Dec. 9):1915.

Tossavainen, Antti. 2004. "Global Use of Asbestos and the Incidence of Mesothelioma," *International Journal of Occupational and Environmental Health* 10, no. 1 (Jan/March):22–25.

Urbina, Ian. 2003. "New Jersey Health Officials Warn of Lead in Mexican Grasshopper Treats." *New York Times*, Nov. 21.

Weisskopf, Michael. 1987. "Japanese Town Still Staggered by Legacy of Ecological Disaster." *The Washington Post*, April 18.

Weitzman, Michael, et al. 1993. "Lead-Contaminated Soil Abatement and Urban Children's Blood Lead Levels." *Journal of the American Medical Association* 269, no. 13 (April 7).

Xintaras, Charles. 1992. "Impact of Lead-Contaminated Soil on Public Health." Agency for Toxic Substances and Disease Registry, U.S. Dept. of Health and Human Services (May).

PESTS AND PESTICIDES

> Rats!
> They fought the dogs and killed the cats,
> And bit the babies in the cradles,
> And ate the cheeses out of the vats
> And licked the soup from the cooks' own ladles.
>
> —Robert Browning
> "The Pied Piper of Hamelin" (1845)

The tale of the mythical rat catcher of Hamelin, who rid that medieval town of its plague of rodents—and subsequently of its children as well—has been told and retold for centuries. Whether based on historical fact or not, the legend accurately conveys the sense of dismay and helplessness experienced by preindustrial societies when confronted with disastrous pest outbreaks. History records countless incidents of the devastating impact that certain insects, rodents, fungi, and so forth, can have on human health and well-being. Such organisms are typically referred to as "pests," a term derived from the Latin word *pestis* ("plague"), which was applied to a number of deadly epidemic diseases that periodically swept through the ancient world.

What Is a Pest?

Biologically speaking, there is, of course, no such thing as a "pest"; no classification system divides living things into categories labeled "good species" and "bad species." The term "pest," then, is a purely human concept and refers broadly to any organism—animal, plant, or microbe—that adversely affects human interests. Pest species comprise only a small percentage of the total number of organisms on earth, the vast majority being either beneficial or, more commonly, neutral so far as their impact on humans is concerned. Pests are not restricted to any one taxonomic group; representative species can be found among such invertebrates as insects, mites, ticks, and nematodes. Several bird species such as starlings, pigeons, and English sparrows can be considered pests, as can some mammals—rats, mice, moles, rabbits, and, in some situations, deer, coyotes, or even elephants! Many types of microorganisms, such as disease-causing bacteria, viruses, rickettsia, and fungi, are pests, as are weeds—any "plant out of place," growing where it's not wanted.

Problems Caused by Pests

Conflict between people and pests has existed since time immemorial and is generated primarily when such organisms compete with humans for the same resources, cause us discomfort, or are vectors of disease. The need to protect human interests by limiting pest damage has created a demand for better methods of combating such problems and constitutes the chief justification for the development and use of chemical pesticides. Although the use of such toxic compounds has, for a variety of reasons, come under increasing scrutiny and criticism in recent years, it is important to review the types of problems caused by pests in order to understand why suggestions to limit or abolish the use of chemical pesticides generates such controversy.

Resource Competition

According to some experts, insects, weeds, and plant pathogens (fungi, nematodes, bacteria and viruses) are responsible for the loss of an estimated 35–42% of the global harvest each year, despite more than 50 years of escalating chemical warfare against agricultural pests (Pimentel, 1997). Insect problems are particularly severe on cotton, tobacco, and potatoes, as well as on most fruit and vegetable crops. Fungal diseases cause significant losses primarily to fruits and some vegetables, while yield reductions due to weed infestations are most pronounced on acreage devoted to corn and soybean production. In addition to such losses in the field, about 6% of the annual harvest in the United States (and a substantially larger share in developing nations) is lost to pests while in storage or transit.

A reduction in current pesticide use would undoubtedly result in a further increase in crop loss due to pest depredation—a cause for concern both to farmers and to humanitarians worried about feeding a hungry world. The extent of such loss is hotly disputed, however. Some scientists estimate that without pesticides or alternative protective measures, U.S. agricultural production would drop by 24–57%, depending on the particular crop. Farm exports would be cut by half and American consumers would see their annual grocery bill rise by almost $230 (NRC, 2000). Others, however, calculate that preharvest losses of all crops resulting from a significant reduction in pesticide use would be minimal. A noted entomologist at Cornell University estimates that if American farmers were to adopt a variety of nonchemical control techniques they could cut current levels of agricultural pesticide use by 50% without experiencing any decline in yields. Under this scenario, substituting nonchemical for chemical controls would result in food price increases of less than 1% (Pimentel, 1991).

Although loss in farm production is the major example of resource competition between humans and pests, many other instances of conflict can be cited: **termites** cause incalculable damage to structures, especially in the tropics; in the United States alone, controlling termites and repairing the damage caused by these wood-destroying pests cost property owners an estimated $11 billion each year (Raloff, 2003). **Cockroaches**, the bread-and-butter of the structural pest control industry, are found worldwide and are universally despised for contaminating food and materials in homes, restaurants, supermarkets, cruise ships, warehouses—literally every place where careless humans provide them with a source of food and water. **Rats and mice** cause enormous economic losses, consuming as much as one-third of the world's harvest and rendering many stored food supplies unusable due to contamination with rodent hairs, droppings, and urine (Mallis, 1997).

Sources of Discomfort

Itching, buzzing, creeping, and crawling may not seem like serious concerns, but the creatures responsible have been driving people to distraction for millennia and have been the targets of a great deal of pesticide use in recent decades. Some of the major villains involved in producing acute human discomfort, if not illness, include the following.

Lice. Head lice, body lice, and crab lice are all human parasites that can cause severe itching, secondary infections, and scarred or hardened skin. Lice are typically associated with people living in crowded conditions where opportunities for bathing and laundering clothes are limited. With the introduction of DDT following World War II, the incidence of lice infestations dropped to low levels. As the use of this insecticide became restricted, however, cases of head lice among schoolchildren have been increasing.

Fleas. Aside from the flea species that transmit the deadly plague bacterium (see next section), fleas commonly found on domestic animals can cause severe irritation, loss of blood, and discomfort. Although most fleas prefer to feed on their animal host, they frequently bite humans if the normal host is absent. Such bites can be extremely painful and may cause swelling and a reddening of the skin.

Mites. These tiny insect relatives are responsible for the serious skin condition known as scabies, as well as a number of other forms of dermatitis such as "grocers' itch," acquired by handling mite-infested grain products, cheese, dried fruits, and so on. Mites that normally live as ectoparasites on birds may become very serious pests of humans when they migrate in large numbers into homes after starlings or sparrows leave their nests. For this reason, householders should discourage birds from nesting on eaves or windowsills or other locations in close proximity to homes. **Chiggers,** a type of mite inhabiting many parts of the southern or midwestern United States, can cause extreme skin irritation lasting for a week or more when they attach themselves to a human host, usually around the waist or armpits.

Bedbugs. During the day these small, lentil-shaped insects are seldom seen, hiding among bedsprings or the tufts of mattresses, in cracks in the bedframe or headboard, under loose wallpaper or area rugs—indeed, any place that is dark, secluded, and in close proximity to a blood meal. At night bedbugs emerge to feed on an unwary sleeper, leaving large, intensely itchy welts on sensitive victims and bloodstains on sheets when an engorged bug is inadvertently crushed as its human host rolls over in bed. Once a common pest almost everywhere, bedbugs largely disappeared in more affluent societies after World War II, due in part to the widespread use of DDT, but also thanks to fashion trends toward less elaborate bedroom furniture (i.e., fewer hiding places) and better vacuum cleaners (more efficient cleaning = fewer bedbugs). In recent years, however, bedbugs—like head lice—are making a comeback, owing in large part to the surge in international trade and travel. Since bedbugs can live for half a year or more without food, they can easily stow away in luggage or shipping crates, emerging hale and hungry in hotels, university dorms, hospitals, and homes half a world away. The old bedtime admonition, "Sleep tight, don't let the bedbugs bite!" has new relevance in this age of globalization; fortunately, bedbugs are not known to transmit any diseases.

Spiders. Although many people harbor an irrational antipathy toward spiders, the vast majority of these eight-legged creatures are quite harmless to humans. Even the fearsome-looking tarantula—the loathsome villain in many a B-grade Hollywood thriller—is actually rather docile. Now widely sold as pets, tarantulas can be handled with ease and rarely bite; even when they do, their venom is of little harm to most people. Only three U.S. species present any real danger: the **black widow** (female only), the **brown recluse** (both sexes), and the **aggressive house spider** (males are more venomous and more likely to bite than females). The black widow, though more abundant in warmer regions of the country, can be found throughout the United States; primarily an outdoor spider, the black widow is typically found around piles of wood or other debris where the female spins a nondescript-looking web. Black widow venom acts as a nerve poison, but while bites may be quite painful they are very seldom fatal, even in the absence of medical attention. Contrary to popular myth, the diminutive male black widow is *not* devoured after mating by his much larger bride—unless she is unusually hungry!—but generally spends a parasitic post-nuptial existence in the vicinity of her web, waiting for any leftovers that may come his way. The brown recluse spider, whose range covers much of the south-central and southeastern United States as far north as Missouri, Illinois, and Indiana, is most often encountered within dwellings where it hides in attics, closets, and other dark, seldom-disturbed places. It is a shy species that bites only when provoked—usually when rolled on at night or when clothes are taken out of storage. The poison injected by the bite of a brown recluse differs from that of a black widow in that it is *cytotoxic*, causing tissue death in the vicinity of the wound. Scarcely noticeable at first, the bite gradually becomes very painful and frequently develops into an open ulceration that persists for weeks and eventually leaves a large ugly scar. The aggressive house spider (alternatively referred to as the "hobo spider"), a European immigrant whose range in North America is currently limited to British Columbia and five states in the northwestern U.S., has only recently been identified as the source of spider bites long attributed to the brown recluse (which doesn't live in that part of the country). Like brown recluse venom, that of the aggressive house spider is a cytotoxin. *Unlike* the brown recluse, however, aggressive house spiders are true to their name and tend to bite without provocation. Large (40 mm in length) and fast running, these spiders tend to live in or near houses, often in rock walls, along foundations, or in woodpiles (many bites occur when firewood is being carried inside). Large numbers of males enter basements and ground floor rooms of homes in the autumn and dogs and cats are frequently bitten on the face as they attempt to investigate, occasionally dying as a result. These are *not* nice spiders! (Akre and Myhre, 1994).

In addition to the above, the buzzing of flies, mosquitoes, gnats, cicadas, June bugs, or wasps—even when these insects are not carrying disease organisms—can provoke extreme annoyance. Certain plant species, particularly poison ivy and its relatives, also have been prime targets of chemical herbicides because of the intensely irritating rash which contact with these plants can produce.

Vectors of Disease

Public health practitioners, along with farmers, were among the first to greet the introduction of synthetic chemical pesticides with great enthusiasm. Compounds such as DDT were viewed as perhaps the ultimate weapon in freeing humanity from the threat of a number of insect-or rodent-borne diseases responsible for millions of deaths and illnesses each year. Quite appropriately, the first use to which DDT was put involved the wartime dusting of refugees in Italy to curb an outbreak of typhus fever. The success of this effort led to extensive spraying campaigns in many parts of the world against the vectors of such dreaded killers as malaria, yellow fever, river blindness, bubonic plague, and encephalitis. Although the medical community's high hopes for complete eradication of the carriers of these diseases have proven overly optimistic, pesticide use has played a significant role in lowering death rates and improving public health in many parts of the world. Some pests of particular public health importance include mosquitoes, flies, body lice, rat fleas, and ticks.

Mosquitoes. Mosquitoes have probably been responsible for more human deaths than any other insect, though their role as disease-carriers was not recognized until late in the 19th century. Worldwide, even today millions of people become ill each year due to such mosquito-borne ailments as malaria, yellow fever, dengue, filariasis, and encephalitis. In the past, there have been major outbreaks of all these diseases, particularly malaria and yellow fever, in parts of the United States. In recent years, entry of large numbers of infected immigrants or returning tourists from regions where **malaria** is still endemic have been responsible for 1,000–1,200 cases of malaria acquired abroad but diagnosed and reported in the United States each year. Since the mosquito vectors responsible for transmitting malaria in the U.S. are common species (*Anopheles quadrimaculatus* and *A. freeborni*), the opportunity still exists for future outbreaks.

Until recently, **dengue fever** and **dengue hemorrhagic fever**, carried by *Aedes aegypti*, also the vector of yellow fever, were considered relatively mild ailments. However, in recent years dengue has emerged as a major cause of death and disease throughout the world's tropics, particularly among children. Dengue is now considered the most important mosquito-borne viral disease of humans (malaria is caused by the *Plasmodium* parasite), sickening tens of millions of people annually. Reasons for the sudden emergence of dengue as a serious public health problem are complex, but according to the Centers for Disease Control and Prevention (CDC), widespread discontinuance of effective mosquito control efforts in the early 1970s due to concerns about the environmental impacts of chemical pesticides played a significant role in fostering the reestablishment of *A. aegypti* populations.

In the United States and Canada, **West Nile Virus** today constitutes the most serious mosquito-borne health threat. Mosquitoes pick up the virus when they feed on the blood of infected birds, subsequently transmitting the pathogen to a human victim. In its most serious form (less than 1% of cases), West Nile Virus causes a fatal inflammation of the brain (encephalitis). The vast majority of cases are far less severe,

Figure 8-1   2004 West Nile Virus Activity in the United States

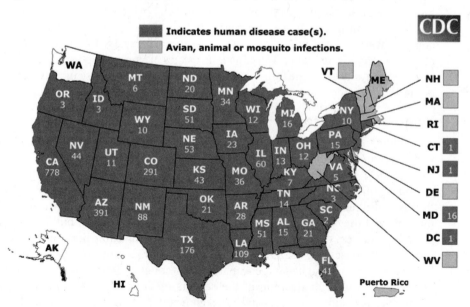

Note: Reported to CDC as of January 11, 2005

Source: Centers for Disease Control and Prevention (CDC).

Box 8-1 Avoiding the Bite

In summers past, many a child took perverse pleasure in allowing a hungry mosquito to alight on his or her arm and begin feeding, slowly swelling up like a tiny red balloon until given a triumphant whack, splattering blood in all directions! Since the arrival of West Nile Virus (WNV) in the United States a few years ago, however, such "fun" now entails considerable health risk. Mosquito-borne West Nile disease has made the avoidance of mosquito bites an important aspect of summertime preventive health care. West Nile Virus was first reported in the United States in the summer of 1999, with most cases occurring in the New York metropolitan area. Since then, the virus has spread rapidly across the country, with Illinois, Colorado, and California reporting the highest number of cases in 2002, 2003, and 2004, respectively. By the end of 2004, human cases of WNV had been reported to the CDC from 45 states and the District of Columbia.

While insecticidal spraying or fogging to reduce populations of adult mosquitoes may occasionally be justified in areas where disease outbreaks are severe, doing so is of limited usefulness and can itself raise health and environmental concerns. A much safer and more effective approach to reducing the risk of mosquito-borne disease is to focus on two complementary strategies: (1) **reducing the size of the mosquito population** and (2) **using repellents to avoid being bitten.** The former primarily involves removing, to the greatest extent possible, any standing water around the house or yard where mosquitoes can lay their eggs. Some potential breeding places are fairly obvious:

- infrequently changed birdbaths or ornamental garden ponds (unless these contain larvae-devouring fish)

- neglected wading pools or swimming pool covers that have collected rainwater

Other egg-laying sites may not be so readily apparent:

- drainage saucers under well-watered planters

- pet water bowls

- leaf-clogged rain gutters that fail to drain adequately

- hollow stumps or tree holes

- rain-collecting tires or debris lying around the yard

- a child's wagon or wheelbarrow that hasn't been moved since the last downpour

While eradication of breeding sites can substantially reduce the number of hungry mosquitoes in an area, it's unlikely to eliminate them altogether, making the judicious use of repellents another important approach for avoiding mosquito bites. Many products claim to be effective repellents, but CDC has long advised that only those containing the chemical compound popularly known as **DEET** keep mosquitoes at bay for any length of time; in 2005 CDC expanded its list of recommended mosquito repellents to include those containing the chemical picaridin or the oil of lemon eucalyptus. Plant-based mosquito repellents such as citronella have very limited effectiveness, deterring mosquitoes, on average, for only 3–20 minutes following application; one soybean-oil-based repellent is a bit better, providing protection up to about one hour. The much-touted moisturizer, *Skin-So-Soft Bath Oil*®, keeps mosquitoes away for less than 10 minutes. Wristbands impregnated with repellent, despite advertising claims, don't work at all, nor do "ultrasonic" devices or Vitamin B.

By contrast, DEET-containing products give complete protection against bites for several to many hours, depending on the concentration of the active ingredient. Rising concentrations of DEET are directly proportional to the duration of the bite-free period, with products containing 6–7% DEET protective for about 2 hours, 20% DEET for 4 hours, 24% DEET an average of 5 hours. Beyond 50%, increasing concentrations of the active ingredient do not further extend the length of protection.

Although in the past some pediatricians warned that the concentration of DEET in formulations used on young children should never exceed 10% (some advised against using DEET on small children at all), an extensive safety evaluation of DEET by the Environmental Protection Agency in 1998 concluded that, when used in accordance with label directions, DEET can be safely used by people of all ages and at all concentrations. Certain safety precautions should, of course, be followed:

- When used directly on skin, apply only to exposed areas, avoiding the mouth, eyes, or any place where the skin is broken. DEET may also be sprayed on clothing, but should not be applied to skin underneath; clothing treated with DEET should be laundered before being worn again.

- When repellent is used on a child, it should be applied by an adult; avoid child's eyes, mouth, and hands (since children tend to put hands in their mouths) and use sparingly around the ears.

- Don't over-apply; a small amount, when evenly spread is adequate for protection. Wash off repellent with soap and water after coming indoors.

Mosquito repellents can be used in conjunction with sunscreen but a single combination sunscreen/repellent lotion is *not* recommended because DEET shouldn't be applied as frequently as is necessary for sunscreen. The CDC advises that sunscreen be applied first, followed by a DEET-containing repellent. Sunscreen can subsequently be reapplied without reapplying repellent.

For optimum protection, insect repellent should be used whenever a person is going to be outdoors in a situation where mosquito bites are likely, especially at dusk or dawn when the largest numbers of hungry females are present. Mosquitoes have always been a summer presence; their new threat as vectors of West Nile Virus makes it more important than ever that we take active precautions to keep them as far away from us as possible!

Reference

Fradin, Mark S., and John F. Day. 2002. "Comparative Efficacy of Insect Repellents against Mosquito Bites." *The New England Journal of Medicine* 347, no.1 (July 4):13–18.

generally manifested as a mild, flu-like ailment that persists for only a few days. Although the first human cases were diagnosed only in 1999 in the U.S. and 2002 in Canada, by 2003 West Nile disease was being reported from coast-to-coast, with the number of people affected soaring to 9,000 confirmed cases and 240 fatalities. Public health officials were braced for even more bad news in 2004, but the number of cases declined that year to slightly under 2,500 cases and 87 deaths. Several other forms of viral encephalitis transmitted from infected birds to humans via mosquito bites occur occasionally during the summer months and early fall. Of these, Eastern equine encephalitis exhibits the highest mortality rates (50–60%), but cases are quite rare, averaging just four per year. A few dozen cases of St. Louis encephalitis, LaCross encephalitis, and Western encephalitis occur sporadically each year, primarily in midwestern states; fatality rates for these diseases are low, but victims may experience long-term central nervous system damage. U.S. Public Health Service officials striving to prevent outbreaks of vectorborne disease fear their task may be complicated by the arrival in the late 1980s of *Aedes albopictus*, the **Asian tiger mosquito**. A number of these alien invaders entered the port of Houston as stowaways in a shipment of used tires. They quickly spread from Texas throughout much of the eastern U.S., presumably hitchhiking on the truckloads of used tires that ply the interstate highway system (the female lays her eggs just above the waterline in tree holes or artificial containers—like tire casings). Because tiger mosquito eggs can overwinter, *A. albopictus* has had no difficulty in becoming established in northern states as well as in warmer regions of the country. Unlike many other mosquito species, it thrives in close proximity to people and can live inside houses year-round, breeding in pet water dishes and in the saucers under houseplants. The tiger mosquito is a vicious biter and, in its Asian homeland, is an important disease vector. Although as yet no outbreaks have been attributed to the newcomer, researchers have determined that the tiger mosquito has the ability to pick up and transmit the viral pathogens for dengue fever and encephalitis and fear that it has the potential to become the most important carrier of mosquito-borne diseases in the United States.

Flies.   Many species of flies, particularly the common housefly, are important carriers of serious gastrointestinal diseases such as **typhoid fever**, **cholera**, **dysentery**, and **parasitic worm infections** due to their habit of feeding on human and animal wastes. If such wastes contain pathogenic organisms, the fly can pick these up either

Figure 8-2

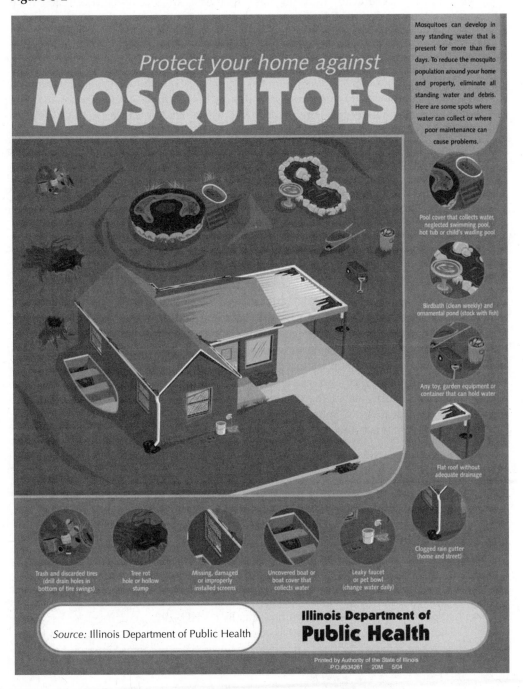

Source: Illinois Department of Public Health

on the sticky pads of its feet or on its body hairs or mouthparts and mechanically transmit them to humans when it alights on food materials. Fly vomitus and feces also frequently contain pathogenic bacteria that can inoculate human food, multiply rapidly in the food medium, and subsequently result in outbreaks of intestinal diseases when the food is consumed by people.

Cockroaches. Contrary to common belief, cockroaches have not been implicated as important vectors of infectious disease, even though laboratory studies have repeatedly shown these insects harbor a wide range of pathogenic microbes on their feet and can mechanically transmit these organisms to food. Some researchers have attributed cases of *Salmonella* food poisoning and other diarrheal illnesses to the presence of large numbers of cockroaches in or near food preparation areas, but the evidence for a cause-and-effect relationship is inconclusive. Undisputed, however, is the fact that heavy cockroach infestations can cause severe allergic reactions and precipitate asthma attacks. Secretions produced by roaches can induce symptoms ranging from skin irritations and runny nose to difficulty in breathing. Acute reaction to cockroach allergens has recently been recognized as the leading cause for the high incidence of **asthma** among inner-city children in the U.S. These findings suggest that vigorous cockroach control programs should be an integral part of public health efforts to combat asthma, the incidence rates of which have been dramatically rising worldwide (Rosenstreich et al., 1997).

Body lice. As mentioned in the previous section, body lice can be a source of intense discomfort, but they are of special public health concern because they are vectors of several serious epidemic diseases. **Typhus fever**, characterized by elevated temperature, severe headache, and a rash, has been a major killer in past centuries, particularly during wartime when perhaps as many soldiers died from typhus as from swords or bullets. The rickettsial pathogen responsible for the disease is passed from louse to human by the feces of the insect, not its bite. When a person infested with lice scratches the affected area, minor abrasions on the skin permit entry to the rickettsia. Other lice subsequently feeding on a person infected with typhus ingest the pathogen and spread it as they move from person to person. This method of transmission explains why typhus outbreaks are most prevalent when people are living together in crowded, unsanitary conditions. Insecticidal dusting of louse-infested persons has proven to be an effective method for controlling the spread of typhus fever. Two other louse-borne diseases, also most common during wartime but with much lower fatality rates than typhus, are trench fever and relapsing fever.

Rat fleas. Aside from the enormous economic damage caused by rats, these pests are of great public health concern because they are vectors of a number of diseases, the most deadly of which is **plague** (the "Black Death" of medieval times). In September 1994 the first major plague outbreak in half a century terrorized residents of the Indian city of Surat, killing more than 50 people. Even before the Surat incident, plague rates had been steadily rising worldwide since the early 1980s. The vast majority of recent plague victims have been in Africa, predominantly in the nations of Madagascar and Tanzania, while Brazil, Peru, Myanmar, and Vietnam account for most of the remainder. Since the late 1980s, the World Health Organization (WHO) has reported the average annual number of plague cases worldwide at about 2,500, with approximately 200 plague deaths annually (WHO, 1997).

The plague bacterium actually is carried by fleas on rats, not by the rats themselves. When infected fleas feed on their rat hosts, the rats too sicken and die. If rats are living in close proximity to humans, a flea whose host has died may then hop onto a person for a blood meal and thus spread the plague organism to human populations. Because of the tendency of fleas to substitute hosts when necessary, rat-poisoning campaigns should always be preceded by insecticidal spraying of rat-infested areas to kill the fleas first. If this precautionary measure is not taken, one runs the risk of transferring rodent diseases to humans.

While most Americans tend to think of plague as a "long-ago and faraway" type of disease, rat fleas infected with the plague bacterium were introduced into California early in the 20th century and quickly became endemic among wild rodent populations in the region. Since that time the focus of plague infection has expanded steadily eastward; today plague-infected rodent populations have been identified in 13 western states and in southwestern Canada. Each year an average of 10–15 human cases of plague are reported from this region, mostly in scattered rural areas. The incidence of plague outbreaks in the United States seems to be increasing, as rapid suburbanization results in growing numbers of people living in close proximity to wild rodent habitat. A worrisome trend noted in recent years is a rise in the number of human cases in which domestic cats were the source of infection. Because cats typically are allowed to roam freely, those living in areas where plague-infected rodents are common have ample opportunity to contract the disease and subsequently transmit the ailment to their human companions (CDC, 1994). People living, camping, hiking, or hunting in areas where plague is endemic should take precautions to avoid contact with wild rodents and rodent burrows (where infected fleas may be present) and should never approach or handle obviously sick or dying wild animals. Even recently dead rodents can present a disease hazard: one plague death in the Southwest involved a housewife who picked up a dead ground squirrel that her cat had proudly deposited on the doorstep. She presumably was bitten by a hungry flea who found her an acceptable alternative host and subsequently contracted a fatal case of bubonic plague.

Ticks. Among our most common parasites, ticks are a source of profound annoyance to campers, hunters, dog owners, and livestock raisers who frequently discover themselves or their pets providing a blood meal to these tiny pests. Ticks are far more than a nuisance, however. They are vectors of several serious human diseases such as **Rocky Mountain spotted fever**, a condition that frequently results in death within two weeks and which, contrary to its name, is not restricted to mountainous areas but is found throughout the continental United States, with the largest number of cases being reported from North and South Carolina.

The most common tick-borne ailment in the United States today is **Lyme disease**, with cases reported from every state except Montana, as well as from various locations along the border in Canada. In spite of its wide geographic distribution (researchers hypothesize that birds are carrying the tick from one region of the country to another, since tick larvae frequently feed on avian hosts), Lyme disease poses a significant risk of infection in only 100 or so counties in the northeast and upper Midwest, where 95% of all cases have been reported. Caused by the spirochete bacterium *Borrelia burgdorferi*, Lyme disease is transmitted to humans by the bite of an infected black-legged tick, *Ixodes scapularis*; on the West Coast a related species, *I. pacificus*, is the vector. The black-legged tick, once inaccurately referred to as the "deer tick," is a tiny arthropod that feeds on the blood of birds, small mammals like the white-footed mouse, deer, and—if they happen to be around—humans who venture into the ticks' woodland habitat. Because the tick is so small and inconspicuous, human victims may not even realize they've been bitten until disease symptoms appear, generally several days to a month later. The first and most characteristic symptom of Lyme disease, observed in 60–80% of patients, is a circular, spreading red rash resembling a rosy "bull's eye" because of

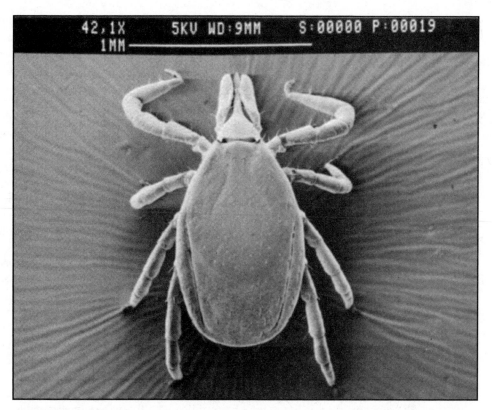

The diminutive black-legged tick (*Ixodes scapularis*) carries the bacterium that causes Lyme disease. [*Mathew Nadakavukaren*]

the pale area of skin in the center. This rash, which usually develops on the torso of the body, though not necessarily at the location of the tick bite, is often accompanied by a splitting headache, fever, chills, backache, and extreme fatigue. At this stage the disease can be effectively treated with antibiotics, which generally produce a quick and complete cure. If not caught at this stage, Lyme disease can progress to a second stage characterized by nervous system dysfunction and muscle pains; the onset of arthritis, usually in the knees or other large joints, typifies the third stage of the disease and can be very painful. Unfortunately, antibiotics may not be particularly effective in combating these later stages of Lyme disease—perhaps as many as 50% of patients who develop chronic symptoms don't respond to antibiotic therapy. In 1998 the first vaccine for preventing Lyme disease, *LYMErix,* was approved by the FDA. Although this product was both safe and efficacious, the manufacturer withdrew it from the market in 2002 due to low consumer demand. The lack of a vaccine increases the importance of personal protective measures for hikers, campers, or those living in tick-infested areas.

The same tick species that carries the Lyme Disease pathogen can also transmit a sometimes fatal bacterial ailment known as **ehrlichiosis** (there are actually two forms of this disease, one of which is carried by the black-legged tick, the other by the Lone Star tick). Approximately 600 cases of ehrlichiosis, most of them in the northeastern U.S., have been confirmed by medical authorities since the disease was first recognized in the mid-1980s; however, this figure may be unrealistically low, since medical experts suspect that many cases have been misdiagnosed or gone undetected. The geographic range of ehrlichiosis continues to expand and the number of people infected is correspondingly increasing. Q-fever, relapsing fever, tularemia, and tick paralysis are just a few of many ailments that can be transmitted by ticks. Species that most commonly feed on humans generally are found in areas of wild vegetation such as woods, high grass, parks, and along paths frequented by wild animals. Here they lie in wait for a potential human or animal host, clinging to bushes or tall weeds, ready to latch onto an unwary passer-by (contrary to popular belief, they don't drop onto victims from trees). People planning outdoor activities in tick-infested areas should take such precautions as applying tick repellent to exposed areas of skin, wearing socks and long trousers, and avoiding sitting on the ground or on logs. They should also be diligent about checking their bodies for the presence of ticks at least twice a day and immediately removing them, since most tick-borne diseases are transmitted only after the creature has been feeding for several hours.

Although the previous discussion is by no means a complete listing of the human health problems caused by various pest species, it should convey some realization of the need for pest control and an understanding of why many public health officials feel that abandoning chemical pesticides would entail the risk of increased mortality and morbidity rates due to vector-borne disease.

Pest Control

Early Attempts at Pest Control

Human efforts to control pest outbreaks date back to the development of agriculture approximately 10,000 years ago, when relatively large expanses of a single crop and sizeable numbers of people living close together in unsanitary conditions favored an increase in pest populations that wouldn't have been possible among small, scattered societies living a nomadic, hunter-gatherer type of lifestyle. Early attempts to reduce pest damage included purely physical efforts—stomping, flailing, and burning—as well as the offering of prayers, sacrifices, and ritual dances to the local gods. A few effective measures were discovered even at such early dates, however. The Sumerians, in what now is Iraq, successfully employed sulfur compounds against insects and mites more than 5,000 years ago; over 3,000 years ago the Chinese were treating seeds with insecticides derived from plant extracts, using wood ashes and chalk to ward off insect pests in the home, and applying mercury and arsenic compounds to their bodies to control lice. Among the Chinese is found the earliest example of using a pest's natural enemies to control it: by AD 300 the Chinese were introducing colonies of predatory ants into their citrus groves to control caterpillars and certain beetles.

During the peak of Greek civilization, records indicate that some of the wealthier citizens used mosquito nets and built high sleeping towers to evade mosquitoes. They also used oil sprays and sulfur bitumen ointments to deter insects. The Romans designed rat-proof granaries, but relied largely on superstitious practices such as nailing up crayfish in different parts of the garden to keep away caterpillars. In medieval Europe people increasingly relied on religious faith to protect them from pest depredations; as late as 1476, during an outbreak of cutworms in Switzerland, several of the offending insects were hauled into court, proclaimed guilty, excommunicated by the archbishop, and banished from the land!

Not until the 18th and 19th centuries did efforts at pest control make any meaningful progress. This was a time when European farming practices were becoming more productive and scientific, and help in combating agricultural pests was eagerly sought. Botanical insecticides such as pyrethrum, derris (rotenone), and nicotine were introduced at this time. Heightened interest in improved pest control methods was generated during the mid-19th century by several of the worst agricultural disasters ever recorded—the potato blight in Ireland, England, and Belgium in 1848, caused by a fungal disease; the fungus leaf spot disease of coffee in Ceylon (now Sri Lanka), which completely wiped out coffee cultivation on the island; and the outbreak of both powdery mildew and an insect pest, grape phylloxera, which nearly destroyed the wine industry in Europe. Such problems led to the development of new chemical pesticides and ushered in a whole new era of pest control. Two of the first such compounds, Bordeaux mixture (copper sulfate and lime) and Paris Green (copper acetoarsenite), were originally employed as fungicides but were subsequently found to be effective insecticides as well. Paris Green became one of the most widely used insecticides in the late 19th century and Bordeaux mixture even today is the most widely used fungicide in the world. Early in the 1900s arsenic-containing compounds such as lead arsenate, highly toxic to both insects and humans, became the most widely sold insecticides in the United States and retained their leading position until the advent of DDT after World War II (Flint and VandenBosch, 1981).

In 1939, Paul Müller, a Swiss chemist working for the Geigy Corporation, discovered that the synthetic compound dichlorodiphenyltrichloroethane (referred to as DDT for obvious reasons!) was extremely effective in killing insects on contact and retained its lethal character for a long time after application. Müller had simply been looking for a better product to use against clothes moths, but the outbreak of war in Europe gave far wider significance to the new chemical. Military authorities, recognizing that extensive campaigns would be carried out in the tropics where insect-borne disease threatened high troop losses, made the search for better insecticides a top priority. DDT, highly lethal to every kind of insect yet harmless to humans when applied

A woman sprays DDT in the bedroom of her child, circa 1945. Use of DDT spread quickly after World War II until it was banned by the EPA in 1972. [© Bettmann/Corbis]

as a powder, was just what the military needed. Initially, production of DDT was exclusively for use in the armed forces where it was employed first as a louse powder and later for mosquito control. At the end of the war DDT was released for civilian use, both in agriculture and for public health purposes. Its use quickly spread worldwide, amidst high expectations of complete eradication of many diseases and greatly reduced crop losses due to insects. Müller was awarded the 1948 Nobel Prize in Physiology and Medicine in recognition of his contribution. The enthusiastic reception given to DDT encouraged chemical companies in their search for new and even more effective synthetic pesticides. By the mid-1950s at least 25 new products that would revolutionize insect control practices were put on the market, among the more important of which were chlordane, heptachlor, toxaphene, aldrin, endrin, dieldrin, and parathion (Perkins, 1982). The age of chemical warfare against pests had begun.

Types of Pesticides

Pesticides, substances that kill pests, are subdivided into groups according to target organism. For example, insecticides kill insects, herbicides kill weeds, rodenticides kill rats and mice, nematicides kill nematodes, and so forth. Within each of these groups there may be further subdivisions based on such characteristics as route of intake of the poison or physiological effect on the target organism. A brief survey of some of the most common groups of pesticides currently in use would include the following.

Insecticides. The largest number of pesticides is employed against a wide variety of insects and includes **stomach poisons** (taken into the body through the mouth; effective against insects with biting or chewing mouthparts, such as caterpillars); **contact poisons** (penetrate through the body wall); and **fumigants** (enter insect through its respiratory system).

The earliest insecticides were **inorganic compounds**, most containing heavy metals or arsenic, and acted as stomach poisons. This meant that they were effective only against pests such as beetles or caterpillars that ingested the insecticide while feeding on treated crops, or against insects like cockroaches that might ingest pesticidal dusts while grooming themselves. Many of these products were quite toxic to humans as well, posing serious health hazards to the applicator and to farm workers; under certain environmental conditions they could also damage crop foliage, and they were relatively expensive. For all these reasons, when the new synthetic organic insecticides became commercially available soon after World War II, they were enthusiastically welcomed by pesticide users. All of the new compounds—the **chlorinated hydrocarbons, organophosphates, carbamates,** and **pyrethroids**—acted as contact poisons, making them, unlike the inorganic insecticides, **broad-spectrum** poisons capable of killing virtually any insect they touched. These new weapons meant that a farmer no longer needed a shelf full of various chemicals to combat the pests in his fields—one insecticide would kill them all. The chlorinated hydrocarbons have an additional feature that initially seemed like a major plus—once applied, they are **persistent** in the environment, leaving a residue that breaks down very slowly, providing protection for a long period after the initial application. For the farmer, persistence meant that he didn't need to worry about re-treating his fields every time it rained—the DDT or aldrin or heptachlor would still be there. Chlordane, a member of this group that for many years was the structural pest control industry's termiticide of choice, was so persistent that, once applied around the perimeter of a home, it provided up to 40 years of protection from these wood-destroying insects. Unfortunately, persistence was found to have a serious down-side as well; because the long-lasting residues are not water-soluble, they accumulate in fatty tissues when taken up by living organisms and may remain in the body indefinitely, becoming increasingly concentrated over time. For this reason, and because of human health concerns associated with this group of pesticides, most of the chlorinated hydrocarbons have been banned in the United States and many other countries. An international

---

Box 8-2   Malaria Resurgent: Can a Case Be Made for DDT?

Environmentalists cheered when the UN-sponsored Stockholm Convention on Persistent Organic Pollutants (a.k.a. the "POPs Treaty") came into force in May 2004. The agreement commits signatory nations to eliminate or reduce as much as possible the production, use, and release of 12 organochlorine compounds known as the "Dirty Dozen," 9 of them insecticides widely used since the late 1940s (see table 8-1). The treaty contains one major exemption, however—the right to continue using DDT against insect vectors of disease.

Why the determination among a sizeable minority of signatory nations to retain a chemical weapon that has been outlawed in the U.S. and many other industrialized countries for more than 30 years? The answer can be summarized in one word: malaria. Throughout the tropics, this debilitating and often fatal disease has reemerged as a major public health problem and an enormous obstacle to economic development. Rightly or wrongly, government officials in affected nations have concluded that use of DDT against mosquitoes is a weapon they simply can't afford to banish from their arsenal.

Disease statistics are truly alarming. Health officials estimate that 300,000–500,000 new cases of malaria are contracted annually, with as many as 7,000, mostly children, dying of the disease every day. While the number of countries affected by malaria is substantially less than it was prior to the mid-20th century (in the past, large areas of southern and southeastern Europe were malarious, as was the Mississippi River Valley and all of the southeastern U.S.), fully 40% of the world's people today live in regions where the threat of malaria is ever-present. On the Indian subcontinent, in Southeast Asia, and in tropical South America the incidence of malaria has been rising rapidly since the 1980s, when government-sponsored mosquito abatement efforts were curtailed. In Africa, however, the disease is taking its heaviest toll—today fully 90% of all malaria victims live in sub-Saharan Africa. At a time when HIV/AIDS dominates the health news from that part of the world, malaria is the cause for 10% of hospital admissions and 20–30% of all doctors' visits. Public health workers in Africa have noted that malaria outbreaks are now occurring even in previously malaria-free regions such as the highlands of Kenya, where the elevation and cooler climate were assumed to discourage disease-carrying mosquitoes.

That one of humanity's most ancient plagues should resurge in the early 21st century seems tragically ironic, considering the high hopes that greeted the "Global Malaria Eradication Program" launched by the newly created World Health Organization (WHO) in 1955. With a powerful new weapon—DDT—and more than 60 nations providing financial support for establishing factories to produce the insecticide in poor countries, the worldwide assault against mosquitoes was initiated amid optimistic assertions that malaria would soon be banished forever. From the beginning, realists conceded that killing every last mosquito was an impossibility. However, it was believed that if populations of the insects could be reduced enough to limit the frequency of bites (and thereby transmission of the malarial parasite), within a few years the parasite would die out among the human population. After that, so it was reasoned, a resurgence in mosquito numbers would represent nothing more than an irritation, since the insects would no longer harbor the malaria pathogen. For several years the strategy seemed to be working brilliantly. By 1961 the incidence of malaria had plummeted in 37 countries; in some areas—notably Taiwan, Jamaica, and Sardinia—the disease was totally eliminated and they remain to this day malaria free. However, by 1969 problems with insecticide resistance among some mosquito populations and growing concerns about health and environmental side effects of DDT use led the WHO to abandon its campaign.

Over the next several decades, in spite of growing evidence that the disease was making a comeback, malaria control remained relatively low on the list of international public health priorities. Policymakers, distracted by new concerns, lost interest in malaria years ago and have drastically cut funding for control efforts and basic research. The dwindling cadre of malaria specialists attribute today's resurgence of the disease in part to the malaria parasite's widespread resistance to chloroquine, for years the medication of choice for malaria victims. Inexpensive, fast-acting, safe, and available over-the-counter, chloroquine has been so overused that it is now largely ineffective due to the development of drug resistance. Replacement drugs like sulfadoxine/pyrimethamine are far more expensive and are already beginning to suffer the same resistance problems as chloroquine. At the same time as anti-malarial drugs are becoming less effective, the insecticides used against the mosquito vectors of the disease are similarly losing their potency. However, in certain locales mosquito populations are still susceptible to DDT and some officials advocate its renewed use in emergency situations.

Among the various options for easing human suffering caused by malaria, the most obvious solution and one long sought by medical researchers is a malaria vaccine. Unfortunately, for a variety of reasons, this appears to be a distant dream, though the recent decoding of the parasite's genome may offer valuable information to assist in this effort. In the meantime, efforts to combat the disease focus primarily on vector control, utilizing strategies aimed at reducing the number of mosquitoes or, alternatively, preventing the insects from getting close enough to bite. Such strategies include promoting the use of pyrethrin-treated bednets, installing screens over windows and doors, and eliminating sources of mosquito breeding near homes (e.g., open water tanks, rooftop cisterns). Unfortunately, such effective and commonsense approaches may be difficult to implement on a wide scale in rural Third World settings where many families can't afford the cost of a bednet and where homes are built in such a way that screening all openings is a near impossibility. Similarly, the regular use of mosquito repellents, while strongly recommended for those traveling to areas where malaria is prevalent, is an unaffordable option for local residents.

These limitations suggest that emergency use of DDT can be justified in situations where mosquito populations are still susceptible and people are dying. As currently employed for malaria control, DDT is sprayed only on interior walls of homes and the backside of furniture, leaving a residual that can kill adult mosquitoes alighting on such surfaces for a period of several months after application. Outdoor spraying of DDT, regardless of circumstances, is no longer considered appropriate due to environmental hazards and to the fact that there are now very effective biological agents available for control of mosquito larvae. Although other more widely approved insecticides (i.e., chemicals not on POPs' "Dirty Dozen" list) *could* be used, they are much more expensive than DDT—a critical consideration in the poverty-stricken areas most afflicted by malaria. Thus it is understandable that many public health officials strongly insist that, POPs Treaty notwithstanding, they must reserve the right to use DDT— the proper usage of which has resulted in few, if any, confirmed human health problems—to prevent premature death and disability caused by malaria.

Over the long term, most health experts agree, reducing malaria's fearsome toll will require concerted action on many fronts, including increased funding for medical research, improved environmental sanitation, a strengthening of community health systems, increased public awareness and use of personal protection methods such as bednets and, perhaps most important, anti-poverty programs that make it possible for people to improve living standards and quality of housing, thereby breaking the cycle of poverty and disease. Hopefully, if the world community can muster the political commitment and financial resources to realize these goals, control of malaria may at last become a reality and whatever rationale exists for continuing to use DDT will disappear.

References

Malaria Foundation International. 2004. http://www.malaria.org/. Accessed March 2, 2004.

McGinn, Anne Platt. 2003. "Combating Malaria." *State of the World 2003*. New York: Worldwatch Institute/W.W. Norton.

treaty ratified in 2004 obligates signatory nations to discontinue the production and use of nine chlorinated hydrocarbon insecticides included on the "Dirty Dozen" list of proscribed **Persistent Organic Pollutants ("POPs")**. Additional chemicals in this group are likely to be added to the list in future years.

Organophosphate and carbamate insecticides, unlike DDT and its kin, are not persistent in the environment, usually breaking down two weeks or less after application. However, some of these products are acutely toxic to humans and must be used with great care (those available to the general public, such as malathion and carbaryl have relatively low human toxicity and shouldn't cause problems when used according to label directions). These chemicals now dominate the insecticide market, along with the increasingly popular pyrethroids, synthetic chemical analogs of pyrethrum, a natural insecticide derived from chrysanthemum flowers. Providing quick knockdown of insects, the pyrethroids are probably the best choice for home or garden use because of their very low toxicity to humans and domestic animals. For this reason, they are among the few insecticides that can be safely used indoors, even in the kitchen. While these products are generally somewhat more expensive than other insecticides, they can be used effectively at much lower rates of application. If it is necessary to use an insecticidal dust, shampoo, or flea collar on young puppies or kittens, a product containing one of the pyrethroids is recommended.

Natural pyrethrum *(Pyrocide)* is still available, as is rotenone *(ChemFish)*, a poison derived from a tropical legume. **Neem**, an extract of a South Asian tree of the same name, is another botanical insecticide registered for use on ornamental plants and vegetables. Valued in India since ancient times for both insecticidal and medicinal properties, neem seeds and leaves contain nine or more different liminoid compounds that exhibit potent repellent and pesticidal properties effective against at least 200 different species of insects. Like the other botanicals, neem is quite safe for humans—in fact, for centuries South Asians have used neem extensively for dental hygiene and a variety of other medical purposes (National Research Council, 1992).

Table 8-1   The "Dirty Dozen"

aldrin[1]	hexachlorobenzene[1] [2] [3]
chlordane[1]	mirex[1]
DDT[1]	polychlorinated biphenyls (PCBs)[2] [3]
dieldrin[1]	polychlorinated dibenzo-p-dioxins (dioxins)[3]
endrin[1]	polychlorinated dibenzo-p-furans (furans)[3]
heptachlor[1]	toxaphene[1]

[1] Pesticide
[2] Industrial chemical
[3] By-product
Source: Environmental Protection Agency, www.epa.gov/oppfead1/international/pops.htm

Herbicides.   Weeds in a field may not appear as threatening as hordes of insects, yet the economic losses caused by these unwanted species can be very high. Weeds compete with crop plants for vital mineral nutrients and water, thus reducing crop yields; they make harvesting more difficult and some species, when consumed, poison livestock.

Wide scale application of chemicals for weed control is a relatively new phenomenon. Although a few inorganic compounds such as iron sulfate and sodium arsenite were used against broadleaf weeds as long ago as 1896, hand-weeding, mechanical cultivation, tillage, crop rotation, and the use of weed-free seeds were the most common methods of reducing crop losses due to weed infestations. After World War II, the first synthetic herbicide (2,4–D) was introduced and has been followed by a succession of more than a hundred different chemical weed killers. Today herbicide use has considerably surpassed insecticide use; in 1997, herbicidal applications on American farms, lawns, and gardens accounted for 568 million pounds of active ingredients, compared to 161 million pounds of insecticides and 165 million pounds of fungicides (Aspelin and Grube, 1999). Reliance on chemical herbicides for weed control has risen steadily. For corn and soybeans, the two most herbicide-dependent crops, the percent of crop acres treated has risen from 50% and 27%, respectively, in the mid-1960s to 96% and 97%, respectively, in the 1990s (Lin et al., 1995).

Although herbicides are used most extensively for agricultural purposes, they also are used by public health workers to control weeds that harbor insects and rodents, and to eradicate nuisance plants such as ragweed or poison ivy.

Herbicides may be classified in various ways, including how and when they are applied or by their mode of action. The first of these categories include **preplanting** herbicides—products applied to the soil before a crop is planted; **pre-emergents**—herbicides applied to the soil shortly before weeds are expected to germinate; and **post-emergents**—those applied to the soil or directly onto the foliage of the weeds after the crop and/or the weeds have sprouted. A familiar example of a pre-emergent herbicide is Preen® (trifluralin), widely used by home gardeners to prevent weeds from germinating in their flowerbeds. Grouped by mode of action, herbicides can be categorized as **selective**—those that kill only certain types of plants (usually broad-leafed dicotyledonous species, a group to which many of the common weeds belong); **contact**—poisons that kill any actively growing plant part with which they come into contact; and **translocated**—herbicides that are absorbed from the soil via the roots or through the foliage into the plant's vascular system, through which they are carried to all parts of the plant. The numerous 2,4–D-containing products used for decades to kill dandelions and other turfgrass weeds while leaving the lawn undamaged are prime examples of selective herbicides (they also could be classified as post-emergents, since they are sprayed directly on the growing weeds). In recent years, sales of the contact herbicide glyphosate (Roundup®) have soared, due to its usefulness in "burning down" weeds prior to planting in no-till fields and for clearing vegetation from roadsides, fencerows, cracks in the sidewalk, or any place where complete plant removal is desired. The recent proliferation of "Roundup Ready" crops has created a steadily expanding agricultural market for this contact herbicide.

Although most herbicides are thought to be only slightly toxic to humans, in recent years there have been several studies suggesting that herbicide exposure can cause genetic mutations, cancer, and birth defects. Farm workers occasionally blame health problems such as weight loss, nausea, vomiting, and loss of appetite to contact with herbicides. In 1986 researchers reported that Kansas farmers who used 2,4–D for more than 20 days per year had a six times greater risk of non-Hodgkin's lymphoma than did a control group with no exposure to herbicides (Blair et al., 1987). In 1991 the *Journal of the National Cancer Institute* reported that dogs, too, are at risk from 2,4–D. If their owners apply the weed killer four times or more each summer, canines are twice as likely to develop malignant lymphoma as are dogs whose owners abstain from herbicide use. More recently, several studies have reported an association between herbicide exposure and the development of persistent asthma among infants under one year of age (Salam et al., 2004) and between mixing and applying herbicides and infertility in women (Greenlee, Arbuckle, and Chou, 2003). Pregnant women who use herbicides during their first trimester triple their risk of bearing a child with a specific type of severe congenital heart defect (Loffredo et al., 2001). Countering these assertions, in June 2004 the EPA released a draft health and environmental risk assessment that concluded 2,4-D does not present a risk to human health nor is there evidence that would implicate the herbicide as a cause of cancer.

During the late 1970s and early 1980s a great deal of public controversy surrounded the use of 2,4,5–T and silvex, selective herbicides that contained traces of dioxin formed as an unavoidable contaminant during the manufacturing process. Notorious as a component of **Agent Orange,** the chemical defoliant used by U.S. military forces during the Vietnam War, 2,4,5–T (actually, the dioxin contaminating 2,4,5–T) was blamed for a wide range of physical and emotional problems among South Vietnamese living in the target areas, as well as among American servicemen who had come into contact with the herbicide during their tour of duty. Although independent studies of veterans' complaints have never been able to confirm an association between the alleged health effects and Agent Orange exposure, production of 2,4,5–T and silvex was terminated in the early 1980s, and in 1984 seven chemical companies agreed to an out-of-court settlement for $180 million with a veterans' group claiming health damage. Rapid growth in the commercial lawn care industry has provoked a vociferous response in many communities by antipesticide activists who warn of the dangers posed to people, pets, and wildlife by toxic lawn chemicals ("Dandelions won't kill you— pesticides do!"). The increasingly common use by lawn care firms of post-application warning signs, accompanied by recommended safety precautions, has been a positive, if limited, industry response to citizen concerns.

Rodenticides. Although good sanitation and rat-proofing of buildings and food storage facilities provide the only effective long-term control of domestic rodents, use of poisons is an important additional tool in keeping rat populations low. Because some rodenticides used in public health work are extremely toxic to humans as well as to rodents, their use in the United States is restricted to certified applicators. The hazard these chemicals pose to humans is evident in news accounts from China, where rat poison has become the murder weapon of choice in a land where private ownership of guns is illegal; readily available rodenticides also are blamed for a significant percentage of suicides in that country. According to the World Health Organization, intentional or accidental poisoning ranks among the top 10 causes of death among young Chinese (Yardley, 2003).

General-use rodenticides, chemicals that should not present a serious hazard either to the user or to the environment when used in accordance with instructions, can be purchased by the public. Even these may not be entirely safe, however; the same study that indicated a tripling of risk for congenital heart defects among children born to women using herbicides during their first trimester of pregnancy showed a *quadrupling* of risk for that same abnormality for women using rodenticides (Loffredo et al., 2001).

The rodenticides most commonly recommended for use by householders act as anticoagulants—compounds that, when consumed over a period of several days, cause internal hemorrhaging, causing the rodents to bleed to death painlessly. These poisons provide excellent control of both rats and mice, although up to two weeks may be required to get an effective kill.

Environmental Impact of Pesticide Use

In the early 1950s, bird-watchers in both the United States and Western Europe were confronted with a baffling mystery—a sudden, inexplicable decline in the populations of bald eagles, pelicans, and peregrine falcons appeared to threaten the very survival of these well-loved species. Investigations into the unanticipated population "crash" ultimately revealed that the villain was not a disease, nor overkilling, nor a scarcity of food, but rather was the presence of startlingly high concentrations of the new insecticide DDT in the tissues of these birds. Although DDT did not appear to have a direct lethal effect on the adult birds, it interfered with their ability to metabolize calcium, thereby resulting in the production of eggs with shells so thin they broke when the nesting parents sat on them. Thus, pesticide-induced reproductive failure—the inability of the birds to produce viable offspring—was ultimately shown to be the factor responsible for the population decline.

This episode represented one of the first glimmerings of awareness on the part of the scientific community at least, that the advent of the new wonder chemicals was not an unmitigated blessing. The public at large, however, remained largely unaware and unconcerned about such matters until the publication in 1962 of Rachel Carson's literary bombshell, *Silent Spring*. This best seller represented a scathing indictment of pesticide misuse and for the first time made the average American aware of the havoc such chemicals could wreak on the environment and on human well-being. In retrospect, the publication of *Silent Spring* made "ecology" a household word and was probably the most important single event in launching the environmental movement of the 1970s. Carson and many subsequent researchers clearly demonstrated that extensive use and near-total reliance on chemicals for pest control have been accompanied by unanticipated and undesired side effects, many of which have raised problems serious enough to threaten the continued usefulness of these products.

Development of Resistance

Those who dreamed that the new pesticides might completely eradicate certain insect or other pest species were obviously ignorant of the principles that govern how the forces of natural selection act upon chance variations occurring within any population—particularly insect populations, whose long evolutionary history demonstrates the remarkable ability of these organisms to evolve and adapt rapidly to changing environmental conditions. The widespread, frequent, and intensive application of chemicals such as DDT in the years following the war was initially successful in drastically reducing pest populations, but eventually was responsible for providing the selective forces that would produce new strains of "super bugs," rendering the original poisons worthless. The mechanism by which this occurs can be visualized by considering a hypothetical population of, say, boll weevils ravaging a field of cotton. Aerial insecticide spraying may kill perhaps 99% of the weevils, but a few will survive, either by chance (perhaps an overhanging leaf shielded them from the spray) or because something in the genetic make-up of a particular individual somehow made it less vulnerable to the poison. Such a hereditary trait might be the production of a particular enzyme capable of detoxifying the pesticide, a less permeable type of epidermis which prevented penetration of the contact poison, a behavioral characteristic that allowed the individual to avoid fatal exposure, or some other factor of this nature. In a pesticide-free environment (the type of situation prevailing prior to the introduction of DDT) such a genetic trait would confer no special advantage to the individual carrying it, so the frequency of such a gene within that population would remain low. Once DDT came into widespread use, however, the boll weevils' environment was radically altered and those few individuals possessing the gene for immunity suddenly enjoyed a tremendous selective advantage. As the accompanying diagram indicates, successive sprayings largely eliminated boll weevils susceptible to the insecticide, but promoted the build-up of a population in which the vast majority carried the gene (or genes) conferring resistance to the chemical. Those seeking to control pest outbreaks were thus forced to turn to newer and more powerful chemicals, only to witness the same cycle of events.

Since pesticide resistance had appeared as a localized problem even with the old-fashioned insecticides, it shouldn't have come as a total surprise when insects resistant to DDT began to appear in the late 1940s and early 1950s. Among the first species to display immunity were certain populations of houseflies and mosquitoes which, as early as 1946, could no longer be controlled with DDT. In 1951, during the Korean War, military officials were alarmed to discover that human body lice, vectors of typhus, had become resistant to DDT. Among agricultural pests, spider mites, cabbage loopers, codling moths, and tomato hornworms developed resistance to several of the common insecticides; by the mid-1950s when the boll weevil became resistant to many of the chlorinated hydrocarbons, the need for alternative control methods became obvious (Perkins, 1982).

At present, more than 500 species of insects and mites are resistant to common pesticides—more than double the number that were resistant just a few decades ago. Largely due to problems of pesticide resistance, crop losses due to insects are nearly twice as high now as they were when DDT was first brought onto the market, in spite of a quantum increase in pesticidal applications by farmers over the past half century. In the public health field, as in agriculture, growing pesticide resistance is causing serious concern. Worldwide, incidence of malaria is now on a sharp upswing as approximately 64 species of mosquitoes have become resistant to insecticides, according to World Health Organization officials.

Problems of pesticide resistance are not restricted to species of arthropods. Some rat populations, particularly those in cities with long-established rodent control programs, no longer respond to warfarin, the most extensively used rodenticide in the world. More than 150 species of plant pathogens (fungi and bacteria) are now resis-

Figure 8-3 Cycle of Pesticide Resistance

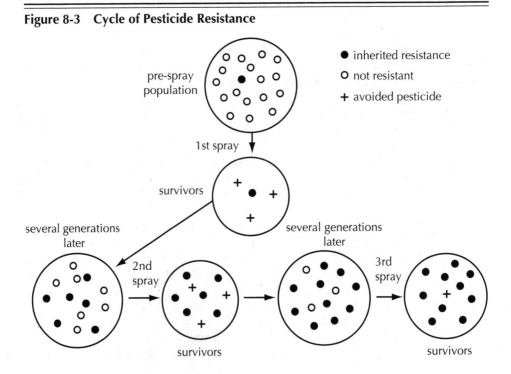

tant to at least one pesticide, as are 286 weed biotypes (GAO, 2001; WSSA, 2004). Although herbicide resistance is a relatively recent development and has received considerably less attention among agricultural experts than has insecticide resistance, weed scientists warn that the phenomenon is already widespread. In Australia, wheat growers by the early 1980s were reporting the emergence of new weed biotypes resistant to every selective herbicide that can be used on wheat. Even more ominous was the discovery in 1996 that Australian ryegrass had developed resistance to glyphosate (*Roundup*®), the world's best selling herbicide. Since then, several more glyphosate-resistant weed populations have emerged in such disparate areas of the world as Chile, Malaysia, California, and in scattered locations in the midwestern, eastern, and southeastern United States. This news is particularly worrisome to farmers because new commercial varieties of wheat, cotton, potatoes, sugar beets, canola, and soybeans have now been genetically engineered to survive direct field applications of glyphosate intended for weed control. Many agricultural researchers are convinced that in areas where glyphosate is used intensively, it is inevitable that an increasing number of weeds will develop resistance to the herbicide. To reduce the rate at which this is happening, they advise against using glyphosate on the same acres every year, instead recommending an annual rotation of both crops and herbicides. At the same time, they point out that fears of the emergence of "superweeds" resulting from excessive glyphosate use are exaggerated, since effective alternative herbicides are available for most weed species (Hartzler and Owen, 2003).

Killing of Nontarget Species

Only a small percentage of insect species are considered pests, yet the most widely used synthetic insecticides are broad-spectrum poisons, killing both friend and foe alike. The destruction of many beneficial predator insect species as well as the target pest has led to two related types of problems. The first of these, referred to as **target pest resurgence,** occurs when an insecticide application that initially resulted in a drastic reduction in the pest population is quickly followed by a sudden increase in pest numbers to a level higher than that which existed prior to the spraying. This occurs because the natural enemies of the pest, which formerly kept its numbers under control, were also heavily decimated by the spraying. Since any predators that survived the pesticide would subsequently starve or migrate, the pests would then confront ideal conditions—no natural enemies and an abundance of their favorite food (i.e., the crop that had been sprayed). As a result, their populations can increase in size very rapidly, above and beyond the original level.

A second situation, known as **secondary pest outbreak,** involves the rise to prominence of certain plant-eating species which, prior to the spraying, were unimportant as pests because natural enemies kept their populations below the level at which they could cause significant economic damage. After pesticides eliminated most of their predators, such insects suddenly experience a population explosion and become major pests in their own right. In 1995 Texas cotton growers in the lower Rio Grande Valley experienced a devastating outbreak of several secondary pests after some 200,000 acres were targeted for aerial spraying with malathion to control boll weevils. Predictably, the spraying decimated beneficial insects along with the target pest, resulting in an unanticipated outbreak of cotton aphids that spread rapidly through the fields. Shortly afterwards, a beet armyworm infestation mushroomed as well, causing severe losses to the cotton crop. The armyworms were followed by whiteflies, which further reduced yields. In spite of as many as 25 insecticidal sprayings on some farms, many growers lost their entire crop and cotton yields in the area that year plunged 80%, from an average harvest of 300,000 bales to just 54,000 (Meister, 1996).

Beneficial insects are not the only nontarget species adversely affected by broad-spectrum poisons. Many kinds of birds, small mammals, fish, and other aquatic organisms are extremely sensitive to chemical pesticides and die immediately after coming into contact with such substances. Indeed, the numerous examples of mass die-offs of robins and other songbirds, squirrels, house cats, salmon, and many other well-loved species vividly documented by Rachel Carson provided the emotional images that explain *Silent Spring*'s profound impact on the national psyche. No one could read passages such as the following and remain unmoved:

> It was a spring without voices. On the mornings that had once throbbed with the dawn chorus of robins, catbirds, doves . . . there was now no sound; only silence lay over the fields and woods and marsh. (Carson, 1962)

Environmental Contamination

Liberal use of pesticides on a worldwide basis has resulted in a more thorough contamination of the biosphere than anyone in 1945 would have dreamed possible. Today pesticide residues, especially those of the chlorinated hydrocarbons, are found virtually everywhere in the tissues of creatures as diverse as Antarctic penguins, fish in deep ocean trenches, decomposer bacteria, and every human being. Since no one deliberately sprayed pesticides in Antarctica or in the middle of the Pacific, how could this have happened? Because the chlorinated hydrocarbons are persistent pesticides (meaning that they break down very slowly), they can circulate through the ecosystem for a long time, often traveling long distances from their point of origin. When such chemicals are aerially sprayed on forest, field, or pastureland, less than 10% of the pesticide actually hits the target; the remainder is carried off by air currents and is subsequently deposited miles away where it will eventually be washed into waterways or taken up by living organisms in the food they eat. Even when carefully applied according to label directions, pesticides can vaporize into the air, be washed off the land into lakes and streams during heavy rains, or percolate downward through the soil. The results of this unintended contamination include the following.

Indirect killing via depletion of food or habitat. When pesticides are targeted against insects, plants, or rodents that serve as a major food source for another group of organisms, the long-term effect can be just as devastating as direct poisoning would be. In New Jersey, populations of certain forest bird species declined by 45–55% after carbaryl spraying for gypsy moth control deprived the birds of their supper. Herbicide use similarly reduces both forage and habitat for many plant-eating insects and can have a "domino effect" when plummeting populations of arthropods adversely impact the food supply of insectivorous birds. On the high plains of Wyoming, a population of native sparrows crashed after herbicidal spraying of sagebrush to enlarge pasture-lands for grazing. Unfortunately for the sparrows, the sagebrush supplied essential cover and nesting sites without which the birds couldn't survive (Parker, 1994).

Groundwater contamination. The discovery in 1979 that 96 wells on Long Island were contaminated with a highly toxic carbamate insecticide, aldicarb, came as unwelcome news to a public that assumed that however polluted our rivers and lakes might be, groundwater supplies were safe from chemical contamination. Any hopes that the New York situation might be an isolated aberration were shattered by the revelation that 3,000 miles to the west, more than 2,000 wells in the fertile San Joaquin Valley were tainted with the nematicide DBCP, a chlorinated hydrocarbon that had earlier made headlines for causing sterility among male pesticide workers exposed to the chemical. In the late 1980s the EPA launched a nationwide survey to determine the extent of pesticide contamination of groundwater supplies. In 1990 the agency released a report showing that 14% of all public and private drinking water wells sampled had measurable levels of at least one pesticide. Two years later the agency reported new results indicating that nearly one-third of rural wells sampled showed unsafe levels of pesticide contamination, with aldicarb and the herbicides atrazine (*Aatrex®*) and alachlor (*Lasso®*), both suspected human carcinogens, posing the most widespread problems. Agency surveyors reported finding nearly 100 different pesticides in groundwater supplies and concluded that heavy agricultural pesticide use was the main cause of the problem ("EPA Study," 1992; Curtis, Profeta, and Mott, 1993). Additional studies carried out in the late 1990s found pesticide residues in over half the samples of well water taken at over 1,000 locations, both rural and urban. While numerous different chemicals were detected, their concentrations in most cases were quite low. Of those for which EPA has established drinking water standards, only one pesticide at one of the many locations sampled exceeded the allowable level. The fact that pesticides were detected almost as often in urban wells as in those from rural areas is an indication that pesticide contamination of groundwater is not a problem confined to agricultural areas. Although such studies show that the problem is widespread, the fact that concentrations are relatively low makes assessment of the potential human health threat problematic and indicates that this is a topic that needs further investigation (NRC, 2000).

Due to concerns over groundwater contamination, several European countries have banned the use of atrazine—one of the world's most popular herbicides—and in 2003 the EU withdrew regulatory approval for this chemical. That same year, the Environmental Protection Agency made the opposite decision, re-approving registration of atrazine in the United States despite the opposition of environmentalists (but to the relief of farmers worried about losing an effective and relatively cheap herbicide). In the developing nations, where the rate of pesticide use is increasing even faster than in the industrialized world, virtually no groundwater monitoring is being carried out at present; it is quite likely that current agricultural activities may be seriously degrading underground water supplies over vast areas without anyone recognizing the potential threat to future generations (Nash, 1993).

Indirect contamination via food chains. Since the chlorinated hydrocarbons are not water-soluble, they are not excreted from the body when ingested but instead are stored in fatty tissues such as liver, kidneys, and fat around the intestines. Toxic substances present in minute amounts in the general environment can thus become quite concentrated as they move along a food chain, sometimes reaching lethal doses in organisms at the highest trophic levels. This process, known as **biomagnification**, was the phenomenon responsible for the reproductive failure in the various birds of prey referred to earlier in this chapter. Eagles, pelicans, and falcons are all top carnivores, fish-eaters, at the end of relatively long food chains. As such, they had accumulated amounts of DDT sufficiently high to interfere with important bodily processes.

A classic example of biomagnification occurred at Clear Lake, California—a favorite fishing spot about 90 miles north of San Francisco. Recreational anglers had long been annoyed by the swarms of nonbiting gnats that were frequently present at Clear Lake. The new synthetic pesticides seemingly offered an easy solution, so in 1949 officials decided to spray Clear Lake with a dilute solution of DDD (a chemical cousin of DDT which is less toxic to fish). After the first spraying, gnat populations dropped to barely detectable levels, but by 1951 the pesky insects were back in bothersome numbers, so the spraying was repeated. Several more sprayings followed in succeeding years as the gnat populations displayed increasing resistance to the poison.

Then some strange side effects became apparent. By 1954 visitors to Clear Lake began reporting significant numbers of carcasses of the Western grebe, a type of waterfowl, around the lake. By the early 1960s, the grebe population at Clear Lake had plummeted from 1,000 nesting pairs to almost none. Suspecting that the repeated pesticide applications might somehow be related to the birds' demise, biologists began to measure DDD concentrations in various components of the lake ecosystem. Although the lake water itself contained traces of DDD in barely detectable amounts (0.02 ppm), concentrations of the pesticide increased dramatically when the tissues of living organisms were examined. The facts they uncovered are entirely consistent with the basic principles of a food chain:

Organism	DDD Concentration in Tissues (ppm)
Phytoplankton (producers)	5
Herbivorous fish (primary consumers)	40–300
Carnivorous fish (secondary consumers)	up to 2500
Western grebes (secondary consumers)	1600

The pesticide that had been sprayed on the lake, in what everybody at the time assumed was a safely dilute amount, was absorbed and concentrated by the plankton, which were the producer organisms of Clear Lake. When these were consumed by the herbivorous fish (primary consumers), the DDD became more concentrated. By the time these fish were eaten by grebes or by bullheads, the DDD had become sufficiently concentrated to cause the death of the birds.

By the late 1960s the futility of spraying to control the now-resistant gnats became obvious and a gnat-eating fish was introduced into the lake in what subsequently proved to be a very successful method of biological control. As pesticide levels gradually dropped, the grebes returned to Clear Lake and today are once again thriving at approximately their pre-1954 population levels. Numerous other examples of biomagnification involving other chlorinated hydrocarbons and heavy metals (methyl mercury at Minamata, for example) have since been described and illustrate the unanticipated effects that toxic substances can have as they move through ecosystems.

Hazards to Human Health

Although pesticides are used specifically to kill pests, many of them are quite toxic to humans as well. In 1999 the EPA estimated that a minimum of 10,000–20,000 pesticide-related illnesses and injuries were being diagnosed among American farm workers every year, most of them due to contact with organophosphate insecticides. Poison control centers in the U.S. report over 100,000 pesticide poisonings each year, with 23,000 victims sick enough to visit hospital emergency rooms. Approximately 20 Americans, mostly children, die annually from accidental pesticide poisoning (Benbrook, 1996).

On a global basis, pesticides take a much higher toll: the World Health Organization estimates that in the Third World alone, acute poisonings among agricultural workers may be as high as 25 million annually (3% of the workforce), with 1% dying as a result of their exposure (Jeyaratnam, 1990). Even these figures may be overly conservative, since field laborers in developing countries seldom seek medical treatment when they feel ill on the job and thus many cases of pesticide poisoning go unreported. While increased emphasis on pesticide safety and improved application equipment has contributed to a marked decline in acute pesticide-related deaths and serious illness in the industrialized nations, such is not the case in most developing countries. Few Third World farm workers receive any training in proper use of farm chemicals,

Box 8-3   The Dark Side of Beautiful Blossoms

Few gifts say "I love you" as effectively as a bouquet of fresh roses, and those wishing to convey such sentiments now have easy year-round access to their favorite blooms at the nearest supermarket, Costco, or Wal-Mart. The current abundance and affordability of fresh flowers in the North American market-place is not due to an explosion in entrepreneurial backyard gardening, but to the boom in commercial flower production in two South American nations. The high-altitude savanna plain west of Bogotá, Colombia, and the fertile region surrounding Quito, Ecuador, are blessed with ideal soil and climate conditions for growing roses, carnations, and other commercially desirable flowers. Colombian farmers have been exporting blooms since the early 1960s, but only in the 1990s did the two countries begin to reap the full economic benefits of their "flower power." In 1991, in an attempt to give growers in the region an alternative cash crop to coca and opium poppies, the U.S. dropped tariffs on Colombian and Ecuadorian blooms. As a result of new economic opportunities afforded by this Andean Trade Preferences Act, flower cultivation in the two countries soared. Colombia is now the world's second-largest exporter of cut flowers (the Netherlands remains #1), while Ecuador has climbed to fourth place. Over 70% of the cut flowers sold in the U.S. today were grown in South America, with one out of every two blooms coming from fields near Bogotá (78% of Colombia's crop is exported to the U.S., the remainder to Europe). The economic benefits to both Colombia and Ecuador have been considerable. Over 100,000 jobs have been created in this once-impoverished region and the national economies have been boosted by hundreds of millions of dollars.

All of this, however, has come at a heavy price to the health of agricultural workers—70% of them women—whose labor makes this bounty possible. Few First-World purchasers realize the impact their demand for blemish-free, perfect blossoms is having on those who grow, cut, wrap, and box tens of thousands of flowers each day. Problems center around workers' exposure to more than 120 different pesticides, three of which (captan, aldicarb, and fenamiphos) are regarded by the World Health Organization

as extremely toxic. Approximately one-fifth of the products used are ones that have been taken off the market in the U.S. and Canada—or never registered for use in the first place—because of the hazard they present to human health. Even those pesticides that can be legally applied in the U.S. are frequently used in an unsafe manner, thanks to inadequate regulatory oversight in both Andean countries. Reports abound of greenhouses being fumigated while workers are still present, even though the health impact of pesticide exposure is three times higher in such a closed environment than it would be outdoors (Colombia's pesticide regulations have no special requirements for greenhouses). Workers doing the fumigation frequently wear no protective clothing and only a small percentage have been taught proper pesticide application methods; a survey conducted in Ecuador by the International Labor Organization (ILO) found only 22% of the workers in that country had received such training. The ILO also reported that approximately one-fifth of Ecuador's 60,000 floriculture workers are children, a troubling finding since children are significantly more vulnerable to pesticide-related health problems than adults.

Among workers of all ages, reports of pesticide poisonings are commonplace; an estimated two-thirds of all floriculture workers in Colombia and Ecuador suffer from job-related health problems. Frequent complaints include headaches, blurred vision, nausea, and fatigue—all classic symptoms of poisoning with organophosphate insecticides. Higher-than-average numbers of miscarriages are experienced by female workers. One 34-year-old woman who had been employed on a flower farm for four years told an interviewer that her hair had begun falling out and commented that, "I am young, but I feel very old." Workers who visit company doctors are routinely told there's nothing wrong and are sent back to work. Care at local hospitals is often unaffordable for laborers who earn only slightly more than minimum wage.

Occasionally, episodes of acute mass poisonings make the headlines. In late November 2003, several hundred workers at a flower company near Bogotá were poisoned when they inhaled fumes of an organophosphate nerve poison. Although the workers began experiencing symptoms such as severe headache, nausea, diarrhea, and swelling soon after arriving at work, company supervisors refused to contact medical authorities until mid-morning, when dozens of workers were fainting. At that point they finally called ambulances to transport the affected women to area hospitals. All recovered relatively quickly, but a few were incapacitated for several days. Company officials have never informed either the public or their employees as to the cause of the accident, but investigators from Colombia's Public Health Ministry subsequently visited the facility and found numerous violations of pesticide management procedures. Their report noted that the tools used for measuring chemicals were inaccurate, procedures for mixing chemicals weren't clearly spelled out, some of the pesticides were stored in containers formerly used for other chemicals, and the dilapidated condition of the work area likely could contribute to falls or spills. Following the incident, officials tried to downplay its seriousness and, in spite of a lingering strong chemical smell in the facility, insisted that employees return to work the following day.

Such problems, as well as concerns regarding labor rights, have prompted a "Fairness in Flowers" campaign by the International Labor Rights Fund (ILRF), a Washington-based organization. This initiative aims to raise awareness among Americans about the challenges facing floriculture workers in Ecuador and Colombia and seeks improvements through action in both the U.S. and Latin America. Among the reforms sought are agreements to use only EPA-registered pesticides (or those approved by an equivalent European regulatory body); to record pesticide use data and make it readily available to workers and the public; to train workers regarding proper use of pesticides; to ensure that no fumigation of greenhouses is carried out while workers are inside; to provide all workers with free, waterproof protective gear; and to establish workplace committees to deal with safety and hygiene issues.

Campaign organizers hope that consumer pressure on the U.S. retailers who sell imported cut flowers will motivate the latter to demand change from their Latin American suppliers. By raising such issues through e-mail messages to corporate headquarters, letters to the editor of local newspapers, etc., consumers can help ensure that when they "Say It With Flowers," they aren't contributing to further pesticide poisoning of workers in distant lands.

References

Pesticide Action Network North America (PANNA). 2004. "Send a Valentine for Colombia Flower Workers." *Pesticide Action Network Updates Services* (Feb. 12). Accessed at http://www.panna.org.

Thompson, Ginger. 2003. "Behind Roses' Beauty, Poor and Ill Workers." *New York Times*, Feb. 13, A27.

which are commonly misused and overapplied. Adequate protective gear is seldom worn or even provided. Worse yet, workers often manually apply pesticides (sometimes by reaching bare-handed into a container of pesticidal dust and broadcasting it onto the target area) or spread them by tractor, affording ample opportunity for dusts, mists, or vapors to be inhaled or absorbed through the exposed skin of the applicator. Since field workers seldom have access to running water while working, quick removal of pesticides spilled on garments or on the skin is not possible and workers frequently wear contaminated clothing home, exposing their children, pregnant wives, or elderly parents (those most vulnerable to health damage from these poisons).

Additional exposure to family members may occur when workers, unaware of the danger, bring home empty pesticide containers to use for storing food or water. Although strict adherence to label directions could prevent some of the problems associated with improper handling, storage, and application practices, in fact Third World farm workers seldom read the label instructions, either because they are illiterate or because labels are printed in a language they don't understand (the latter situation poses a safety concern even in the United States where many agricultural laborers read only Spanish and are thus unable to heed warnings printed in English). Even worse, in many developing countries pesticides are often transferred from the original container to another unlabeled receptacle so that the user, even if literate and multilingual, has no way of knowing what hazards the material might present—or even its identity. Finally, a future threat that hasn't received the attention it deserves is the question of what to do with sizeable stocks of outdated or unusable pesticides—many of them persistent chlorinated hydrocarbons such as dieldrin and DDT—more than 15 million pounds (7 million kg) of which have accumulated in 35 developing countries. In many cases the containers in which these are stored are unlabeled, corroded, and leaking, posing serious pollution and health problems. Yet, the countries involved have no proper means for disposing of such toxins nor the resources for cleaning up contamination that has already occurred (World Resources Institute, 1994).

To cause harm, a pesticide must be taken internally through the mouth, skin, or respiratory system. Most oral exposure is due to carelessness; for example, leaving poisons within reach of young children, smoking or eating without washing hands after handling pesticides, using the mouth to start siphoning liquid pesticide concentrates, eating unwashed fruit that was recently sprayed, or accidentally drinking pesticides that were poured into an unlabeled container. Deliberate ingestion of highly toxic pesticides for the express purpose of committing suicide is responsible for a significant percentage of pesticide-related fatalities (NRC, 2000).

Exposure through the skin can occur when pesticides are spilled on the body or when wind-blown sprays or dusts come into contact with skin. Reentering a field too soon after pesticide application or careless handling of discarded containers can also

---

Figure 8-4   Dermal Absorption Rates as Compared with the Forearm

The seriousness of absorbing pesticide through the skin depends on the dermal toxicity of the chemical, the size of the contaminated skin area, the length of time the material is in contact with the skin, and the rate of absorption through the skin. As the diagram indicates, different parts of the body have very different rates of skin absorption.

Scalp (3.7)

Ear canal (5.4)

Forehead (4.2)

Abdomen (2.1)

Forearm (1.0)

Palm (1.3)

Scrotal area (11.8)

Ball of foot (1.6)

Source: Illinois Pesticide Applicator Study Guide, Univ. of Illinois Cooperative Extension Service.

result in absorption of pesticides through the skin. The larger the skin area contaminated and the longer the duration of contact, the more serious the results. Theoretically, dermal exposure could be reduced significantly through the use of protective clothing and equipment. In practice, however, such precautions are frequently ignored. Such gear is often expensive, cumbersome, and uncomfortable, especially during hot weather. All too often, applicators who know better fail to comply with safety recommendations and have been observed, in some instances, plying their trade wearing little more than bathing suits! Poisoning due to inhalation is most common in enclosed areas such as greenhouses but also can occur outside when pesticide mists or fumes are inhaled during application or if the applicator is smoking.

Symptoms of **acute** exposure (i.e., "one-time" cases) include headache, weakness, fatigue, or dizziness. If poisoning is due to one of the organophosphate insecticides, the victim may experience severe abdominal pain, vomiting, diarrhea, difficulty in breathing, excessive sweating, and sometimes convulsions, coma, and death. In contrast, **chronic** pesticide poisoning (low-level exposure over an extended time period) is characterized by vague symptoms that are difficult to pinpoint as having been caused by pesticide exposure (Bever et al., 1975). The greatest concern regarding chronic pesticide exposure, particularly to chlorinated hydrocarbons, is their potential for causing cancer or reproductive problems.

For many years **cancer** was the prime focus of concern regarding chronic effects of pesticide exposure. Extensive testing during the 1980s revealed that, on the basis of amounts applied, 60% of all herbicides, 90% of fungicides, and 30% of insecticides are either carcinogens or potentially carcinogenic (NRC, 1987). Beginning with its prohibition on the use of DDT in 1972, the EPA has gradually banned or restricted most of the chlorinated hydrocarbon pesticides, including endrin, aldrin, dieldrin, mirex, heptachlor, chlordane, and so on, largely because tests showed them to be carcinogenic to laboratory animals. The environmental consequences of this phaseout have been dramatic. In the United States, concentrations of these persistent pesticides in animal tissues have been steadily declining since the 1970s; certain bird populations that had nearly vanished by the late 1960s due to bioaccumulation of chlorinated pesticides have now largely rebounded. DDT levels in human breast milk also have plummeted by 90% since the EPA ban took effect (Schneider, 1994).

The impact of pesticide exposure on cancer incidence is still provoking debate among the experts (in California, the largest case-control study to date, published in April 1994, contradicted results of previous research by finding no association between breast cancer and DDT exposure). Meanwhile, a growing body of evidence supports the contention that **disruption of the endocrine and immune systems**, not cancer, constitutes the most serious long-term pesticide-related health concern. Since the endocrine hormones regulate a wide spectrum of bodily functions, including fertility and fetal development, compounds that interfere with such hormones have the potential for serious reproductive effects even at low levels of exposure. Scientists have now identified a number of pesticides, including many of the chlorinated hydrocarbons as well as some synthetic pyrethroids and triazine herbicides, as potent hormone disruptors. Studies of wildlife populations have shown that exposure to these compounds can lead to abnormal sexual behavior (especially feminization of males), birth defects, and impaired fertility among the offspring of pesticide-exposed parents (Curtis et al., 1993). Several of the more notorious pesticide-related tragedies have involved problems caused by the reproductive effects of chronic pesticide exposure. The nematicide DBCP (1,2–dibromo-3–chloropropane), for example, is known to have caused sterility among men in the California factory where it was manufactured, as well as among 1,500 male banana plantation workers in Costa Rica.

Immune system dysfunction can be provoked by either acute or subchronic exposure to many commonly used pesticides, including the herbicide 2,4–D and the insecticides malathion, parathion, aldicarb, carbofuran, and most of the chlorinated hydrocarbons (though most of these are no longer used in the United States, their residues persist in the environment). Young children, especially when malnourished, as well as elderly adults appear most vulnerable to pesticides' immuno-suppressive effects and tend to contract infectious diseases more frequently than individuals not exposed to pesticidal compounds. Pesticide-induced immunotoxicity may also be manifested as allergic contact dermatitis, a skin inflammation caused by immune system response to a foreign substance—in this case to pesticide exposure. Allergic reactions to contact with even minute amounts of pesticides can become chronic and in some cases have resulted in farm workers becoming permanently disabled due to chemical intolerance.

The adverse health and reproductive effects induced by endocrine-disrupting pesticides are further compounded when exposure to two or more such chemicals occurs simultaneously. The insecticides endosulfan and DDT, for example, interact synergistically to produce estrogenic effects 160–1,600 times greater than those of either pesticide alone. Inasmuch as humans are constantly exposed to numerous endocrine-disrupting chemicals (including PCBs and dioxins as well as pesticides) in air, food, and water, levels of exposure until now regarded as "safe" may need to be reassessed (Arnold et al., 1996).

The human health impact of **dietary exposure** to pesticides via residues on food has attracted intense public scrutiny since the 1987 publication of a study by the National Research Council (NRC), estimating that traces of carcinogenic fungicides,

Figure 8-5   Percentage of Fruits, Vegetables, and Grains with Detectable Residues of Organophosphate Pesticides

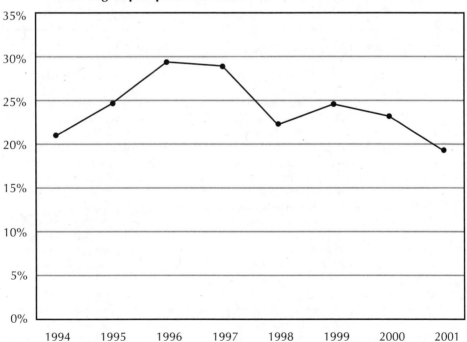

Source: U.S. Environmental Protection Agency, 2003. *America's Children and the Environment: Measures of Contaminants, Body Burdens, and Illnesses*. www.epa.gov/envirohealth/children, based on data from U.S. Department of Agriculture, Pesticide Data Program.

insecticides, and herbicides on the nation's fruits, vegetables, and meat could result in an additional 20,000 cancer deaths per year in the United States. These findings were hotly disputed by agrichemical interests but generated intense public concern over how pesticides are regulated. Demands for reform received added impetus following publication in June 1993 of a long-awaited study by the NRC on pesticides in the diets of infants and small children. NRC scientists were critical of the EPA's outmoded approach for setting pesticide tolerance levels on agricultural produce (a system based on the estimated amount of any given pesticide the "average person"—i.e. an adult—is likely to consume as part of a typical American diet), and concluded that the youngest members of society are at enhanced risk because they consume more calories per unit of body weight and because their diet is less varied than that of adults. Immediately after publication of the NRC report, a second study dealing with the same issue was released by the Environmental Working Group (EWG), a nonprofit research organization, stating that up to 35% of an individual's lifetime dose of dietary pesticides occurs before the age of 5, largely because young children consume proportionately far more residue-laden fruits and vegetables than do adults (EWG, 1998). Preschoolers, for example, eat six times the amount of fruit consumed by their parents and drink 31 times more apple juice in relation to their body weight than do adults. Thus pesticide residue safety levels based on presumed "average" diets may greatly underestimate the actual amount of exposure received by a young child. These reports also emphasized the fact that most foods contain residues of several different pesticides (a laboratory analysis performed on one pear identified 11 different pesticidal compounds), not just one, and that the sources of pesticide exposure are not restricted to food, but frequently include drinking water, lawn chemicals, and household insecticides as well.

All of these factors suggested that the existing regulatory framework for ensuring food safety was inadequate to protect infants and children (NRC, 1993; Curtis et al., 1993). In response to these concerns, the U.S. Congress in 1996 enacted comprehen-

Box 8-4 "EPA-Registered"—Synonymous with "Safe"?

The war against insects, rodents, and weeds is waged as vigorously on the home front as it is on the farm. An estimated 85% of American households harbor pesticidal products—three to five different chemicals, on average—that are used in prodigious amounts. Unfortunately, unlike farmers and structural pest control operators who are required to pass competency examinations, the average householder purchasing such pesticides has little or no idea of the health and environmental hazards such chemicals pose. After all, the reasoning goes, the label says "EPA-Registered." If the government permits them to be sold, they must be safe! This conviction reflects a dangerous ignorance of how pesticides are regulated and leads to a degree of complacency on the part of the general public that isn't warranted by the facts.

Early laws regulating pesticides focused almost exclusively on protecting farmers from untested, ineffective products, requiring truthful labeling but ignoring issues pertaining to human health or environmental impacts. By the late 1940s, as pesticide use began to grow rapidly, Congress enacted legislation requiring that chemical companies register their pesticide labels with the designated federal agency (originally with the U.S. Department of Agriculture; in 1970 that role was transferred to the newly created Environmental Protection Agency). Thus the fact that a particular product is government-registered simply means that it is legal to sell and use in the United States—nothing more.

By 1972, mounting evidence of human poisonings and environmental damage convinced policymakers that a shift in regulatory focus was needed. In that year, the old Federal Insecticide, Fungicide, and Rodenticide Act (FIFRA) was amended to incorporate health and environmental considerations into the regulatory process for the first time. These amendments mandated that henceforth chemical manufacturers must submit health and safety test results for new pesticides when they seek EPA registration for those products. Basic risk-benefit standards were developed for evaluating data submitted, the intention being to exclude high-risk pesticides from the market. Also in 1972, EPA canceled the registration of DDT, thus ending its legal use in the U.S., and shortly thereafter the agency took similar action with eight additional chlorinated hydrocarbon insecticides.

With this seemingly protective regulatory framework in place for over 30 years and with most of the notorious cancer-causing insecticides banned from the U.S. marketplace, why shouldn't average citizens assume that pesticides currently in use pose negligible health risks? Several reasons:

1. The requirement for safety testing prior to registration was not retroactive; hundreds of acutely hazardous pesticides were already registered for use at the time the new law was enacted. The vast majority of these remain on the market. Only through a lengthy process of collecting scientific data and proving that these "grandfathered" chemicals pose "unreasonable adverse effects" can EPA end their legal use.

2. Safety testing data is required only for the active ingredients in a given pesticidal product, yet the largest part, by volume, of many pesticides is made up of so-called "inert" ingredients, for which no safety testing is required. Some of these inerts are themselves known to be toxic, yet label requirements don't even require that they be identified by name. Pesticide legislative reform efforts regularly target the issue of inert ingredients, so far to no avail.

3. Many pesticides introduced since 1972 obtained EPA approval on the basis of fraudulent testing data. A scandal that made headlines in the early 1980s revealed that the largest independent laboratory in the nation, Industrial Bio-Test (IBT), had contracts with a number of chemical companies to supply the toxicological test data required for EPA registration. Only after more than 200 pesticides had been registered on the basis of falsified test results did it become known that the company had perpetrated the most massive scientific fraud ever committed in the United States. The IBT executives involved in the deception eventually received prison sentences, convicted of conducting and distributing fake scientific research and then attempting to cover-up their crimes. Nevertheless, many of the products registered during this period remain on the market today. A 1988 amendment to FIFRA requires EPA to speed up the re-registration process for pre-1972 pesticides and for those originally tested by IBT, but that project is far behind schedule and isn't expected to be completed until sometime after 2010.

4. Pesticides like DDT and chlordane, which were removed from commercial use due to concern for their *chronic* health effects, particularly cancer, were replaced largely by organophosphate or carbamate products that were often more acutely toxic than the chemicals they replaced, and are thus more dangerous to use. A number of these compounds are still commonly purchased for home or garden use, largely because they are cheaper than the less toxic pyrethrins.

In spite of many decades of pesticide regulation, overall use of chemical poisons continues to increase and the health and environmental risks they pose are as great as ever. Following common-sense safety precautions certainly can reduce the chance of injury or illness: follow label directions when using pesticides; keep pesticides in their original containers; keep them out of reach of children and pets; always wear protective clothing when applying chemicals; and avoid spraying when conditions are windy. Nevertheless, the decision to use chemical poisons always entails some degree of risk. Undeniably, pest problems need to be managed, but where nonchemical IPM approaches are equally effective, they represent the wiser, safer choice.

References

Benbrook, Charles M. 1996. *Pest Management at the Crossroads*. Consumers Union.

Schneider, Keith. 1983. "Faking It." *Amicus Journal* no. 4 (Spring).

sive legislation to reform and modernize the nation's laws dealing with food safety and the setting of pesticide tolerance levels. The **Food Quality Protection Act of 1996** now requires that when the EPA sets tolerance levels for pesticide residues on food, it must take into account available information on consumption habits of infants and children, as well as the neurological differences between adults and children that make the latter uniquely sensitive to the harmful effects of pesticide exposure. The law also requires EPA to take into account the cumulative effect of multiple residues when establishing pesticide tolerance levels in food, incorporating an additional tenfold margin of safety to protect children, infants, and babies *in utero* (Benbrook, 1996). As required by the Food Quality Protection Act, EPA has reevaluated all food tolerances to ensure they meet the law's "reasonable certainty of no harm" standard, particularly in regard to children's health. The agency points out that although 19–29% of food samples tested between 1994 and 2001 contained detectable levels of organophosphate pesticide residues (the highest rates were detected in 1996 and 1997), during that same period the amounts of insecticides used on the foods most frequently eaten by children dropped by 44%. In 1999–2000, out of concern for children's pesticide exposure, EPA imposed new restrictions on the use of several organophosphate poisons on certain food crops, as well as in and around the home (EPA, 2003).

Alternatives to Chemical Pest Control

As increasing numbers of pest species become resistant to available chemicals and as concerns over the long-range effects of pesticide exposure on human health and the environment continue to grow, the advisability of continuing to rely exclusively on chemicals for pest control is increasingly being questioned. In recent years a different philosophy of pest control has gained support, a strategy known as **Integrated Pest Management (IPM).** After ascertaining that a pest problem does indeed exist, IPM practitioners combine various compatible methods to prevent pest populations from reaching economically damaging levels while causing the least harm to human health and the environment. In 1977 the U.S. Department of Agriculture (USDA) adopted an official policy of encouraging IPM practices, sponsoring numerous research, development, and demonstration projects to promote IPM. In 1993 USDA set a goal, not yet achieved, of implementing IPM on fully 75% of total U.S. crop acreage by 2000 in order to reduce pesticide use and the environmental health risks posed by overreliance on chemicals for pest control (GAO, 2001).

While the emphasis in IPM is on utilizing natural controls such as predators, food deprivation, or weather to increase pest mortality, it also can include pesticide application, but only after careful monitoring of pest populations indicate a need. Unlike the total chemical control approach, IPM recognizes the extraordinary adaptability of insects and does not attempt to eradicate a particular pest entirely, but rather aims to keep pest populations below the threshold level at which they can cause significant economic loss. Among the methods that could be included in an IPM strategy are the following.

Natural Enemies

Many of our most serious insect and weed pests (such as Japanese beetle, gypsy moth, fire ant, kudzu, water hyacinth, and so on) are foreign imports that rapidly multiplied here in the absence of their natural enemies. Other native pests have caused serious problems only after their predators were eliminated by indiscriminate use of pesticides. Since the late 1800s, the government has imported more than 500 insect predators in an attempt to control alien species; more than 70 of these are now providing significant control of several important insect pests and weeds (Vail et al., 2001). Laboratory breeding of large populations of insect predators in hopes of overwhelming certain pests is also being conducted. Great success in controlling scale insects and mealybugs in citrus orchards was obtained by mass rearing and release of vedalia beetles and certain parasitic wasps. Home gardeners and organic farmers can assist natural predators in keeping pest insects at low levels by avoiding the use of broadspectrum insecticides and by planting a diverse assemblage of species that provide alternative food sources and habitat for beneficial insects (see box 8-5). It is *not* recommended, however, that IPM enthusiasts purchase insect predators such as ladybird beetles or praying mantises for release in their home gardens. Doing so is basically a waste of money because commercially sold ladybirds, once released, typically disperse and fly elsewhere, providing minimal levels of control for the purchaser; praying mantises are general feeders and will eat other beneficials (even each other!) as well as pests. In addition, because of their low survival rates and territorial nature, mantids have a negligible impact in controlling pest outbreaks.

Microbial Pesticides

A further step in biological warfare against insects involves introducing various disease agents into a pest population. A number of microbial pathogens are now being marketed commercially and more are in the research and development stage. To date, the most successful and widely used is the bacterium, *Bacillus thuringiensis (Bt)*, an organism that produces a toxin fatal to over 100 species of caterpillars. Use of *Bt*-based biopesticides has been increasing rapidly in response to consumer concerns about pesticide residues on food, as reflected in mounting demand for organically grown produce. In addition to *Bt*'s use on food crops, variants of this pathogen are widely employed against a number of other insect pests. *Bt kurstaki (Btk)* is the most widely used insecticide against forest pests such as the gypsy moth, spruce budworm, and tent caterpillar; *Bt tenebrionis (Btt)* is being targeted against various beetles such as the Colorado potato beetle, an insect now resistant to virtually every chemical pesticide; and *Bt israelensis (Bti)* is quite effective as a mosquito larvicide.

Fungal pathogens also have been enlisted in the war against insect pests. These organisms produce spores capable of penetrating the insect's exoskeleton, growing inside the host and digesting its tissues, resulting in death within a few days. One of these, *Metarhizium anisopliae*, is used extensively in Brazil for control of spittlebugs on sugar cane. Another, *Verticillium lecanii*, has been employed against greenhouse pests such as whiteflies, thrips, and aphids that are now resistant to almost all the chemical insecticides registered for use in greenhouses.

Pathogenic viruses also offer a promising method of pest control, since viral diseases in nature are frequently devastating to pest populations. A number of companies are currently conducting research on insect viruses that they hope to market against specific pests, but few are commercially available at present. The most widely used viral pesticide currently is a nuclear polyhedrosis virus, *Anticarsia gemmatalis*, used to combat the velvetbean caterpillar on nearly 15 million acres of Brazilian soybean fields (NRC, 2000). Researchers with the Canadian Forest Service are hopeful about developing an insect virus effective against the spruce budworm, pine sawfly, and other pests that periodically devastate Canadian forests.

A naturally occurring protozoan, *Nosema locustae,* has been successfully employed to control grasshoppers and Mormon crickets. When *Nosema* spores sprayed on a wheat-bran bait are consumed, they germinate inside the insect's stomach, multiply rapidly, and devour the pest from inside.

Sex Attractants

Certain chemical stimulants (pheromones) control many aspects of insect behavior, including mating. Sex pheromones may be excreted by the female to attract the male, or vice-versa. Some of these female pheromones have been synthesized in the lab and used to bait traps that can attract males from miles around. When the males enter the trap, expecting to encounter a receptive female, they are caught by a sticky substance on the bottom or sides of the trap. A variation on this method has yielded encouraging results in efforts to manage the codling moth, an insect whose larvae cause serious economic losses to pear and apple growers. To disrupt mating of adult moths, farmers place 10-inch-long twist-ties impregnated with female moth pheromone high in the branches of their orchard trees. When approximately 400 of these devices are used per acre, the "come hither" scent so pervades the area that male moths are thoroughly confused, not knowing in which direction to fly to find a mate. In this situation, most females remain unmated, lay infertile eggs, and over time the pest populations decline (Benbrook, 1996). The increasingly popular Japanese beetle trap marketed for home gardeners is baited with both a sex pheromone to attract males and a floral lure to entice female beetles. Although they are quite effective in doing just that, agricultural advisers recommend that homeowners not use them. Because they attract beetles from far and wide, many of which wouldn't have come otherwise, and because many of the arriving beetles evade the trap, gardeners who use these devices often experience more plant damage than they would have incurred without them.

Because the use of sex attractants as just described is effective only against adult insects, the technique is of limited effectiveness, since much crop damage is caused by insect larvae. In addition, because most pest species concentrate on a single crop, the market demand for any particular pheromone is relatively small. If the prospects for sales profits are not sufficiently attractive, manufacturers have no interest in producing them! Therefore, in recent years the prime strategy regarding sex attractants has shifted from using them to capture or confuse pest insects to employing pheromones to lure "good bugs" (i.e., predator species) into problem areas where they will then encounter—and eat—the "bad bugs." Since most predators eat a wide variety of pests, the same predator species could be a useful control agent in many different situations, a fact that significantly enhances the market demand for its pheromone. A recently patented product (The RESCUE®) being marketed through nurseries and hardware stores features a pheromone attractive to the spined soldier bug—a predator of approximately 100 different insect pests (ARS, 2004).

Insect Growth Regulators (IGRs)

Sometimes referred to as "biorational" insecticides, IGRs are chemicals that are identical to or closely mimic growth substances produced by the target pest. IGRs act either as **chitin inhibitors,** preventing proper development of the exoskeleton after molting, or, more commonly, as **juvenoids.** When the larvae of insects with a complete metamorphosis (fleas or mosquitoes, for example) contact or ingest juvenoids, these synthetic analogs of natural insect hormones prevent them from emerging as adults after pupating, thus effectively disrupting their life cycle. For insects characterized by a gradual metamorphosis (such as cockroaches) in which there is no pupal stage, nymphs may progress to adulthood but are abnormal in appearance and incapable of reproducing.

Several IGRs are now widely used in structural and public health pest control operations (usually in combination with standard insecticidal formulations to provide a "double whammy"), offering long-term control of such troublesome pests as cockroaches, fleas, ants, and floodwater mosquitoes. An obvious limitation to the use of insect growth regulators is that they are only useful against insects that cause damage as adults; many of the worst agricultural pests are larvae (such as caterpillars and grubs) against which IGRs are ineffective.

Sterile Insect Technique

This method relies on the mass rearing and release of huge numbers of male insects that have been sterilized by chemicals or radiation, usually gamma rays or X-rays. Subsequent mating of a normal female with a sterile male thus results in the production of infertile eggs. If the ratio of sterilized males to normal males is sufficiently large, most matings will be unsuccessful and over several generations pest populations will die out (the technique is most effective against target pest species in which the females mate only once). This technique was employed with great success on Zanzibar's Unguja Island to eradicate a tsetse fly population that for decades had caused devastating losses to livestock herds. Over a two-year period, from 1995–1997, an average of 50,000 male flies, mass-reared in laboratories and sterilized with a 28-second dose of gamma radiation, were released from airplanes across the island. With sterile males outnumbering the natural population of normal males by 50 to 1, induced sterility among females increased rapidly and the density of fly populations steadily dropped. The ultimate result was the total elimination of tsetse flies from the island (Kinley, 1998). Earlier SIT programs had been similarly successful in eradicating the screw-worm fly from Curacao, Florida, and parts of Central America, as well as the Mediterranean fruit fly from Chile, Mexico, and California. Not applicable in every setting, SIT is most effective when the pest population is geographically isolated, making reinvasion of the area with normal males unlikely.

Host Plant Resistance

Selective use of crop plant species that exhibit genetic resistance to pests is probably the most ecologically sound method for reducing losses due to plant diseases and nematodes. Practical applications of this IPM technique are numerous. For example, savvy home gardeners, as well as commercial growers, insist that the tomato seeds or plants they purchase be varieties bearing code letters that indicate resistance to several important tomato pathogens (e.g., the designation "**VFNT**" informs a prospective buyer that the plant in question is resistant to **V**erticillium wilt, **F**usarium wilt, **N**ematodes, and **T**obacco mosaic virus, and thus is unlikely to require chemical pesticide applications to keep the plant disease-free). Host resistance also has been successfully employed against insect pests such as the Hessian fly, grape phylloxera, spotted alfalfa aphid, rice stem borer, and corn earworm.

More recently, genetic engineering has provided new and faster techniques for introducing desired characteristics from one species into another. In 1995, EPA approved the first **transgenic** corn variety engineered for resistance to the European corn borer (ECB), a moth whose larvae cause significant crop losses throughout the Corn Belt each year. Scientists spliced a gene for toxin production from the bacterium *Bt* into the DNA of corn, creating a hybrid plant that can poison an invading corn borer larva on the first bite. A crop that "fights back," killing its enemy before sustaining damage itself, offers big benefits to farmers in terms of increased yields, reduced exposure to chemical toxins, and reduced expenditures for insecticides. Environmental benefits are obvious as well, since pesticide contamination of streams and groundwater in agricultural areas should be significantly reduced on *Bt*-crop acreage. However, most observers concede that there is a serious potential problem associated with the rapid proliferation of *Bt* crops; that is, the near-certainty that within a few years widespread

Box 8-5   IPM in Your Own Backyard

Although agriculture accounts for approximately three-fourths of all pesticide use in the United States, sales of herbicides and insecticides for home lawn and garden use have soared in recent decades. Millions of homeowners and backyard gardeners each year purchase and apply prodigious amounts of toxic chemicals to their property with little or no understanding of how to use, store, or dispose of such products in a safe manner. Increasing parental concerns about potential harm to children and pets from dangerous pesticide residues, confrontations among neighbors when "spray drift" from one property kills the flowers next door, and recognition that bird and butterfly populations plummet where insecticide use is profligate have prompted some to look for a better way to control weeds and insects in residential areas.

Integrated Pest Management (IPM) is a concept initially developed within the context of commercial agriculture, but its basic precepts are equally applicable and practical for the home gardener. Admittedly, it *is* much more demanding than conventional reliance on chemical pesticides, requiring an understanding of the life cycle and habits of the target pest. In the long run, however, IPM is a safer, more effective, and more sustainable approach to managing pest populations than conventional chemical treatment.

In a home lawn and garden environment, IPM is a process consisting of several steps:

1. **Determine whether a problem actually exists.** There's no point in automatically treating a lawn for grubs or spraying roses for aphids if none are present. Regular, systematic monitoring for the presence of pests prior to taking action is an essential component of any IPM program. This requires careful visual inspection of plants for signs of insect or disease problems or can involve the use of traps to determine whether certain pests are in the vicinity.

2. **Accurately identify the pest causing the problem.** Remember, not every insect present on a plant is a pest, nor is every discolored leaf evidence of a disease. Determination of the cause of damage can, in some cases, be tricky; injury due to herbicide spray drift, adverse weather conditions, or nutrient deficiency may produce symptoms similar to those of insect damage. Brown patches in the lawn, for example, may have many possible causes: drought, chemical burn, grubs, sod webworms, inadvertent spraying of dandelions with *Roundup®* (it happens!), or urination by a female dog. Determine the cause before taking appropriate action. If insects are spotted on a plant, note whether they appear to be causing any damage (chewing on leaves? sucking plant juices?); they may simply be harmless species "passing through" or a predator insect waiting to pounce on one of the "bad guys." Some knowledge of insect life cycles is important, since many pest species are damaging only during their larval stage or only as adults; attempting to control an insect at the wrong stage is generally a waste of effort. Similarly, spraying to control an insect that isn't a pest is environmentally bad and a waste of time and money—and may result in a worse problem if the victim happens to be a "good bug" who was helping to keep the pest population in check. Novices who don't feel capable of identifying presumed pests accurately can generally obtain help without charge at their county extension office or from a local Master Gardener group.

3. **Decide if the problem is serious enough to warrant action.** Once the problem is correctly identified, a decision must be made as to whether the pest is causing enough damage to warrant the effort and expense of controls. In an outdoor residential setting, this involves a subjective determination of the "aesthetic threshold"—how bad does a tree, lawn, or garden have to look to make rescuing it worthwhile in terms of time, money, and potential health risks due to pesticide exposure? It must be kept in mind that some types of infestations (e.g., spittlebugs or columbine leaf miners) may look threatening but really aren't significantly harming the plant. Decisions on whether or not to take action should also be influenced by the time of year when the infes-

tation occurs; for example, insects defoliating trees in late spring represent a much more serious problem than would defoliation in late summer when the tree has already accumulated food reserves for winter and will soon lose its leaves anyhow. Application of pest control measures are probably appropriate in the former situation, but may not be recommended in the latter, even when the extent of leaf damage is the same. In some cases, weather conditions alone may take care of the problem—infestations of turf-destroying sod webworms may be completely eliminated during cool wet springs, thanks to a fungal pathogen of webworms that thrives under those climatic conditions. It should also be kept in mind that healthy, vigorous plants can sustain a considerable amount of insect feeding without much lasting damage. For all these reasons, doing *nothing* is one valid option in an IPM program.

4. **If the pest problem is deemed severe enough to warrant control, utilize a combination of methods best suited to the specific pest in question.** Such controls include many of the same strategies relied upon by farmers—planting cultivars that are resistant to pests or diseases known to be a problem in the area (e.g. scab-resistant crabapple trees, mildew-resistant *Phlox* 'David'); maintaining plants in good health by proper fertilization and watering practices; and, when all else fails, judicious chemical pesticide applications, using the "littlest gun" that will do the job, applied in a manner least likely to harm nontarget organisms.

A number of additional IPM strategies have been successfully practiced by home gardeners for generations.

Mechanical controls include hand-picking, stomping, and squashing (it's unlikely bugs will ever evolve resistance to being stepped on nor weeds to being ripped from the ground!). Floating row covers can protect young plants from flea beetles, cabbage moths, and a host of other flying insect pests, while stiff paper collars or bottomless coffee cans around tender transplants can effectively deter cutworms. Similarly, the use of nets or chicken wire to block access to plants may offer the only reliable

approach to keeping birds and rabbits away. Pruning off infested plant parts (e.g., cutting off the ends of tree branches harboring fall webworm nests, removing infected iris rhizomes when dividing overgrown clumps, using scissors to cut bagworms off tree branches before the eggs hatch in the spring) can be far more effective than pesticide spraying in certain situations.

Cultural practices include adjusting the planting time of certain crops (e.g., potatoes) so that critical periods in plant development (in this case, blossom initiation) don't coincide with peak pest populations. Another highly recommended practice, especially in vegetable gardens, is the removal of all plant debris at the end of the season to reduce overwintering habitat of such common insect pests as squash bugs, flea beetles, and iris borers. A thorough fall cleanup also helps prevent fungal problems the following year; the main strategy for combating *Botrytis* blight, the most serious disease of peonies, is to cut the old plants down to ground level at the end of the season and remove all dead foliage and debris from around the base of the plant. During the growing season, fungal diseases in general can be minimized by spacing plants far enough apart to maintain good air circulation; watering in the early morning rather than in the evening so that wet foliage will dry quickly also helps to avoid conditions favorable for fungal pathogens. To suppress weed growth, a 1–2" layer of organic mulch (shredded bark, leaf mold, grass clippings straw, etc.) applied around the base of plants in early spring is quite effective in preventing weed seeds from germinating and smothering young weed seedlings; weeds that do manage to grow through the mulch are easily removed by hand. Black plastic can also be used to control weeds, especially in vegetable gardens where transplants can be inserted and grown through slits in the plastic cover.

Biological controls involve using natural enemies to keep pest populations at tolerable levels. The most important way to do this is to avoid, wherever possible, the use of chemical insecticides, since most of those on the market are broad-spectrum poisons that make no distinction between harmful and beneficial species. In addition, to encourage the "good guys" to take up residence in close proximity to where the pests are, gardeners need to provide harborage and alternative sources of nutrition for these species (have you ever considered what ladybugs eat in the early spring before the aphids arrive?—dandelion pollen, among other things!). This can be done quite easily by planting a variety of flowers nearby; some of the best species for this purpose include members of the mustard family (*Cruciferae*) like sweet alyssum and dame's rocket; members of the carrot family (*Umbelliferae*), including dill, coriander, and Queen Anne's lace; various legumes such as alfalfa and sweet clover, and many members of the aster family (*Asteraceae*)— marigolds, coneflowers, goldenrod, and, yes, even dandelions! "The more, the merrier" in terms of species in a garden seems to be the best approach to a chemical-free method of managing garden pests.

Inevitably there comes a time when gardeners must make a choice between allowing some plants to be destroyed by an out-of-control pest explosion or the judicious application of chemical pesticides (under an IPM regimen, unlike true organic gardening, chemical use is permitted as a last resort). However, adherence to an IPM program will minimize the need for such painful decisions and will result in a healthier backyard environment for plants and gardeners alike.

resistance to the *Bt* toxin will develop among populations of target insects. To slow down what is generally regarded as an inevitable consequence of widespread exposure to *Bt*, farmers are being urged to reserve approximately 20% of their total acreage for non-*Bt* crop varieties. By doing so, it is hoped, pests within the reserve won't be under selective pressure to develop resistance; if resistant individuals from outside the reserve subsequently encounter and mate with one of these nonresistant pests, large-scale resistance within the population can at least be delayed. Unfortunately, anecdotal evidence from farm country suggests that the majority of growers are not setting aside enough of their cropland to make a significant difference. Hence it is likely that *Bt*'s unquestioned value for organic growers and large commercial farmers alike will be short-lived, undermined by increasing *Bt*-resistance within pest populations.

Sanitation

For control of insect and rodent pests in residential areas or business establishments, the most effective way to reduce pest numbers and keep them low is to apply the basic principles of sanitation. To survive and multiply, pests need a source of food, water, and harborage. If these are in short supply, large pest populations cannot be maintained. Strict observance of the rules of good housekeeping—promptly cleaning up spilled food, storing foods in tightly sealed containers, keeping garbage cans covered, avoiding use of mulch immediately adjacent to building foundations, mowing tall grass or weeds near structures, locating woodpiles at some distance from dwellings, regularly collecting and disposing of animal feces—will be far more effective in eliminating flies, rodents, and roaches over the long term than will pesticidal spraying. Similarly, structural alterations such as screens, metal or cement barriers, and caulk applied to cracks and crevices can assist in "building out" certain household pests. Habitat modification such as changing water in birdbaths frequently, keeping roof gutters free of twigs and leaves to permit complete drainage of rainwater, and maintaining premises free of discarded articles that could collect water can be very effective in reducing mosquito breeding. Pesticide use can provide a "quick fix," but without adherence to good sanitary practices, control will be temporary at best.

None of the above methods alone is the total answer to effective pest management. However, in the proper combination after an accurate assessment of a specific pest situation, IPM techniques promise a safer, more ecologically sound, and ultimately more successful approach to limiting pest damage than does total reliance on chemicals.

References

Agricultural Research Service (ARS). 2004. *Technologies in the Marketplace: Better Traps, Fewer Bugs.* Accessed at http://www.ars.usda.gov/business/docs.htm?docid=769 (March 16).

Akre, Roger D., and Elizabeth A. Myhre. 1994. "The Great Spider Whodunit." *Pest Control Technology* 22, no. 4 (April).

Arnold, S. F., D. M. Klotz, B. M. Collins, P. M. Vonier, L. J. Guillette, Jr., and J. A. McLachlan. 1996. "Synergistic Activation of Estrogen Receptor with Combinations of Environmental Chemicals." *Science* 272 (June 7):1489–1492.

Aspelin, A. L., and A. H. Grube. 1999. *Pesticide Industry Sales and Usage.* 733–R-99–001. Washington, DC: U.S. Environmental Protection Agency, Office of Pesticide Programs.

Benbrook, Charles M. 1996. *Pest Management at the Crossroads.* Yonkers, NY: Consumers Union.

Bever, Wayne, et al. 1975. *Illinois Pesticide Applicator Study Guide.* Cooperative Extension Service, University of Illinois College of Agriculture, Special Publication 39.

Blair, Aaron, et al. 1987. "Cancer and Pesticides Among Farmers." *Pesticides and Groundwater: A Health Concern for the Midwest.* The Freshwater Foundation.

Carson, Rachel. 1962. *Silent Spring.* Boston: Houghton Mifflin.

Centers for Disease Control and Prevention (CDC). 1994. "Human Plague—United States, 1993–1994." *Morbidity & Mortality Weekly Report* 43, no. 13 (April 8).

Curtis, Jennifer, Tim Profeta, and Laurie Mott. 1993. *After Silent Spring: The Unresolved Problems of Pesticide Use in the United States.* New York: Natural Resources Defense Council.

Environmental Protection Agency (EPA). 2003. *America's Children and the Environment: Measures of Contaminants, Body Burdens, and Illnesses.* 2nd ed. EPA 240–R-03–001, Office of Children's Health Protection (Feb).

Environmental Working Group (EWG). 1998. "Same As It Ever Was." Press Release, May 21.

"EPA Study Links Pesticide Use with Ground Water Contamination." 1992. *Environmental Health Letter,* Jan. 28.

Flint, M. L., and R. VandenBosch. 1981. *Introduction to Integrated Pest Management.* New York: Plenum Press.

General Accounting Office (GAO). 2001. *Management Improvements Needed to Further Promote Integrated Pest Management.* GAO-01-815, Agricultural Pesticides (Sept. 28). Washington, DC: U.S. GPO.

Greenlee, A. R., T. E. Arbuckle, and P-H. Chou. 2003. "Risk Factors for Female Infertility in an Agricultural Region." *Epidemiology* 14:429–436.

Hartzler, Bob, and Mike Owen. 2003. "Status and Concerns for Glyphosate Resistance." *Integrated Crop Management.* Ames: Department of Entomology, Iowa State University (March 17).

Jeyaratnam, J. 1990. "Acute Pesticide Poisoning: A Major Global Health Problem." *World Health Statistics Quarterly* 43.

Kinley, David H. 1998. "Aerial Assault on the Tsetse Fly." *Environment* 40, no. 7 (Sept).

Lin, B. H., M. Padgitt, H. Delvo, D. Shank, and H. Taylor. 1995. *Pesticide and Fertilizer Use and Trends in U.S. Agriculture.* Agricultural Economic Report No. 717, Economic Research Service. Washington, DC: U.S. Department of Agriculture.

Loffredo, C. A., et al. 2001. "Association of Transposition of the Great Arteries in Infants with Maternal Exposures to Herbicides and Rodenticides." *American Journal of Epidemiology* 153 (6):529–536.

Mallis, Arnold. 1997. *Handbook of Pest Control.* 8th ed. Mallis Handbook and Technical Training Company.

Mansur, Mike. 1994. "The Food Chain." *The 1994 Information Please Environmental Almanac.* World Resources Institute. Boston: Houghton Mifflin.

Meister Publishing Co. 1996. *Ag Consultant Magazine* (March).

Nash, Linda. 1993. "Water Quality and Health." In *Water in Crisis: A Guide to the World's Fresh Water Resources,* edited by Peter H. Gleick. New York: Oxford Univ. Press.

National Research Council (NRC). 2000. *The Future Role of Pesticides in U.S. Agriculture.* Washington, DC: National Academy Press.

———. 1993. *Pesticides in the Diets of Infants and Children.* Washington, DC: National Academy Press.

———. 1992. *Neem: A Tree for Solving World Problems.* Washington, DC: National Academy Press.

National Research Council (NRC). 1987. *Regulating Pesticides in Food: The Delaney Paradox.* Washington, DC: National Academy Press.

Parker, Tracey. 1994. "Recent Studies Document the Complex Ways Pesticides Affect Birds." *Journal of Pesticide Reform* 14, no. 1 (Spring).

Perkins, John H. 1982. *Insects, Experts, and the Insecticide Crisis.* New York: Plenum Press.

Pimentel, David, ed. 1997. *Techniques for Reducing Pesticide Use: Economic and Environmental Benefits.* New York: John Wiley & Sons.

———, et al. 1991. "Environmental and Economic Impacts of Reducing U.S. Agricultural Pesticide Use." *Handbook of Pest Management in Agriculture.* CRC Press.

Raloff, Janet. 2003. "Munching Along." *Science News* 164, no. 22 (Nov. 29):344–346.

Rosenstreich, David L., Peyton Eggleston, Meyer Kattan, Dean Baker, Raymond G. Slavin, Peter Gergen, Herman Mitchell, Kathleen McNiff-Mortimer, Henry Lynn, Dennis Ownby, and Floyd Malveaux. 1997. "The Role of Cockroach Allergy and Exposure to Cockroach Allergen in Causing Morbidity Among Inner-City Children with Asthma." *New England Journal of Medicine* 336, no. 19:1356–1363.

Salam, M. T., Y-F. Li, B. Langholz, and F. D. Gilliland. 2004. "Early Life Environmental Risk Factors for Asthma: Findings from the Children's Health Study." *Environmental Health Perspectives* 112, no. 6 (May):760–765.

Schneider, Keith. 1994. "Progress, Not Victory, on Great Lakes Pollution." *New York Times,* May 7.

Vail, P. V., J. R. Coulson, W. C. Kauffman, and M. E. Dix. 2001. "History of Biological Control Programs in the United States Department of Agriculture." *American Entomologist* 47, no. 1 (Spring).

Weed Science Society of America (WSSA). 2004. http://www.weedscience.com/. Accessed March 15.

World Health Organization (WHO). 1997. "Human Plague in 1995." *Weekly Epidemiological Record* 46 (Nov. 14):289.

World Resources Institute. 1994. *World Resources 1994–1995.* New York: Oxford Univ. Press.

Yardley, Jim. 2003. "Rat Poison: Murder Weapon of Choice in Rural China." *New York Times,* Nov. 17.

FOOD QUALITY

> It was no uncommon occurrence for a man to find the surface of his pot of coffee swarming with weevils after breaking up hardtack in it, which had come out of the fragments only to drown; but they were easily skimmed off and left no distinctive flavor behind. If a soldier cared to do so, he could expel the weevils by heating the bread at the fire.
> The maggots did not budge in that way.
> —John Billings ("Hardtack and Coffee," 1887)

A Civil War veteran's reflections on the insect-infested fare common to both Yankee and Confederate armies during that historic conflict give evidence that concerns about food contamination and food quality in general are nothing new. From time immemorial, humans have grappled with the problem of protecting stored food supplies from insects, molds, and rodent infestations; they learned through sad experience about natural toxins in certain foods and found they could minimize risk of food poisoning through proper processing and cooking practices. Until the mid-1800s however, problems related to food quality were relatively limited and localized because most people raised their food at home or purchased it from local producers. Consumers carefully inspected purchased items for signs of insect infestation, sniffed meat and fish to detect spoilage, and in general served as their own food inspectors. Government regulation of food quality prior to the 20th century was extremely limited, focusing primarily on commercially baked bread. Early bread laws were designed to standardize the weight of loaves in relation to the price of wheat; i.e., they were essentially price-fixing laws. Other regulations prohibited adding foreign substances such as ground chalk or powdered beans to flour. Subsequent laws provided for inspection of weights and flour quality (Janssen, 1975).

In the United States, prior to the 1900s the federal government had no role in regulating food safety, that issue being regarded as solely a prerogative of state or local authorities (NRC, 1998). However, in the decades following the Civil War, the close-to-home food production, distribution, and marketing systems that had prevailed virtually everywhere in the world up to that time began experiencing revolutionary change. The explosive growth of cities and the expansion of transportation networks—especially the railroad—during these years gave birth to an organized food industry that became national, and eventually global, in scope. The subsequent introduction of refrigerated railcars (and later refrigerated trucks and air freight) made possible the shipment of hitherto unavailable fresh meat and produce to markets thousands of miles distant from their place of origin. This rapid development, in the

275

absence of regulation, was marred by deplorably unhygienic conditions and frequently unethical practices.

The biggest scandal of 19th-century food establishments involved the widespread practice of **adulteration**—the deliberate addition of inferior or cheaper material to a supposedly pure food product in order to stretch out supplies and increase profits. Adulteration has undoubtedly been practiced on a small scale for millennia by unscrupulous merchants when they thought they could get away with it, but the anonymity of large, unregulated corporations selling foodstuffs to faceless consumers hundreds of miles away gave great impetus to the proliferation of this age-old practice. Substances used as adulterants in some cases were harmless ingredients, cheating consumers only in a financial sense; in other instances, the adulterants consisted of toxic substances that posed a serious health threat to those consuming the adulterated products. Some foods commonly adulterated during the 18th and 19th centuries included: (1) black pepper commonly mixed with such materials as mustard seed husks, pea flour, juniper berries, or floor sweepings; (2) tea, adulterated on a large scale with leaves of the ash tree which were dried, curled, and sold to tea merchants for a few cents per pound. Green China tea was often adulterated with dried thorn leaves, tinted green with a toxic dye; black Indian tea was more easily adulterated by collecting used tea leaves from restaurants, drying and stiffening them with gum and then tinting them with black lead, also toxic, to make them look fresh; (3) cocoa powder "enriched" with brick dust; (4) milk supplies extended with water; (5) coffee blended with ground acorns or chicory.

Perhaps even more alarming were revelations in the late 19th century that many of the food colors and flavorings in widespread use were poisonous; e.g., pickles colored bright green with copper, candies and sweets brightly tinted with lead and copper salts, commercially baked bread whitened with alum, beer froth produced by iron sulfate. By the turn of the century, over 80 synthetic agents were being used to color foods as diverse as mustard, jellies, and wine. Many had never been tested for adverse health effects and all were being used without any monitoring or regulatory controls; amazingly, some of these chemical additives had been developed as textile dyes and were never intended to be used in food products! Not surprisingly, contemporary accounts document a number of human illnesses and a few deaths attributable to consumption of toxic food colorants in those years (Tannahill, 1973; Henkel, 1993).

A growing awareness of such problems led to congressional passage in 1906 of the **Pure Food and Drugs Act**, one of the first federal laws intended to protect consumers against adulteration, mislabeling of foods, and harmful ingredients in food. As a result of this act and of subsequent food quality legislation, instances of adulteration in the United States are now much rarer, though regulations have had to be instituted from time to time to prevent the gradual degradation of foods, such as the increase in fat or ground bone content of hot dogs or the decrease in fruit content of jams or fruit pies. However, occasionally flagrant abuses still occur. In the fall of 1993 the Flavor Fresh Foods Corporation of Chicago, as well as 11 of its corporate officials, pled guilty to charges of defrauding consumers of more than $40 million through sales of adulterated orange juice. For 12 years Flavor Fresh had been marketing a product labeled as "100% pure orange juice from concentrate," selling it widely throughout the Midwest. In reality, the juice contained 55–75% beet sugar, along with other adulterants added to conceal the substitution. The two-year investigation, which culminated in the convictions of those responsible, demonstrated that unscrupulous attempts to make a quick dollar are still a threat more than a century after the adulteration scandals of the late 1800s (Ropp, 1994).

Within recent years the focus of public attention regarding food quality has shifted from adulteration to a concern over contaminants and additives in our food supply. The fact that few people today produce their own foods at home means that almost all of us, to a greater or lesser degree, have no choice but to rely on foodstuffs produced by a massive food industry—foods that contain many kinds of additives and, in some cases, contaminants over which we have very little control. The widespread interest in "health foods" is due, in no small measure, to the feeling of many people that industrially produced food is somehow less safe and less nutritious than the "natural" foods of yesteryear. Representatives of the food industry and, indeed, many scientists, counter that chemical additives are both safe and essential to ensure an abundant supply of food at affordable prices to a still-growing population. In an attempt to understand the nature of the debate and the rationale behind existing or proposed regulations, it is helpful to distinguish between those substances accidentally introduced into foods and those deliberately added to prevent deterioration or to enhance taste or attractiveness.

Food Contaminants

Substances accidentally incorporated into foods are called **contaminants.** Such contaminants include dirt, hairs, animal feces, fungal growths, insect fragments, pesticide residues, traces of growth hormones or antibiotics, and so on, that are introduced into food during the harvesting, processing, or packaging stage. They serve no useful purpose in the finished product and are presumed to be harmful unless proven otherwise. (In many cases, however, common food contaminants constitute an aesthetic affront to consumers rather than an actual health threat; for example, the thought of eating a fly wing hidden among the oregano leaves on a frozen pizza may be repugnant, but it won't make you sick—at least not if you don't see it!) Certainly every

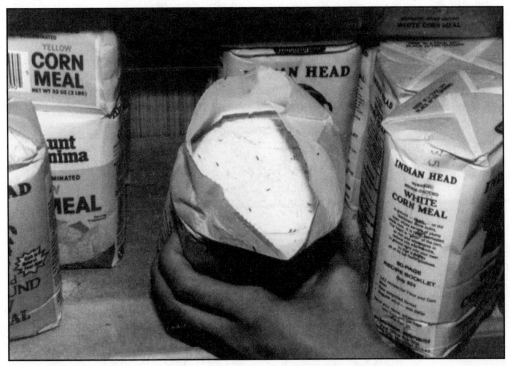

What consumer wouldn't be repulsed by the sight of rodent feces in a package of corn meal? [*NYS Department of Agriculture and Markets, Division of Food Safety and Inspection*]

effort should be made to keep our foods as free from contamination as possible; however, it has never been, and probably never will be, possible to grow, harvest, and process crops that are totally free of natural defects. In order to ensure that foods are never contaminated by even a few insects, rodent hairs, or droppings, etc., we would have to use much larger amounts of chemical pesticides and would thus risk exposing consumers to the potentially greater hazard of increased levels of toxic residues. Current philosophy holds that it is wiser to permit aesthetically unpleasant but harmless natural defects rather than pouring on more synthetic chemicals. For this reason, the Food and Drug Administration (FDA) has established what it terms **defect action levels**, specifying the maximum limit of contamination at or above which the agency will take legal action to remove the product from the market. It is important to understand that such defect action levels are not average levels of contamination—the averages are considerably lower—but represent the upper limit of allowable contamination. Defect action levels are set at that point where it is assumed there is no danger to human health. Some examples of existing defect action levels are shown in table 9-1.

Several groups of food contaminants that are less visible but more worrisome are the traces of antibiotics (see box 9-1) and growth hormones in meat products and toxic pesticide residues on fruits and vegetables. The issue of hormone-treated meat has been rankling relations between the European Union (EU) and major meat-exporting countries (primarily the U.S., Canada, Australia, and New Zealand) since 1989, when

Table 9-1 Examples of Food Defect Action Levels

Product	Defect	Action Level
Apricots, canned	Insect filth	Average of 2% or more by count insect-infested or insect-damaged
Beets, canned	Rot	Exceeds average of 5% by weight of pieces with dry rot
Broccoli, frozen	Insects and mites	Average of 60 aphids, thrips, and/or mites per 100 grams
Cherries, maraschino	Insect filth	Average of over 5% rejects due to maggots
Corn, canned	Insect larvae (corn ear worms, corn borers)	Two or more 3 mm or longer larvae, cast skins or cast skin fragments of corn ear worm or corn borer, the aggregate length exceeding 12 mm in 24 pounds
Curry powder	Insect filth	Average of more than 100 insect fragments per 25 grams
	Rodent filth	Average of more than 4 rodent hairs per 25 grams
Olives, pitted	Pits	Average of more than 1.3% by count of olives with whole pits and/or pit fragments 2mm or longer measured in the longest dimension
Peanut butter	Insect filth	Average of 30 or more insect fragments per 100 grams
	Rodent filth	Average of 1 or more rodent hairs per 100 grams
	Grit	Gritty taste and water insoluble inorganic residue is more than 25 mg per 100 grams
Tomatoes, canned	Drosophila fly	Average of 10 fly eggs per 500 grams; or 5 fly eggs and 1 maggot per 500 grams; or 2 maggots per 500 grams

the EU banned imports of meat from animals treated with growth hormones. Such hormones, illegal in Europe, are widely used by American beef producers, administered in the form of slow-release pelleted implants inserted under the skin on the backside of the earflap. Approximately 90% of feedlot cattle in the U.S. are implanted, as are a smaller percentage of sheep (neither hogs nor chickens receive hormone implants). Beef producers have used hormones for decades to hasten weight gain of their animals while using less feed and to produce meat with a lower fat content. The EU justifies its prohibition of hormone-treated meat as a consumer safety measure, fearing that lingering traces of hormones in meat at the time of slaughter could pose human health risks. However, scientific studies in both the United States and Europe conclude there is no evidence of such a threat from the five hormones the FDA has approved for use in U.S. livestock (estradiol, testosterone, progesterone, trenbolone acetate, and zeranol). Because humans daily produce several thousand times larger quantities of these hormones through their own metabolic activities than they are exposed to via meat consumption, health authorities conclude hormones in meat present negligible risk. The Codex Alimentarius Commission, an international group that makes recommendations on food safety questions, has given its support to the use of natural hormones in meat production; similarly, a group of 15 European scientists presented findings to the British Veterinary Association concluding that use of growth-promoting hormones in cattle presents no human health threat. Nevertheless, for reasons U.S. negotiators suspect are due to domestic economic and political considerations, the 15 nations comprising the EU continue to defy a ruling by the World Trade Organization stating that their ban on imports of hormone-treated meat is a violation of free trade rules. Since European public opinion is strongly supportive of the ban, resolution of this dispute appears unlikely in the near future (Hanrahan, 1996).

Early in 1994 a genetically engineered growth hormone intended to boost milk production was introduced onto the market by Monsanto, a move that provoked an outpouring of concern from some consumer groups (as well as from some dairy farmers worried about milk surpluses and falling prices). The hormone, alternatively known as **rBGH** (recombinant Bovine Growth Hormone) or **BST** (Bovine Somatotropin), is injected into dairy cows every 14 days, resulting in a 10–20% increase in milk production. After extensive studies evaluating its safety and efficacy, the FDA approved sale of the hormone, making rBGH the first commercially important product of agricultural biotechnology to be incorporated into the nation's food supply. In spite of FDA assurances that there is no human health risk associated with rBGH, many consumer groups remain wary. Critics charge that, by raising milk output per cow, the hormone puts additional stress on the animals, increasing the likelihood of udder infections and thereby necessitating more use of antibiotics. This, they fear, could result in lingering traces of antibiotics in milk and contribute to the selection of antibiotic-resistant bacteria in milk-drinking humans. The FDA insists the government has safeguards in place to monitor milk supplies for traces of antibiotics and bacteria and will destroy any milk that is tainted. In 1998, after examining new evidence, the Joint Expert Committee on Food Additives, comprised of representatives of the United Nations' Food and Agriculture Organization (FAO) and World Health Organization (WHO), reconfirmed its position that use of rBGH is safe. Nevertheless, the United States remains the only major country to permit use of the hormone and many American consumers, still unconvinced, are paying premium prices for organically produced milk (Nestle, 2003; FAO, 1998).

Pesticide residues in food occur when crops are sprayed directly or when livestock consume pesticide-contaminated fodder, traces of which can then be translocated into meat, eggs, or milk. EPA has established **tolerance levels** for all pesticides used on

Box 9-1   Abusing a Valuable Resource

Antibiotics represent one of the great medical advances of the 20th century, relegating once-dreaded bacterial killers to the status of easily curable diseases. Unfortunately, overuse and misuse of these valuable pharmaceutical resources are contributing to the build-up of antibiotic resistance in an ever-increasing number of bacterial populations. Blame for this current state of affairs is widely shared by physicians and patients alike. For years microbiologists have criticized the overuse of antibiotics to treat conditions that would soon be resolved without medication, as well as the misuse of these drugs against viral infections or other health problems that don't respond to antibiotic treatment. The need for more judicious medical use of antibiotics in the face of increasing bacterial resistance is gradually being accepted by doctors and by the general public, but few people are aware that another source of microbial exposure to these drugs is posing a major human health threat.

For decades the widespread use of antibiotics in the livestock and poultry industries has sparked bitter controversy between agropharmaceutical interests and food safety experts. Over 40% of the antibiotics manufactured in the United States each year are used in poultry, pork, and beef production. Of this amount, about one-fifth is administered for veterinary purposes, to treat animal diseases, while the remainder is incorporated in subtherapeutic amounts into animal feed and trough water to enhance growth and weight gain. Both of these uses have the potential for fostering development of antibiotic resistance among bacterial populations, yet livestock producers have vigorously—and successfully—lobbied against regulatory controls. Claiming that antibiotic use is necessary to produce affordable meat and poultry, industry spokespersons long argued that no scientific evidence exists to show the practice has adversely affected human health. That argument can no longer be made; since the late 1990s, irrefutable proof of humans infected with antibiotic-resistant foodborne microbes has been traced to drug-resistant bacterial strains in animals.

In 1998, CDC researchers reported that one strain of Salmonella (DT104) had acquired resistance to five of the antibiotics commonly used against it: ampicillin, chloramphenicol, streptomycin, tetracycline, and the sulfonamides. In just seven years—from 1989 to 1996—the percentage of DT104 samples testing positive for multi-drug resistance climbed from 0.6 to 34%, even though the number of human Salmonella infections remained relatively constant during the same time period. Although the majority of Salmonella infections run their course without need for medication, a small percentage (3–10%) result in bacteremia (i.e., bacteria invading the bloodstream), requiring antibiotic treatment. If the causative pathogens fail to respond to such treatment, the situation could become life-threatening.

Further evidence of a cause-and-effect relationship between human disease and antibiotic use in meat production made news in 1999 when resistant bacterial isolates from people stricken with Campylobacter food poisoning were shown to have the same "DNA fingerprint" as Campylobacter strains found on chicken products. Currently the most common form of bacterial food poisoning in the U.S., Campylobacter infections are generally treated, when necessary, with fluoroquinolone antibiotics such as ciprofloxacin. In the early 1990s, fluoroquinolone-resistant Campylobacter was quite rare—slightly over 1% of all reported cases—and virtually all of these were acquired during foreign travel. In 1995, the use of fluoroquinolones to treat respiratory infections in poultry flocks was approved by the FDA over the vigorous objections of CDC scientists concerned about the wide-scale exposure of chickens to a relatively new human drug that the medical community hoped would remain effective for many years. Their worries appeared well-founded, since similar approval of fluoroquinolones for veterinary use in Spain in 1990 had resulted in resistant human Campylobacter isolates soaring from almost 0% in 1989 to 30–50% in 1991. As the CDC had feared, within a year after licensure of fluoroquinolone for use on poultry farms, cases of domestically acquired ciprofloxacin-resistant human Campylobacter infections began to climb in the U.S., reaching 14% by 1998. By 2001, researchers sampling meats from local supermarkets reported finding antibiotic-resistant bacteria in packages of chicken, beef, and pork. These pathogens could still be found 1–2 weeks later in the intestines of consumers who ate them. If they had been present in sufficient numbers to induce illness, treatment with antibiotics would have been useless. Since pharmaceutical companies have no new wonder drugs currently in the pipeline, health authorities are increasingly worried that the livestock industry's profligate use of the same antibiotics needed to treat human disease is a reckless squandering of a vital resource (of the 17 classes of antibiotics used as growth promoters in food animals, 6 are also used to treat human diseases).

In response to increasingly vocal concerns being expressed by medical authorities, environmental organizations, and concerned consumers, some segments of the food industry have begun to take action on this issue. In 2001 McDonald's Corporation told its poultry suppliers to phase out use of fluoroquinolones in the chickens it purchased from them; the following year, without any fanfare, two large poultry producers began reducing the use of growth-promoting antibiotics. Most significant, however, was McDonald's declaration in June 2003 that it was calling on its direct suppliers worldwide to phase out use of all animal growth-promoting antibiotics that are also used in human medicine; indirect suppliers are similarly encouraged to eliminate these drugs and to reduce other antibiotic usage as well. Certification of compliance with the new standards must be provided each year and suppliers must maintain records of antibiotic use and make them available for company audit and review. The importance of McDonald's policy shift reflects the company's marketplace dominance; as the world's largest fast-food chain, McDonald's uses over 2.5 billion pounds of meat and chicken annually. When McDonald's

speaks, meat producers listen. The impact will be greatest in the poultry industry, where suppliers such as Tyson Foods directly control the stages of production where decisions about antibiotic use are made. Tyson supported McDonald's decision, as did Cargill, another major supplier, and both promised vigorous efforts to comply with the new standards. Whether other fast-food chains decide to follow McDonald's lead remains to be seen; several have said such action is being considered.

At the governmental level, FDA's stance is that the use of antibiotics in farm animals is both safe and effective; nevertheless, agency officials concur that "less is better." The situation is quite different in Europe, where increasing numbers of human illnesses blamed on use of antibiotics for meat production led to a ban on this practice by the European Union; the World Health Organization also has recommended a phaseout. Although a number of consumer groups and some members of Congress have repeatedly called for a prohibition on all nontherapeutic antibiotic use in U.S. farm animals, political pressures and seeming public indifference have stymied passage of legislation requiring such action.

References

Glynn, M. K. et al. 1998. "Emergence of Multidrug-Resistant Salmonella Enterica Serotype Typhimurium DT104 Infections in the United States." *New England Journal of Medicine* 338, no. 19 (May 7):1333–1338.

McDonald's Corporation Press Release. June 19, 2003.

Smith, K. E. et al. 1999. "Quinolone-Resistant Campylobacter jejuni Infections in Minnesota, 1992–1998." *New England Journal of Medicine* 340, no. 20 (May 20):1525–1532.

food crops representing the maximum quantity of a pesticide residue allowable on a raw agricultural commodity. Such tolerances constitute the federal government's principle means of regulating pesticide residues in food. These levels are based on results of field trials performed by pesticide manufacturers and reflect the maximum residue concentrations likely when farm chemicals are applied properly. In essence, tolerance levels are set on the basis of good agricultural practices and not on considerations of human health. In 1987 the National Research Council (NRC) of the National Academy of Sciences published an alarming report estimating a significant increase in can-

Mounting evidence indicates that routine use of antibiotics in the poultry and livestock industries is creating antibiotic-resistant bacteria that also cause disease in humans. Concern over the health implications prompted McDonald's Corp. to ask its meat suppliers to phase out use of growth-promoting antibiotics that are also used in human medicine. [*AP photo / April L. Brown*]

cer mortality among American consumers due to ingestion of certain pesticide residues on food, even when the amounts of such chemicals are within the established tolerance levels. A subsequent NRC report issued in 1993 questioned whether existing tolerance levels, established on the basis of estimated adult food consumption patterns, were sufficiently protective of children's health. The report pointed out that youngsters consume more chemically tainted fruit in relation to their body size than do adults and, because of their rapid rate of growth and development, they are more vulnerable than older people to toxic chemicals in food (NRC, 1993; 1987). These concerns led Congress to include a provision in the 1996 **Food Quality Protection Act** that EPA consider the consumption habits and unique vulnerability of children when setting tolerance levels and must be able to guarantee that any tolerance level approved by the agency is safe for children (Merrill, 1997).

While the findings contained in the 1987 and 1993 NRC reports demonstrate the need for strict controls, the National Academy of Sciences contends that under the current U.S. regulatory system, pesticide residues on food pose a negligible health threat to the general population. In a 1996 report, the NRC pointed out that although traces of pesticide residues are detectable in food and water virtually everywhere, the amounts present on U.S.-grown crops are typically very low and do not present a significant risk of cancer or other health problems. In recent years both the concentration of pesticide residues in food and the frequency with which they are found has steadily declined, due in part to the pesticide industry's shift to chemicals that break down quickly and hence are no longer present at harvest time. Since many of the newer chemicals are effective against pests at much lower concentrations than those applied in years past, the absolute quantity of residues present on pesticide-treated crops today is one-tenth or less that found on crops sprayed with the chemicals formerly used in U.S. agriculture (NRC, 2000; 1996).

Nevertheless, public perception of risk has given added impetus to a burgeoning consumer demand for organically grown food. Although the health benefits of organic foods have yet to be scientifically proven, organic foods represent the most rapidly growing segment of the food market. While they still represent a small portion of total U.S. food production, organic foods are increasing their market share by 20% annually (in contrast to a 1% per year growth rate for conventionally grown foods). Some observers predict that by 2010 organic foods could comprise 20% of all food in the U.S. marketplace. In response to a request by organic farmers that Congress establish standards for designating food as organic, the federal government several years ago promulgated a list of practices that would be regarded as incompatible with the "organically grown" label. In addition to requiring chemical-free production methods, the new standards also prohibit application of the term "organic" to animals fed antibiotics, to any genetically modified foods, foods that have been irradiated, or those grown in soils amended with sewage sludge ("biosolids"). Incorporating the latter three criteria provoked a great deal of controversy; they were not included in the rules as originally proposed but were subsequently added in response to an unprecedented

Box 9-2 Global Supermarket

Within a generation, America's food system has become international in scope. Food imports to the United States have increased dramatically in recent years, particularly such high-value products as seafood, red meat, cheese, fruit juices, and fresh produce. This booming trade is spurred in part by lower costs of production in many developing countries, but primarily is due to a growing demand by health-conscious consumers for a year-round supply of fresh fruits and vegetables. Federal officials estimate that since the late 1990s, approximately one-third of all the fresh fruit eaten by Americans is imported, as is 60% of all seafood. Mexico alone supplies as much as 79% of particular off-season crops and the percentage of fresh produce from other developing countries has been rapidly increasing as well.

This burgeoning international food trade has brought many nutritional and gustatory benefits to American consumers, but it has brought some unexpected problems as well. Whereas most foodborne disease outbreaks in the past were associated with contaminated meat or dairy products, recent years have witnessed a sharp increase in food poisoning incidents linked to fresh produce, much of it imported from countries where standards of health and hygiene are less rigorous than those in the U.S. Since fresh fruits are seldom cooked and many fresh vegetables likewise are eaten raw, consumers have little defense against invisible microbial hazards. Though most foodborne disease problems go unreported, several outbreaks during the past ten years were large enough to prompt major investigations: in both 1996 and 1997, imported Guatemalan raspberries were linked with over 2,300 cases of foodborne diarrhea caused by a previously little-known protozoan parasite, cyclospora, that inhabits Guatemalan waterways. Those same years also witnessed outbreaks of salmonellosis, affecting hundreds of people in 24 states, and ultimately traced to alfalfa sprouts whose seeds originated in Uganda and Pakistan; a food-poisoning outbreak at a 1991 convention in Minneapolis was caused by Peruvian carrots contaminated with a new pathogenic strain of E. coli bacteria; and a 1991 cholera outbreak was blamed on tainted frozen coconut milk from an unlicensed processing plant in Thailand. In 1997 Japan experienced a food-poisoning outbreak caused by contaminated radish sprouts from Oregon-supplied seeds, and in 2003 the largest-ever U.S. outbreak of hepatitis A food poisoning was traced to green onions from Mexico.

Microbial hazards are not the only food quality concern associated with imported foods. The presence of toxic pesticide residues on produce entering the U.S. has been a long-standing issue among consumer advocacy groups. Since the mid-1970s, when EPA prohibited U.S. farmers from using a number of persistent pesticides on American agricultural crops, many consumers assumed their exposure to these chemicals had ceased. Unfortunately, many of the chemicals now banned in North America, Europe, and Japan are still being produced and are sold to developing nations, whose growers use them in prodigious amounts to produce crops for export to U.S. and other foreign markets. China, a leading exporter of fresh vegetables, is encountering problems marketing its produce in the E.U., Japan, and the United States because of excessively high levels of pesticide residues on these crops. In 2001 the Chinese government itself found that 47% of vegetables grown in that country exhibited residues in excess of government standards. The same tolerance levels set to regulate pesticide residues on domestic produce apply to imported fruits and vegetables, but since only 2% of the nearly 6 million food shipments arriving in U.S. ports each year are ever sampled, violations are seldom detected. On the rare occasion when a sample is taken and sent for laboratory analysis (a process that may require several weeks), the shipment in question isn't detained at the port of entry; therefore even when illegal residues are detected, it is usually too late to prevent marketing and consumption of the product. Also, negative test results don't necessarily mean the product is free of chemical residues, since many of the pesticides used by farmers in developing countries can't be detected by the analytical methods currently available to FDA personnel.

At the same time that safety concerns about imported foods have been mounting, federal efforts to detect problems are severely compromised by tight budgets, an inadequate number of inspectors to handle the overwhelming workload, and an archaic food safety regulatory system. Authority for regulating food imports is split between USDA, which exercises jurisdiction over incoming meat and poultry, and FDA, which enforces standards on all other food products. Although both agencies maintain the position that imported food should meet the same standards of safety, composition, and labeling as U.S.-produced foods, their ability to ensure that such standards are met are sharply limited. While FDA inspectors can impound suspect imports, they cannot automatically block importation of food shipments from countries whose food safety system is known to be sub-standard (USDA *can* do so). FDA officials are not permitted to inspect foreign processing facilities and are not allowed to travel abroad to investigate an ongoing food-poisoning outbreak unless invited to do so by the host government. FDA was given a little more clout and a modest increase in funding when new regulations under the 2002 Bioterrorism Act took effect in December 2003. These rules require foreign exporters to notify FDA in advance of food shipments to the U.S. and mandate foreign facilities that manufacture, process, pack, or hold food for consumption in the U.S. to register with FDA.

International efforts to remove trade barriers, thereby creating a "global economy," have further complicated food safety initiatives. Just as American farmers and ranchers charge that European bans on genetically altered seed or hormone-treated beef are efforts to limit competition rather than true safety issues, so growers in developing countries view U.S. scrutiny of their products as a thinly veiled form of protectionism. As one federal food safety official remarked, "Where *we* see a safety issue, *they* see a trade issue."

In the long term, safeguarding the quality of food imports can only be achieved through international efforts to develop uniformly high food safety standards in every country and to assist developing nations in improving methods of food production and drinking water quality. Until then, consumers are well-advised to wash fruits and vegetables well, or to cook them, before eating.

References
National Research Council. 1998. *Ensuring Safe Food From Production to Consumption*. Washington, DC: National Academy Press.

Nestle, Marion. 2003. *Safe Food: Bacteria, Biotechnology, and Bioterrorism*. Berkeley: Univ. of California Press.

deluge of negative public comments following publication of the proposed, less restrictive criteria (Nestle, 2003).

On rare occasions chemicals may contaminate foods through sheer carelessness or criminal neglect by processors. One of the largest and most costly incidents of chemical food contamination in recent years created havoc in Belgium in 1999, when dioxin-contaminated oil was mixed with animal fat added to livestock feed. The tainted fodder was subsequently distributed to more than a thousand farms throughout Belgium and fed to poultry, hogs, and cattle. The problem was only discovered when chickens stopped laying eggs and subsequently died. Laboratory analysis of the feed revealed the presence of dioxin, but Belgian government officials failed to notify the public or the European Union of this fact and took no immediate action. When the news finally broke more than a month later, pandemonium erupted and virtually every food that might possibly have been contaminated was stripped from grocery shelves. Throughout Europe a ban on Belgian pork, beef, poultry, and eggs was imposed; even the U.S. and some Asian countries refused to accept certain Belgian farm products. Losses to the Belgian agricultural sector, heavily dependent on exports, were estimated at more than $850 million. Although no human illnesses appear to have occurred among unknowing consumers who ate tainted meat or eggs, the incident prompted demands throughout the European Union for stronger food safety measures (the EU has no equivalent to the United States' Food and Drug Administration) to prevent such problems in the future.

Food Additives

More controversial than the accidental, often unavoidable, food contaminants are the approximately 2,800 food **additives,** substances intentionally added to food to modify its taste, color, texture, nutritive value, appearance, resistance to deterioration, and so forth. The years since the end of World War II witnessed explosive growth of the food chemical industry, as food processors responded to public demand (or occasionally created public demand) by promoting a host of new products—convenience foods, frozen foods, dehydrated foods, ethnic foods, low-calorie foods. Many of these products could not exist in a world free of additives. Nevertheless, a great many people are automatically suspicious of additives with long, often unpronounceable names. However, there's nothing inherently evil about using additives, provided that the chemical in question has no adverse effect on human health and performs a useful function. Many substances that can technically be termed "additives" have been in use for thousands of years—sugar, salt, and spices are just a few examples. Some additives come from natural sources; lecithin, derived from soybeans or corn, is used as an emulsifier to achieve the desired consistency in products such as cake mixes, non-dairy creamers, salad dressings, ice cream, and chocolate milk. Other food additives are factory made but are chemically the same as their natural analogs. The synthetic vitamins and minerals added to foods to improve nutritive value are examples of these; identical in chemical composition to natural vitamins and minerals found in food, they are preferentially used because they are less expensive and more readily available. Such synthetic additives frequently are more concentrated, more pure, and of a more consistent quality than some of their counterparts in the natural world. The use of synthetic vitamins and minerals in food over the past half century has had a profound impact on public health in the United States, virtually eliminating certain deficiency diseases that formerly afflicted large numbers of Americans. The addition of vitamin D to milk, iodine to table salt, and niacin to bread has relegated rickets,

Table 9-2 Common Types of Food Additives

Group	Purpose	Examples
Antioxidants	prevent fats from turning rancid and fresh fruits from darkening during processing; minimize damage to some amino acids and loss of some vitamins	BHA, BHT, propylgallate
Bleaching Agents	whiten and age flour	benzoyl peroxide, chlorine, nitrosyl chloride
Emulsifiers	to disperse one liquid in another; to improve quality and uniformity of texture	lecithin, mono-and diglycerides, sorbitan monostearate, polysorbates
Acidulants	maintain acid-alkali balance in jams, soft drinks, vegetables, etc., to keep them from being too sour	sodium bicarbonate, citric acid, lactic acid, phosphoric acid
Humectants	maintain moisture in foods such as shredded coconut, marshmallows, and candies	sorbitol, glycerol, propylene glycol
Anti-caking compounds	keep salts and powdered foods free-flowing	calcium or magnesium silicate, magnesium carbonate, tricalcium phosphate, sodium aluminosilicate
Preservatives	control growth of spoilage organisms	sodium propionate, sodium benzoate, propionic acid
Stabilizers	provide proper texture and consistency to ice cream, cheese spreads, salad dressings, syrups	gum arabic, guar gum, carrageenan, methyl cellulose, agar-agar

goiter, and pellagra, respectively, to nearly nonexistent status in this country. Other additives perform such useful functions as retarding spoilage, preventing fats from turning rancid, retaining moisture in some foods and keeping it out of others.

Most people don't quarrel about additives used for these purposes. What does concern many scientists and consumers is that a not-insignificant number of chemicals are used as food additives for purely cosmetic purposes—and many of these have been shown to be toxic, carcinogenic, or both.

Until 1958, food processors wishing to use a new additive were free to do so unless the FDA could prove that it was harmful to human health. With the passage of the Food Additives Amendment to the Food, Drug, and Cosmetic Act in that year, the situation was reversed: the manufacturer of any proposed food additive or new food-contact chemical (e.g., packaging materials, equipment liners) now has to satisfy the FDA that the product is safe before it can be approved for use. Proof of safety must include such considerations as: (1) the amount of the additive that is likely to be consumed along with the food product, (2) the cumulative effect of ingesting small amounts of the additive over a long period of time, and (3) the potential for the additive to act as a toxin or a carcinogen when consumed by humans or animals (Foulke, 1993). Approval can be rescinded by the FDA at any time if new information indicates that the additive is unsafe.

While protection of public health is the main intent of the Food Additives Amendment, the law is also designed to prevent consumer fraud by prohibiting the use of preservatives that make foods look fresher than they really are. A case in point is the regulation forbidding the use of sulfites on meats, since these restore the red color, deceptively lending a just slaughtered appearance to a variety of meat products. On the other hand, sodium nitrite, another additive recognized for its ability to "fix" the red color of fresh meats, can legally be added to meat, fish, and poultry because its primary purpose is to act as a preservative, deterring both spoilage and botulism, a deadly disease caused by the presence of a bacterial toxin. Because it is now known that nitrites can react with other compounds in food to produce **nitrosamines,** substances known to be carcinogenic, food processors wishing to use the additive must take precautionary measures to severely limit nitrosamine formation (Foulke, 1993).

Undoubtedly the section of the Food Additives Amendment that has generated the most heated controversy in recent years is the **Delaney Clause,** which flatly prohibits the use in food of any ingredient shown to cause cancer in animals or humans. (People who question why the FDA bans certain moderately carcinogenic food dyes yet takes no action against cigarettes have to be reminded that the Delaney Clause pertains solely to carcinogenic food additives, not to carcinogens in general; if a food processor should propose to add cigarette smoke as a flavoring to, say, cured meats, this would undoubtedly be prohibited under the Delaney Clause.) While many environmental groups feel that the Delaney Clause constitutes the public's sole line of defense against the deliberate addition of carcinogens to the nation's food supply, critics charge that the "zero tolerance" standard implicit in this mandate is unrealistic and an example of regulatory overkill which fails to recognize enormous advances in analytical techniques. Whereas the best efforts at chemical analysis during the 1950s yielded results in the parts per million range, today's monitoring devices routinely detect the presence of chemical residues in the parts per trillion. New evidence for the existence of threshold levels of exposure for at least some carcinogens has added fuel to the debate as well (when the Delaney Clause was enacted in 1958 it was presumed that *any* amount of exposure to a carcinogen, no matter how small, could result in cancer). The Food Quality Protection Act attempted to address these concerns to a limited extent when it amended the Delaney Clause in 1996 by excluding pesticide residues in processed food from regulation as food additives. The revised mandate now permits EPA to approve a tolerance level for residues of a carcinogenic pesticide so long as the agency determines that doing so presents a "negligible risk" (defined as no more than one cancer death per one million population) to consumers. For all other food additives, the "zero tolerance" standard explicit in the Delaney Clause remains intact (Merrill, 1997).

Since many hundreds of food additives were already in widespread use at the time the 1958 amendment was passed, a portion of this legislation exempted such substances from the rigorous safety testing demanded for new additives. Instead, additives already in common usage were designated "generally regarded as safe" and placed on what is referred to as the **GRAS list.** In order to remove a food additive from the GRAS list, the FDA must demonstrate that the substance is harmful. Original screening of existing food additives to determine whether they should be placed on the GRAS list was done rather haphazardly, and by the 1970s it was recognized that long-time usage is no firm guarantee of safety. More thorough studies of certain substances included on the GRAS list have resulted in withdrawal of approval for the use of such once-common food additives as cyclamates (artificial sweeteners suspected of being carcinogenic); safrole (mutagenic and carcinogenic extract of sassafras root, formerly used to give root beer its characteristic flavor); and a number of coal-tar dyes (long used as food colorings but delisted because they were shown to be carcinogenic or to cause organ damage).

Numerous other additives still on the GRAS list are considered of dubious safety by many researchers, yet remain in use due to lack of conclusive evidence or because of industry pressure on FDA regulators. Critics of current policy insist that food additives require a higher standard of care than other environmental chemicals and shouldn't be used if they present a health risk. They base this judgment on the fact that everyone is exposed to chemicals in food, not only those who voluntarily assume the risk. Varying levels of susceptibility among individuals and the effects of simultaneous exposure to other chemicals, including synergistic effects, have to be taken into consideration. Both MSG (monosodium glutamate), a flavor enhancer that can cause the headache, dizziness, nausea, and facial flushing sometimes referred to as "Chinese Restaurant Syndrome," and a group of sulfur-containing compounds known collectively as "sulfites" or "sulfiting agents," added to certain foods, drugs, and wine to prevent discoloration and spoilage, are examples of food additives that serve a useful purpose and pose no danger to the majority of consumers but which can provoke severe allergic reactions among a sizeable minority of sensitive individuals. Because of the vast processed food market, any miscalculation of risk can have far-reaching implications. Nevertheless, although some health authorities recommend avoiding foods containing nonessential additives (such as artificial colors and flavorings) wherever possible, little evidence exists at present to indicate that the health of Americans is suffering due to the chemical food additives currently in use.

Foodborne Disease

Ironically, while questions dealing with the safety of chemical additives or pesticide residues generate most of the public's concern regarding food quality these days, most cases of illness or death due to food involve a number of old-fashioned foodborne diseases commonly referred to as "food poisoning." Food poisoning can result from a variety of causes.

Natural Toxins in Food

The widely prevalent notion that all "natural" foods are safe and nutritious is a dangerous misconception. There are many common plants, both wild and cultivated, that are poisonous, capable of causing ailments ranging from mild stomach disorders to a quick and painful death if consumed by the unwary. In addition, certain marine fish and shellfish species may contain toxins that induce severe illness or death. Some examples of plants or animals capable of causing a toxic reaction if eaten include the following.

Mushrooms. Mushrooms constitute a gourmet's delight, provided, of course, that the item in question is a nonpoisonous variety. Unfortunately, there is no simple rule of thumb for distinguishing between those wild forms that are safe and those that are not. Although only a relatively few of the thousands of species found in North America are poisonous, they may look very much like nonpoisonous species and frequently even grow together. One of the most poisonous types, the amanitas (one species of which is called the "Death Angel"), grows commonly in "fairy rings" in woods and on lawns. Just one or two bites of these alkaloid-containing amanitas can be fatal to an adult and, in fact, the vast majority of deaths due to mushroom poisoning are caused by these.

Water hemlock (*Cicuta maculata*). Sweet-tasting but deadly, this relative of carrots, parsley, celery, and parsnips (to which it bears a strong resemblance) is the most toxic of all native North American plants. Because it is found throughout the continent, is quite similar in appearance to edible plants for which it is commonly mistaken, and is lethal even in small amounts, water hemlock is responsible for more deaths due to misidentification than is any other plant species. **Cicutoxin,** the poison-

Box 9-3 Beware of Mad Cows

In December 2003, American beef-lovers got news they never expected to hear—a dairy cow in Washington State had tested positive for **bovine spongiform encephalopathy (BSE)**, commonly called **"mad cow disease."** Following similar identification of a case in Alberta, Canada, in May of the same year, dismayed federal officials and beef industry representatives were forced to admit that what they had assured the public was a European problem now threatens North America as well. Though the numbers were small—one cow each in Canada and the U.S. (three additional BSE-infected cows were detected by mid-2005; two in Canada and one in Texas)—the health and economic implications of BSE's trans-Atlantic emergence were enormous and prompted a rapid (some would argue belated and still insufficient) regulatory response in both countries to strengthen existing safeguards against further spread of the disease.

BSE was largely unknown to the general public until 1986, when large numbers of British cattle began to stagger and collapse as the slowly progressing infection took its toll. By 1988 the British government had made BSE a reportable disease and by 1999 at least 175,000 infected cows had been reported (some authorities estimate that the total number of affected animals in the U.K. may exceed one million). Although "mad cows" were a new phenomenon in Britain, a similar malady known as "scrapie" had been observed there for centuries as a disease of sheep. While fairly common, scrapie didn't seem to affect any other species and was assumed to be a problem restricted to sheep. A search for the cause of BSE eventually revealed a surprising link between scrapie and mad cow disease. For a number of years it has been the practice in many countries, including the U.K., to add rendered meat-and-bone meal and other animal protein to livestock feed as a cheap dietary supplement. Such products are derived by cooking the otherwise unusable parts of dead animals (offal) using solvents and high-pressure steam to kill any pathogens that might be present. Scrapie-infected sheep carcasses went into this mix and seemed to cause no problems. In the late 1970s, cost-cutting measures in the British meat-rendering industry led it to adopt techniques that utilized lower cooking temperatures. By the early 1980s the new practice had spread throughout the U.K. and shortly afterwards the first cases of mad cow disease were reported.

In retrospect, researchers concluded that the lower rendering temperatures, while effective in destroying bacteria and viruses, failed to inactivate previously unrecognized infectious proteins called *prions*. These agents are now regarded as the cause of several fatal nervous system disorders called *spongiform encephalopathies*—conditions that produce sponge-like holes in the brains of both animals and humans. BSE thus appears to have originated as a "species jump" of pathogenic prions from scrapie-infected sheep to cattle when material from inadequately rendered offal was incorporated into cattle feed. Belated recognition of what was happening prompted the British government in 1988 to ban the use of offal in cattle feed, to report all BSE cases, and to destroy any cows suspected of harboring the disease. At the same time, government officials repeatedly assured the public that mad cow disease presented no human health threat and that British beef was perfectly safe to eat.

Some scientists, however, harbored doubts about human immunity to the BSE pathogen, fearing that infectious prions could, indeed, be transmitted to people who ate contaminated meat. Their apprehensions were confirmed in 1996 when physicians diagnosed ten young beef-eating Britons as suffering from a previously unknown form of **Creutzfeldt-Jakob Disease (CJD),** a rare, always-fatal ailment that occurs sporadically among human populations, generally affecting the elderly and progressing to death in five months or less. By contrast, the newly identified variant form **(vCJD)** is primarily a disease of young people (average age of victims is 28) and kills more slowly, the duration of illness averaging 13–14 months. By early 2004, 156 cases of vCJD had been reported worldwide, the vast majority in the United Kingdom. Since symptoms of the ailment are not manifested until years after eating prion-contaminated meat, some medical authorities in Britain fear that future cases could number in the thousands. No longer is there any doubt that prions can cross the species barrier, first from sheep to cattle and, more recently, from cattle to humans.

USDA officials were determined to prevent the growing BSE epidemic in Britain from infecting American cattle, and in 1989 imposed a ban on the importation of live cattle, sheep, and their derived products from the United Kingdom and several other countries experiencing BSE outbreaks (the ban was extended to all of Europe in 1997). In 1990, USDA launched a limited surveillance program to detect BSE-affected cows, performing laboratory analyses on a small percentage of animals exhibiting signs of brain damage. During the 1990s, only a few hundred cattle were tested each year, a figure that by 2003 had risen to slightly over 20,000 out of approximately 35 million slaughtered. Demands from food safety activists that USDA greatly expand testing of slaughtered cattle for BSE were strongly resisted by the federal agency. Although most western European countries test all cattle over two years old and Japan tests every cow slaughtered regardless of age, USDA continued to insist that doing so would be prohibitively expensive and largely unnecessary, given the existing safeguards against infection of U.S. herds. By 1997, after the first cases of human disease associated with eating prion-contaminated British beef made headline news around the world, both the United States and Canada imposed bans on using animal protein, such as meat-and-bone meal, in feed intended for cattle or other ruminant animals such as sheep or goats.

Having assured the public and ranchers that these regulatory "firewalls" guaranteed that BSE would never threaten North American cattle herds or the beef-consuming public, the 2003 discovery of a "mad cow" in Canada and in the U.S. left government officials scrambling to explain how such a thing could have happened and led to a further strengthening of regulatory precautions.

Immediately following USDA's announcement regarding the BSE-positive cow, the herd from which the animal had come was placed under a state hold order and a recall of its meat was ordered. The cow's infectious brain and spinal cord were traced to several rendering plants, which placed a voluntary hold on them; this quick action fortunately prevented commercial distribution of any potentially infectious products. In the meantime, USDA's Animal and Plant Health Inspection Service, working with the Canadian Food Inspection Agency, traced the birth of the infected Washington cow to a ranch in Alberta, the same province where Canadian authorities had discovered their single mad cow case earlier in the year. Eventually it was learned that both animals were over 6 years old and hence had been born prior to the 1997 ban on rendered animal protein in cattle feed—the presumed source of their subsequent BSE infection.

Seeking to reassure the public that the government was taking effective measures to protect human and animal health, the USDA and the Food and Drug Administration (FDA) announced in December 2003 that henceforth all "downer cattle" (those unable to walk) would be banned for human consumption. In addition, specified high-risk organs and tissues (e.g., brain, eyes, spinal cord) from cattle older than 30 months, as well as small intestine from animals of any age, cannot be used in human food, since these are parts of the cow most likely to harbor infectious prions. Nervous system tissue in certain meat products obtained by "advanced meat recovery" (AMR)—a process whereby machines extract the last remaining bits of meat on a carcass—was also banned. Responding to public fears as well as to the demands of overseas purchasers of U.S. beef, USDA announced in June 2004 that it would expand surveillance for mad cow disease on a one-time basis for the following 12–18 months, during which time approximately 220,000 animals were targeted for testing. While the majority of these cattle would be non-ambulatory animals ("downers") or ones who died on the farm, a random sampling of apparently healthy older cows would be included also. Although critics argue that even this level of testing is insufficient, given the millions of cattle entering the food supply each year, USDA contends that the enhanced program is capable of detecting BSE at a 99% confidence level even if only a tiny minority of cows is harboring the pathogen.

Since doubts persist regarding the adequacy of current levels of testing to detect very low levels of BSE in U.S. cattle, precautions such as the recent prohibition on inclusion of high risk tissues and organs from human food assume added importance. Doing so is more difficult than it sounds, however, because meats produced through the advanced meat recovery process not infrequently contain bits of spinal cord. Meat products derived from AMR systems are not required to be labeled as such and are difficult to distinguish from other meats, with which they are often blended.

Unlike bacterial or viral contamination, thorough cooking does not reduce the risk of contracting vCJD because the causative prions are not destroyed by normal cooking temperatures. Nevertheless, the extremely low health risk of eating U.S. or Canadian beef can be reduced even further by choosing cuts of beef least likely to contain potentially infectious nervous system tissue. Safest of all are boneless muscle cuts such as steaks and roasts; equally risk-free are milk and dairy products and any meat from grass-fed or organically raised cattle, since these animals have never been exposed to rendered protein in their feed. Cuts containing bones, such as T-bone or porterhouse steaks, beef ribs, standing rib roast, or bone-in pot roast present a very slight risk due to the possibility, albeit remote, that they might contain nervous system tissue. Of greatest concern are cow brains, neck bones, head-cheese, cheek meat, and ox-tail. Similarly, meat containing AMR ground beef products such as hot dogs, taco fillings, pizza toppings, sausages, and ground beef itself (unless known to have been ground from whole muscle cuts) are included in the "potentially risky" category due to the all-too-frequent presence of spinal cord material in such meats.

Though hopefully an aberration in an otherwise safe beef supply, North America's mad cow scare has been a wake-up call for federal agencies and the beef industry to reconsider livestock production methods, while tightening safeguards to prevent an emerging pathogen from gaining a foothold here.

References

Bren, Linda. 2004. "Agencies Work to Corral Mad Cow Disease." *FDA Consumer* (May/June).

DeWaal, Caroline Smith, and Leora Vegosen. 2003. "Bovine Spongiform Encephalopathy: The Importance of Precautionary Measures to Protect the Food Supply." *Food and Law Journal* 58, no. 4:536–548.

Nestle, Marion. 2003. *Safe Food: Bacteria, Biotechnology, and Bioterrorism*. Berkeley: Univ. of California Press.

ous substance in water hemlock, is a neurotoxin present in all parts of the plant and at every stage of development. Concentrations of the toxin are at peak levels in springtime and are highest in the root. In the fall of 1992, a 23-year-old Maine resident died three hours after taking just three bites from the root of a water hemlock plant he had collected in the woods (CDC, 1994). Children have occasionally suffered fatal poisonings after playing with toy whistles made from the hollow stems of water hemlock. Since there is no antidote for cicutoxin, about 30% of reported poisonings have resulted in the death of the victim.

Castor bean (*Ricinus communis*). This attractive shrublike plant is commonly grown as an ornamental foundation planting as well as commercially for its oil. The leaves of the plant are only slightly toxic, but the colorful mottled seeds can be deadly, containing a toxin called **ricin.** Children who chew on the seeds experience intense irritation of the mouth and throat, gastroenteritis, extreme thirst, dullness of vision, convulsions, uremia, and death. Only one to three seeds can kill a child; four to eight are generally required to cause fatality in adults.

Jimsonweed *(Datura stramonium)*. This common weed contains toxic alkaloids in all parts of the plant. The seeds and leaves are especially dangerous; children have been poisoned by sucking nectar from the flowers, eating the seeds, or drinking liquid in which the leaves have been soaked. A very small amount can be fatal to a child.

Ergot (*Claviceps purpurea*).   This fungus, which frequently infects cereal grains, especially rye, produces a toxic alkaloid, ergotamine, responsible for the serious type of food poisoning known as ergotism or "St. Anthony's Fire." When the fungal sclerotia growing on the rye grain are ground up with flour and subsequently consumed in bread, violent muscle contractions, excruciating pain, vomiting, deafness, blindness, and hallucinations can follow. One type of ergotism is characterized by severe constriction of the blood vessels, development of gangrene, and a painful death. Outbreaks of ergotism resulting in thousands of deaths were common until the 20th century, when the decrease in home milling and institution of quality control in commercial mills reduced the level of flour contamination. Even so, small outbreaks of ergotism are still reported from time to time. Interestingly, federal controls do not apply to rye grown for the organic foods market (Klein, 1979).

Aflatoxin.   Another mycotoxin (fungal poison) already discussed in chapter 6, aflatoxins are produced by the mold *Aspergillus flavus*, which grows on a wide variety of nuts, grains, and peanuts. When consumed, they can cause serious liver damage and are some of the most potent carcinogens known.

Certain fish and shellfish.   Several different types of food poisoning are associated with eating various marine organisms. **Ciguatera fish poisoning**, responsible for numerous food poisoning outbreaks in Florida and Hawaii, is caused by eating certain large reef-dwelling fish such as barracuda and red snapper containing a potent algal toxin and is one of the most common seafood-related illnesses in the United States. **Scombroid poisoning**, generally associated with deep-sea fish such as tuna and mackerel, is caused by ingestion of a toxin produced by certain bacteria acting on the flesh of fish that aren't handled properly after catching. Onset of symptoms such as a flushing of the skin, headache, dizziness, a burning sensation in the mouth, hives, and the usual gastrointestinal discomfort, generally occurs very quickly, averaging 1/2 hour after eating. **Paralytic Shellfish Poisoning (PSP)** results from eating shellfish such as oysters, clams, or scallops contaminated with saxitoxin, a nerve poison produced by microscopic dinoflagellates (algae). PSP is characterized by numbness in the mouth and extremities, gastroenteritis, and in severe cases, difficulty in speaking and walking; such symptoms occur within 30 minutes to 3 hours after eating. In a small percentage of cases death may result. Protection of the public against PSP depends on effective shellfish sanitation and inspection programs in the states where harvesting occurs.

Microbial Contamination

Microbial pathogens are responsible for the vast majority of food poisoning incidents; in the United States alone, the Centers for Disease Control and Prevention (CDC) estimates that 76 million people each year contract a foodborne illness, 325,000 are hospitalized as a result, and 5,000 die; economic costs to society from microbial foodborne disease are difficult to quantify but have been estimated in the billions of dollars. Since CDC's estimates are based on a voluntary reporting system, many health experts are convinced that the actual number of cases is considerably higher (Nestle, 2003). Whatever the case, authorities agree the problem is a serious one, as evidenced by numerous well-publicized food-poisoning outbreaks and food recalls in recent years. Although the toll in human suffering is immense, food-poisoning cases are often misdiagnosed by victims ("I just had a touch of 24-hour flu"), stoically endured (". . . it'll pass in a day or two"), and, due to the nature of symptoms, often not reported (who wants to discuss the details of a bout with diarrhea!). As a result, this entirely preventable malady fails to arouse the public attention it deserves and is perpetuated by widespread carelessness and ignorance of safe food-handling principles. Although food poisoning can, and frequently does, occur with foods prepared and consumed at home, public health officials are most concerned with the potential for large-scale poisoning inherent in the current trend toward more frequent eating outside the home and with the rapid growth and sheer size of the food service industry in the United States today (the National Restaurant Association reports that each year over 54 billion meals are served at 844,000 commercial food establishments in the U.S. and that 44% of adult Americans eat at a restaurant on a typical day). Institutions such as day care centers and nursing homes, as well as congregate feeding centers for the indigent or homeless, also serve meals to large numbers of people on a daily basis. Diners at these facilities comprise many of those most vulnerable to foodborne disease: the very young, the very old, the ill, the immunocompromised. As the number of meals eaten away from home increases, the task of preventing foodborne disease grows more challenging.

It should be noted that food *spoilage* is not the same thing as food poisoning. Spoilage involves the decomposition of foods due to the action of natural enzymes within food, to chemical reactions between food and containers, or to the activities of certain types of bacteria, fungi, or insects, resulting in unpleasant odors, taste, or appearance of the food. However, spoilage organisms do not produce toxins that would cause human illness if they were consumed, nor does eating food containing such live organisms induce sickness. The same cannot be said of food-poisoning bacteria, whose presence is not betrayed by the appearance, smell, or taste of the food. The old term "ptomaine poisoning" often used in reference to food poisoning is a misnomer—there is no such thing. Ptomaines are foul-smelling chemical compounds produced by bacterial decomposition of proteins. Eating food containing ptomaines will not produce any illness.

The microbial culprits responsible for food poisoning can be grouped into three general categories: bacteria, viruses, and parasites.

Bacteria. Of the various foodborne diseases, the greatest number of outbreaks can be traced to ingestion of food containing certain pathogenic bacteria or bacterial toxins preformed in the food before it was eaten. Bacterial foodborne diseases are classified either as **infections** or **intoxications,** depending on whether illness is caused by consuming large numbers of live organisms or by ingesting preformed bacterial toxins, respectively. The more common types of bacterial food poisoning have rather similar symptoms: diarrhea, abdominal pain, vomiting, dehydration, prostration, and often fever and chills in the case of bacterial infections (not, however, with intoxications). Onset of such symptoms usually occurs within 1–24 hours after eating the contaminated food, depending on the type of bacteria involved and the amount of food ingested. Examples of foodborne bacterial infections include the following.

Salmonellosis. Often referred to by more descriptive appellations such as "Delhi Belly" or "The Tropical Trots," salmonellosis is one of the most common bacterial foodborne diseases in the United States, second only to *Campylobacter.* Its incidence, however, has been gradually declining since 1996, presumably as a result of a new food safety system imposed on slaughterhouses and meat processing plants in 1997 (see box 9-5). Caused by a number of species of the genus *Salmonella,* the disease is typically associated with eating poultry, meat, or eggs harboring large numbers of the rod-shaped bacterium. Nevertheless, numerous outbreaks have been traced to foods not generally associated with the disease: the largest salmonellosis outbreak in U.S. history, affecting an estimated 200,000 people (16,000 laboratory-confirmed cases, many more unreported) in Illinois and several other Midwest states in the spring of 1985, was traced to milk. Although potentially an excellent medium for the growth of *Salmonella* and other foodborne pathogens, milk today is considered one of our safest foods due to pasteurization and high standards of sanitation in the dairy industry; less than 1% of all foodborne disease outbreaks in recent years have been traced to contaminated milk. Alfalfa sprouts tainted with *Salmonella* have caused widespread food poisoning outbreaks in recent years. Though many people regard raw sprouts as a healthy and nutritious food item, sprouts seeds can be contaminated on the farm with *Salmonella*-tainted water, animal feces, improperly composted manure used as fertilizer, or dirty harvesting or processing machines. The same conditions that promote seed germination are also ideal for the multiplication of *Salmonella* organisms. As a result, government food safety agencies recommend that sprouts always be cooked before eating to reduce the risk of illness (CDC, 2002a). Another unpleasant surprise has been the emergence since the mid-1980s of *Salmonella enteritidis* infections associated with whole, uncracked eggs. Contamination occurs when the bacteria are transmitted from infected hens via their ovaries into the developing egg; short of laboratory testing, neither egg producers nor home cooks have any way of identifying which eggs are tainted. It is estimated that one out of every 10,000 eggs (approximately 4.5 million/year) is contaminated. Although the problem was originally confined to the northeastern U.S., it is now nationwide. As a result, today eggs are at or near the top of the list as prime contributors to food-poisoning outbreaks in the United States. For this reason, much to the dismay of Caesar salad and homemade eggnog lovers, health agencies now strongly advise against the consumption of raw or undercooked eggs—hard-boiled is the only guarantee of safety!

Inside the small intestine, colonies of *Salmonella* continue to grow and invade the host tissue, irritating the mucosal lining. Sudden onset of disease symptoms most commonly occurs within 12–24 hours after eating the contaminated food, with 18 hours being the most common time interval; discomfort may persist for several days and some victims may remain carriers for months after all outward symptoms have disappeared, shedding bacteria in their feces and remaining capable of infecting others. Severity of the disease ranges from very mild to very severe, with young children, the elderly, and travelers often the most adversely affected. Among otherwise healthy adults, fatalities due to salmonellosis are rare (victims only *wish* they were dead!). However, salmonellosis can be life-threatening to the elderly, to patients in hospitals and nursing homes, and to people whose immune systems are compromised. Hundreds of Americans, most of them from one of these highly vulnerable groups, die of salmonellosis each year.

In addition to the obvious short-term effects of the ailment, salmonellosis sufferers may also develop serious chronic disorders as a result of their infection. About 2–3% of victims later contract chronic arthritis, while a much smaller percentage develop painful septic arthritis when the *Salmonella* bacteria invade the joints.

Campylobacter jejuni. One of several ailments often referred to as "Traveler's Diarrhea" because cases used to be most common among vacationers returning home from abroad, infections caused by *Campylobacter jejuni* have become the most common form of bacterial food poisoning in the United States. Like salmonellosis, however, *Campylobacter* incidence has begun to decline in recent years and for the same reason—improved food safety practices in the facilities that kill and process poultry. *C. jejuni* infections are characterized by high fever and bloody diarrhea, along with the nausea and abdominal pain typical of most foodborne ailments; symptoms generally persist for about a week but may last much longer. Most worrisome is the fact that as many as 10% of sufferers develop serious, long-term complications such as Guillain-Barré syndrome, arthritis, or meningitis. Undercooked chicken or turkey is by far the leading source of *C. jejuni* infections, since the organism is almost always present on poultry carcasses. The marked shift from beef to chicken consumption in the U.S. over the past 30 years has been accompanied by a rapid increase in *Campylobacter* foodborne disease. Other sources of infection include raw clams and other shellfish, inadequately cooked pork, and unpasteurized milk.

E. coli 0157:H7. Among the most dangerous foodborne pathogens, this nasty relative of the harmless *E. coli* strains that are normal inhabitants of the human gut was first recognized as a newly emerging public health problem in 1982. Several sporadic outbreaks occurred during the 1980s, but it was only in 1993 that the disease hit the headlines when four children died and hundreds of people became ill after eating hamburgers at several Jack-in-the-Box restaurants in the Pacific Northwest. Since then, numerous outbreaks have occurred in at least 30 countries around the world. In the summer of 1996, the largest outbreak to date killed three and sickened over 12,000 Japanese, mostly schoolchildren, in Sakai City near Osaka (Task Force, 1997). Estimates for the number of pathogenic *E. coli* infections occurring annually range from 10,000–20,000, resulting in approximately 50–100 deaths.

E. coli 0157:H7 normally inhabits the intestinal tract of healthy cattle and is excreted with fecal material. It frequently is found on the udders of cows and thus can be readily transferred to raw milk or to milking equipment. When people come into direct contact with fecal material harboring the pathogen or with fecal-contaminated food or water, infection can result. Unlike most foodborne pathogens that must be

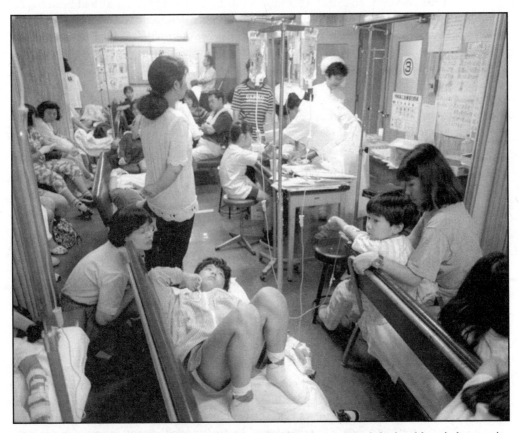

Victims of the 1996 food-poisoning outbreak in Sakai City, Japan crowd the local hospital to receive treatment. The outbreak, which sickened more than 12,000 people, was traced to *E. coli 0157:H7.* [*AP photo/Yomiuri Shimbun*]

present in very large numbers to cause illness, the infective dose for *E. coli 0157:H7* is extraordinarily low—as few as 50 organisms have been shown capable of inducing disease symptoms. Once ingested, *E. coli 0157:H7* multiplies within the human digestive tract, producing a potent toxin that damages cells of the intestinal lining. These lesions permit blood to leak into the intestines, giving rise to the bloody diarrhea that generally develops within several days of eating contaminated food and is one of the characteristic symptoms of *E. coli* infection. Sufferers may also experience abdominal pains, vomiting, and nausea; only rarely will fever be present, however. In most cases the disease runs its course in 5–10 days and the victim recovers completely without treatment. Administration of antibiotics does nothing to improve a patient's condition and may cause kidney problems. Similarly, the use of antidiarrheal medicine is not advisable. For 2–7% of victims the consequences of infection are much more dangerous. If bacterial toxins pass through the damaged intestinal wall and enter the bloodstream, they travel to the kidneys where they can cause **hemolytic uremic syndrome (HUS)**, a serious ailment in which red blood cells are destroyed, leading to kidney failure and possible death. Such patients often require blood transfusions and kidney dialysis. Even with intensive care, 3–5% of patients who develop HUS die.

In the U.S., undercooked hamburgers were initially identified as the food most often implicated in *E. coli 0157:H7* outbreaks. Accordingly, public health agencies renewed their warnings to commercial food establishments and home cooks to cook beef to 160°F until no traces of pink remain in the center and juices run clear. By the late 1990s, however, an even larger number of *E. coli* food poisonings had been traced to such seemingly harmless foods as alfalfa sprouts, lettuce, and unpasteurized fruit juices (in Japan as well, the Sakai City outbreak was ultimately linked to tainted radish sprouts). In all these cases, poor sanitation at some stage of production or processing allowed food to become contaminated with *E. coli*-contaminated cow manure. Since the foods mentioned above are seldom cooked prior to consumption, live pathogens were present on the food when it was eaten. As a result of these incidents, people at high risk of serious consequences if they contract food poisoning (e.g., young children, the ill or elderly, AIDS patients) are being advised simply to avoid eating sprouts and unpasteurized juice.

Listeriosis. Caused by *Listeria monocytogenes*, a pathogen associated with an extremely wide range of hosts (mammals, birds, fish, ticks, crustaceans) and commonly found in food-processing environments, this disease, once considered rare in human populations, has become a subject of increasing concern in recent years. Listeriosis outbreaks have most frequently been associated with contaminated cold cuts, hot dogs, milk, soft cheeses, and other refrigerated products generally eaten without further cooking. Listeriosis is particularly dangerous in pregnant women, where infection often results in septicemia, miscarriage, or stillbirth. Apparently healthy babies born to infected mothers may develop meningitis within a few days or weeks after birth. Newborns infected with *Listeria* have high fatality rates, as do older victims suffering from diabetes or compromised immune systems (AIDS victims or people receiving corticosteroids, chemotherapy, radiation therapy, etc.). Listeriosis, fortunately, is much less common than salmonellosis or *C. jejuni* diarrhea; on average, less than 2,000 people in the U.S. fall victim to listeriosis each year; fatality rates are high, however—of those stricken, approximately 20% die. Recognition that *Listeria*, unlike other microbial pathogens, grows vigorously at low temperatures makes this organism a subject of serious concern to regulatory agencies and to the food industry in general, since refrigeration provides no assurance against bacterial multiplication. The FDA has set a "zero tolerance" requirement for presence of *Listeria* in foods.

Vibrio vulnificus. First described as a cause of human illness only in 1979, this free-living marine bacterium lives in unpolluted warm ocean waters. It is commonly found along the Gulf Coast in the southeastern U.S. where it may contaminate oysters and other shellfish. Most human illnesses result from consuming raw oysters, since the bacteria are readily killed by cooking. *V. vulnificus* infections are especially dangerous for individuals with preexisting liver disease resulting from alcoholism, viral hepatitis, or other causes, and for those with compromised immune systems (CDC, 1993).

Among bacterial foodborne intoxications the most important are:

Staphylococcus aureus. Sometimes known as "Roto-Rooter Disease" because of its violent onset, *Staphylococcus* intoxication is caused by a common bacterium present in pimples, boils, hangnails, wound infections, sputum, and sneeze droplets. People thus constitute the prime source of these organisms, which flourish in such proteinaceous foods as cooked ham, sauces and gravies, chicken salad, egg salad, cream pies and pastries, and so on. Growth of the bacteria within the food medium results in production of an enterotoxin (poison of the intestinal tract) that is not destroyed when the food is cooked. When consumed, the toxin causes irritation and inflammation of the stomach and intestine, resulting in vomiting and diarrhea. Since illness is produced by a poison already in the food at the time of eating rather than by bacterial growth within the victim's intestine, the effects of bacterial intoxication appear more rapidly than do those of an infection. People consuming *Staphylococcus* toxin may experience the sudden onset of vomiting and diarrhea within as little as 30 minutes after eating, although a period of 2–4 hours is more common. As is the case with most foodborne illness, individual differences in susceptibility will result in some people becoming quite ill after eating the tainted food, while others may be unaffected (Koren, 1980). Due to the nature of the symptoms and the fact that the illness is relatively brief, seldom persisting for more than a day or two, sufferers of staph intoxication frequently blame their miseries on "the 24-hour flu" rather than on the true culprit—contaminated food. Deaths from this foodborne disease are extremely rare and most victims recover quickly without any complications.

Botulism. The most serious of all bacterial foodborne diseases, botulism is caused by the spore-forming soil bacterium *Clostridium botulinum,* which, growing

---

Table 9-3 Microbial Foodborne Ailments

Because many people assume that food poisoning always occurs within a few hours after eating contaminated food, they frequently misdiagnose the cause of their illness or lay the blame on some innocent menu item in the last meal consumed before disease symptoms appear. In fact, most microbial foodborne ailments manifest themselves 24 hours or more after tainted foods are eaten. The time required before a food poisoning victim feels sick varies depending on the pathogen involved and the amount of contaminated food consumed. Listed below are the time periods typically required for signs of illness to appear for a representative group of foodborne ailments:

Pathogen	Time Frame for Onset of Symptoms
Campylobacter	1 to 10 days (usually 3 to 5 days)
Clostridium botulinum	12 to 36 hours
E. coli 0157:H7	1 to 10 days (usually 3 to 5 days)
Hepatitis A	1 to 7 weeks (usually 25 days)
Listeria monocytogenes	4 days to several weeks
Salmonella	6 hours to 3 days (average 18 hours)
Staphylococcus aureus	2 to 7 hours
Vibrio vulnificus	1 to 3 days

under anaerobic conditions, produces a deadly neurotoxin, the most poisonous substance known. Outbreaks of botulism have been most frequently associated with home-canned, low-acid foods such as beans, corn, beets, spinach, and mushrooms. This is because many home canners fail to realize that a long processing time (or a shorter time at high pressure in a pressure cooker) is necessary in order to kill the heat-resistant bacterial spores. If the spores survive, they can germinate and, in the absence of oxygen, multiply within the food medium, producing the deadly poison. If food contaminated with the botulism toxin is boiled for 15–20 minutes, the poison will be destroyed, but all too frequently such food is eaten uncooked or only briefly warmed, with disastrous results.

Commercially processed foods, mostly smoked fish or vacuum-packed items, occasionally have been identified as the cause of botulism outbreaks, as have some highly atypical sources. In the fall of 1983, one of the worst botulism outbreaks in U.S. history resulted in the hospitalization of 28 victims (one of whom subsequently died) who had eaten "patty melt" sandwiches at a restaurant in Peoria, Illinois. Surprised investigators ultimately identified sautéed onions as the cause of the problem. Contaminated with *C. botulinum* spores from the soil in which they grew, the onions were fried in margarine, which provided a protective air-free shield for germinating bacteria. The bacteria proceeded to multiply in the incubating temperatures provided by the warming tray in the restaurant kitchen. By the time the onions were consumed many hours later, enough of the deadly botulinum toxin had been formed to cause the disease outbreak. In an unrelated incident in Baton Rouge, Louisiana, the following year, a restaurant patron was stricken with botulism after eating a foil-wrapped baked potato, warmed up from the previous day. The foil wrapping had provided the anaerobic conditions that permitted growth of bacterial spores on the potato skin, while remaining at room temperature overnight allowed the organism to multiply and produce the toxin (Miller, 1984).

Botulism is first evidenced by the usual gastrointestinal distress, which generally appears within 12–36 hours, followed by the onset of such neurological symptoms as double vision, stammering, and difficulty in breathing. If untreated, botulism can result in death due to respiratory paralysis. Another manifestation of the disease that has now become the most common form of human botulism in the United States affects only children under one year of age and is referred to as "infant botulism." This condition can occur when babies are fed honey (or when infant pacifiers are dipped in honey) containing *C. botulinum* spores. When these spores germinate inside the baby's intestinal tract, they release a nerve poison that may cause a weakening of the infant's muscles, resulting in a condition called "floppy baby." Other symptoms of infant botulism include excessive drooling, difficulty in swallowing, droopy eyelids, lack of facial expression, weak cry, constipation, and sometimes respiratory arrest. The condition often requires a lengthy period of hospitalization. Because infant botulism can be provoked by as few as 10–100 *C. botulinum* spores, parents are advised never to feed babies honey (Tarr and Doyle, 1996).

Viruses.   Since viruses are unable to multiply outside a living host cell, these pathogens do not increase in number when they are introduced into food materials. Virus-contaminated foods simply serve as a route of transmission—a means by which virus particles can be transported from one host to another. Nevertheless, because the infectious dose needed to cause a viral disease is thought to be quite small, perhaps as low as 10–100 particles, viruses should never be allowed to contaminate food in the first place. Because the viruses associated with foodborne illness are of fecal origin, poor hygienic practices on the part of food handlers or food contact with sewage-polluted water are the most frequent causes of outbreaks. Since viruses are not utilizing the food as a growth medium, *any* type of food is a potential reservoir (i.e., pathogenic foodborne viruses, unlike bacteria, do not have any particular nutritional requirements for survival and hence are not restricted to certain "potentially hazardous foods"). Two of the more prevalent foodborne illnesses of viral origin are:

Noroviruses. Formerly called "Norwalk-like viruses," noroviruses cause more cases of acute gastroenteritis—about 23 million annually—than any other foodborne pathogen. As with *Staphylococcus* intoxication, victims often attribute the sudden and violent onset of nausea, profuse vomiting, cramps, and diarrhea to "stomach flu." Low-grade fever, chills, headache, muscle pains, and a general malaise also can occur. Fortunately, the illness generally lasts only a day or two and has no long-term health consequences. Fecal contamination of food or water is the primary means of transmission, with salads and shellfish the foods most often implicated in outbreaks, particularly when consumed raw or undercooked (Pierson and Corlett, 1992). Highly contagious, noroviruses can spread easily from person-to-person through direct contact (e.g., via airborne particles of vomitus) or by hand-to-mouth contact with virus-contaminated objects such as doorknobs. In recent years the cruise ship industry has been plagued by repeated norovirus outbreaks, demonstrating the environmental persistence of the organism and the difficulty of controlling it through routine sanitary measures (CDC, 2002b).

Hepatitis A (HAV). Most commonly associated with the consumption of raw clams or oysters harvested from sewage-tainted coastal waters, hepatitis A outbreaks also have been traced to foods as diverse as glazed doughnuts, strawberry sauce, sandwiches, orange juice, and salads. Uncooked green onions were identified as the cause of the United States' largest-ever outbreak of HAV in the fall of 2003, when over 550 patrons of a Chi-Chi's restaurant in western Pennsylvania were sickened and three died. Symptoms of the disease, which include jaundice (an indication of liver infection) as well as the usual gastrointestinal distress, generally don't appear until 10–50 days after eating the contaminated food. An infection typically persists for weeks or even months, and can, in some cases, lead to permanent liver damage. An individual suffering from HAV can easily transmit the virus to others if he or she isn't conscientious about good hygienic practices, since the virus is shed in urine and feces. A victim is most contagious 10–14 days before the onset of disease symptoms and remains infectious until about a week after jaundice appears; thus rigorous adherence to routine hand-washing practices is of critical importance in preventing the transmission of HAV. A number of hepatitis A outbreaks have been attributed to direct person-food-person transmission, when an infected food handler failed to wash his/her hands after using the toilet, subsequently touched food that received no further cooking, and then served it to a customer (Applied Foodservice Sanitation, 1985). Although this was initially suspected as the cause of Pennsylvania's HAV outbreak, traceback investigations revealed that contamination of the onions likely occurred due to contact with HAV-infected fieldworkers or HAV-polluted water on the farm in Mexico where the onions were grown and processed prior to shipment (CDC, 2003).

Parasites. Certain parasitic protozoan diseases such as amoebic dysentery or giardiasis are typically associated with ingestion of sewage-contaminated drinking water but have been known to occur when infected food service workers transmitted the microbes to food as a result of faulty hand-washing practices. Certain parasitic roundworm infections can occur when untreated sewage ("nightsoil") containing worm eggs is used to fertilize certain vegetable crops. If such produce is consumed raw, the eggs subsequently hatch inside the human host and perpetuate the cycle of infection. Other sources of helminthic (i.e., worm) foodborne ailments include the consumption of raw or undercooked fish. In recent years the United States has witnessed a small but increasing number of foodborne helminthic ailments traced to the growing popularity of ethnic specialties such as *sushi* or *ceviche*. Tapeworm infections are the most commonly reported problems, occurring predominantly along the West Coast where most victims admit to having eaten raw fish, mainly salmon. Symptoms of tapeworm infections, as well as time of onset, vary greatly from one person to another: some victims report experiencing severe cramps, nausea, and diarrhea almost immediately after eating; others may not develop symptoms for weeks or months. However, most victims experience no symptoms at all and only realize they have an infection when they pass the tapeworm, or segments of it, in their stool. Tapeworm infections can be eradicated with drugs, but roundworm infections (anisakiasis) are much more serious since there is no effective medication available. Such infections are very painful and may require surgery to remove the parasite. Consumers can easily avoid such problems simply by thoroughly cooking fish until it is flaky (internal temperature should be at 145°F for five minutes) or by freezing it at –4°F for 3–5 days before eating in order to kill the worms.

Trichinosis, another foodborne illness caused by a parasitic roundworm, results primarily from the consumption of undercooked pork products (occasionally outbreaks are traced to bear meat or other wild game), which may harbor the larvae of the pathogen, *Trichinella spiralis*. Inside the human host, larvae mature into adult worms and burrow into the intestinal wall, producing new larvae that travel via the circulatory system to muscle tissue. There they embed themselves and produce the typical symptoms of foodborne disease. Although the presence of *Trichinella* in pork is considerably lower today than in past decades (thanks, in part, to prohibitions on feeding uncooked garbage to hogs—a practice that in years past perpetuated the cycle of reinfection), a potential for infection remains nevertheless. Because *Trichinella* larvae are killed by high temperatures, the surest way to prevent trichinosis is *always* to cook pork until well done. *Trichinella* is also cold-sensitive and will die if exposed to a temperature of 5°F (–15°C) for 30 days.

Preventing Foodborne Disease

You won't be surprised that diseases are innumerable—count the cooks.
—Seneca (1st century AD)

Microbial contamination of foods can occur at any time from the production of food in field or feedlot right up to preparation and serving of the meal. Thus strict adherence to principles of food sanitation are essential at every step from production to processing, transportation, storage, preparation, and service if food-poisoning outbreaks are to be avoided.

In theory, *any* food can be a route of transmission for foodborne disease. However, some foods are implicated in food-poisoning outbreaks much more frequently than others and are therefore designated by the U.S. Public Health Service as **potentially hazardous foods**—those that are capable of supporting rapid and progressive growth of infectious or toxigenic microbes. Most potentially hazardous foods are high-protein animal products such as poultry, meat, fish, dairy products, and eggs. Foodborne pathogens also grow well in cooked rice or beans, baked or boiled potatoes, and tofu. Because bacteria must obtain their nutrients in dissolved form, they can only multiply on moist food media, explaining why *cooked* rice, for example, is considered "potentially hazardous" while raw rice is not. The inability of bacteria to grow in foods with very low water content is the basis for preservation of such food products as beef jerky or dried apricots. Drying foods does not *kill* microbes, however—it merely prevents their multiplication. If these foods become wet, bacterial growth will resume and their consumption could result in foodborne illness. Certain types of moist foods, peanut butter for example, are not considered potentially hazardous because the sugar and salt they contain tie up the water through chemical bonding, making it unavailable to support microbial growth. Food-poisoning bacteria also have specific pH requirements. Most species grow best at pH levels ranging from 4.6 to 9; highly acidic foods such as citrus fruits, tomatoes, most fresh fruits (low-acid berries and cantaloupe are exceptions to the rule), and pickles are seldom implicated in bacterial foodborne disease outbreaks.

The bacterial pathogens that cause foodborne disease are common inhabitants of the intestinal tracts of humans and domestic animals, present in healthy and sick individuals alike; some are naturally present in boils as well. When discharged in fecal material, these organisms can survive for long periods in litter, feces, trough water, and soil. Livestock feed is often contaminated with *Salmonella* organisms introduced when infected animal by-products are rendered and added to the feed mixture. Animals can become infected from any of these sources and thus bring such pathogens into slaughterhouses and poultry-processing plants. Just one infected organ or carcass or animal feces can contaminate cutting equipment or workers' hands and thereby can transfer the bacteria to other carcasses or foods, a process referred to as **cross-contamination.** Once in a processing plant or food establishment, pathogenic organisms can survive on the surface of equipment for long periods and thus constitute sources of food contamination over an extended time period. For this reason, cleaning and sanitizing of grinders, choppers, slicers, and other equipment after each use and frequent hand washing are important measures in preventing cross-contamination.

Foods, particularly those of animal origin, often contain pathogens such as *Salmonella* and *Campylobacter jejuni* when they enter the kitchen. Once in the kitchen, additional opportunity for contamination is presented by the food handlers themselves. The primary reservoir of the *Staphylococcus* organism is the human nose; if kitchen workers cough or sneeze near foods, the bacteria are readily transferred to an appropriate growth medium. If food handlers have infected cuts on their hands, boils, bad cases of acne, or other skin eruptions, *Staphylococcus* bacteria likewise can be transferred to food. Similarly, since approximately 40% of all healthy people carry *Salmonella* organisms in their gastrointestinal tract and regularly shed the live bacteria when they defecate, kitchen workers who do not wash their hands thoroughly after using the bathroom can contaminate foods with this pathogen. The low pay, lack of health benefits, limited education, and minimal employment opportunities that characterize the average food service worker complicate efforts to instill a strong commitment to safe food-handling practices.

Since so many foods contain at least *some* disease-causing bacteria, it is fortunate that the number of bacterial cells or concentration of bacterial toxins within the ingested food must be relatively high to induce the symptoms of most bacterial foodborne diseases (listeriosis and *E. coli 0157:H7* food poisoning are exceptions to this general rule). Thus the approach to preventing foodborne disease outbreaks must be two-pronged: (1) to the greatest extent possible, avoid microbial contamination of food in the first place through rigorous adherence to rules of good sanitation and hygiene; and (2) maintain environmental conditions that inhibit the multiplication of bacteria that may be present in small numbers within the food medium.

Box 9-4   Irradiating Foodborne Microbes

Reason and scientific facts triumphed over fear-mongering and misinformation in February 2000 when the federal government added raw beef and lamb to the list of foods that can be irradiated to control foodborne pathogens. This action followed FDA's determination in 1997 that irradiation does not make meat unsafe to eat, change its taste or smell, nor significantly alter its nutritional value. Subsequently, in 1999, USDA's Food Safety Inspection Service gave its approval, allowing irradiated hamburger to make its debut the following year. USDA had already approved regulations governing irradiation of pork (1986) and of poultry (1992), but the action on raw beef marked a major milestone in gaining official acceptance of this technology. It should be noted that USDA's action does not *require* that meat be irradiated, but merely permits it for producers or marketers who desire to utilize the technology as an effective weapon against foodborne disease. The Centers for Disease Control and Prevention (CDC), most public health officials, private groups such as the American Council on Science and Health and the Food Safety Consortium, and food industry representatives, all hailed the government's action as an important step toward reducing the incidence of foodborne illness in the U.S. Some authorities liken the approval of food irradiation to the advent of pasteurized milk in terms of its potential benefit to public health.

Approval of meat irradiation came after many years of controversy over the advisability of using ionizing radiation to kill microbial pathogens or insect pests in food products and to delay spoilage of fresh foods. Irradiation was approved in 1963 to control mold in wheat flour and in 1964 to inhibit sprouting of potatoes. By the 1980s FDA had given the go-ahead to use irradiation to kill trichina worms in fresh pork, to control insects and to slow ripening in fruits and vegetables, and to kill pests in dry herbs, spices, and tea. As the range of food products approved for irradiation expanded, vociferous objections arose from some consumer and environmental groups fearful of possible health implications. Their concerns, expressed in a torrent of negative comments to the FDA in the late 1990s, were reflected in that agency's subsequent exclusion of irradiated products from its official definition of what foods can be marketed as "organic."

Public opinion elsewhere in the world appears to be more accepting of food irradiation. By 2003, the process had been approved in over 50 countries and was being successfully used on several types of food in more than 30. Many of these nations, including Canada, Japan, and most European countries, have a long history of high standards on food safety issues. Moreover, food irradiation has been endorsed by the World Health Organization, the American Medical Association, and a number of public health organizations. Nevertheless, until the early 1990s, efforts to expand the range of U.S. products approved for irradiation were stymied by perceived public opposition. Marketing research confirmed the impression of consumer reluctance to embrace the technology; a 1998–99 survey conducted by FoodNet, a division within the CDC, found that only 49.5% of respondents said they were willing to buy irradiated meat or poultry, a percentage that fell to about 24% if the irradiated products cost more than non-irradiated products—as they inevitably do, due to the expensive technology involved. FoodNet researchers concluded that, in the absence of extensive public education on the food safety benefits of irradiated food, demand is likely to remain weak.

The event that galvanized supporters of food irradiation and sparked new interest in the issue was the 1993 *E. coli 0157:H7* outbreak. Food scientists are convinced that,

Source: USDA

other than thorough cooking, irradiation is the only method known that can completely eliminate pathogenic *E. coli* in raw meat. Numerous food-poisoning outbreaks and meat recalls due to contamination with *E. coli* and *Listeria* in the late 1990s reinforced the conviction among food safety experts that food irradiation's time had come (federal food safety agencies are now considering whether to approve irradiation of ready-to-eat processed meats such as cold cuts and hot dogs for *Listeria* control).

Government approval doesn't guarantee that irradiated foods will be widely accepted in the U.S., however. Widespread public ignorance and misinformation about the technology has resulted in little demand for irradiated foods; by 2005 over 4,000 supermarkets nationwide were selling irradiated meat, up from just 84 in 2000 but still a small minority of U.S. supermarkets. Irradiated chicken is purchased mainly by some hospitals and nursing homes where sick or elderly patients are more vulnerable than the general population to foodborne illnesses. Some consumers avoid irradiated food products due to erroneous ideas about what the process entails. The most common irradiation methods employ gamma rays (generally from a cobalt-60 source), X-rays, or electron beams which, unlike pesticides, accomplish the task for which they were intended without leaving any residue and without rendering the food itself radioactive (just as people receiving dental X-rays or luggage passing through an airport metal detector don't become radioactive themselves as a result). The alleged "unidentified radiolytic products" raised as a concern by anti-irradiation activists have never been found by independent researchers. Ideally, the product is irradiated after it is packaged and sealed, thus preventing any opportunity for recontamination. Consumers handling or eating irradiated food are exposed to no radiation whatsoever. To ensure safe operations, food irradiation facilities must adhere to strict regulations promulgated by the Nuclear Regulatory Commission and the Occupational Safety and Health Administration. Nearly 50 years of experience using irradiation to sterilize medical devices, a process very similar to food irradiation, have demonstrated that the technology has performed extremely well in terms of safeguarding employee health and transporting radioactive material.

One consumer advocacy group, the Center for Science in the Public Interest, worries that widespread adoption of irradiation to control foodborne pathogens might tempt meat producers to become lax in maintaining high sanitary standards in processing facilities. Proponents, however, insist that irradiation will never be a substitute for hygienic processing and handling of food; indeed, they stress that irradiation's microbiocidal efficiency depends on the cleanliness of the food being treated. Similarly, they emphasize the importance of safe food-handling practices after the irradiated food package is opened, since recontamination then becomes a possibility. Contrary to much of the negative publicity surrounding the issue, irradiation is simply one additional tool—along with production of healthy animals, sanitary processing plants, and proper cooking—to ensure wholesome, pathogen-free food.

References

American Council on Science and Health. 2003. "Irradiated Foods." Accessed at www.acsh.org/publications/pubID.198/pub_detail.asp (June 7, 2004).

Frenzen, P., A. Majchrowicz, B. Buzby, B. Imhoff, and the FoodNet Working Group. 2000. "Consumer Acceptance of Irradiated Meat and Poultry Products." *Agriculture Information Bulletin* 757:1–8.

Sanitation

High standards of cleanliness and personal hygiene among those who handle or prepare food are of the utmost importance in preventing outbreaks of foodborne disease. Regulations that local and state public health agencies impose on more than a million retail food establishments in the United States highlight the responsibility of food service personnel for observing good sanitary practices—practices equally relevant to food preparation at home. In its model *Food Code,* a compilation of recommendations that state and local health departments can adopt when developing or updating their own regulatory requirements, the FDA recommends that food service workers be held accountable for lapses in personal hygiene. The *Code* places a special obligation on employees to notify supervisors if they are experiencing any symptoms of gastrointestinal illness or if they are suffering from boils, dermatitis, or other infections on the hands, wrists, exposed portions of the arms, or other parts of the body, unless covered by a proper bandage (such pus-filled infections are prime sources of *Staphylococcus* bacteria). Thus informed, a supervisor is required to restrict sick employees from direct contact with food or to exclude them from the establishment altogether until health problems have been resolved.

Perhaps the most important of all sanitary practices in protecting food quality is frequent and proper hand washing. The FDA cites germ-laden hands as a major vehicle of disease transmission, a situation resulting largely from negligence on the part of food handlers. Emphasizing that *rigorous hand-washing practices represent the single most effective means for breaking the chain of infection*, public health authorities recommend that immediately before handling food, food service workers and home cooks alike should engage in a vigorous 20-second scrub using soap and running water, followed by thorough rinsing under clean water. This procedure should be repeated as often as necessary during food preparation to remove soil and to prevent cross-contamination when changing tasks or after handling soiled equipment. Good hand-washing procedures, including using a fingernail brush to clean the fingertips and under the nails, are especially important after food handlers use the toilet, cough, sneeze, smoke, eat, or drink.

Good sanitation of course involves attention to more than employee health and hygiene. General cleanliness of the facility, routine sanitization of cutting tools and food preparation equipment, safe food storage practices, effective dish-washing procedures, proper waste disposal and trash storage—all are important for ensuring that dangerous microbes and food never have a chance to meet.

Time-Temperature Control

When certain environmental preconditions such as optimum pH, moisture, essential nutrients, and temperature are met, populations of pathogenic bacteria in food multiply in accordance with the sigmoidal growth pattern described in chapter 2: after an initial lag phase of about one hour, during which there is negligible increase in numbers while the organisms adjust to new conditions, a period of extremely rapid increase in population size continues until the supply of essential nutrients diminishes and toxic by-products accumulate. At this stage, growth levels off and the number of organisms remains relatively constant until eventually a progressive die-off of cells occurs. Perhaps the most crucial element in determining the rate of bacterial multiplication during this sequence of events is *temperature*. The bacteria responsible for the majority of foodborne disease outbreaks multiply most rapidly within a temperature range referred to as the **Danger Zone,** defined under the FDA's *Food Code* as **41°–140°F (5°–60°C).** Temperatures above 140°F will kill most actively growing bacteria, though bacterial spores and a few thermophilic species may survive. At temperatures below 41°F, growth of the bacterial populations associated with common foodborne illnesses either ceases entirely or is extremely slow; however, the organisms are not killed by cold temperatures and can remain viable for long periods of time, resuming multiplication when temperatures rise. Therefore, the most effective way to prevent buildup of bacterial numbers is to keep foods refrigerated, especially those proteinaceous foods that most frequently harbor pathogenic bacteria. Heating such foods thoroughly will kill bacteria

Box 9-5 HACCP—Preventive Approach to Food Safety

In confronting the challenge of how best to ensure the safety of food supplies from biological, chemical, or physical hazards, government regulators and food industry personnel alike traditionally relied on an approach that involved periodic inspections of food-processing facilities (e.g., mills, slaughterhouses, canneries, bakeries, supermarkets, restaurants, etc.) and random end-product analyses. The mandated inspection system for meat and poultry still relies heavily on visual examination, the inspector touching and sniffing carcasses to detect signs of disease or spoilage. Most food safety experts decry this approach as outdated and completely useless for identifying the presence of the foodborne pathogens that constitute today's most urgent food quality concerns. In recent years a paradigm shift has been occurring in the way regulatory agencies approach foodborne disease prevention. Moving away from a century-old reactive food safety strategy, regulators are turning instead to a science-based concept called the **Hazard Analysis and Critical Control Point** system, or **HACCP** (pronounced "hassip").

So what *is* this radical new approach? Essentially HACCP is a preventive system of quality control which, when properly applied, can be used to control any point in the food system that might contribute to a hazardous situation. The concept originated with the space program in the late 1950s, when NASA asked the Pillsbury Company to produce a food that could be eaten by astronauts in orbit. Such an undertaking presented a number of challenges, none more daunting than the imperative of ensuring that any food developed be 100% free of microbial, chemical, or physical contamination. The potentially disastrous consequences of a food-poisoning outbreak inside a space capsule had to be avoided at any cost. Pillsbury scientists realized that only a proactive preventive system could provide the high degree of safety assurance required. Pillsbury spent the following decade developing and refining its concept and in 1971 adopted the HACCP approach in its own facilities. That same year the FDA awarded Pillsbury a contract to conduct classes for its employees on the HACCP system, and in 1973 the company published the first comprehensive document on HACCP principles as a training manual for FDA personnel. By the early 1980s a number of U.S. food companies had established their own HACCP programs, but HACCP's wider application in the public sector remained extremely limited. In 1980, several federal agencies requested that the National Academy of Sciences examine the potential applications for microbiological criteria in food. The result was a 1985 NAS publication that strongly recommended the application of HACCP in regulatory programs, stating that HACCP "provides a more specific and critical approach to the control of microbiological hazards in foods than that provided by traditional inspection and quality control approaches."

Following this ringing endorsement by NAS, an increasing number of federal, state, and local agencies have been redesigning their regulatory approach in conformance with HACCP principles. In 1994 the FDA embraced HACCP as the best method for ensuring food safety, promulgating voluntary HACCP rules for seafood and shellfish (1997), raw sprouts and eggs (1999), and fresh juices (2001). USDA has instituted a mandatory HACCP requirement for meat and poultry, with rules specifically targeted toward reducing microbial levels in these products. The HACCP rules developed by these two federal agencies for the various segments of the food industry each regulates (meat, poultry, and processed eggs by USDA, all other foods by FDA) differ in several respects, most notably in USDA's requirement that the firms under its jurisdiction test for the presence of bacteria, while FDA has no such mandate. In addition, while USDA's HACCP requirements pertain to all meat and poultry operations, FDA has promulgated HACCP rules on a food-by-food basis, leaving many foods it regulates without any proposed controls. It should be mentioned that, even without government prodding, several large food companies have developed and implemented pilot HACCP systems for products as diverse as breakfast cereal, cheese, bread, and salad dressing. Results have been what food safety experts would have predicted: HACCP controls are quite effective in helping companies detect—and then correct—food safety problems.

While food producers must develop individualized HACCP systems tailored to their own processing and distribution conditions, each HACCP program consists of seven basic steps:

1. **Analyze hazard,** identifying potential hazards associated with the food in question, based on close observation of how the food is grown, processed, and distributed—right up to the point of consumption; an assessment is then made of the likelihood of those hazards occurring and preventive measures for controlling such hazards are identified.

2. **Determine critical control points (CCPs)** to minimize or eliminate the hazards identified; CCPs comprise operational steps or procedures such as cooking, chilling, sanitizing, employee hygiene, etc.

3. **Establish critical limits or tolerances** that must be met to ensure that the CCP is under control; some of the criteria most often used include temperature, time, pH, humidity, salt concentration, etc.

4. **Establish a monitoring system** through scheduled testing or observation to ensure that CCP is being controlled.

5. **Establish the corrective action** to be taken when monitoring indicates a deviation from appropriate controls; because of the wide range of possible critical control points, a specific corrective action plan must be developed for each one.

6. **Establish effective record-keeping systems** that document the HACCP plan.

7. **Establish verification procedures** that demonstrate that HACCP is working correctly; such procedures require minimal end-product sampling (due to safeguards built into the system), relying instead on frequent reviews of plan procedure and affirmation that the plan is being followed correctly. Both the food producer and the appropriate regulatory agencies have a role to play in verifying HACCP plan performance.

Implementing a HACCP program in any given setting is neither quick nor easy. HACCP is a technically sophisticated system requiring extensive site-specific research, discussion, and preparation prior to application. Intensive training of both in-plant personnel and regulatory agency inspectors, a high degree of industry/government cooperation, and rigorous enforcement efforts by the regulatory agency inspectors are essential prerequisites to the success of any HACCP plan. Nevertheless, ultimate results are well worth the effort. According to the NAS analysis, effective use of HACCP in food production systems is the one approach by which meaningful reductions in the incidence of foodborne disease can be achieved.

References

National Research Council. 1998. *Ensuring Safe Food From Production to Consumption.* Washington, DC: National Academy Press.

Nestle, Marion. 2003. *Safe Food: Bacteria, Biotechnology, and Bioterrorism.* Berkeley: Univ. of California Press.

that may be present in the food; the higher the temperature above 140°, the shorter the time the bacterial population will be able to survive (normal cooking times and temperatures are not sufficient, however, to break down *Staphylococcus* toxin).

To ensure complete heat penetration throughout the item being cooked, it is advised that internal temperatures reach the following USDA-recommended minimum levels to guarantee that any pathogens present within the food are killed:

Ground Poultry	165°F (74°C)
Ground beef, veal, lamb, pork	160°F (71°C)
Roast beef or lamb	145°F (63°C)
Roast pork	160°F (71°C)
Ham, fresh	160°F (71°C)
Ham, pre-cooked	140°F (60°C)
Roast chicken, turkey	180°F (82°C)
Chicken or turkey breast	170°F (77°C)
Stuffing	165°F (74°C)

It should be noted that the internal temperature of the item being cooked, rather than the temperature of the oven or burner, is the crucial factor. In many instances, large roasts of beef, ham, or turkey still harbor viable pathogens after cooking because they weren't in the oven long enough for temperatures at the center of the roast to reach the recommended level. In the same way, large pieces of cooked meat held in the refrigerator for cooling frequently have internal temperatures well within the growth range, even though the refrigerator thermostat registers at or below 41°F as advised. To promote rapid cooling, cooked meat should be sliced into thin layers and placed in shallow pans before being refrigerated.

The most effective methods that food handlers can follow to prevent foodborne disease, be it in the home, in restaurants, or at large public gatherings, is to complete the processing of food within an hour or two while the bacteria remain in the lag phase of growth and to cool foods rapidly if they are not to be consumed immediately.

Unfortunately, although good sanitation and proper time-temperature controls are relatively simple preventive concepts, they are all-too-frequently neglected by homemakers and commercial food establishments alike. Thus bacterial food poisoning, which fundamentally is a result of improper food-handling practices and should not even exist in affluent modern societies, will undoubtedly remain our most prevalent food-related health problem.

References

Applied Foodservice Sanitation. 1985. John Wiley & Sons in cooperation with the Educational Foundation of the National Restaurant Association.

Centers for Disease Control and Prevention (CDC). 2003. "Hepatitis A Outbreak Associated with Green Onions at a Restaurant—Monaca, Pennsylvania, 2003." *Morbidity & Mortality Weekly Report* 52 Dispatch (Nov. 21).

———. 2002a. "Outbreak of *Salmonella* Serotype Kottbus Infections Associated with Eating Alfalfa Sprouts—Arizona, California, Colorado, and New Mexico, February–April, 2001." *Morbidity & Mortality Weekly Report* 51, no. 1 (Jan. 11).

———. 2002b. "Outbreaks of Gastroenteritis Associated with Noroviruses on Cruise Ships—United States, 2002. *Morbidity & Mortality Weekly Report* 51, no. 49 (Dec. 13).

———. 1994. "Water Hemlock Poisoning—Maine, 1992." *Morbidity & Mortality Weekly Report* 43, no. 13 (April 8).

———. 1993. "*Vibrio vulnificus* Infections Associated with Raw Oyster Consumption—Florida, 1981–1992." *Morbidity & Mortality Weekly Report* 42, no. 21 (June 4).

Food and Agriculture Organization of the United Nations (FAO). 1998. "Expert Committee: No Danger to Humans from Milk and Meat from BST-Treated Cows." *News & Highlights* (March 5).

Foulke, Judith E. 1993. "A Fresh Look at Food Preservatives." *FDA Consumer* (Oct).

Hanrahan, Charles E. 1996. "The European Union's Ban on Hormone-Treated Meat." *Congressional Research Service Report for Congress,* 96–122 ENR (Feb. 8).

Henkel, John. 1993. "From Shampoo to Cereal: Seeing to the Safety of Color Additives." *FDA Consumer* (Dec).

Janssen, Wallace F. 1975. "America's First Food and Drug Laws." *FDA Consumer* (June).

Klein, Richard M. 1979. *The Green World: An Introduction to Plants and People.* New York: Harper & Row.

Koren, Herman. 1980. *Handbook of Environmental Health and Safety.* Vol. 1. Oxford: Pergamon Press.

Merrill, Richard A. 1997. "Food Safety Regulation: Reforming the Delaney Clause." *Annual Review of Public Health* 18:313–340.

Miller, Roger W. 1984. "How Onions and a Baked Potato Became Sources of Botulism Poisoning." *FDA Consumer* (Oct).

National Research Council (NRC). 2000. *The Future Role of Pesticides in U.S. Agriculture.* Washington, DC: National Academy Press.

National Research Council (NRC). 1998. *Ensuring Safe Food from Production to Consumption.* Washington, DC: National Academy Press.

———. 1996. *Carcinogens and Anti-Carcinogens in the Human Diet.* Washington, DC: National Academy Press.

———. 1993. *Pesticides in the Diets of Infants and Children.* Washington, DC: National Academy Press.

———. 1987. *Regulating Pesticides in Food: The Delaney Paradox.* Washington, DC: National Academy Press.

Nestle, Marion. 2003. *Safe Food: Bacteria, Biotechnology, and Bioterrorism.* Berkeley: Univ. of California Press.

Pierson, Merle D., and Donald A. Corlett, Jr., eds. 1992. *HACCP: Principles and Applications.* New York: Chapman & Hall.

Ropp, Kevin L. 1994. "Juice Maker Cheats Consumers of $40 Million." *FDA Consumer* (Jan/Feb).

Tannahill, Ray. 1973. *Food in History.* New York: Stein and Day.

Tarr, Phillip I., and Michael Doyle. 1996. "Food Safety: Everyone's Responsibility." *Pediatric Basics* no. 78 (Fall):2–13.

Task Force on the Mass Outbreak of Diarrhea in School Children of Sakai City. 1997. *Report on the Outbreak of E. coli 0157:H7 Infection in Sakai City* (Dec).

RADIATION

The human race has today the means for annihilating itself—either in a fit of complete lunacy, i.e., in a big war, by a brief fit of destruction, or by careless handling of atomic technology, through a slow process of poisoning and of deterioration in its genetic structure.

—Max Born, *Bulletin of Atomic Scientists* (1957)

There is no evil in the atom; only in men's souls.

—Adlai Stevenson (1952)

Late in the autumn of 1895, a German physics professor, Wilhelm Roentgen, was busily pursuing a line of research that would soon revolutionize medical science and transform our understanding of the nature of matter and energy. Roentgen was experimenting with a cathode-ray tube, a device perfected by the English scientist Crookes two decades earlier that consisted of a glass vacuum tube through which flowed a high voltage electric current. By chance, Roentgen noticed that emissions from the tube caused a nearby sheet of paper coated with a fluorescent chemical to glow, and he observed that these emanations could be blocked to varying degrees by materials of different densities. Calling his wife to place her hand on a photographic plate, Roentgen turned on the cathode ray tube; when the plate was subsequently developed, Roentgen amazed the world with a picture of his wife's bones inside her hand. Realizing that he had stumbled upon a form of radiation whose existence was hitherto completely unsuspected, Roentgen appropriated the mathematical symbol for the unknown and called his discovery "X-rays." Within a few days after publication of his findings, the medical profession put the fluoroscope and "roentgenogram" to use—the shortest time gap between announcement of a major medical discovery and its practical application yet recorded.

The implications of Roentgen's announcement far transcended the field of medicine, however. Upon hearing of Roentgen's findings, the noted French scientist Henri Becquerel became intrigued by the relationship between X-rays and fluorescence and thereupon directed his attention to naturally phosphorescent minerals. In February of 1896, just two months after publication of Roentgen's report, Becquerel placed some crystals of a uranium compound on a photographic plate wrapped in black paper and demonstrated that the emanations from the uranium exhibited the same characteristics as Roentgen's X-rays. Becquerel's work was quickly picked up by Marie and Pierre Curie who termed the mysterious phenomenon "radioactivity" and who soon succeeded in isolating two new radioactive substances, polonium and radium, from uranium ore (Kevles, 1997). Thus the independent discovery of both artificial and nat-

World's first X-ray: this is the "roentgenogram" that Wilhelm Roentgen took of his wife's hand thereby demonstrating the existence of the mysterious emanations that he named "X-rays."

ural radioactivity within a three-month time span quickly led to the birth of a whole new field of scientific inquiry with far-reaching implications in physics, biology, medicine, and, unfortunately, warfare.

Ionizing Radiation

Early investigations of radioactivity quickly revealed that the observed emissions were of several different kinds. Some consisted of subatomic particles—protons, neutrons, or electrons—released when atoms spontaneously decay; these came to be known as **particulate radiation**, a group that includes **alpha** and **beta particles**. Other emissions, such as Roentgen's X-rays and naturally occurring **gamma rays,** were shown to consist of highly energetic short wavelengths of electromagnetic radiation, a form of energy that also includes ultraviolet light, visible light, infrared waves, and microwaves. Alpha and beta particles, as well as X-rays and gamma rays, are today referred to as **ionizing radiation** because the particles or rays involved are sufficiently energetic to dislodge electrons from the atoms or molecules they encounter, leaving behind ions, i.e., electrically charged particles. While certain forms of non-ionizing radiation such as ultraviolet light and microwaves can have an adverse effect on living organisms and will be discussed later in this chapter, ionizing radiation's ability to destroy chemical bonds gives it special significance in relation to both human health and environmental pollution. It is recognized today that when certain particularly vulnerable cells (e.g., fetal cells, sex cells) are exposed to ionizing radiation, birth defects or mutations can result; in any cell, radiation-induced alteration of DNA can lead to cancer. Although discovery of ionizing radiation was immediately hailed as a momentous medical and scientific event, subsequent investigations regarding what is frequently called our "most studied and best understood pollutant" have revealed the importance of extreme caution in dealing with radioactive materials.

Radiation Exposure

Exposure to ionizing radiation is an inescapable circumstance of life on this planet. Every individual, to a greater or lesser extent, comes into contact with ionizing radiation from three general types of sources: naturally occurring, naturally occurring but enhanced by human actions, and human generated.

Natural sources.   Although the fact was not realized until Becquerel's discovery in 1896, earth, air, water, and food all contain traces of radioactive materials that constitute a ubiquitous source of naturally occurring, or "background," radiation. Some of the more significant sources of background radiation include the following:

Cosmic radiation.   High-energy particles composed primarily of protons and electrons continually stream toward the earth both from outer space and from the sun following episodes of solar flares. An appreciable amount of such cosmic radiation is blocked by the layer of atmosphere surrounding the globe, so that exposure to cosmic radiation is considerably less at sea level than at high altitudes (annual exposure to cosmic radiation approximately doubles with each 2,000-meter increase in altitude above sea level). For this reason, residents of Denver receive about twice as much cosmic radiation as do inhabitants of Los Angeles or Miami; the one million residents of La Paz, Bolivia, receive annual radiation exposures fully 7.5 times higher than do people living at sea level (Bennett, 1997). Flying long distances in an airliner also results in higher-than-average exposure to cosmic rays for those aboard. In fact, flight crews on airliners flying more northerly routes receive annual radiation doses in excess of those experienced by most hospital radiologists; as a result, they are classified as radiation workers by a number of European countries (Hall, 2000). While the natural tendency is to assume that something which has always been with us must be harmless, some biologists assert that perhaps 25% of all spontaneous mutations are caused by cosmic radiation.

Radioactive minerals in the earth's crust.   Radioactive compounds of uranium, thorium, potassium, and radium are found in soils and rocks in many parts of the world. For example, people living along the Kerala coast in southwestern India, the Morro de Ferro and Meaipe regions of Brazil's Atlantic coast, and in Yangjiang, Guangdong Province in China are all exposed to significantly higher-than-average levels of background radiation due to emissions from thorium-rich monazite sands. Similarly, Floridians living near radioactive phosphate deposits, and residents of New Hampshire, the Rocky Mountain region of the United States, and parts of Sweden— all granite-rich areas—are constantly exposed to external radiation from the soils and rocks around them. In some localities, notably Badgastein in Austria and Mahallat and Ramsar in Iran, high levels of background radiation exposure are received inter- nally due to the ingestion of naturally occurring radioactive minerals in drinking water and to the inhalation of radon gas when bathing in the hot springs for which these regions are famous (Sohrabi, 1998).

Coal deposits frequently contain a number of radioactive elements that are released into the atmosphere when the coal is burned. Ironically, the growing appeal of low-sulfur western coal as an economical approach to reducing sulfur emissions ignores the fact that western coal contains about 10 times more radionuclides than do eastern or midwestern coal deposits (Carter, 1977).

Radionuclides in the body. A number of radioactive substances enter the body by ingestion of food, milk, water, or by inhalation and are incorporated into body tissues where their concentration may be maintained at a steady state or gradually increase with age. Plants growing in soil containing radioactive minerals readily take up potas- sium-40, a radioactive isotope believed to make a not-insignificant contribution to human radiation exposure. Some authorities hypothesize that potassium-40 ingested with food may be one source of human mutations (Hall, 2000). In regions where groundwater is in contact with radioactive rock strata, well water used for domestic drinking supplies may constitute a significant source of indoor exposure to radioactive radon gas. Another unavoidable source of radiation exposure is carbon-14, a naturally occurring isotope of carbon, which is inhaled with the air we breathe and is incorpo- rated into the tissues of all living organisms (a fact that has useful implications for sci- entists who employ C-14 dating techniques to ascertain the age of ancient plant and animal remains).

Enhanced natural sources. This category of sources, while not fundamentally different from the group just discussed, is considered separately because of the impact human activities have on levels of exposure that would, under other conditions, be much lower. Examples of enhanced natural sources include uranium mill tailings, phosphate mining, and jet airline travel (due to increased exposure to cosmic radia- tion at high altitudes). Experts consider radon gàs, our single most significant source of radiation exposure, to be an enhanced natural source because, although naturally occurring, it reaches potentially dangerous concentrations only in enclosed environ- ments such as houses and mine shafts ("Ionizing Radiation," 1987). For more infor- mation on radon, see the section on "Indoor Air Pollutants" in chapter 12.

Human-generated sources. Human beings have evolved and multiplied in an environment where constant exposure to low levels of ionizing radiation is a universal experience. With the exception of indoor radon concerns that are currently the subject of a great deal of attention and remedial action, most naturally occurring radiation is relatively constant and cannot be controlled or reduced in any feasible way. However, human-created sources of ionizing radiation have multiplied at exponential rates dur- ing the years since Roentgen first exhibited the X-ray of his wife's hand to an astonished world. It is these artificial sources, which *can* be controlled, that constitute the focus of a growing concern today about the impact of ionizing radiation on human health.

Medical applications. By far the greatest source of exposure to artificial ionizing radiation for the average American comes from the use of medical X-rays and radio-

Figure 10-1   Contribution of Various Radiation Sources to the Total Average Effective Dose Equivalent in the U.S. Population

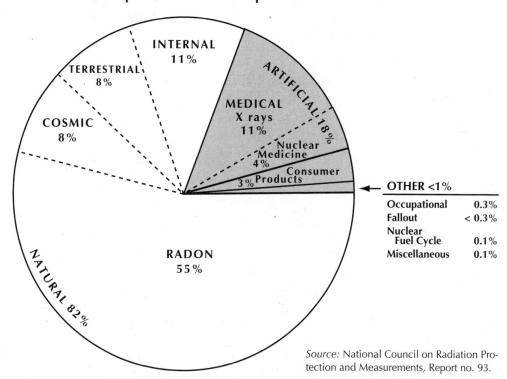

Source: National Council on Radiation Protection and Measurements, Report no. 93.

pharmaceuticals for both diagnostic and therapeutic purposes. Today approximately 75% of all Americans receive one or more medical or dental X-rays annually. Radioactive isotopes of phosphorus, technicium, iodine, iron, chromium, cobalt, and selenium are widely employed in hospitals for therapy and diagnosis, with as many as one-fourth of all patients in some hospitals receiving applications of some form of nuclear medicine. In addition to X-ray machines and radionuclides, the health professions utilize other such radiation-producing devices as Computerized Axial Tomography machines (CAT scans), teleradioisotope units and accelerators (e.g., cyclotrons, linear accelerators) to generate subatomic particles for radiotherapy. While radiation has provided medical science with an extremely valuable tool, its occasional misuse has been accompanied by some serious health problems; thus a thoughtful weighing of risks versus benefits should precede any decision regarding the application of ionizing radiation for medical purposes.

Nuclear weapons fallout.   Since the explosion of the first atomic bomb in 1945 until the signing of the Limited Test-Ban Treaty in 1963, atmospheric testing of nuclear weapons by several of the major powers, primarily the United States and the former Soviet Union, resulted in significant amounts of radioactive fallout worldwide. Such fallout consists of a number of atomic fission products, including strontium-90, iodine-131, cesium-137, and radioactive krypton. Weapons fallout is not always evenly distributed, however. Local fallout close to the test site can be quite intense for about a day following the explosion, a fact that became obvious after the March 1, 1954, detonation of a multimegaton U.S. bomb over Bikini Atoll in the

Pacific. Heavy fallout of large radioactive particles and dust contaminated several inhabited islands nearby, as well as a Japanese fishing boat sailing in the vicinity. Many of the Marshall Islanders and the fishermen developed burns, skin lesions, and loss of hair as a result of radiation exposure, and one of the islands, Rongelap, had to be evacuated and remained unoccupied for a number of years following the incident. In some cases air currents or rainstorms can cause radioactive particles and gases to precipitate unevenly. The greatest concern about weapons fallout is focused on those isotopes that enter the human system in food and are incorporated into body tissues. Of these, the most significant health threat is the increased risk of thyroid cancer posed by exposure to iodine-131 in milk from cows or goats that grazed on pasture-

Official military observers watch the mushroom cloud form after an atomic artillery shell was fired in the Nevada desert in 1953. Such tests resulted in significant amounts of radioactive fallout. [*AP/Wide World Photos*]

lands exposed to fallout (Institute of Medicine and National Research Council, 1999). During the peak period of weapons testing, an average individual's radiation exposure due to bomb fallout was 13 millirems annually, a figure that has been steadily falling since 1963 (Eisenbud, 1973). According to the National Council on Radiation Protection and Measurements (NCRP), annual fallout exposure currently averages less than 0.01 mSv (1 mrem) and, barring a resumption of atmospheric testing of nuclear weapons, will continue to decline. Having reached such negligible levels, nuclear weapons fallout need no longer be taken into account in calculating total human radiation exposure.

Nuclear power plant emissions. Public opposition to construction of nuclear power plants often centers around fears concerning radioactive emissions both to the air and in wastewater released from such plants. Radioisotopes such as tritium (H3), iodine-131, cesium-137, strontium-90, krypton, and others are indeed released into the environment during routine operation of a nuclear power generator, but the quantities involved are extremely minute—the average annual dose to individuals living within a 50-mile radius of the plant being less than one millirem, an amount considerably lower than that received from background radiation ("Ionizing Radiation," 1987).

Consumer products. In addition to the sources mentioned above, very small amounts of exposure are received from luminous instrument dials (radium, tritium), home smoke detectors (americium), static eliminators (polonium), airport security checks (X-rays), and tobacco products (polonium). Of these sources, the most significant is tobacco; the radioactive polonium particles in cigarette smoke lodge primarily in the bronchial epithelium of the upper airways—the site of most lung cancers—thereby further contributing to the health risk posed by other carcinogenic and toxic substances in tobacco smoke (NCRP, 1987).

Since radon exposure alone constitutes approximately 55% of the average American's annual radiation burden, background (including enhanced) sources, contributing 82% of total radiation exposure, are far more significant than the 18% from artificial sources (NCRP, 1987). For any one individual, of course, the ratio can vary widely. A person living in an area of unusually high natural radioactivity (e.g., Salt Lake City, Denver) or sleeping in a basement bedroom where radon levels are exceptionally high might receive an even larger portion of his or her total exposure from background sources, while a person undergoing radiation therapy or working inside a nuclear power plant would receive a disproportionate share from artificial sources.

Health Impacts of Ionizing Radiation

The advent of X-ray technology for diagnosing and treating human maladies, so eagerly and immediately seized upon by the medical profession, was soon shown to be a double-edged sword so far as its impact on human health was concerned. The first reported case of X-ray induced illness involved an American physician, Grubbe, who began self-experimenting with a homemade cathode ray tube. Within a few weeks he reported acute irritation of the skin on his hand; later cancer developed and eventually his hand had to be amputated. Grubbe's case was not an isolated one. By 1897, scarcely a year after the new technology came into use, 69 cases of X-ray induced injuries had been documented from various clinics and laboratories in different parts of the world (Eisenbud, 1973). One of the most famous early radiation victims was Clarence Dally, Thomas Edison's chief assistant, who "died by inches" after just a few years of working with X-rays. In 1896 Dally had begun experimenting with Roentgen's new device in Edison's West Orange, New Jersey, laboratory, frequently holding his hand in front of the tube to make sure X-rays were being produced. Dally soon noticed slight burns and hair loss, but continued his work. By 1902 he was suffering from oozing ulcers on his hands and eventually had his left hand amputated; cancerous sores then appeared on his right hand and four fingers were amputated, followed by both arms. In such acute pain he couldn't even lie down, Dally died in agony in 1904 (Kevles, 1997). Reports of health damage due to radiation from natural sources were not long in following. Becquerel himself reported a reddening of the skin on his chest as a result of carrying a vial of radium in his vest pocket. He and the Curies subsequently used a radium extract to produce a skin burn on the forearm of a male volunteer, thereby demonstrating that X-rays and natural radioactivity have essentially identical biological effects (Cooper, 1973).

In spite of an increasing awareness of the hazards, as well as the usefulness, of ionizing radiation, the first few decades of the 20th century witnessed numerous cases of radiation-induced illness or death resulting from carelessness, faulty equipment, or simple ignorance. As early as 1903 a dangerous misconception of radiation's curative powers catapulted both X-rays and radium into prominence as the latest medical fads, regarded as modern panaceas for a wide range of ailments. Over a period of approximately 20 years, first in Europe and later in the U.S. as well, radiation treatments were prescribed to hopeful patients both for destroying unwanted external tissue (e.g., warts, birthmarks, excess facial hair) and as an internal medicine. Many researchers during this period were convinced that radiation selectively destroyed diseased cells while actually promoting the growth of healthy ones. Some claimed that the radioactive element radium had germicidal properties, leading one scientist to propose the inhalation of radioactive gas as a treatment for tuberculosis! The discovery during this period that the mineral waters at many health spas were radioactive reinforced the notion that radioactivity must confer health benefits and encouraged promoters of such popular resorts as Saratoga Springs, New York, and Hot Springs, Arkansas, to claim their waters had the power to cure ailments ranging from rheumatism to malaria, alcoholism, chronic skin disease, anemia, and female sterility!

More surprising in retrospect was the medical practice, widespread during the 1910s and 1920s, of administering intravenous injections of radium salts as a treatment for such maladies as high blood pressure, arthritis, leukemia, sexual dysfunction, and senility; rather than curing such ills, the treatment all too often provoked the development of anemia or cancer (Clark, 1997). Outside physicians' offices, a wide variety of radium-based consumer products—candies, liniments, creams, and so on— were being marketed to a gullible public with assurances that the effects of radiation in trace amounts were beneficial to health, perhaps even necessary! One such bogus cure-all, "Radithor," was advertised as a panacea for impotence, high blood pressure, indigestion, and more than 150 other ills. Sold in the United States for over six years, Radithor was taken off the market only after it had induced fatal cancer in a well-known socialite, a Radithor devotee who was reported to have consumed 1,000 to 1,500 bottlefuls of the radium solution between 1927 and 1931. The legal restrictions on sales of radiopharmaceuticals currently prevailing in the United States were a direct result of the outrage provoked by the Radithor scandal almost 75 years ago (Macklis, 1993). To cite another example of a practice that in retrospect seems inconceivably misguided, starting in about 1925, some doctors began irradiating children's scalps to treat ringworm, their heads and throats for enlarged tonsils and adenoids, and their faces to banish acne. Even as late as the 1960s some physicians used low-voltage X-rays to shrink the thymus gland (located in the neck) of infants in the erroneous belief that such treatments would cure colds. Unfortunately, such X-rays could not be precisely focused. As they spread out they irradiated not only the target tissue but the thyroid gland as well. The thyroid is one of the most radiation-sensitive organs

Box 10-1 "See Alice Glow!"—Tragedy of the Radium Dial-Painters

The agonizing deaths suffered by scores of young female workers in the radium dial-painting industry in the 1920s and 1930s constitute the most infamous example on record of fatal carelessness in the handling of radioactive materials. The tragedy that befell these first victims of occupational radiation poisoning had its origin in the development, in 1915, of radium-containing luminous paint—a product that promptly found use in the watch-making industry for producing "glow-in-the dark" wristwatches. To supply the demand for this latest consumer fad, between 1917 and 1925 dial-painting factories were established in Orange, NJ; Waterbury, CT; and Ottawa, IL, cumulatively employing 3,000–4,000 workers over the years they were in operation.

Offering what they touted as "ideal working conditions," firms such as U.S. Radium in New Jersey and Radium Dial Company (later replaced by Luminous Processes) in Illinois selectively recruited a workforce composed of women in their late teens and early twenties, regarding such employees as particularly well-suited for jobs requiring little physical strength but considerable manual dexterity. From moderately prosperous working-class families, these women felt fortunate to find employment in firms offering above-average wages in pleasant surroundings. They also found it exciting to be in daily contact with a substance as magical as radium. In more playful moments they applied the luminous paint to their fingernails, eyelids, and buttons; one particularly vivacious girl in New Jersey laughingly painted her teeth with radium to surprise her boyfriend with a glow-in-the-dark smile! Dial-painters often returned home from work with their hair and clothes liberally speckled with luminous powder and would sometimes amuse friends and family by standing in a dark closet where they cast off a ghostly glow.

The dial-painters' most ill-advised practice, however, was lip-pointing. As instructed by supervisors, each worker used her lips to maintain a fine point on the brush as she painted the tiny numbers on the watch dial; in doing so, she inadvertently swallowed small amounts of radium each time the brush touched her mouth. Although most of the ingested radium was subse-quently excreted, some was absorbed into the bloodstream and eventually accumulated in the bones where it constituted a chronic source of internal radiation exposure. Knowing little about the properties of radium themselves, the women were reassured by management that the substance with which they were working was quite harmless. In the Ottawa plant one worker interviewed years later recalled a supervisor telling her that radium would "put a glow in our cheeks"! Since radium in those years also was being marketed for medicinal use, such statements were readily believed. Unfortunately, they were untrue.

In 1922, a young New Jersey woman who had worked at U.S. Radium for only three years became the first dial-painter to die of radium poisoning; by then several of her coworkers were gravely ill and within a few years they were dead also. Each of these early deaths involved necrosis of the jawbone, followed by rampant infections that proved uncontrollable in that pre-antibiotic era. Several died of anemia, while other women experienced debilitating weakening of their bones, often resulting in arms or legs breaking from even modest pressure. The largest number of dial-painter fatalities, however, was due to bone cancer or multiple myelomas, which began to appear in the late 1920s. Word of the mysterious ailments plaguing their coworkers began to spread among dial-painters who were increasingly convinced they were confronting a new occupational disease. By 1925, after the death of a 21-year-old employee at the Waterbury plant, managers instituted a ban on lip-pointing, even though the company never officially acknowledged radium as the cause of this tragedy. With definitive scientific proof still lacking, neither industry, government regulators, nor medical researchers were ready to concede that radium was the culprit causing the health problems that were now appearing with increasing frequency.

By 1927, however, the mounting evidence could no longer be ignored; in that year a physiologist hired by industry to refute evidence of radium's harmful effects came to the conclusion that "radium is partially if not the primary cause of the pathological condition described." While the radium industry, much like modern-day tobacco company spokespersons, continued to deny any adverse health effects associated with its product, the medical and scientific community at last recognized radium as a major occupational hazard. With this acknowledgment, the focus of attention shifted to that of winning financial compensation for dying workers and their families. By contemporary standards, such compensation was surprisingly meager. In general, the dial-painters who were affected the worst and the earliest received most of the money awarded; many victims were given nothing at all. While records indicate that altogether 84 dial-painters died of radium-induced cancer and an undetermined but smaller number perished from jaw necrosis or anemia, compensation was awarded to just 13 women in Illinois, 16 in Connecticut, and 10 or 11 in New Jersey. The highest amount received was $5,700; most awards were for considerably lower sums.

During the 1920s, as the women desperately sought recognition for their plight, they received little support from male-dominated labor organizations; the State Health and Labor Department officials who might logically have been expected to espouse their cause instead supported the politically influential radium industry; scientists and medical researchers likewise tailored their reports to please the corporate sponsors who funded their research or paid their salaries. Nevertheless, publicity surrounding the mounting toll of dying and disabled workers raised general awareness of the problem and eventually resulted in improved worker safety precautions in the dial-painting facilities. The scientific investigations launched in response to an obvious problem gave birth to a new field of study—health physics—and in time yielded the information that formed the basis of health standards for a new generation of industrial workers, scientists, medical personnel, and patients.

Reference

Clark, Claudia. 1997. *Radium Girls: Women and Industrial Health Reform, 1910–1935.* Chapel Hill: Univ. of North Carolina Press.

in the body, and about 10 or more years following exposure (19 years seemed to be the peak period) significant numbers of these now-teenagers or young adults developed thyroid cancer (Norwood, 1980).

One segment of the population at special risk during the early years of work with radiation was the medical community itself, particularly radiologists whose enthusiastic use of their new machines exposed not only their patients but also themselves to large amounts of radiation on a daily basis. A questionnaire sent to all American radiologists in 1928 revealed that a shockingly high percentage of respondents had been unable to father children and the rate of defective births among those who did have offspring was double that considered normal. Radiologists' mortality rates due to cancer, particularly leukemia, were several times higher than those of their colleagues in other areas of medicine, and the gloved or amputated hand became a macabre symbol of the radiologists' profession. Organizers of a 1920 banquet at a radiologists' convention blundered badly by including chicken on the menu because most of the guests present had lost at least one hand and were unable to cut their meat (Kevles, 1997).

Observations of radiation-induced health problems such as those just described led to extensive research into safer methods of utilizing this valuable but dangerous tool. Since the early 1940s, improvements in equipment design and increasingly stringent standards relating to allowable exposure have significantly reduced the incidence of overt cases of radiation damage. Nevertheless, concerns regarding unnecessary use of X-rays for diagnostic purposes and new understanding regarding long-term effects of low-level exposure require that individuals must be alert to the dangers implicit in any degree of radiation exposure and take an active role in deciding whether such exposure is justified.

A child looks through a fluoroscopy machine at a shoe store to see if his shoes fit. This and other ill-advised practices were gradually discontinued as the deleterious health effects of radiation exposure became known. [*FDA Consumer*]

Types of Ionizing Radiation

Although any exposure to ionizing radiation is potentially dangerous, the degree and nature of harm varies depending on the type of radiation involved. Early studies of radioactivity revealed that ionizing radiation comprises several different types of emissions, the most biologically significant of which include the following.

Alpha particles. Basically helium nuclei consisting of two protons and two neutrons, alpha particles are relatively massive particles that are the most energetic type of radiation, yet are the least penetrating. Such flimsy barriers as a sheet of paper, clothing, or even human skin can stop them. The greatest threat to health involving alpha radiation occurs when alpha-emitting particles (e.g., plutonium, radium, radon) are inhaled, ingested with food or water, or taken into the body through a cut or wound. Once in contact with delicate internal tissues, alpha radiation can cause intense damage within a localized area. Theoretical projections of large numbers of lung cancer deaths following a nuclear power plant meltdown are based on assumptions of pulmonary damage caused by inhalation of alpha-emitting plutonium dust.

Figure 10-2   Penetrating Power of Alpha and Beta Particles and Gamma Rays

Radiation Source

Alpha Particles

Stopped by a
piece of paper

Beta Particles

Stopped by a layer of clothing
or by a few millimeters of a
substance such as aluminum

Gamma Rays

Stopped by several
feet of concrete
or a few inches of lead

Organic
tissue

Source: Environmental Protection Agency.

Beta particles.   Consisting of single electrons, beta particles are more penetrating than alphas, capable of passing through the skin to a depth of about a half-inch. Like alphas, however, they are most dangerous when ingested. Since several beta emitters (e.g., strontium-90, iodine-131) are chemically similar to naturally occurring bodily constituents, they may substitute for those elements and concentrate in living tissues (e.g., bones, thyroid), where they continue to emit radiation for an extended period of time, increasing the risk of cancer or mutations. Most fission products in spent fuel rods or in reprocessed nuclear wastes are beta-emitters.

Gamma rays.   These are the most penetrating form of ionizing radiation and generally accompany beta radiation. Shielding with a dense material such as lead is necessary to prevent gamma radiation from penetrating the body and harming vital organs. Short-lived beta emitters such as krypton-85 generally exhibit the highest levels of gamma radiation.

X-rays.   Though slightly less penetrating, X-rays have basically the same characteristics as gamma rays.

Dosage

Since ionizing radiation can neither be seen nor felt, human exposure is measured in terms of the amount of tissue damage it causes. Under the International System of Units, the term **gray (Gy)** is the unit of absorbed dose, used to quantify the amount of energy from ionizing radiation absorbed per unit mass of material (the gray is replacing the term "rad" which is still in temporary use; a gray is equivalent to 100 rads). The most common unit for measuring effective radiation dose in humans, however, is the **sievert (Sv),** a figure obtained by multiplying the absorbed dose in grays by a factor called the **relative biological effectiveness (RBE).** This measurement reflects the fact that the health impact of radiation depends not only on the amount of energy absorbed, but also on the form of that energy. For example, X-rays and gamma rays that pass through tissue striking only occasional molecules along their path have an RBE of 1; beta particles have RBEs ranging from 1 to 5, depending on their energy level, while the relatively massive alpha particles have an RBE of 10, indicating their greater potential to damage living tissue. For practical purposes, human radiation exposure standards are set in terms of **millisieverts (mSv),** an amount one-thousandth of a sievert, since these represent levels of exposure most commonly encountered by the average individual. Just as the gray is a relatively new term for what formerly was called the rad, sieverts and millisieverts are gradually replacing units, still used in many references, called "rems" and "millirems" (mrem). Under the new system a sievert is equivalent to 100 rems. The average amount of whole-body radiation exposure for a person in the U.S. from all sources is estimated to be 3.6 mSv (360 mrem) a year or 0.01 mSv (1 mrem) per day.

There is little evidence that present average levels of exposure to ionizing radiation are having any adverse effect on the health of the general public. It is well known, however, that higher doses can be extremely injurious to living tissues. Types of radiation-induced biological damage include mutations, birth defects, impairment of fertility, leukemia and other forms of cancer, infections, hemorrhage, cataracts, and reduced lifespan. Humans, and mammals in general, are far more sensitive to ionizing radiation than are lower forms of life. The same degree of damage that a dose of 0.5 Sv (50 rems) can cause in a mammalian cell requires 1,000 Sv (100,000 rems) exposure in an amoeba or 3,000 Sv (300,000 rems) in a paramecium. The frequent reference in horror films to cockroaches inheriting the earth in the aftermath of all-out nuclear war is reflective of the fact that insects also have a very high level of tolerance to ionizing radiation.

Dose **rate,** the quantity of radiation received within a given unit of time, is thought to be very significant in determining the extent of tissue damage incurred, perhaps even more important than total dose. The prevailing view holds that radiation absorbed over an extended period is less harmful than the same amount delivered during a brief time span, due to the existence of bodily repair mechanisms. Furthermore, not only does the risk of damage (e.g., cancer) fall as the dose rate is decreased, but also the latency period becomes longer (Goldman, 1996). A contrary conclusion has been advanced by two noted British epidemiologists who argue that, at least in relation to carcinogenesis, numerous small doses of radiation exposure are *more* likely to induce cancer than is a single large dose. Basing their conclusions on a study of health records of 35,000 nuclear bomb production workers at the federal government's Hanford Reservation in Richland, Washington, these researchers hypothesize that large doses of radiation *kill* cells, while smaller doses simply *damage* the genetic material, giving rise to mutations that increase the likelihood of cancer (Kneale and Stewart, 1993).

High-Level vs. Low-Level Radiation Exposure

Health effects of ionizing radiation can be subdivided into those types of damage caused by high-level and low-level exposure, respectively. **High-level radiation exposure** is defined as a whole-body dose of 1 Sv (100 rems) or more, delivered within a relatively short period of time—minutes or hours. As soon as a few hours after exposure or as long as several weeks later, people receiving a dose of high-level radiation begin to exhibit obvious symptoms of radiation sickness, ranging in severity from nausea, vomiting, or hair loss to bloody diarrhea, convulsive seizures, and death. These effects are referred to as "deterministic," a term used to describe effects observed only after a threshold level of exposure has been exceeded and whose severity is directly proportional to the dosage received (Hall, 2000). Levels of ionizing radiation capable of inducing the above-mentioned effects would most likely occur only in such extreme situations as a nuclear bomb explosion, a nuclear power plant meltdown, or in severe industrial accidents involving mishandling of radioactive materials. Such effects are

Box 10-2   Half-Life

Not all radioisotopes are dangerous for the same length of time. Each radioactive element is characterized by its own unique half-life (T$\frac{1}{2}$)—a period of time during which half of the amount originally present, undergoing radioactive decay, is transformed into something else. The concept of half-life, in essence, is the reverse of exponential growth. Assume, for example, that one has a gram of cesium-137 whose half-life is 30 years. After 30 years there would remain $\frac{1}{2}$ gram of cesium-137 and $\frac{1}{2}$ gram of cesium's nonradioactive daughter product, barium-137; the radiation now being emitted is only half the original value. After 60 years the radioactivity would be only $\frac{1}{4}$ the original amount; in 90 years $\frac{1}{8}$ the original value, and so on.

Obviously the term half-life is not synonymous with safety—$\frac{1}{2}$ gram of cesium-137 still presents a hazard. Indeed, highly radioactive substances may have to go through 10 or more half-lives (i.e., 300 years in the case of cesium) before their level of radioactivity is low enough to pose no significant health threat. However, the half-life concept has considerable relevance in assessing relative hazards and in devising waste management strategies.

Isotopes with very short half-lives are intensely radioactive initially; that is, they are experiencing a very high number of disintegrations at any one point in time. However, within a few days or weeks they go through so many half-lives that they no longer present a significant risk. The best management strategy for such wastes is simply to isolate them from human contact during the brief period when they are dangerous. Isotopes with extremely long half-lives will be radioactive virtually forever, but the level of emissions at any one point in time is relatively low; one can briefly handle a piece of long-lived uranium or thorium ore with little concern for radiation injury. The most difficult management problems involve those isotopes with intermediate-length half-lives, elements such as plutonium which, with a half-life of 24,000 years, remains hazardous for hundreds of thousands of years. Human contact with such radioisotopes must be accompanied by stringent safety precautions and ultimate disposal of such material must be carried out in such a way that it remains isolated from the general environment for extremely long periods of time.

Some representative half-lives

Element	Half-life
Radon-222	3.8 days
Iodine-131	8.1 days
Phosphorus-32	14 days
Krypton-85	11 years
Tritium	12 years
Strontium-90	29 years
Cesium-137	30 years
Radium-226	1,600 years
Carbon-14	5,800 years
Plutonium-239	24,000 years
Uranium-235	710,000,000 years
Thorium-232	14,000,000,000 years

largely reflective of cell death which, if extensive, can be fatal to the organism. Human effects of high-level exposure have been determined from studies of victims of the Hiroshima-Nagasaki atomic bomb explosions, from experience with radiation therapy, and from observations of the results of nuclear accident victims. The 135,000 unfortunate Ukrainians and Byelorussians exposed to large amounts of radioactive debris resulting from the 1986 disaster at Chernobyl constitute a particularly valuable study group for radiation biologists because the radiation doses they received were measured at the time of the accident, unlike the wartime situation in Japan where exposures were estimated after the event. As one British radiation specialist remarked, "The human experiment has now been done. At last we can test our hypotheses" (Hawkes et al., 1987).

Low-level radiation exposure, encompassing dosage levels below 1 Sv (100 rems), seldom results in immediately apparent health damage. It can, however, produce "stochastic" effects—problems whose ultimate severity (e.g., death due to cancer) is not related to dosage received but whose likelihood of occurring at all increases with increasing dose. It is assumed for purposes of regulation that there is no threshold for stochastic effects, although, as will be explained shortly, that assumption is no longer universally held. Because of its potential to *damage* the cell rather than to kill it outright, low-level radiation has the potential to induce mutations, congenital abnormalities, and cancer. Since almost everyone experiences low-level exposure at one time or another, the human health effects of low doses of radiation have been a prime focus of radiation research for many years.

Radiation-Induced Mutations

Exposure even to very low levels of ionizing radiation can result in gene mutations; indeed, experiments to date indicate that there is no threshold level below which no mutations would be expected (however, at very low levels of exposure the mutation rate will correspondingly be quite low). There is, rather, a direct linear relationship between increasing radiation dosage and an increased number of mutations, either at the gene or chromosomal level. Both diagnostic X-rays and radioactive isotopes used for treating various ailments have been shown to damage chromosomes. Nuclear power plant workers and medical personnel, particularly radiotherapy nurses, who receive small doses of radiation on a daily basis have been shown to exhibit a marked increase in the frequency of mutations in their chromosomes (these can be observed as breaks or changes in chromosome number when chromosome smears are made from a sampling of white blood cells). The number of such abnormalities is generally highest among individuals who have been occupationally exposed to radiation for a number of years, indicating that the damaging effects of radiation exposure are cumulative.

Of greatest concern from a genetic standpoint, of course, are the mutations that accumulate in the gonadal cells, which are the precursors of eggs and sperm. The number of new mutations that an individual passes on to his or her children depends on the amount of radiation the sex organs have absorbed from the time of conception up to the moment each of his or her children are conceived. Most radiation-induced mutations are recessive; hence even though most are of a harmful nature, they are likely to persist in the human gene pool, increasing in frequency over several generations before carriers of the recessive gene mate, producing offspring who exhibit the mutant characteristic. Studies recently conducted on populations living downwind from the former Soviet Union's nuclear bomb test site at Semipalatinsk in Kazakhstan found that more than half the children of parents exposed to radioactive fallout during the early 1950s exhibit germline mutations—clear evidence that genetic damage caused by radiation can be passed on from one generation to the next (Dubrova et al., 2002).

In addition to inducing mutations in sex cells, X-ray exposure also has been shown to be capable of causing chromosomal damage in developing fetuses. Because the majority of such instances involved diagnostic X-rays of women in the very early stages of pregnancy who were not yet aware of their condition, it is now recommended that irradiation of reproductive-age women be limited to the first ten days after the onset of their last menstrual cycle to prevent exposure of an unsuspected embryo. Males and females alike should insist on being provided with a gonadal shield (e.g., lead apron) to reduce the risk of sex-cell mutations whenever X-rays are administered.

Radiation and Birth Defects

Laboratory experiments with animals, as well as direct observations of unintended consequences of humans exposed to ionizing radiation during fetal or embry-

Box 10-3 "Loose Nukes" and "Dirty Bombs"

Of all the security threats confronting the United States, none is more nightmarish than the prospect of a terrorist group exploding a nuclear device in the middle of a large American city. In what later proved to be a false alarm, warnings in October 2001 that Al Qaeda operatives inside the U.S. possessed a 10-kiloton weapon prompted alarming calculations of the damage a bomb that size could wreak. Easily transportable in an ordinary passenger vehicle, a 10-kiloton nuclear bomb, upon detonation, would vaporize everything within a radius of one-third mile; beyond that point to three-quarters of a mile away, buildings would be reduced to rubble; raging fires and massive levels of ionizing radiation would extend in a third circle out to 1½ miles from ground zero. Hundreds of thousands of people would be killed within minutes by collapsing buildings and fires. Within days many more would perish of radiation sickness. The blast-generated electromagnetic pulse would wipe out all forms of electronic communication and the ability of rescue personnel and medical facilities to deal with such a crisis would be overwhelmed. Over the long term, survivors would have to be evacuated and resettled, since the resulting radioactive contamination of the area would render it uninhabitable for years to come. And evacuation of the survivors wouldn't end their suffering—tens of thousands would inevitably die prematurely due to radiation-induced cancer.

Though most of us find it hard to imagine such a catastrophe actually occurring, a number of nuclear antiterrorism experts reluctantly conclude that "it's not a matter of *if*; it's a matter of *when*." Their pessimism stems from a realization of how many unsecured sources of weapons-grade material exist around the world (Russia, Pakistan, and North Korea constitute particularly worrisome potential sources) and how readily available, both on the Internet and in libraries, is the information necessary for any reasonably intelligent person to build a nuclear bomb.

Once obtained, there are numerous ways in which a bomb or nuclear material could be smuggled into the country and transported to its intended target. Many terrorism experts suggest that the most likely method would be to pack it inside one of the approximately 20,000 shipping containers that arrive at U.S. ports every day—fewer than one in 20 of which is inspected upon arrival. Another option might be airfreight, courtesy of FedEx or UPS. With less than 10% of air cargo on passenger and all-cargo flights subject to screening, the chances of a concealed bomb being detected are not great. Nuclear weapons inside shipping containers also could enter the U.S. by truck at one of approximately 300 crossing points along the 4,000-mile land border with Canada or the 2,000-mile Mexican border. Here again, chances of detection are slight; by land, sea, or air, incoming shipments on commercial carriers have about a 5% chance of being inspected—rather good odds for a terrorist. Of course other options exist in addition to commercial carriers. As criminal smugglers of drugs and illegal immigrants well know, there are many places to sneak across U.S. borders on land; backpacks can easily carry enough plutonium for making a bomb. Similarly, thousands of miles of unguarded coastline offer ample opportunity for small boats to bring deadly cargo ashore, even in full public view, since Customs officials routinely inspect fewer than 10% of noncommercial private vessels.

Although acquisition and detonation of a small nuclear bomb represents the ultimate horror, obtaining enough fissile material to make one could present some difficulties. For this reason, terrorists seeking to use radiation as a weapon might opt instead for a **radiological dispersion device (RDD)**, popularly referred to as a "dirty bomb." Designed to scatter radioactive materials throughout a localized area without a nuclear explosion, dirty bombs could take one of several forms. The simplest, and perhaps the most likely, might consist merely of several sticks of dynamite packaged with a small amount of radioactive material such as cesium-137; it could also take the form of a large truck packed with a fertilizer-based explosive wrapped in cobalt-60. In both cases, detonation of the explosive would pulverize the radioactive material, dispersing it into the surrounding environment.

With this type of dirty bomb, the explosion itself would announce the terrorist attack, prompting a rapid evacuation of the area and thus limiting human exposure to the radioactive materials released. A more stealthy approach—and one likely to result in higher casualties—would be the nonexplosive release of certain radioactive isotopes via burning, vaporization, or by dissolving them in a solvent and spraying the liquid around an area. The threat represented by the latter tactic would be less immediately obvious, so widespread radiation exposure could occur before the danger was recognized.

Unfortunately, the ingredients for a dirty bomb are much easier to obtain than are the plutonium or highly enriched uranium needed to build a nuclear device; approximately 2 million sealed radiation sources exist in the United States alone. The radioactive isotopes whose physical properties render them capable of causing immense harm (e.g., cesium-137, cobalt-60, strontium-90, radium-226, iridium-192) are used for a wide range of medical, industrial, and commercial purposes and are readily and legally available. They also can be stolen or simply scavenged when equipment containing radioactive sources is carelessly discarded. Many experts fear that lax monitoring and inadequate regulatory controls of these materials poses a serious threat, both to public health and national security, since there is little to prevent a determined terrorist from accessing such widespread, carelessly guarded sources. The General Accounting Office (GAO) reported more than 1,300 incidents between 1998–2002 in which sealed radioactive sources in the U.S. were abandoned, lost, or stolen; it's doubtful whether the record in more than 100 other countries utilizing such materials is any better. The International Atomic Energy Agency reported 27 sources of cesium-137 disappearing in Croatia during the war in the Balkans in the mid-1990s; in 2003 after the U.S. invasion of Iraq, cobalt and cesium sources were stolen from a nuclear research center south of Baghdad. Numerous "orphaned" materials in regions of the world plagued by war, civil unrest, or organized crime constitute additional potential sources of supply for terrorists wanting to fashion a dirty bomb.

The closest the world has come yet to a RDD attack occurred in 1995 when Chechen separatists called a Russian television station to say they had placed a radiological weapon containing dynamite and cesium-137 in a Moscow park. Although they didn't detonate their crude bomb, the act vividly demonstrated the capability of a dedicated terrorist organization to wreak havoc in the heart of their enemy's largest city. It was once assumed that such groups would be deterred from making a large RDD because, in doing so, those involved would themselves receive a lethal dose of radiation. Such assumptions no longer appear valid, given the willingness of many terrorists to sacrifice their own lives for their cause.

While a dirty bomb attack would cause far fewer human deaths and radiation-induced cancers than a nuclear explosion, it would have a devastating economic and psychological impact on the affected area. Several variables, including the size of the bomb, the type of radioactive material used, and whether the release occurs within a confined space or in the open air, can affect the number of casualties and the subsequent extent of radioactive contamination. The largest number of deaths, if any, is likely to be caused by the blast itself, not by the ensuing radiation exposure. Those who survive the initial explosion presumably would flee the affected area quickly enough to escape damaging doses of external radiation exposure. If they subsequently wash their bodies, hair, and clothing thoroughly, their chances of developing health problems related to radiation exposure are minimal.

A far greater threat than external exposure is the possibility of internal contamination if radioactive particles are inhaled (as could occur if large amounts of dust are generated) or ingested. Individuals who experience internal exposure themselves become radioactive, their body wastes and everything they contact becoming contaminated. People ministering to their needs must take special precautions and use shielding to protect themselves from the patient. Long-term elevated cancer risk in the affected region is difficult to predict, but since virtually everyone would be evacuated from areas where contamination levels are excessive and hence would not be subject to prolonged exposure, most health authorities doubt that the few additional radiation-induced cancers that might occur 20 or 30 years later could be identified among the 2,000 out of every 10,000 Americans who die annually of cancer from nonradiation related causes.

Experts estimate that, under the worst circumstances, fatalities due to a radiological dispersion device would number in the tens to hundreds; although such deaths would be tragic to the families involved, the most damaging societal impact of a dirty bomb attack would be economic. Due to the EPA's extremely stringent cleanup standards following a radioactive release (set with small-scale laboratory accidents in mind), after-the-fact decontamination efforts would be enormously expensive, probably requiring the removal of contaminated buildings and soil. Simply finding a location to dispose of enormous volumes of low-level radioactive wastes would pose an immense challenge, given the public's overwhelmingly negative "not in my backyard" response to the siting of such disposal facilities. Economic activities would necessarily be suspended for many months following a dirty bomb attack and large numbers of people would have to be evacuated and resettled, perhaps permanently. Since virtually all insurance policies explicitly exclude radiation damage, losses suffered by businesses or homeowners would not be compensated, imposing great financial hardship on those involved. The fear created by radiological contamination would, in all likelihood, far exceed the actual danger and could severely hamper efforts to revive commerce, tourism, or agriculture in the affected area even after successful cleanup efforts.

Unarguably, the consequences of either a "loose nuke" or "dirty bomb" would be catastrophic and every effort should be made to prevent such an eventuality. Far more could be done to ensure that nuclear weapons and radioactive materials in the former Soviet Union and elsewhere are secured, out of reach to terrorists and criminal gangs. Tighter U.S. border controls, including more stringent inspections of incoming shipping containers, are urgently needed, as are tougher licensing requirements for those legally buying and selling radioactive materials. Serious consideration should be given to increasing the allowable level of residual radiation following cleanup of a dirty bomb attack; doing so would reduce the otherwise astronomical costs of remediation with minimal impact on human health. Finally, civil defense authorities should be much more proactive in providing the public with accurate information about what to do in the event of an attack. In particular, they should educate citizens as to the difference between a nuclear weapon and a dirty bomb, assuring them of the high likelihood of surviving the latter without serious injury and with little additional cancer risk if they avoid panic and evacuate in a timely fashion. If we're lucky, the ultimate nightmare can be avoided, but more vigorous governmental efforts to reduce the odds are overdue.

References

Allison, Graham. 2004. *Nuclear Terrorism: The Ultimate Preventable Catastrophe*. New York: Times Books, Henry Holt.

Zimmerman, Peter D., and Cheryl Loeb. 2004. "Dirty Bombs: The Threat Revisited." *Defense Horizons*, no. 38. Center for Technology and National Security Policy, National Defense University.

onic development, provide ample evidence of radiation's teratogenic effects. The most tragic and widely studied cases of radiation-induced birth defects involve the Japanese children irradiated *in utero* at the time of the atomic bomb explosions over Hiroshima and Nagasaki and of children who received X-ray exposure while still in the womb. While these sources of fetal/embryonic exposure are now, hopefully, relics of the past, other less acute sources of radiation exposure still pose safety concerns. Among these are natural radionuclides (potassium-40, carbon-14, radon and its daughter products) that can be inhaled or ingested by a pregnant woman with food or water. Radioactive fallout products, such as those released after the nuclear power plant explosion at Chernobyl, constitute another potential source of exposure. Occupational activities of the mother could result in exposure of the unborn child if her work involves production, distribution, or use of radiopharmaceuticals or the treatment and handling of patients undergoing nuclear medicine procedures. Similarly, administration of radiopharmaceuticals to pregnant patients for diagnosing or treating health problems may pose a radiation risk to the embryo/fetus (NCRP, 1998).

Sensitivity to radiation is many times greater during fetal development than at any subsequent period of a person's life, since rapid development and differentiation of tissues is occurring during this time (the more actively cells are dividing, the more vulnerable they are to radiation). In terms of *lethal*, as opposed to *teratogenic* effects, the radiosensitivity of the embryo/fetus steadily decreases during the period before birth. However, the nature and extent of fetal injury (i.e., congenital abnormalities as opposed to death) caused by radiation vary widely, depending not only on the dose absorbed but also on the precise stage of development. Because the fetal tissues are constantly growing and differentiating, the developmental response to radiation exposure on any given day may be quite different from what it would have been the day before or the day after. In addition, there are individual genetic differences in sensitivity to radiation that make it unlikely that any two fetuses would respond in precisely the same manner, even when the doses are identical. In general, radiation exposure during the first 10 days after conception will either kill the fetus or, conversely, have no discernible teratogenic effect at all. Exposure during the following period of organ formation (organogenesis), extending through the eighth week of pregnancy, can result in severe malformations. Both the skeletal system and the central nervous system are especially radiosensitive, thus exposure to X-rays or other sources of ionizing radiation can result in babies being born with abnormally small heads (microcephaly), spinal deformities, eye problems, and permanent growth retardation (the latter effect can be produced by exposure at any time during prenatal development but is most pronounced when exposure occurs during organogenesis). After the second month of pregnancy, radiation does not cause major structural defects but can provoke severe mental retardation, since the third and fourth months of pregnancy mark a period of rapid brain development. Studies of Japanese children irradiated at Hiroshima revealed that the period of highest risk for mental retardation from *in utero* exposure is between the 8th and 15th weeks of pregnancy, with another slightly less sensitive period occurring between the 16th and 25th weeks. Late-term radiation exposure has not been linked to structural problems or functional disturbances, but has been shown to increase the risk of developing childhood cancer.

The severity of the effects described increase with increasing radiation dosage; however, the existence of a threshold dose (i.e., a "safe level" of exposure below which no teratogenic effects have been observed) in the range of 0.2 to 0.4 Gy is now generally accepted (Streffer, 1997).

Radiation-Induced Cancer

The potential for health damage as a result of radiation exposure was first recognized in connection with the development of skin cancers among early radiologists, of whom nearly 100 fell victim to this disease within 15 years following the discovery of X-rays. Since then other forms of cancer, most notably leukemia, bone cancer, lung cancer, and thyroid cancer, also have been linked to radiation exposure.

Leukemia is perhaps the classic example of X-ray-induced malignancy. As early as 1911 a report of 11 cases of leukemia among radiation workers suggested a connection between the disease and their occupational exposure. Subsequently, epidemiological studies among radiologists, Japanese survivors of Hiroshima and Nagasaki, patients treated with X-ray therapy, and children who were irradiated in the womb when their mothers received diagnostic X-rays, all confirm the association between exposure to ionizing radiation and the induction of leukemia. Leukemia, like other forms of cancer, is characterized by a latency period following the initial exposure, with development of disease symptoms in this case occurring, on the average, after 5–7 years (some as early as just 2 years after irradiation).

Evidence on the amount of radiation required to induce a malignancy is scarce, particularly at doses less than 0.5 Sv (50 rems). Radiation protection policies since the early 1950s have been based on the assumption that *all* radiation exposure, no matter how low, is harmful; low doses are regarded as having the same effects as high doses, though at a lower rate of incidence (a concept known as the **linear no-threshold theory**). The validity of this belief has been challenged in recent years by a growing body of evidence indicating that an exposure threshold for radiation-induced cancer does, in fact, exist and that, more surprisingly, exposure to very low levels of ionizing radiation may actually reduce the risk of cancer and enhance longevity, a phenomenon known as "hormesis." The scientific rationale for this point of view is that the ability of cells to repair minor genetic damage is stimulated by low-dose radiation, thus increasing the effectiveness of the DNA damage-control biosystem. Proponents of this argument point to the millions of people living in regions of higher-than-normal background radiation (e.g., those areas in India, Brazil, China, Austria, and U.S. described in an earlier section of this chapter) whom several epidemiologic studies have shown to have lower rates of cancer than people living outside those areas. A study conducted in 1993 on Japanese atomic bomb survivors revealed significantly greater longevity among those exposed to radiation than among unexposed Japanese; a 1991 report on U.S. nuclear shipyard workers showed a statistically significant decrease in mortality rates for deaths from all causes among men occupationally exposed to gamma radiation when compared with unexposed workers. These studies suggest to their authors that while there is no question that at doses of 1 Gy or above cancer risk increases with increasing dosage, doses of radiation under 0.2 Gy are not carcinogenic. Indeed, they argue that very low levels of radiation not only present no health threat, but may actually be beneficial (Jaworowski, 1999; Pollycove, 1997).

However, in 2005 the Nuclear and Radiation Studies Board of the National Research Council took issue with such reasoning and, citing data generated over the last 15 years, reaffirmed the linear relationship between radiation exposure and human cancer incidence. According to Board Chairman Richard Monson, "The scientific research base shows that there is no threshold of exposure below which low levels of ionizing radiation can be demonstrated to be harmless or beneficial." Currently, federal standards set 1 mSv/year (100 mR/year), excluding medical exposure, as the upper limit for annual effective dose equivalent for continuous or repeated exposure for members of the general population as a whole, no more than 0.25 mSv (25mR) of which should come from a nuclear power facility. Individuals may receive up to 5 mSv/year (500 mR/year) as the maximum permissible annual effective dose equivalent when exposure is infrequent. Workers in radiation-related occupations are allowed average yearly exposures of 50 mSv (5 rems). People under the age of 18 are permitted no occupational exposure whatsoever (Hall, 2000). Such standards have been set for the intended purpose of protecting human health against the long-term radiation effects of cancer and genetic defects. These standards do not reflect levels of absolute safety but rather attempt to strike a balance between possible adverse effects of low-level exposure and the known benefits of nuclear power and other uses of radioactive materials. In the late 1980s the safety of current exposure limits was called into question by new interpretation of data on exposure received by Japanese survivors at Hiroshima and Nagasaki. Post-war estimates of likely radiation levels at varying distances from ground zero, correlated with observed health effects, have formed the basis for radiation standards since the end of World War II. Results from studies conducted during the 1980s suggested that the original data overestimated the radiation dosage received by people in the affected area. Some researchers now believe that the observable health damage experienced by survivors was caused by approximately one-half the amount of radiation exposure calculated previously. These findings, if correct, imply that current radiation protection standards should be at least twice as stringent as they are now in order to protect public health.

It should be noted that the above-mentioned consequences of low-level radiation exposure may also be manifested at higher rates among survivors of high-level radiation doses. Mutations, birth defects among offspring, a significantly heightened risk of leukemia and other cancers, as well as cataracts and a general shortening of life span due to premature aging, are realistic possibilities confronting individuals who have recovered from overt symptoms of radiation sickness.

Radiation and Nuclear Power Generation

While medical uses of X-rays and radioisotopes constitute by far the largest amount of non-background radiation exposure, it is not these sources but rather the perceived health and safety threat from nuclear power plants that has received the lion's share of public attention in recent years. Since 1957 when the first commercial nuclear power plant in the United States came on line in Shippingsport, Pennsylvania (the world's first civilian nuclear plant opened in 1954 in the former USSR), the percentage of electricity generated by nuclear energy in the United States grew rapidly until the mid-1970s, much more slowly since then. No new commercial nuclear reactors have been ordered by U.S. utility companies since 1978 and construction on the last was completed in 1995. At present, approximately 20% of the electrical energy in the United States is generated by 103 nuclear power plants at 66 locations. Canada ordered the last of its 22 nuclear reactors in 1973 (17 of which were operating in 2005, the remaining 5 undergoing refurbishment), but is considering construction of a new plant in Ontario, possibly by 2008. Although the 40-year licenses of currently operating U.S. plants begin to expire in 2009, by mid-2005 the Nuclear Regulatory Commission had granted 20-year license extensions to 32 plants. With 41 additional plants expected to have their licenses renewed, it appears certain that nuclear power will continue to be an important part of the U.S. energy mix for decades to come. Concerns about global warming caused by fossil-fuel-burning power plants, plus the sharply rising cost of natural gas, are prompting support in some quarters for a new generation of advanced-design nuclear plants to meet future energy needs. Several utilities are considering applying for licenses to build and operate new reactors, but most observers doubt that any plant construction is likely to begin before 2010, if then. Whether society should increase reliance on nuclear power or shift to other energy sources continues to be a subject of intense controversy.

Even before the serious accident in 1979 at the Three Mile Island power plant near Harrisburg, Pennsylvania, and the catastrophe at Chernobyl in the USSR in 1986, concerns about the safety of nuclear power had given rise to an active and vocal antinuclear movement. Internationally, antinuclear groups have become a powerful political force, echoing the "Hell, no, we won't glow!" sentiments of their American colleagues two decades earlier. Following the 1998 national elections in Germany, the victorious coalition of Social Democrats and the environmental activist Green Party promptly initiated a program to close all 19 German nuclear power plants within 10 years, even though these plants accounted for one-third of Germany's electricity. Widespread antinuclear sentiment in western Europe is not echoed, however, in Asia and eastern Europe, where more than 30 nuclear reactors are under construction. In

2004 China had 8 nuclear power plants and expects to build at least 20 more by 2020; industry experts predict that over the coming decade nuclear power generation will grow more rapidly in China than anywhere else in the world (Buckley, 2004). Japan, already reliant on nuclear power from 52 operating plants for almost one-third of its electricity, views the expansion of nuclear power as vital to efforts to reduce the CO_2 emissions that contribute to global climate change. Although public sentiment in Japan against nuclear power has been mounting in recent years, fueled by a series of widely publicized accidents, the government still hopes to build 11 more nuclear plants by 2010 and increase the percentage of electricity produced by nuclear power to 40% (Brooke, 2004). Elsewhere, India, South Korea, Ukraine, Iran, Russia, Slovakia, the Czech Republic, Romania, and Argentina have nuclear reactors under construction.

Nevertheless, in many countries opposition to nuclear power continues to stymie or delay efforts to build new facilities. Arguments by proponents that nuclear power is urgently needed to curb greenhouse gas emissions are discounted by a public concerned about the absence of safe methods for permanent radwaste disposal, aware that "accidents can happen," and harboring a visceral fear of anything labeled "radioactive." Given the emotionalism involved, it is important that citizens clearly understand the extent to which nuclear power generation contributes to the overall radiation burden experienced by the general public. Although most attention is focused on the power plants themselves, nuclear power production is dependent upon a number of activities, collectively referred to as the **nuclear fuel cycle**. The three main components of this cycle, along with their environmental health impacts, are described in the following sections.

Front-end. Prior to the generation of power inside a nuclear reactor, the nuclear fuel itself must be mined, processed, and fabricated into fuel rods. Uranium-235 constitutes the fissionable fuel in most nuclear reactors and is mined in a number of locations around the world, including Australia, Canada, parts of eastern Europe, and several western states in the U.S. In the past, when uranium ore was obtained primarily from underground mines, the most significant radiation hazard was the increased risk of lung cancer among uranium miners, caused by the inhalation of alpha-emitting radon gas and radon daughters (radioactive isotopes of polonium and lead) attached to tiny particles of mine dust. Between 1950–1990, more than 500 miners, the majority of whom were Navajos recruited by the government to work for the nuclear weapons industry but never warned about the known health risks, died of lung cancer resulting from their occupational exposure—a death rate 4–5 times higher than that prevailing among the general population. Similarly, at least 20,000 East German miners, mobilized in the late 1940s and early 1950s to supply uranium for the former Soviet Union's nuclear arsenal, have died or are dying of lung diseases caused by their exposure to radioactive gases and dust (Kahn, 1993). Open-pit uranium mining avoids the occupational health risks entailed by underground mining; however, like stripmining for coal, it is environmentally disruptive and often results in soil erosion and contaminated runoff.

The uranium ore extracted from underground or open-pit mines must subsequently be crushed and processed to produce the form of uranium dioxide known as "yellowcake." These milling operations and the enormous piles of sandlike tailings they create (for every ounce of uranium extracted from ore, 99 ounces of waste tailings are generated) constitute by far the most significant source of public exposure to ionizing radiation related to nuclear power production. In the United States, more than 140 million tons of radioactive tailings were left at abandoned mill sites scattered across seven western states, releasing radon into the air and leaching radium into the subsoil. In 1979, the rupture of an earthen dam at a uranium mine and mill site near Churchrock, New Mexico, released 1,100 tons of tailings sludge and 90 million gallons of radioactively contaminated water into a stream running through the Navajo reservation. Considered the worst radwaste spill ever to occur in the United States, this accident resulted in traces of radioactive materials being carried at least 75 miles downstream across the Arizona border. In Grand Junction, Colorado, mine tailings were incorporated into concrete that was used for foundations of homes, churches, and schools. For nearly 20 years until the problem was recognized, approximately 30,000 people living in those dwellings were exposed to levels of radon up to seven times the maximum allowable level for uranium miners; subsequent cleanup efforts at the Grand Junction mill site and over 4,000 nearby properties cost the government close to $700 million. A number of other western communities, including Denver and Salt Lake City, also have used radioactive tailings in constructing roads and the foundations of buildings. Because of the radiation hazards posed by mill tailings (radiation levels 40–400 times above normal background levels), Congress in 1978 passed legislation authorizing the U.S. Department of Energy to remediate 50 uranium-processing sites, as well as nearby contaminated properties. While a number of mills were still active in 1978 when the law was passed, all are now closed and cleanup of surface contamination has been completed. In most cases site remediation involved enclosing the tailings in a containment cell, covering the cell with compacted clay to prevent the release of radon, and, finally, topping the area with vegetation or rocks. Cleanup of contaminated groundwater at these sites is ongoing and isn't expected to be finished until at least 2014 (Steinhardt, 1996).

Similar environmental problems associated with uranium milling operations continue to plague a number of European countries. In eastern Germany, Hungary, and the Czech Republic, large areas are today littered with abandoned piles of uranium tailings and other radioactive wastes, confronting the leaders of those countries with massive cleanup challenges.

Today almost all production of uranium in the United States, and in many places elsewhere in the world, utilizes an extraction process called **in-situ leaching (ISL)**. ISL is a closed-loop mining system whereby uranium is dissolved in place by a leaching agent—usually sulfuric acid—that is injected into the ore deposit, with the liquid subsequently being pumped to the surface where the uranium is recovered out of solution. After processing, the fluid is returned to the well field to continue the leaching cycle. Unlike underground or open-pit mining, ISL methods eliminate worker exposure to radioactive gases, minimize surface disruption, and produce no tailings whatsoever; the only surface wastes associated with the process are small evaporation ponds. Nevertheless, while in-situ leaching is often described by advocates as an "environmentally benign" method of mining uranium, it isn't problem-free. The injection of massive amounts of acid into rock deposits can result in extensive groundwater contamination if proper precautions aren't followed. At an in-situ leaching site that has been operating for more than 25 years in the Czech Republic, highly contaminated liquids have migrated from the leaching zone, seeping along faulty wells to an upper-level aquifer. As a result of this, some 76 million cubic meters of drinking water in northern Bohemia's largest aquifer are now polluted (Perera, 1997).

Transforming the milled yellowcake into nuclear fuel requires several additional steps. First, the uranium is converted into gaseous uranium hexafluoride, then enriched to increase the concentration of the fissionable U-235 isotope from its original 0.7% (the bulk of uranium ore is U-238, a nonfissionable isotope) to 2–4%, the level necessary to sustain a fission reaction. Finally, at a fuel fabrication facility, the enriched uranium hexafluoride gas is converted into solid uranium dioxide pellets that are then loaded into fuel rods. Cumulatively, these processes have very minimal environmental health impacts, entailing the venting of small, regulated quantities of radioactive emissions into the air and very limited discharges of diluted liquid wastes; occupational exposure among workers in the plants where these activities are carried out likewise is very low.

In summary, the front-end of the nuclear fuel cycle is characterized by relatively low levels of radioactive emissions and minimal public exposure to radiation, the major exception to this being those people living in the vicinity of improperly managed uranium mill tailings and the unfortunate uranium miners whose untimely deaths due to lung cancer can be attributed largely to their workplace exposure to radioactive gases in underground mines.

Power production. Under normal operating conditions, radiation exposure to the general public emanating from nuclear power plants comes primarily from the deliberate release of controlled amounts of radioactive gases to the atmosphere. Gaseous fission products such as tritium and krypton build up in the fuel rods, leak through the cladding into the reactor building, and must be periodically vented. In addition, small amounts of radioactive materials may be discharged with wastewaters. Overall, the radiation hazard to people living in the vicinity of a normally operating nuclear reactor is minimal, considerably less than that from natural background sources.

The main fear among those opposed to further reliance on nuclear power, of course, is the potential, however remote, of catastrophic release of radioactive materials should a major accident occur. Although most people today realize that it is physically impossible for a nuclear power plant to explode like a bomb (for this to occur the U-235 fuel would have to be enriched to a concentration far above the level necessary to sustain a fission reaction for power production purposes), a **core meltdown,** which represents a worst-type accident scenario, would be nearly as devastating. Overheating of the reactor core, such as might occur if water should cease to circulate among the fuel rods (a "loss-of-coolant" accident), could result in melting of the fuel rods and breaching of the containment vessel. The massive release of highly radioactive isotopes into the atmosphere, such as occurred at Chernobyl, or into groundwater supplies could cause widespread human exposure to lethal doses of radiation, contamination of the general environment with radioactive fallout, and would initiate numerous leukemias and other cancers that would be manifested years later. Although

Box 10-4   Aftermath of Chernobyl

Two decades after the name "Chernobyl" became an internationally recognized synonym for nuclear catastrophe, the full impact of that disaster remains a subject of research and controversy. What *is* clear, however, is that the death tally of 31 persons killed in the explosion, as initially reported by Soviet authorities in the weeks following the accident and still recognized as the official figure by certain international organizations, grossly understates the accident's true human health and environmental toll.

When reactor #4 of the nuclear power complex near the Ukrainian town of Cher-nobyl experienced a steam explosion and core meltdown on April 26, 1986, the resulting massive release of radioactive materials contaminated the environment with fallout equivalent to that of a hundred Hiroshima-type bombs. The graphite core of the reactor burned uncontrollably for nine days in spite of heroic efforts by firefighters to quench the blaze and prevent its spread to the three nearby reactors. Of the 31 fatalities attributed to the accident by Soviet officials, 28 were among these men who knowingly braved lethal doses of radiation, standing their ground even as their boots stuck to the melting tar of the reactor roof.

By this time the radioactive plume rising from the stricken reactor had spread over much of Europe. Due to the wind direction at the time of the accident, approximately 70% of the radioactive fallout from Chernobyl was deposited in the neighboring republic of Belarus, where 21% of the national territory remains contaminated nearly 20 years later. Significant fallout also affected northern Ukraine in the area surrounding Chernobyl, as well as in nearby regions of Russia.

Evacuation of the population living in the vicinity of Chernobyl was delayed for about 36 hours following the explosion due to administrative confusion and indecision, but eventually resulted in the permanent relocation of about 135,000 people from within a 19-mile (30 km) radius of the plant. The evacuated region, officially designated as the "Scientific Exclusion Zone" (but commonly referred to as the "Dead Zone"), now constitutes a living laboratory where scientists can study the long-term ecological effects of radioactive contamination on biotic communities.

Ukrainians and Belarussians also are subjects of interest to researchers, human "guinea pigs" whose incidence rates of cancer and other radiation-related illnesses will be studied for years to come. Government agencies in Russia, Ukraine, and Belarus cite 25,000 post-accident deaths among the 800,000 "liquidators" who participated in cleanup operations following the explosion; a committee representing members of this group put the figure as high as 100,000. Other observers dispute the contention that these deaths were a direct result of radiation exposure, saying most were caused by diseases the victims' bodies could no longer control because their immune systems had been weakened by radiation. In Ukraine alone, approximately 2.4 million people, including some 640,000 children, continue to live in areas regarded as contaminated, thus the eventual human health toll from radiation exposure will be considerable (amazingly, at least 800 people, most of them elderly villagers, have now moved back into their homes in the "Dead Zone," in spite of official prohibitions on doing so).

It is known that many of the liquidators, as well as surviving workers at the power plant, received high radiation doses. Workers who suffered symptoms of radiation sickness such as hair loss or skin lesions have since recovered. Nevertheless, although the death rate among those who received high doses of radiation is currently no higher than that of the general population, they tend to get sick almost three times as often and experience the sorts of illnesses usually associated with old age before they reach 45. Medical authorities in Belarus and Ukraine fear that over the next 20–30 years they may see an upsurge in urogenital, lung, and stomach cancer among the liquidators and other male inhabitants of severely contaminated regions. An increase in breast cancer already has been acknowledged in the highly contaminated area around the Belarussian city of Gomel, where the number of cases doubled between 1989–1999.

Thyroid cancer rates also have soared in contaminated areas. Of all the documented health problems associated with radiation exposure at Chernobyl, the dramatic upswing in thyroid malignancies, particularly among children, is the most significant. As cattle grazed on pasturelands contaminated by radioactive fallout during the weeks immediately following the accident, iodine-131 traveled via milk to children's thyroid glands where it concentrated to levels 100 times higher than in other tissues. Youthful thyroid glands are 25 times more sensitive to radioactive iodine than are those of adults and within four years of the disaster, cases of childhood thyroid cancer began to be reported with increasing frequency. The Gomel area exhibits the greatest increase in childhood thyroid cancers, with over 50% of its victims under the age of 5 at the time of the accident. The World Health Organization predicts that fully one-third of Gomel area residents who were 0–4 years old in 1986 will contract thyroid cancer at some point during their lifetime. Nor is Gomel the only region affected; several UN agencies cite a dramatic rise in thyroid cancer among children in Ukraine also. Adult cases are increasing as well; in 2004 a British researcher documented a 12-fold increase in thyroid cancer among adult women in Belarus. Although thyroid cancer is generally curable, the cases now occurring as a result of the Chernobyl accident represent an atypically aggressive form of the disease, with metastasis frequently occurring even in the early stages. In a large number of cases, nearby lymph nodes have been affected and in a small minority of cases the malignancy has spread to other organs. The unfortunate victims have to undergo regular checkups at special clinics and will be on medication throughout their lives.

The environmental and economic costs of the Chernobyl tragedy are mounting as well. Extensive areas of agricultural and forest lands have been heavily contaminated by radioactive fallout; relatively immobile and with a 30-year half-life, cesium-137 is especially problematic because it will persist near the soil surface in the root zone of plants for many decades to come. Radioactive contamination of forest plants utilized by villagers for food raises serious public health concerns. In Belarus, wild mushrooms have long been a national dish, and even though fallout contaminated mushrooms in half the country, villagers continue to collect and eat them. Cattle and goats bioaccumulate radioactive isotopes present on pasture grasses and incorporate these materials into milk and meat, while fish from contaminated lake waters present yet another source of dietary radiation exposure. Close to 30% of Ukraine's entire annual budget is spent on problems relating to Chernobyl—significantly more than it spends on health, education, or culture. The financial impact on Belarus has been equally severe—one expert estimates that in the years since the accident, Belarus' economic losses have been ten times greater than the country's annual budget.

Unfortunately, there's no end in sight to Ukraine's Chernobyl-related problems. Perhaps most urgent, the damaged reactor continues to pose serious health and environmental threats. The concrete "sarcophagus" built immediately after the accident to contain further radioactive releases from the molten core was hastily constructed without a structural margin of safety. Experts fear that the sarcophagus, which has already developed hundreds of dangerous cracks, could collapse if overburdened with heavy snow—a disquieting prospect, since engineers have confirmed the presence of some 34 tons of radioactive dust within the sarcophagus. Adding to concerns is the fact that the basement of the sarcophagus is flooded with about 3,000 cubic meters of radioactively contaminated water, due to infiltration of precipitation and routine spraying for dust suppression. There are fears that this water has the potential to contaminate groundwater, the level of which has been rising under the reactor since 1993. Pollution of groundwater in the vicinity is made even more problematic by the existence of large amounts of intensely radioactive wastes buried in shallow trenches on plant grounds and at various locations within the exclusion zone. These hastily constructed burial trenches are situated just 4 meters above the water table and lack waterproof barriers. Inside the sarcophagus, high humidity and standing water are dissolving fission products in the radioactive debris, causing it to crumble and leading to fears that a burst of neutrons (a "criticality incident") could result due to the increasing concentration of fission products.

Acknowledging that the damaged reactor was in desperate need of repair and that outside help was needed, in 1997 the Group of Seven (G7) industrialized countries, plus Russia, the European Union, and Ukraine launched the Shelter Implementation Plan—a project to build a new 20,000 ton structure to enclose the existing sarcophagus. Intended to provide safe confinement of the radioactive materials still inside the damaged reactor for at least 100 years, the new shelter is scheduled for completion in 2008. In the meantime, officials in Russia and Ukraine continue to argue publicly about the condition of the deteriorating sarcophagus, with Russia's top atomic energy official warning that the sarcophagus is in serious danger of collapse while Ukrainian officials insist the problem is under control. Regrettably, Chernobyl's lethal legacy of health and environmental threats will continue to bedevil policymakers, scientists, and the medical community for decades to come.

References

Bradley, Don J. 1997. *Behind The Nuclear Curtain: Radioactive Waste Management in the Former Soviet Union*. Columbus, OH: Battelle Press.

Dobson, Roger. 2004. "Thyroid Cancer Has Increased 12-Fold in Women since Chernobyl." *British Medical Journal* 328, no. 1394 (June 12).

A core meltdown in reactor #4 at the nuclear facility in Chernobyl, Ukraine, in 1986 resulted in a fire that burned uncontrollably for days and released massive amounts of radioactive materials. [© *Kostin Igor/Corbis Sygma*]

physical destruction of buildings and property would not occur, the biological impact of a core meltdown would be nearly as serious as a bomb blast in terms of human health and environmental degradation. The "defense in depth" concept employed in the construction of nuclear plants, characterized by repeated layers of thick shielding materials and multiple safeguards designed to ensure safety even in the event of partial failure, are intended to prevent this situation from ever becoming a reality.

In spite of such precautions, thousands of mishaps have occurred both here and abroad since the advent of commercial nuclear power. Prior to the Three Mile Island incident, two of the most serious U.S. accidents occurred at the Enrico Fermi experimental fast breeder reactor near Detroit, where part of the fuel in the core melted in early October 1966, and at Browns Ferry, Alabama, where in March 1975, a fire ignited by an electrician's candle raged for seven hours, destroying all the emergency cooling systems in one of the reactors at the complex. In both cases, a core meltdown was only narrowly averted. Each major accident has led to a tightening of safety regulations; no accidents resulting in damage to the reactor core have occurred since the partial meltdown at Three Mile Island in 1979, nor have any offsite releases of large amounts of radioactivity taken place. In recent years the number of "safety-significant events" reported to the Nuclear Regulatory Commission has declined significantly; in 1990 they averaged around two per plant each year, but by 2000 had declined to less than one-tenth that number. The next generation of nuclear reactors should have an even better safety record, since new plant designs incorporate features intended to prevent accidents and to minimize the severity of those that occur (Lake, Bennett, and Kotek, 2002).

The operating record of nuclear power plants in Japan and the countries of western Europe roughly parallels that of the United States. Since the breakup of the former Soviet Union, however, numerous concerns have been raised about the deplorable conditions prevailing at a number of nuclear power plants operating in Russia and several of the former Soviet republics. Russian safety experts, nuclear plant workers, and Western scientists have all concluded that the nuclear power industry throughout the former USSR is on the verge of disaster. The tragic accident at Chernobyl in 1986, initially blamed on violations of operating procedures by plant personnel, is now attributed primarily to fundamental design faults in the reactor itself. This conclusion is worrisome because 11 other reactors of similar design are operating in Russia, two more in Lithuania. These plants, in the view of many experts, are "accidents waiting to happen." Neither the Chernobyl-style reactors nor the older Soviet-version pressurized water reactors are enclosed by the concrete and metal radiation containment structures that are a standard feature of reactor design in other industrial countries (Russian reactors built after 1981 do have full containment structures, however). An inventory of nuclear facilities conducted by Russia's State Committee for Nuclear and Radiation Safety Oversight (Gosatomnadzor) in 1993 revealed that many of the nation's older reactors were in dire need of radical reconstruction due to repeated failures of obsolete or worn-out equipment and system components. Some of these older facilities are characterized by such serious design flaws that Committee members concluded they could never be retrofitted to international standards and urged that they be closed. In the Moscow area alone, 50 nuclear reactors were judged to be unsafe and Gosatomnadzor, after concluding its investigation, reported that "Russia's nuclear power plants are incapable of maintaining their equipment in a safe state" (Feshbach, 1995).

Back-end. After a fuel assembly has been in operation for about a year, waste fission products accumulate in the rods to such an extent that the fission reaction can no longer be sustained, necessitating replacement of these "spent" rods with fresh ones. Spent fuel rods, highly radioactive, are initially placed in swimming pool-like cooling tanks where the isotopes with very short half-lives decay within a relatively brief time. The rods are still highly radioactive (and physically hot as well) due to longer-lived fission products still present and also contain appreciable amounts of unused fuel in the form of U-235 and plutonium that formed during the fission process within the fuel rods. To separate these two useful products from the other isotopes that constitute high-level radioactive wastes, **reprocessing** of the material in the spent rods was once envisioned as a vital part of the nuclear fuel cycle. In this process the fuel is removed from the rods and dissolved in nitric acid, the solution then being treated chemically to separate it into uranium, plutonium, and waste components. This operation represents a potential public hazard, since volatile radioisotopes, particularly krypton, are released into the atmosphere and other radioisotopes are discharged with liquid wastes. Workers inside the reprocessing plant also are exposed to higher levels of radioactivity than are nuclear power plant workers, though conceivably safeguards could be taken to reduce this risk.

Although reprocessing was considered an important means to reduce the amount of what would otherwise be considered waste and extend the fuel supply, a moratorium on commercial reprocessing was imposed by President Ford in 1976 and continued by President Carter due to the concern that reprocessing plants would be tempting targets for attack by terrorists intent on obtaining weapons-grade plutonium. Although President Reagan subsequently lifted the ban, financial considerations have deterred private interests from reentering the reprocessing business and at present there is no commercial reprocessing in the United States. Scientists with Harvard University's *Managing the Atom Project* contend that fuel reprocessing makes no economic sense, arguing that for the foreseeable future burying radioactive waste is far more cost-effective than reprocessing.

Nevertheless, France and the United Kingdom continue to reprocess spent fuel from nuclear reactors, for both their own nuclear power industry and for foreign customers. The Japanese have reprocessing facilities at Tokaimura, about 70 miles northeast of Tokyo, and are building another, larger plant at Rokkasho-mura in northern Honshu. Highly controversial and plagued by numerous problems, the facility is scheduled to open in 2006. Russia has three formerly secret reprocessing plants, built primarily to obtain plutonium for weapons production during the Cold War years. In 1957 a high-level waste tank at one of these facilities, the Mayak Production Association near the town of Kyshtym, exploded, releasing about two million curies of radiation over the region. Although the outside world was not told of this event until three decades later, during the year following the accident 11,000 people were evacuated from the area and for many years farming was prohibited on 440 square miles of heavily contaminated land surrounding the site. Today Russia's Mayak reprocessing plant generates badly needed foreign exchange by reprocessing, for a fee, spent nuclear fuel from other countries. In 1993, one of the plants, Tomsk-7 in Siberia, experienced an explosion that contaminated 1,500 square meters of land in the vicinity of the plant; radioactive fallout from the accident was detected over a 120-square-kilometer area, with the most heavily contaminated areas registering gamma radiation readings 20 times above background levels (Perera, 1998). Japan's Tokaimura reprocessing facilities have experienced several serious accidents in recent years. A fire and explosion in March 1997 exposed 37 workers to low levels of radiation and released some plutonium into the environment ("Reprocessing Facility," 1997). In the autumn of 1999, improper handling of enriched uranium at a fuel processing plant resulted in a critical reaction that exposed three workers to life-threatening levels of radiation (one of these men subsequently died). Neutrons escaping from the facility irradiated a number of people outside the plant as well; the government's official count of people experiencing radiation exposure was 69, although some environmental groups insisted the actual number was much higher. Regarded as the worst accident to date in Japan's nuclear program, the incident prompted a temporary evacuation order for residents living nearest the plant, while an additional 310,000 people within a six-mile radius were advised to remain indoors until radiation levels subsided (Landers, 1999). It should be noted that although reprocessing has been touted as a way to solve nuclear waste disposal problems, the nuclear by-products remaining after enriched uranium and plutonium have been removed from the spent fuel are themselves highly radioactive, requiring safe storage and disposal. In addition, when spent, the mixed oxide (MOX) uranium-plutonium fuel produced through reprocessing is even hotter and more radioactive than conventional spent fuel.

While reprocessing facilities may present radiation hazards both to their workers and to the environment, the most significant source of dangerous radioactive emissions from the back-end of the nuclear fuel cycle is the waste material produced by nuclear reactors. Nuclear power production generates large quantities of both high- and low-level wastes, the former primarily in the form of spent fuel from reactors, the latter consisting of contaminated clothing, clean-up solutions, wiping rags, hand tools, etc. **High-level wastes** are extremely radioactive, highly penetrating, and generate a great deal of heat, hence must be handled without direct human contact. Currently, most high-level commercial wastes in the U.S. are being stored in cooling ponds or aboveground containment casks at the power plants where they were produced; a relatively small percentage is in storage at facilities in Morris, Illinois, and West Valley, New York, once intended as reprocessing plants.

Responding to criticism that the lack of any clear-cut policy for permanent disposal of high-level radioactive waste could prove the Achilles' heel of the nuclear power industry, Congress in 1982 enacted the **Nuclear Waste Policy Act.** This legislation delegated responsibility for high-level radwaste management to the federal government and designated the U.S. Department of Energy as the lead agency to coordinate the effort to site, construct, and operate the nation's first permanent repository for such wastes. The politically sensitive search for a location for this facility is now focused on Yucca Mountain, Nevada, where extensive characterization studies are ongoing to determine the site's geologic suitability for deep burial of solidified wastes. Since the fission products in spent fuel rods will be dangerously radioactive for tens of thousands of years, suitability of any site chosen for an underground repository will depend on the ability of surrounding geological formations to absorb heat and to prevent radioactive emissions from escaping into the environment. Issues of special concern at the Yucca Mountain site include the long-term potential for earthquakes or volcanic eruptions in an area of known seismic activity and the possibility of groundwater intrusion into storage caverns in the eventuality of future climatic change. The fact that the area contains numerous mineral deposits raises worries that future generations, ignorant of the hazardous materials entombed on the site, might drill into the repository in search of gas or oil.

In December 1998, the Department of Energy released its long-awaited viability assessment for Yucca Mountain; in its report DOE concluded that although some uncertainties remain, there are no major problems that would disqualify the site from consideration. In February 2002, Secretary of Energy Spencer Abraham recommended that President Bush approve Yucca Mountain as the nation's high-level waste disposal site, stating that the location is "scientifically and technically suitable for the development of a repository." The president promptly did so and several months later, in spite of vehement objections from Nevada lawmakers, Congress voted to approve the site. The State of Nevada, fearful of acquiring the image of a "national sacrifice zone," then vetoed the project, only to see their action overturned by a joint resolution of the U.S. Senate and House of Representatives. The Department of Energy, bolstered by this success, announced its intent to submit a license application to the Nuclear Regulatory Commission by December 2004, and hoped to have Yucca Mountain operational by 2010. Those plans were unexpectedly thwarted in July 2004, when a federal appeals court, acting on a case brought by the State of Nevada and several environmental groups, ruled that the government's radiation protection standards for the Yucca Mountain facility were insufficiently protective. Citing a National Academy of Sciences report that said the peak period for radiation risk from the repository might be hundreds of thousands of years hence, the three-judge panel declared EPA's extension of radiation standards over a 10,000-year period insufficient and ordered the agency to rewrite them. The roadblock posed by this ruling derailed DOE's plans to file a license application in 2004; the agency subsequently announced that its revised license application would be ready for submission by the end of 2005. Yucca Mountain's future was further clouded early in 2005 by evidence that U.S. Geological Survey hydrologists had falsified site study data, generating outrage from critics who charged that the DOE had forfeited public trust in the project's scientific foundations. In addition, government underfunding of work at the site has repeatedly delayed repository operations, further postponing a final decision on Yucca Mountain's ultimate fate. Unfortunately, if the Yucca Mountain site is ultimately rejected, there is no alternative "Plan B." The 1987 law designating the Nevada location as the focus of characterization studies explicitly forbids consideration of any other site; for political reasons Congress, in essence, put all the nation's "eggs in one basket."

In the meantime, spent fuel rods continue to accumulate at power plants across the country, posing a major problem for the federal government as well as for the nuclear power industry. Under terms of the Nuclear Waste Policy Act, Washington has been collecting a one-tenth of a cent fee on every kilowatt-hour of electricity generated by nuclear power since 1983, with these revenues being deposited in a special fund earmarked for development of the permanent repository. In return, Washington made a contractual commitment to the utility companies that it would begin to move spent fuel from reactor sites in 1998. By the time the deadline date arrived, utilities had paid $14 billion into the Nuclear Waste Fund and were furious that the federal government had failed to meet its obligation under the law (a court ruling in November 1997 affirmed DOE's obligation to pick up the spent fuel and stated that the department could be liable for damages if it did not do so). As a consequence, by 2004 65 lawsuits totaling approximately $50 billion had been filed against the government by utilities seeking to recover the costs of waste storage. As an interim measure, more than a dozen reactor complexes where cooling ponds are at or near capacity have begun utilizing dry cask storage, sealing the radioactive wastes inside huge steel containers with 9-inch thick walls and placing them outdoors on a barbed-wire enclosed concrete pad. It is likely that many more utilities will turn to dry cask storage as a default solution for their waste disposal needs in the years immediately ahead.

For a number of years the Department of Energy tried, with very limited success, to attract interest from states, counties, or Native American tribes to host a "temporary," away-from-reactor site where, in return for certain financial benefits, spent nuclear fuel could be stored in aboveground dry casks until a permanent repository is eventually opened. In the mid-1990s the Mescalero Apaches in New Mexico seriously considered such an undertaking, but eventually declined. Subsequently, the small Skull Valley Band of the Goshute tribe in Utah entered into a joint venture with Private Fuel Storage, LLC (PFS)—a consortium of eight utility companies—to develop a storage facility on tribal land 70 miles west of Salt Lake City. Utah state officials are adamantly opposed to the project and are doing all they can to block it. The Goshutes contend that, as a sovereign Indian nation, they are entitled to proceed without state consent if the federal Nuclear Regulatory Commission grants approval. The site, comprising 100 acres within an 820-acre controlled area, will be developed in phases as storage space is required and could eventually accommodate up to 4,000 casks. Having overcome several court challenges filed by the State of Utah, PFS is moving forward with its license application process and estimates the Skull Valley facility could be open by 2007 (PFS, 2004). To the Goshutes, the proposed development offers a way out of poverty on a reservation described by the tribal chairman, Leon D. Bear, as a place that "doesn't grow much of anything." Arguing that Utah's governor and other antinuclear opponents of the project are guilty of "economic paternalism," Mr. Bear defends the initiative as both safe and of great potential benefit to his people. "My ancestors ate grasshoppers," Mr. Bear commented; "I don't want to live like that" (Fialka, 1998).

While controversy over a monitored retrievable storage facility continues to inflame passions in Utah, elsewhere in the Southwest a radioactive waste management success story has unfolded. In March 1999, the **Waste Isolation Pilot Plant (WIPP)** opened its gates and in so doing became the world's first certified deep radwaste facility. Designed as a permanent repository for lower-level **transuranic wastes**—plutonium-contaminated rags, tools, and protective clothing from nuclear weapons production facilities—WIPP is a subterranean complex of shafts, tunnels, and rooms excavated more than 2,000 feet (655 meters) underground in a salt formation 25 miles east of Carlsbad, New Mexico. Site selection was driven by a search for the most secure salt bed in the country, salt considered most desirable because of its solid, impermeable nature and because of its tendency under pressure to flow, sealing up any excavated cavities. Although its development was repeatedly delayed by legal challenges related to technical and safety issues, WIPP has won the approval of scientists, regulators, and citizens of Carlsbad as a safe repository. WIPP's opening was welcome news for the ten national weapons laboratories where nearly 60,000 cubic meters of transuranic wastes have been in "interim" storage for years. While no radwastes from commercial nuclear power plants can be sent to WIPP (by law, the facility is reserved exclusively for defense radwastes), the opening of a final resting place for transuranic wastes marks an important milestone in the federal government's efforts to implement a responsible radioactive waste management program (Kerr, 1999).

Elsewhere in the world, the 29 additional countries currently utilizing nuclear power face a similar radioactive waste disposal challenge. Although none have yet developed a permanent disposal facility, there is unanimous agreement that deep burial of such materials is the best option. Public opposition to such facilities not withstanding, policymakers in many countries are increasingly aware of the vulnerability of aboveground wastes to terrorist attack and view deep geologic repositories as the best way to prevent radioactive disaster. As a result, in more than 20 countries efforts are now underway to identify appropriate locations for such facilities. Their success or failure will, in large part, determine whether the nuclear power industry will experience the renaissance predicted by proponents, since efforts to launch a "second nuclear era" are unlikely to take off until the high-level waste disposal dilemma is satisfactorily resolved (Stone, 2004).

A portion of an underground tunnel at the WIPP facility is shown here, along with a machine used for excavation. [*Courtesy of U.S. Department of Energy*]

Low-level wastes, produced not only by nuclear power plants but also by hospitals, research labs, universities, and industries, exhibit low but sometimes potentially hazardous concentrations of radioisotopes. They differ from high-level wastes in having significantly lower levels of radioactive emissions; they are not physically hot, generally require no shielding, and, unlike high-level wastes that remain dangerous for millennia, most decay to harmless levels within 100–300 years. In the United States during the 1950s, many low-level commercial radwastes were buried on military reservations along with defense wastes or were simply dumped into the ocean—a practice that didn't cease entirely until 1970 (as recently as the fall of 1993, Russia defied world public opinion and infuriated the Japanese by brazenly dumping more than 900 tons of low-level radwastes into a prime squid fishing area in the Sea of Japan). From 1947–1970 at least 47,500 barrels of radwastes, primarily low-level wastes but also including plutonium wastes from atomic research labs, were dumped at three different sites near the Gulf of Farallones National Marine Sanctuary, an ocean wildlife preserve about 25 miles offshore from San Francisco. While the 55-gallon drums containing the wastes had a 10-year life expectancy in seawater and the concrete encasing the wastes was calculated to remain intact for 30 years, the radionuclides themselves have half-lives ranging from 30–24,000 years. By now virtually all of the barrels have reached their functional life span, but it isn't known for certain whether the radionuclides they contained remain deposited in or on nearby sediments or whether they have already been widely dispersed by ocean currents (Suchanek et al., 1996).

By the 1960s, the commercial nuclear industry was relying on shallow land burial for disposal of low-level wastes, utilizing six privately owned facilities specifically licensed for this purpose. By the late 1970s, three of these sites had closed due to migration of radioactive materials from the trenches, though no radioactive contamination was detected outside site boundaries. Because the states in which the three remaining sites were located (South Carolina, Nevada, and Washington) vigorously objected to being the "nuclear dumping ground" of the nation, Congress was persuaded to enact the **1980 Low-Level Radioactive Waste Policy Act.** This legislation placed responsibility for low-level radwaste management on *state* governments (as opposed to *federal* jurisdiction over high-level wastes), which were required to provide a means of safe disposal for all low-level wastes generated within their borders. Any states failing to do so could find their radwastes barred from disposal at existing sites in other states. However, recognizing that construction of 50 separate disposal facilities was neither necessary nor economically feasible, Congress permitted states to negotiate regional **"compact"** agreements among themselves to provide for the establishment, operation, and regulation of low-level radioactive waste facilities within each compact area. Currently 42 states are members of ten regional compacts approved by Congress; eight additional states, the District of Columbia, and Puerto Rico remain unaffiliated. Each regional compact is required to designate one of its members as the **"host state"**—i.e., the state in which the disposal facility is to be located—and to make numerous decisions regarding operational procedures, disposal fees, and type of facility to be constructed.

The original 1986 deadline date for completion of regional facilities was extended to January 1, 1993, but in every compact area, intense public opposition to siting has stymied efforts to carry out the requirements of the law. At the end of December 1992, the small facility at Beatty, Nevada, closed its gates and the Hanford, Washington, landfill restricted access to all but 11 northwestern and Rocky Mountain states; only the facility at Barnwell, South Carolina—the largest of the three—remained open to meet the radwaste disposal needs of generators from the remaining 39 states. A new radioactive waste landfill owned and operated by Envirocare of Utah, Inc., opened in

Box 10-5   Depleted Uranium—Facts vs. Fiction

Ever since the first Persian Gulf War, a coalition of activist organizations in Europe and North America have been vigorously protesting the military use of depleted uranium (DU), first in Kuwait and Iraq by the United States and the United Kingdom in 1991, subsequently by NATO forces in the Balkans in the mid- to late 1990s, and, most recently, in 2003 by U.S. troops invading Iraq. Some of these critics charged that DU might be responsible, at least in part, for the mysterious health complaints, known as "Gulf War Syndrome," reported by thousands of veterans returning from the 1991 conflict.

How valid is the case against DU? An attempt to answer this question first requires an explanation of what depleted uranium is and why military forces in at least 16 countries include DU weapons in their arsenals. Depleted uranium is the waste material left over from the production of enriched uranium used in nuclear fuel rods. Because it contains less U-235 than does natural uranium, its radioactivity is about 40% less than that of the latter and several orders of magnitude lower than that of enriched uranium. However, it has certain chemical and physical characteristics that make it ideal for a number of military and commercial applications. It is even more dense than lead, has a very high melting point, bursts into flame when it fragments, and has a tensile strength similar to steel. Such qualities give DU munitions the offensive capability to penetrate enemy armor more effectively than conventional munitions while also serving defensive purposes in the form of DU shielding in heavy armor tanks.

Following the 1991 Gulf War, the Department of Defense (DOD) conducted a number of studies to determine ways in which U.S. troops might have received harmful exposure to depleted uranium. DOD concluded that the highest levels of exposure probably occurred when soldiers were in or near vehicles that were mistakenly hit by DU munitions (i.e., "friendly fire" incidents) and were struck by DU fragments. Similarly, if they entered vehicles too soon after impact they could have inhaled airborne DU particles. Somewhat lower levels of exposure could have occurred when DU-

contaminated vehicles were being repaired or during cleanup after a large fire at a facility containing DU munitions. It is believed that cleanup crews may have inhaled dust containing DU particles or ingested such particles via inadvertent hand-to-mouth contact. Some of these servicemen, particularly those with embedded DU fragments remaining in their bodies, are now participating in a medical surveillance follow-up study to detect any long-term health impacts. The focus of concern for the anti-DU coalition, however, is on exposed local populations in war zones where uranium weapons have been used and where soils and water supplies have tested positive for low levels of radioactivity. In Iraq these include children playing close to buildings or vehicles struck by DU munitions, people selling food next to burned-out tanks, and scavengers collecting DU-contaminated scrap metal for sale. In Serbia the concern is for residents living in areas where wind or human activities may resuspend DU particles from contaminated soils, resulting in exposure via inhalation, or where DU-tainted water supplies pose ingestion concerns.

Possible health problems related to depleted uranium exposure focus primarily on cancer, due to the ionizing radiation associated with DU, and serious kidney problems related to uranium's chemical toxicity. Responding to concerns about unexplained illnesses among Gulf War veterans, the Department of Veterans Affairs several years ago contracted with the Institute of Medicine to review the scientific literature in an effort to determine if there was any association between known agents to which veterans may have been exposed and their reported health problems. Depleted uranium was one of the agents evaluated, with information culled from extensive animal toxicity research as well as from numerous epidemiological studies of uranium processing mill workers whose occupational exposure to uranium ore is regarded as a reasonably close approximation to depleted uranium exposure. Although much of this research is several decades old and has some limitations in terms of its applicability to the health complaints of Gulf War veterans, the information reviewed by the Institute of

Medicine provided much useful information and enabled the committee to make some tentative conclusions, while encouraging further long-term follow-up studies using more sophisticated statistical analyses.

The committee's most significant findings in terms of DU and veterans' health complaints is that, at the levels of radiation exposure commonly experienced by soldiers (below 200 mSv), the evidence suggests no connection between depleted uranium and subsequent development of lung cancer (at exposure levels above 200 mSv, evidence is insufficient to say whether an association exists). Similarly, even among veterans with embedded DU fragments who have detectable levels of uranium in their urine, there is no evidence of kidney damage or renal dysfunction. In terms of an association between DU and lymphatic cancer, bone cancer, nervous system disease, noncancerous respiratory problems, and a range of other health issues, the committee concluded that there simply isn't enough evidence to indicate the existence of a connection. The committee also stated that any lung cancer cases that developed less than 10 years after participation in the Gulf War must have been caused by something other than DU, due to the characteristically long latency period that typifies lung cancer. They also cited studies of nuclear industry workers whose health was followed over a period of more than 30 years; in spite of having received relatively high levels of exposure during their early years on the job, this group exhibited no higher levels of cancer than the general population.

The Institute of Medicine's conclusions, while cautious, implied that there are few reasons to believe that DU exposure is as health-threatening as members of the international coalition insist. More recent reports by the United Nations Environment Programme (UNEP), the International Atomic Energy Agency (IAEA), and by a number of independent researchers also suggest that public fears are overblown.

In 2002, UNEP, conducting investigations in war-ravaged Bosnia, confirmed that DU from weapons fired by NATO forces in the mid-1990s had contaminated drinking water supplies at one site and could still be detected in airborne dust particles. Investigators reported, however, that the levels of contamination detected were very low and do not present any immediate health or environmental risk. UNEP noted that where ground contamination occurs, radiation levels are low and are usually localized to a 1–2 meter radius from the DU penetrator's point of impact.

The IAEA came to a similar conclusion when it sent a team to Kuwait in 2002 to determine whether DU residues at 11 different locations presented any radiological hazards to the Kuwaiti people. After taking approximately 200 samples of soil, water, and vegetation, the investigators found that radiation doses associated with these locations are lower than those from normal background radiation and present no radiological threat to local people. Independent scientific research published in 2004 came to the same conclusion, its authors stating that ". . . the widely spread information in newspapers and Internet concerning dramatic health deterioration for Iraqi citizens should not be linked directly with their exposure to DU after the Gulf War." Other claims of DU-induced illness among Serbian civilians or increased incidence of leukemia among Swedish military personnel in the Balkans also have been undermined by published research that fails to show a definitive association between DU exposure and disease.

Investigators' recommendations that follow-up studies be performed to evaluate long-term risk among those exposed to uranium weapons are appropriate, as is UNEP's call for regular monitoring of drinking water supplies at or near sites known to be radiologically contaminated. Nevertheless, current evidence strongly suggests that alarmist claims about the hazards of depleted uranium are vastly exaggerated and that, in terms of human health and environmental quality, society has many more important issues to worry about.

References
Bem, H., Bou-Rabee, F. 2004. "Environmental and Health Consequences of Depleted Uranium Use in the 1991 Gulf War." *Environment International* 30, no. 1 (March).

Fulco, Carolyn E., Catharyn T. Liverman, Harold C. Sox, eds. 2000. *Gulf War and Health*. Vol. 1. Washington, DC: Institute of Medicine, National Academy Press.

Figure 10-3

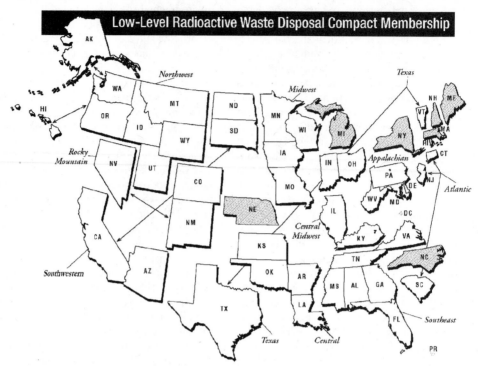

Low-Level Radioactive Waste Disposal Compact Membership

Appalachian Compact
Delaware
Maryland
Pennsylvania
West Virginia

Atlantic Compact
Connecticut
New Jersey
South Carolina

Central Compact
Arkansas
Kansas
Louisiana
Oklahoma

Central Midwest Compact
Illinois
Kentucky

Northwest Compact
Alaska
Hawaii
Idaho
Montana
Oregon
Utah
Washington
Wyoming

Midwest Compact
Indiana
Iowa
Minnesota
Missouri
Ohio
Wisconsin

Rocky Mountain Compact
Colorado
Nevada
New Mexico

*Northwest accepts Rocky
Mountain waste as agreed
between compacts*

Southeast Compact
Alabama
Florida
Georgia
Mississippi
Tennessee
Virginia

Southwestern Compact
Arizona
California
North Dakota
South Dakota

Texas Compact
Texas
Vermont

Unaffiliated States
District of Columbia
Maine
Massachusetts
Michigan
Nebraska
New Hampshire
New York
North Carolina
Puerto Rico
Rhode Island

Source: Produced by the Low-Level Radioactive Waste Forum, Inc.—June 2005. Used with permission.

1988 at a site 80 miles west of Salt Lake City within a 100-square mile hazardous waste zone (neighbors include an Army nerve gas storage site and Dugway Proving Grounds), but facility operations are restricted solely to the management of naturally occurring radioactive materials such as slightly contaminated soil and certain types of low-activity, high-volume wastes.

In 2001, to the dismay of many generators, South Carolina passed legislation requiring that by mid-2008 access to Barnwell be restricted to the three members of the Atlantic Compact (South Carolina, New Jersey, and Connecticut), leaving the remaining 36 states with nowhere to send any but their lowest activity wastes (because of lower disposal costs, most of these are already being shipped to Envirocare). Impending closure of Barnwell to out-of-compact wastes has sparked growing concern among radwaste generators and regulatory officials alike. During a 2005 symposium on the current state of low-level radioactive waste management, Richard Meserve, former Chairman of the Nuclear Regulatory Commission, warned that "The system is headed for a train wreck" ("Low Activity Waste Disposal," 2005). Groups such as the California Radioactive Materials Management Forum, alarmed by the looming disposal capacity crisis, are urging Congress to authorize development of a national low-level waste disposal facility. Others have suggested repealing the 1980 law that established the compact system, thereby motivating development of private sector radwaste management operations or, alternatively, requiring DOE to accept some commercial low-level wastes at its facilities ("Planned Barnwell Closure," 2005).

Low-level radioactive wastes are stored in concrete vaults and then placed in earthen trenches at the Barnwell, South Carolina, facility. When the trenches are full they are covered with an engineered cap of multiple layers of sand, clay, high-density polyethylene, and top soil. [*Courtesy of Chem-Nuclear Systems, LLC*]

In the meantime, those engaged in the struggle to provide radwaste disposal options must continue public education efforts, aware that the contentious issue of where to locate needed facilities will continue to bedevil efforts to manage low-level radioactive wastes in a responsible manner. While most radiation experts contend that low-level wastes, properly managed, pose minimal health or environmental hazards, the public's inability to distinguish between the vastly different risks presented by high-level vs. low-level radwastes contributes to the hysteria surrounding the facility-siting issue, making resolution of the nation's radioactive waste disposal conundrum one of our most difficult public policy issues.

Ultraviolet Radiation

Wavelengths of the electromagnetic spectrum ranging between 40–400 nanometers in length are categorized as ultraviolet (UV) light. Although UV waves longer than 124 nanometers are not of sufficiently high energy to ionize atoms and molecules, certain portions within this range are strongly absorbed by living tissues, particularly by DNA that constitutes the major target of UV damage. Injury to the hereditary material of cells is the reason for the lethal or mutational effects which excess UV exposure can provoke in living organisms. Research has shown that the most detrimental effects to biological systems occur when UV radiation is in the 230–320 nanometer range (referred to as UVB, as opposed to longer-wavelength UVA), peak absorption by DNA occurring at 260 nm. Much of the ultraviolet light naturally present in incoming solar radiation is filtered out by the layer of atmospheric ozone located about 20 miles above the earth's surface (see chapter 11). Living organisms have developed various defense mechanisms to protect themselves against the amounts that do penetrate—shielding devices such as fur, feathers, shells, or darkly pigmented skin, as well as light-avoidance behavior patterns among a variety of species. Of equal importance has been the evolution of enzymatic mechanisms for repairing UV-induced damage to DNA when levels of injury are not excessive. Without this cellular repair ability it is doubtful whether many organisms could survive existing levels of UV exposure. The importance of such mechanisms can be seen in the example of individuals suffering from the genetic disease xeroderma pigmentosum. Lacking the enzyme needed for repair of radiation-damaged DNA, victims of this ailment have to remain indoors throughout daylight hours or risk the development of multiple fatal skin cancers. There appears to be a tenuous balance between continual UV assault on the hereditary material and its biochemical repair. If the cell's capacity to deal with such damage is overwhelmed, the cell will die.

Since ultraviolet light cannot penetrate very deeply into living tissues, the major concern in reference to UV injury to humans involves the induction of skin cancers, particularly in lighter-skinned individuals who lack protective melanin granules in their epidermal skin layers.

Since the late 1940s, when the tyranny of fashion decreed that pale skin was "out" and the bronzed look "in," the apparently irresistible urge among fair-complexioned citizens to spend hours broiling themselves under the sun or at rapidly proliferating tanning parlors has resulted in an alarming increase in the incidence of skin cancer in Western countries due to increased exposure to UV radiation, a known carcinogen and mutagen. According to the American Cancer Society, three major types of skin cancer account for approximately half of all cancer cases diagnosed in the United States each year. The situation is even worse in Australia, where skin cancer rates are the highest in the world; an estimated two out of every three white Australians will be diagnosed with some form of skin cancer by the time they reach age 75.

Skin cancer risk is highest among people with fair complexions and blonde or red hair; malignancies are lowest among African-Americans, who are 20 times less likely than whites to develop skin cancer. **Basal cell carcinoma** and **squamous cell carcinoma** comprise the vast majority of all skin cancers—over a million new cases in the U.S. each year—and are increasing at a 5% annual rate. Chronic exposure to sunlight is recognized as the cause of over 90% of these two cancers. They appear, predictably, on portions of the body receiving the greatest sun exposure—face, neck, ears, back of the hands—and until recently were unusual in people under the age of 50. Now, however, numerous cases have been diagnosed among people in their 20s and 30s and occasionally even in teenagers. Not surprisingly, they are also being found on the legs, chest, and back of victims as the sunbathing mania takes its toll. Fortunately, the majority of such cancers can be treated if detected early, but each year 1,000–2,000 cases prove fatal when their neglect leads to invasion of underlying tissues.

Malignant melanoma is much less common than basal cell or squamous cell carcinomas, but far more deadly. In 2004 an estimated 55,100 new victims were diagnosed with malignant melanoma and almost 8,000 died of the disease. The incidence of malignant melanoma in the U.S. is increasing by 7% annually and is now the most common form of cancer to strike women under the age of 30. Americans born during the 1990s are at 12 times the risk of eventually developing malignant melanoma as are those born in the 1940s, and twice as likely as those born in the 1980s (DeLeo, 1992). The American Cancer Institute now estimates an American's lifetime risk of developing melanoma is 1 in 57 for men, 1 in 81 for women; in Australia, where melanoma rates are the highest in the world, the chances are 1 in 70.

Unlike the nonmelanoma skin cancers, in which risk of contracting the disease is greatest among people receiving repeated UV exposure over a period of many years, malignant melanoma may be triggered by a single severe sunburn during childhood or adolescence. According to the U.S. National Library of Medicine and the National Institutes of Health, one blistering sunburn before the age of 20 doubles an individual's risk of developing malignant melanoma as an adult. Interestingly, while basal cell and squamous cell carcinomas develop only on sun-exposed portions of the body, malignant melanomas frequently occur on areas normally covered. They also tend to occur at a younger age than do the other two forms of skin cancer; although the risk of melanoma increases with age, half of all cases occur among those under 50, with incidence rates rising most rapidly among people below 40 years of age. Because of the suspected link between childhood sunburn and melanoma, groups such as The Skin Cancer Foundation are urging parents to be particularly careful in protecting youngsters from excessive sun exposure.

Ill effects of UV-light exposure are not limited to cancer and sunburn. Premature wrinkling, drying, and mottling of the skin are among the less desirable consequences

Box 10-6 Can Sunscreens Prevent Skin Cancer?

Health educators' efforts to promote sunscreen use among a sun-loving public have met with considerable success in recent years. It is now well recognized that sunscreens with an SPF (sun protection factor) of 15, when used properly, are very effective in preventing sunburn as well as protecting the skin against premature aging and wrinkling. However, their role in preventing skin cancer—the primary concern among most users—has been questioned by some researchers who point to the simultaneous rise in sunscreen sales and skin cancer rates. Some physicians go so far as to suggest that the use of chemical sunscreens is, in large part, responsible for the current skin cancer epidemic, pointing out that the highest rates of melanoma are being reported from countries where the use of chemical sunscreens has been strongly promoted.

Although the vast majority of dermatologists remain strong advocates of sunscreen use, some worry that users of these products may assume they can safely remain in the sun for long periods of time, unaware that sunscreens absorb most, though not all, UVB rays (those that cause sunburn), but are ineffective against UVA radiation, which penetrates more deeply into the skin than does UVB and is strongly absorbed by the cells (melanocytes) that are involved both in tanning and melanoma formation. UVA, like UVB, has been linked with both skin cancer and immune system damage. For this reason, most experts agree that while sunscreen use is both desirable and recommended, it is not enough. Even more important are common-sense strategies such as staying indoors or in the shade during mid-day hours (10 AM to 3 PM) when the sun is most intense and wearing a tightly-woven long-sleeved shirt and trousers with a broad-brimmed hat when exposure is unavoidable.

Such precautions are particularly important for youngsters, who generally spend much more time outdoors than do adults; indeed, it is estimated that fully 80% of a person's lifetime exposure to UV radiation occurs before age 20. Parents should be especially careful not to allow infants or children to become badly sunburned, since childhood sunburns are widely considered to be a triggering factor for subsequent development of malignant melanoma. Extreme care should be taken to minimize sun exposure of infants; babies under 6 months of age have very sensitive skin and should be kept in the shade when outdoors. Conscientious parents will ensure that strollers are fitted with hoods and babies protected with wide-brimmed hats. Baby oil should never be applied to an infant's skin before going outdoors, since it makes the skin more translucent to harmful solar radiation. Toddlers and older children are somewhat less vulnerable than infants, but dermatologists advise that they, too, should wear protective clothing and hats while playing outdoors. Unfortunately, the inconvenience of these precautions makes it unlikely that such advice will be heeded; accordingly, parents need to do the next best thing and insist that their children regularly use sunscreen.

Dermatologists surmise that an additional explanation for the rise in skin cancer incidence among sunscreen users could be due to improper application of these products. For greatest effectiveness, sunscreen should be applied 30 minutes prior to sun exposure so that protective ingredients have time to be absorbed; it should then be reapplied every two hours or whenever perspiration or contact with water removes the original protective layer. Sunscreens should be liberally applied to parts of the body especially prone to sunburn—lips, nose, ears—and should be used on cloudy or hazy days as conscientiously as when the sun is shining brightly. Similarly, sunscreen should be worn when one is out in the snow, particularly at high altitudes. Use of products with an SPF value lower than 15 provides insufficient protection, regardless of skin type (experts are unsure whether *higher* SPF sunscreens offer any additional protection). The best sunscreens are resistant to being washed off by sweating or swimming—a feature that is largely determined by the product's base material. In general, the most water-resistant sunscreens are those that feel the greasiest; clear lotions and gels are the most easily washed off, while creamy lotions rank midway between.

While sunscreens may indirectly increase the risk of melanoma by encouraging people to remain in the sun longer than they should, most experts continue to regard them as a "last line of defense"—not a panacea to prevent skin cancer but an important component in an overall strategy for personal protection from the sun's damaging rays.

References

Epstein, John H. 1998. "Sunscreens and Skin Cancer." *Southern Medical Journal* 91, no. 6 (June).

Fackelmann, Kathleen. 1998. "Do Sunscreens Protect Against Cancer?" *Consumers' Research* 81, no. 8 (Aug):23–26.

Garland, Cedric F., et al. 1992. "Could Sunscreens Increase Melanoma Risk?" *American Journal of Public Health* 82, no. 4 (April).

Napoli, Maryanne. 1998. "Sunscreens—Not the Protection We Thought." *Health Facts* 3, no. 6:1–3.

The much sought-after "bronzed" look can come at a high price: skin cancer, premature wrinkling, and immune system dysfunction.

of UV exposure. In recent years the growing popularity of tanning parlors has been accompanied by claims from the owners of such establishments that they provide a safe alternative to sunbathing because they utilize UVA radiation rather than UVB and hence cannot result in burning. Nevertheless, tanning parlor patrons are exposing themselves to several other serious risks. Not only can UVA, like UVB, induce skin cancer, it also causes premature aging of the skin and development of cataracts. In addition, UVA enhances the effect of sunlight: individuals who sunbathe outdoors shortly after a stint in a tanning parlor frequently suffer extremely severe sunburns. Photosensitive reactions to either tanning parlors or outdoor sunbathing can occur when unwary sun-worshippers expose themselves to UV light while taking antibiotics (especially tetracycline), antihistamines, birth control pills, even certain cosmetics. Such a toxic reaction is generally manifested as an unusually severe sunburn immediately following exposure to UV light.

Exposure to even moderate amounts of ultraviolet radiation can be dangerous for individuals suffering from *lupus erythematosus,* an autoimmune ailment. Between 40–60% of lupus patients experience aggravation of skin disease or systemic symptoms when exposed to either UVA or UVB light. Many researchers contend that the threat of UV damage to the body's immune system should be regarded just as seriously as its ability to induce skin cancer. Studies have shown that ultraviolet radiation from both natural and artificial sources can alter the proportions of various types of white blood cells and depress the activity of natural killer-T cells in the bloodstream. Immune system dysfunction caused by UV exposure is not related to the amount of pigmentation in a person's skin, as is the case with skin cancer. Individuals with black or brown skin are just as likely to suffer immune system damage if they spend too much time in the sun as are fair-skinned people. Unfortunately, most sunscreens do *not* appear to be effective in preventing the type of immune system damage provoked by UVB exposure

(Sontheimer, 1992; "Sunscreens," 1992). Weighing serious long-term health risks against short-term fashion benefits, dermatologists are unanimous in their recommendation that all UV exposure, whether on the beach or at a tanning salon, be avoided to the greatest extent possible.

Ultraviolet light has some beneficial as well as harmful effects. A certain amount of skin exposure is necessary to promote the bodily synthesis of vitamin D, a deficiency of which can result in the development of rickets, a bone deformity. The germicidal properties of UV light have recommended its use in operating rooms to reduce the danger of bacterial or viral infections. Ultraviolet light applications have also been successfully employed to treat such bacterial skin diseases as acne and boils (Schreiber, 1986).

Microwaves

Electromagnetic radiation comprising wavelengths ranging from approximately one millimeter to one meter (intermediate between infrared and short-wave radio wavelengths) is termed microwave radiation. Since microwave energies are so low, such radiations are typically characterized by their frequencies which, in the case of microwaves of biological interest, generally fall between 100 and 30,000 megahertz (MHZ).

Humans today are continuously bombarded with microwaves from such diverse sources as military radar installations, radio and television transmitters, communications and surveillance satellites, radar and radio frequency transmitters at airports and on planes and ships, microwave ovens, telephone and TV-signal relay towers, cell phones, video display terminals, automatic garage door openers, and so on. At the low levels of exposure represented by these sources, most researchers believe that microwave radiation presents a negligible public health threat. Unlike X-rays, microwaves are non-ionizing; instead, when absorbed they cause an increased rate of vibration in the molecules of the absorbing material, resulting in the production of heat. Depending on frequency, microwaves are differentially absorbed by bodily tissues. Those of very low energy (below 150 MHZ) simply pass through the body without being absorbed; those of intermediate frequency (150–1200 MHZ) are absorbed by the deeper tissues without any noticeable heating of the skin. This poses a danger of serious bodily harm, since internal organs can receive highly damaging doses of microwave radiation without the victim realizing that anything is wrong. As microwave frequency increases, tissue penetration decreases and at 3500 MHZ warming of the skin can be felt; above 10,000 MHZ only the surface of the skin is heated and no penetration of the body occurs.

Differential absorption of microwave energy by bodily tissues is to a large degree a function of their water content. Moist tissues such as skin, muscle, and the intestines absorb more microwaves than do bones and fatty tissues. Sensitivity of specific organs to microwaves depends not only on how readily such radiation is absorbed, but also on how effectively blood circulating through the organ can dissipate the excess heat. Experiments have shown that body parts with poor circulation—the eyes, gastrointestinal tract, testes, urinary bladder, and gall bladder—are the areas most susceptible to injury from microwaves (Dalrymple, 1973).

Electromagnetic Fields (EMF)

In 1979 a team of researchers at the University of Colorado Medical Center in Denver reported that children who are exposed to stronger than average magnetic fields, such as those living in the vicinity of power transmission lines, have a two to three times greater risk of developing leukemia than do children living at a distance from such sources. While this study was subsequently discredited because of methodological flaws (e.g., small size of group studied, lack of direct measurements of exposure received), the report sparked intense public alarm about an inescapable component of everyday life. The extremely-low-frequency (ELF) wavelengths produced by the transmission and distribution of electric power, as well as by the plethora of electrical appliances that fill virtually every modern household, are impossible to avoid, so the suggestion that subtle but significant adverse health effects could be caused by electromagnetic fields prompted numerous scientific studies during the 1980s and 1990s. The primary concern of researchers focused on whether exposure to the levels of low-frequency radiation typical of residential environments could, as some investigators claimed, increase the risk of childhood leukemia. The impact of EMFs in provoking birth defects, miscarriages, learning disabilities, or behavioral modifications also received attention. From the beginning, many scientists were skeptical of any cancer-EMF association, simply because the amounts of radiation emanating from power lines and appliances are so minute in comparison with the earth's own magnetic field. Numerous research efforts to verify a possible EMF-cancer connection yielded inconclusive results; some epidemiologic studies showed a slight risk of cancer with EMF exposure, while others revealed no such association. Significantly, experiments using animal models failed to demonstrate any correlation between laboratory exposure to low frequency radiation and the induction or promotion of cancer. Several major studies in the early 1990s found evidence for an association between EMF and cancer inconsistent and inconclusive; in 1995 the American Physical Society, the world's largest group of physicists, entered the fray, saying its members could find no evidence that electromagnetic fields radiating from power lines have any impact on cancer rates. The Society deplored the fact that public fears about an EMF-cancer connection were responsible for the unnecessary diversion of billions of dollars (estimated at $1–3 billion annually in the U.S.) for moving power lines and installing shielding. The scientific debate was effectively resolved (1) when the National Academy of Sciences issued a major report stating that its review of more than 500 scientific papers failed to provide any evidence that electromagnetic fields adversely affect human health (NRC, 1997) and (2) when scientists at the National Cancer Institute convincingly demonstrated no association between electric power lines and leukemia in children (Linet et al., 1997). Although the public fears raised by more than two decades of controversy have not been altogether vanquished, the scientific community regards further investigation into the health impacts of EMF as unnecessary—sleeping under an electric blanket or living near a power line doesn't cause cancer!

References

Allison, Graham. 2004. *Nuclear Terrorism: the Ultimate Preventable Catastrophe*. New York: Time Books, Henry Holt and Company.

Bennett, B. G. 1997. "Exposure to Natural Radiation Sources Worldwide." In *Proceedings of 4th International Conference on High Levels of Natural Radiation: Radiation Doses And Health Effects*, edited by L. Wei, T. Sugahara, and Z. Tao. Beijing, China, October 1996.

Brooke, James. 2004. "Four Workers Killed in Nuclear Plant Accident in Japan." *New York Times*, Aug. 10.

Buckley, Chris. 2004. "Chance to Revive Sales Draws Nuclear Industry to China." *New York Times*, March 10, W1.

Carter, L. J. 1977. "More Burning of Coal Offsets Gains in Air Pollution Control." *Science* 198.

Clark, Claudia. 1997. *Radium Girls: Women and Industrial Health Reform, 1910–1935*. Chapel Hill: Univ. of North Carolina Press.

Cooper, George, Jr. 1973. "The Development of Radiation Science." In *Medical Radiation Biology,* edited by Glenn V. Dalrymple, M. E. Gaulden, G. M. Kollmorgen, and H. H. Vogel, Jr. Philadelphia: W. B. Saunders.

Dalrymple, Glenn V. 1973. "Microwaves." In *Medical Radiation Biology*, edited by Glenn V. Dalrymple et al. Philadelphia: W. B. Saunders.

DeLeo, Vincent, M.D. 1992. Testimony before the Senate Committee on Governmental Affairs, June 5.

Dubrova, Yuri E., Rakhmet I. Bersimbaev, Leila B. Djansugurova, Maira K. Tankimanova, Zaure Zh. Mamyrbaeva, Ritta Mustonen, Carita Lindholm, Maj Hultén, and Sisko Salomaa. 2002. "Nuclear Weapons Tests and Human Germline Mutation Rate." *Science* 295, no. 5557 (Feb. 8).

Eisenbud, M. 1973. *Environmental Radioactivity*. San Diego: Academic Press.

Feshbach, Murray. 1995. *Ecological Disaster: Cleaning Up the Hidden Legacy of the Soviet Regime*. New York: The Twentieth Century Fund Press.

Fialka, John J. 1998. "Goshute Indians' Plan to Store Nuclear Waste for Eight Utilities Is Opposed by Utah Governor." *Wall Street Journal*, Aug. 26.

Goldman, Marvin. 1996. "Cancer Risk of Low-Level Exposure." *Science* 271:1821–1822.

Hall, Eric J. 2000. *Radiobiology for the Radiologist*. 5th ed. Philadelphia: Lippincott.

Hawkes, Nigel, Geoffrey Lean, David Leigh, Robin McVie, P. Pringle, and A. Wilson. 1987. *Chernobyl: The End of the Nuclear Dream*. New York: Vintage Books.

Institute of Medicine and the National Research Council (IOM and NRC). 1999. *Exposure of the American People to Iodine-131 from Nevada Nuclear-Bomb Tests*. Washington, DC: National Academy Press.

"Ionizing Radiation Exposure of the Population of the United States." 1987. National Council on Radiation Protection and Measurements, Report No. 93, Sept. 1.

Jaworowski, Zbigniew. 1999. "Radiation Risk and Ethics." *Physics Today* 52, no. 9 (Sept).

Kahn, Patricia. 1993. "A Grisly Archive of Key Cancer Data." *Science* 259 (Jan. 22).

Kerr, Richard A. 1999. "For Radioactive Waste From Weapons, A Home at Last." *Science* 283, no. 5408 (March 12):1626–1628.

Kevles, Bettyann Holtzmann. 1997. *Naked to the Bone*. New Brunswick, NJ: Rutgers Univ. Press.

Kneale, George W., and Alice M. Stewart. 1993. "Reanalysis of Hanford Data: 1944–1986 Deaths." *American Journal of Industrial Medicine* 23 (March).

Lake, James A., Ralph G. Bennett, and John F. Kotek. 2002. "Next Generation of Nuclear Power." *Scientific American* 286, no. 1 (Jan).

Landers, Peter. 1999. "Uranium Leak Feeds Antinuclear Sentiment in Japan." *Wall Street Journal,* Oct. 4.

League of Women Voters Education Fund. 1993. *The Nuclear Waste Primer*. Lyons & Burford.

Linet, M. S., E. E. Hatch, R. A. Kleinerman, L. L. Robison, W. T. Kaune, D. K. Friedman, R. K. Severson, C. M. Haines, C. T. Hartsock, S. Niwa, S. Wachodler, and R. E. Tarone. 1997. "Residential Exposure to Magnetic Fields and Acute Lymphoblastic Leukemia in Children." *New England Journal of Medicine* 337, no. 1 (July 3):1–7.

"Low-Activity Waste Disposal System About to Crash." 2005. *Nuclear Waste News* 25, no. 4 (Feb. 24): 37–39.

Macklis, Roger M. 1993. "The Great Radium Scandal." *Scientific American* (Aug).

National Council on Radiation Protection and Measurements (NCRP). 1998. "Radionuclide Exposure of the Embryo/Fetus." NCRP Report No. 128. Bethesda, MD: NCRP.

———. 1987. "Ionizing Radiation Exposure of the Population of the United States." NCRP Report No. 93. Bethesda, MD: NCRP.

National Research Council (NRC). 1997. *Possible Health Effects of Exposure to Residential Electric and Magnetic Fields*. Washington, DC: National Academy Press.

"New Study Suggests Recommended Radiation Dose Limit Is Too High." 1992. *Environmental Health Letter*, Feb. 11.

Norwood, Christopher. 1980. *At Highest Risk*. New York: Penguin Books.

Perera, Judith. 1998. "Officials Charged with Misuse of Funds for Tomsk Cleanup." *Nuclear Waste News* 18, no. 14 (April 2):132.

———. 1997. "EU Offers Some Aid for Massive Eastern Europe Uranium Cleanup." *Nuclear Waste News* 17, no. 35 (Sept. 11):335.

———. 1993. "New Radiation Standards Urged for British Workers." *Environmental Health Letter,* June 11.

"Planned Barnwell Closure Sparks NRC Low-Level Waste Review." 2005. *The International Radioactive Exchange* 24, no. 8 (May 2):4.

Pollycove, Myron. 1997. "The Rise and Fall of the Linear No-Threshold Theory of Radiation Carcinogenesis." *Nuclear Waste News* (June):34–37.

Private Fuel Storage, LLC (PFS). 2004. http://www.privatefuelstorage.com/project/project.html. Accessed October 2, 2004.

"Reprocessing Facility Blast Leads to Review of Japan's Nuclear Plans." 1997. *Nuclear Waste News* 17, no. 12 (March 20):115.

Schreiber, Michael M. 1986. "Exposure to Sunlight." *Comprehensive Therapy* 12, no. 5.

Sohrabi, Mehdi. 1998. "The State-of-the-Art on Worldwide Studies in some Environments with Elevated Naturally Occurring Radioactive Materials (NORM)." *Applied Radiation Isotopes* 49, no. 3:169–188.

Sontheimer, Richard D. 1992. "Photosensitivity in Lupus Erythematosus." *Lupus News* 12, no. 2.

Steinhardt, Bernice. 1996. *Uranium Mill Tailings: Status and Future Costs of Cleanup.* United States General Accounting Office, GAO/T-RCED-96-85.

Stone, Richard. 2004. "Deep Repositories: Out of Sight, Out of Terrorists' Reach." *Science* 303, no. 5655 (Jan. 9).

Streffer, Christian. 1997. "Biological Effects of Prenatal Irradiation." *Health Impacts of Large Releases of Radionuclides.* Wiley, Chichester (Ciba Foundation Symposium 203):155–166.

Suchanek, Thomas H., Manuel C. Lagunas-Solar, Otto G. Raabe, Roger C. Helm, Fiorella Gielow, Neal Peek, and Omar Carvacho. 1996. "Radionuclides in Fishes and Mussels from the Farallon Islands Nuclear Waste Dump Site, California." *Health Physics* 71, no. 2 (Aug):167–178.

"Sunscreens May Not Afford Protection." 1992. *Environmental Health Letter,* June 12.

PART 3

ENVIRONMENTAL DEGRADATION

HOW WE FOUL OUR OWN NEST

The first Earth Day celebration on April 22, 1970, helped usher in an era of environmental activism.
[© *Bettmann/Corbis*]

> The fouling of the nest which has been typical of man's activity in the past on a local scale now seems to be extending to the whole system.
>
> —Kenneth Boulding

Air pollution, water pollution, excessive levels of noise, and the accumulation of disease-breeding refuse are not phenomena unique to the modern age. Wherever humans have congregated in appreciable numbers, the burning of fuel, the thoughtless disposal of excreta and material wastes, and the din arising from a multitude of human activities have created conditions that adversely affected the health and well-being of the very people responsible for those conditions. For most of human history, environmental degradation was primarily local in scope, concentrated in the relatively few places where humans established urban centers. The extent of pollution in these cities, however, often far exceeded the levels of filth plaguing our environmentally conscious society of today. Streets and gutters clogged with human body wastes, animal excrement, and garbage were a result of both overcrowding and a transference to the city of more casual rural practices. By the time of the Industrial Revolution in the late 18th and early 19th centuries, belching smokestacks from thousands of factories and the noise of machinery and transport vehicles further degraded the quality of urban life. Indeed, back in the "good old days" health and sanitary conditions due to air and water pollution and to inadequate (or nonexistent) refuse collection and disposal were far worse than anything with which we are familiar today. When repeated epidemic outbreaks of waterborne disease killed thousands of citizens or when smog-laden air caused millions to wheeze, cough, and occasionally die, the more enlightened civic leaders began to question society's shortsightedness in fouling its own nest. Many of the most important reforms in civic life that occurred late in the 19th century involved implementation of public health measures to deal with water pollution, refuse collection, and smoke abatement. However, throughout this period when urban pollution levels were rising, the countryside remained relatively uncontaminated, except for those areas where a local industry—perhaps a metal smelter or pulp mill—created noxious conditions within its own sphere of influence.

The changes that transformed local pollution problems into global concerns have occurred largely in the years since the end of the Second World War. Reverse migration from urban centers into sprawling suburbia was made possible by a quantum increase in the number of automobiles ("infernal combustion engines") whose exhaust fumes guaranteed that air pollution would no longer be restricted to areas of heavy industry. The escalating energy demands of a growing, affluent population were accompanied by construction of massive new power plants, most of them coal-burning and many located in regions previously noted for pristinely clean air. Perhaps most significant was the vast outpouring of new, synthetic chemical products, many of them toxic compounds, which do not break down readily and can be transported immense distances by air currents, water, or in the tissues of living organisms to wreak their havoc far from their place of origin. In spite of the warnings of a few farsighted individuals, several decades of experience were required before society as a whole became aware of the insidious nature and now-massive scope of environmental degradation.

During the decade of the 1970s, a national awakening in the United States regarding issues of ecology and environmental health produced a flood of federal and state legislation aimed at pollution abatement. The battle has been joined and some successes have already been achieved, but it has become increasingly evident that the problem of environmental pollution is far more complex than originally perceived. Issues not even considered until fairly recently—such as acid precipitation, carbon dioxide accumulation, ozone layer depletion, contamination of groundwater with toxic organic chemicals, and the fearsome dilemma of what to do about abandoned chemical waste dumps—present policymakers, scientists, and citizens with thorny technical and political problems. Solutions to older questions pertaining to community waste disposal practices, air pollution abatement measures, or stormwater runoff control are well understood but often fail to be implemented due to fiscal constraints.

The concluding chapters of this book attempt to delineate the nature of the pollution problems confronting society in the early 21st century. They also describe the legislative tools with which we are now attempting to combat the contamination of our nation's air and water resources in order to prevent future generations from perpetuating the "fouling of the nest" which so endangers our health and well-being.

THE ATMOSPHERE

> .. this most excellent canopy, the air, look you, this brave o'er hanging firmament, this majestical roof fretted with golden fire . . .
>
> —William Shakespeare (*Hamlet*)

The airy canopy above Earth which so inspires poets and painters is a physical characteristic of our planet unique in the solar system. Its existence makes possible the rich diversity of life forms found on Earth, making this globe a veritable oasis in space.

Questions regarding the origin of Earth's atmosphere have intrigued scientists for decades. It is generally assumed that Earth formed almost five billion years ago when particles in a gigantic whirling cloud of dust and gases were pulled together into an aggregate body by enormous gravitational forces. This infant planet had an atmosphere consisting primarily of light gases such as hydrogen and helium, very similar to the present-day atmosphere on the larger planets of Jupiter and Saturn. However, due to Earth's smaller size, gravitational forces were insufficient to retain these elements and they subsequently dissipated into space. This original atmosphere was gradually replaced by a secondary atmosphere produced through the outgassing of volatile materials from the interior of Earth as the once-molten orb began to cool. Modern phenomena such as volcanic eruptions provide vivid evidence that such outgassing continues right up to the present day.

While there has long been widespread agreement among scientists that the primitive Earth's atmosphere was significantly different in chemical composition from that of the present, opinions varied as to precisely which compounds were the major constituents of the early atmosphere. For many years it was widely accepted that a mixture of hydrogen, methane, ammonia, and water vapor would have provided the most congenial environment for the origin of life; these must have been the predominant gases in prebiotic times. More recently, however, this assumption has been challenged by observations that gases ejected by volcanoes consist largely of carbon dioxide and water vapor, leading to the conclusion that, unless volcanoes operated very differently in the past than they do today, the main component of Earth's early atmosphere was carbon dioxide, just as it is today on our neighboring planets of Mars and Venus. This concept of a primitive atmosphere composed primarily of carbon dioxide, water vapor, and nitrogen, with mere traces of ammonia and notably devoid of free oxygen, constitutes the consensus of scientific opinion today. The origin of our modern oxygen-rich atmosphere is traced to the evolution of green plants about two billion years ago. The photosynthetic activities of green plants resulted in the uptake of considerable quantities of atmospheric carbon dioxide and the subsequent release of free oxygen—a necessary precursor for the evolution of higher forms of life (Kasting, 1993; Budyko, 1986; Gribbin, 1982).

Although the chemical constituents of the atmosphere have existed in roughly their present proportions for at least several hundred million years, these constituents are in a constant state of flux, reacting with the continents and oceans to form our weather patterns, constantly being removed and recycled (see chapter 1 on "Geochemical Cycles") as a part of great natural processes. The intimate interrelationships between the atmosphere and land, water, and living things make it relevant to refer to such interactions as the **earth-atmosphere system.** This system is essentially a closed one—every material that goes into the air, though it may circulate and change in form, nevertheless remains within the earth-atmosphere system. This fact has disquieting implications for humans who have always viewed the skies as a convenient garbage dump for their volatile wastes—unfortunately, the concept of a pollutant or any other substance "vanishing into thin air" is a physical impossibility.

Composition of the Atmosphere

The modern atmosphere consists of a mixture of gases so perfectly and consistently diffused among each other that pure dry air exhibits as distinct a set of physical properties as is possessed by any single gas. By volume, the composition of dry air can be broken down as follows:

78% Nitrogen (N_2)
21% Oxygen (O_2)
0.9% Argon (Ar)
0.03% Carbon Dioxide (CO_2)
trace amounts—neon, helium, krypton, xenon, hydrogen, methane, and nitrous oxide

Of the four major atmospheric components, only two, oxygen and carbon dioxide, directly enter into biological processes. Oxygen is required by most living organisms for the production of energy, a process known as aerobic respiration; carbon dioxide constitutes the carbon source for photosynthesis—a series of photochemical reactions whereby chlorophyll molecules in green plants absorb sunlight and use its energy to synthesize simple sugars from carbon dioxide and water. Atmospheric nitrogen, on the other hand, can be utilized only by a few species of nitrogen-fixing bacteria and cyanobacteria, while argon is chemically and biologically inert and thus plays no significant role in the biosphere.

Regions of the Atmosphere

Although the composition of its component gases is uniform throughout the atmosphere from sea level to an altitude approximately 50 miles (80 km) above the earth's surface, scientists subdivide this extent into three distinct regions based on temperature zones.

Troposphere. Extending from sea level to an altitude about 8 miles above the earth (slightly less above the poles, more above the equator) is the region known as the troposphere. Virtually all life activities occur within this region and most weather and climatic phenomena occur here. In addition to the usual gases, the troposphere also contains varying amounts of water vapor and dust particles. Within the troposphere temperature steadily falls with increasing altitude, a decrease of 5.4°F per 1,000 feet (10°C/km). The upper limit of the troposphere is known as the **tropopause**.

Stratosphere. Above the troposphere lies the stratosphere, a region distinguished by a temperature gradient reversal. Here the temperature slowly rises with increasing altitude until it reaches 32°F (0°C) at a height of about 30 miles (50 km), the upper boundary of the stratosphere known as the **stratopause.** Unlike the troposphere, the stratosphere contains almost no water vapor or dust. It is the site, however, of the **ozone layer,** a region characterized by higher-than-usual concentrations of the

Figure 11-1   Regions of the Atmosphere

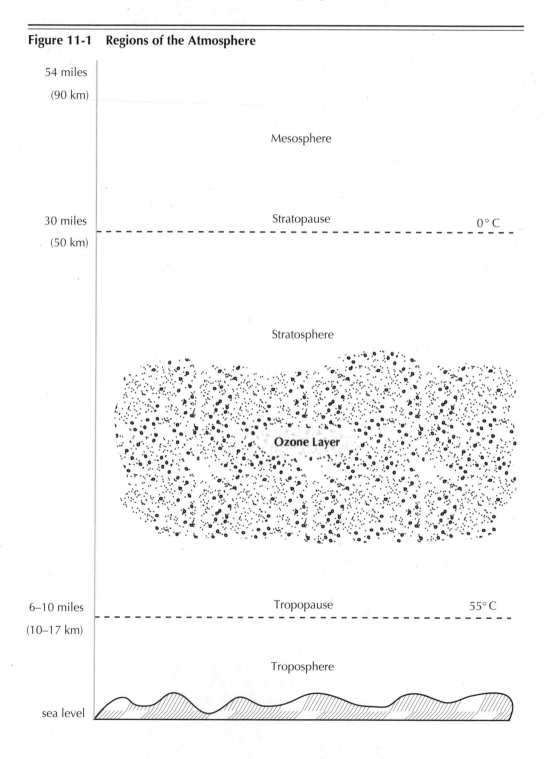

54 miles
(90 km)

Mesosphere

30 miles   Stratopause   0° C
(50 km)

Stratosphere

Ozone Layer

6–10 miles   Tropopause   55° C
(10–17 km)

Troposphere

sea level

rare gas ozone (O_3), an isotope of oxygen (O_2). The ozone layer extends from about 8–15 miles (12–25 km) above the earth's surface, being most concentrated between 11–15 miles. Amounts of ozone vary depending on location and season of the year. Ozone concentrations are lowest above the equator, increasing toward the poles; they also increase markedly between autumn and spring (Parson, 2003).

Mesosphere. Above the stratopause is the region known as the mesosphere, where temperature once again begins to fall with increasing altitude. Since the air becomes progressively more diffuse as the altitude above the earth increases, it is difficult to say precisely where the atmosphere ends. In terms of mass, 99% of our atmosphere lies within 18 miles of the earth's surface—an astonishingly thin blanket nurturing beneath it all the life known to exist in the universe (Strahler and Strahler, 1973).

Radiation Balance

In addition to providing the major source of certain chemical elements necessary for life, the atmosphere performs a vital role in controlling the earth's surface environment by regulating both the quality and quantity of solar radiation that enters and leaves the biosphere.

The source of all energy on earth, of course, is the sun. However, solar energy can be subdivided into several categories, depending on wavelength of the various forms of radiation involved. These categories and their wavelengths are as follows:

Type of Radiation	% of Total Energy	Wavelength (in micrometers)
Ultraviolet rays	9	0.1–0.4
Visible light rays	38	0.4–0.7
Infrared rays (heat)	53	0.7–3000

These forms of electromagnetic radiation travel outward from the sun at a rate of 186,000 miles (300,000 km) per second, taking slightly over nine minutes to reach the earth. Although none of the sun's energy is lost as it travels through space, once it begins to penetrate earth's atmosphere both a depletion and diversion of solar radiation begin to occur.

Most of the ultraviolet radiation present in sunlight is absorbed by the ozone layer as it passes through the stratosphere, though some of the UV wavelengths longer than 0.3 micrometers (the so-called UVB region) manage to penetrate to the earth's surface where they can produce sunburn and skin cancers. The ozone layer itself is actually created by ultraviolet light, since UV radiant energy causes ordinary oxygen molecules to break apart, releasing single atoms of oxygen which then react with intact oxygen molecules to form ozone. Since, as was explained in chapter 10, ultraviolet radiation can have serious adverse effects on living organisms, the existence of the ozone layer is of great biological significance (Panofsky, 1978).

Visible light rays and infrared radiation penetrate through the upper stratosphere unaffected by the ozone layer. However, as the atmospheric gas molecules increase in density closer to the earth, these molecules cause a random scattering of the incoming visible light waves (infrared waves are not so affected and for the most part continue to stream directly toward the earth). Entering the troposphere, additional scattering and diffuse reflection of visible light waves occur due to contact with dust particles and clouds (a clear sky appears blue because the shorter blue wavelengths are scattered to a greater extent than are the longer red wavelengths and thus reach our eyes from all parts of the sky). Additional amounts of incoming solar radiation are lost by reflection from the upper surfaces of clouds, oceans, or from the land (particularly when covered with snow or ice). Energy losses also occur when carbon dioxide and water vapor absorb infrared radiation (heat waves) as sunlight enters the lower atmosphere. This heat absorption results in an increase in air temperature. Although the carbon dioxide content of the air is constant everywhere, the amount of water vapor varies considerably and is the main factor accounting for differences in the amount of infrared absorption in various climatic regions (e.g., arid regions experience greater temperature extremes during a 24-hour period than do more humid areas at the same latitude because the low water vapor content of desert air minimizes the absorption of the infrared waves). Altogether, scattering, reflection, and absorption of sunlight can result in the loss of as little as 20% of incoming solar radiation when skies are clear to

Figure 11-2   Earth's Energy Budget

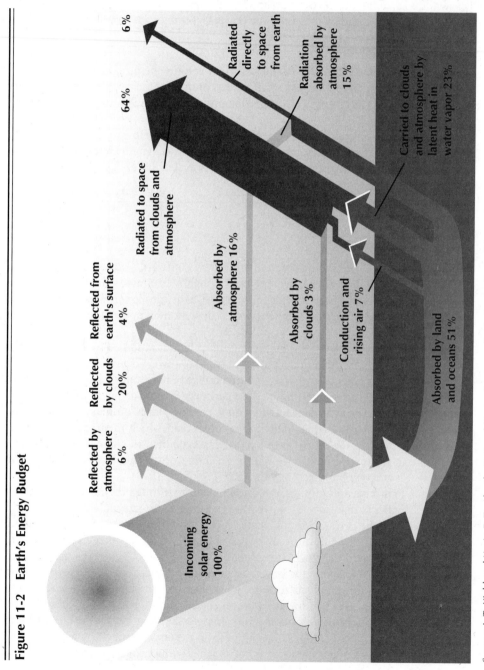

Source: J. T. Kiehl and Kevin E. Trenberth, National Center for Atmospheric Research, Boulder, Colorado. Used with permission.

nearly 100% under conditions of heavy cloud cover. On a global yearly average it is estimated that the earth-atmosphere system absorbs about 68% of the total incoming solar radiation, 32% being lost due to the factors just mentioned.

In order to maintain a global radiation balance, energy absorbed by the earth from incoming sunlight must be equaled by outward radiation of energy from the earth's surface. This so-called "ground radiation" occurs in the form of infrared waves longer than 3 or 4 micrometers (referred to as "long-wave radiation"), which are continually being radiated back into the atmosphere, even at night when no solar radiation is being received. Some of the infrared waves leaving the earth (those in the 5–8 and 12–20 micrometer range) are absorbed by water vapor and carbon dioxide in the atmosphere, a portion of which are reradiated back to the earth's surface, thereby keeping the earth's climate warmer than it would otherwise be. This phenomenon, known as the greenhouse effect, has extremely important climatic implications that will be discussed in more detail later in this chapter.

While incoming and outgoing units of radiation are often not in balance at any one particular time and place (indeed, such imbalances provide the forces behind our constantly changing weather patterns), an equilibrium of such units for the world as a whole during any given year exists, resulting in the maintenance of annual average global temperatures that fluctuate very little from year to year (Strahler and Strahler, 1973). One of the most pressing concerns among atmospheric scientists today is that human activities may be altering the global radiation balance in ways that may have far-reaching climatic consequences.

Human Impact on the Earth-Atmosphere System

Geologic records give ample indication of drastic climatic changes at various times in Earth's long history, the most recent being four successive periods of widespread glaciation (the "Ice Ages"), the last of which ended only 10,000 years ago. Obviously humans had nothing to do with past fluctuations in the global heat balance, but our impact today may no longer be so negligible. Temperature measurements compiled over many decades clearly indicate that possibly significant changes in climate are already underway; the extent to which human activities are provoking or enhancing such trends is presently the topic of heated academic debate.

The major causes of human-induced atmospheric change are:

1. Introduction into the atmosphere of pollutant gases and particles not usually found there in significant amounts

2. Changes in the concentrations of natural atmospheric components

The following sections illustrate two of the most difficult issues we must confront as the impact of human activities on the earth-atmosphere system inexorably intensifies— depletion of the ozone layer and rising levels of atmospheric CO_2 (global warming).

Depletion of the Ozone Layer

Although ozone is one of the rarest of atmospheric gases, its presence in the stratosphere is of vital importance in protecting life on Earth from the damaging effects of solar ultraviolet radiation. As mentioned earlier, the ozone layer is created when UV energy splits the oxygen molecule and the freed atoms rejoin other oxygen molecules to form ozone (O_3). At the same time, the highly reactive ozone is being broken down again to normal oxygen (O_2); thus the ozone layer is maintained in a state of dynamic equilibrium, daytime increases being balanced by nighttime decreases.

In 1974 atmospheric chemists advanced a hypothesis that certain pollutant emissions into the atmosphere had the potential to disrupt this equilibrium, threatening the long-term integrity of the ozone layer. Initially attention focused on the damage potential of nitrous oxides emitted with jet airplane exhausts (particularly from supersonic transports such as the Anglo-French Concorde) and the use of nitrogen fertilizers. It gradually became apparent, however, that a far more serious threat to the ozone layer was posed by the widespread use at that time of a group of synthetic chemicals known as **chlorofluorocarbons (CFCs)**, one of the best known of which was the refrigerant Freon®. Utilized commercially since the 1930s for home and industrial refrigeration, freezing, and air-conditioning, CFC applications expanded in the post-World War II period to include use as propellants in aerosol spray cans. By the 1970s the latter use constituted the single largest portion of CFC production, as hundreds of products from paints and insecticides to hair sprays and deodorants were repackaged in aerosol cans. As new applications for CFCs were developed, world production of these chemicals soared; by the early 1970s, approximately a million tons were being produced each year. Another closely related group of chemicals, the **halons** (bromofluorocarbons), were developed in the 1950s as extremely effective fire suppressants and came into widespread commercial use in the 1960s and 1970s. Unfortunately, the very property of CFCs and halons (collectively referred to as **ozone-depleting substances**) that made them so valuable commercially—their extreme chemical stability—also made them a serious threat to the global environment. When released into the air through vaporization or leakage from enclosed systems, or when directly sprayed from aerosol containers or fire extinguishers, the chemicals don't break down. Instead, they drift upward through the troposphere into the stratosphere where the molecules are finally broken down by UV radiation, releasing atoms of chlorine (CFCs) or bromine (halons) that react with and destroy ozone. The halogen-ozone reaction is a catalytic one; in the case of CFCs, for example, the same chlorine atom can repeat the reaction with tens of thousands of ozone molecules. This, plus the fact that the chlorine atoms will remain in the atmosphere for 100 years or more, explains why CFCs' destructive impact on the ozone layer is so much greater than emission levels might suggest. Bromine is even more problematic; although its atmospheric concentrations are far lower than those of chlorine, bromine depletes stratospheric ozone 45–50 times more efficiently than CFC-derived chlorine atoms.

Depletion of the ozone layer is worrisome from a human health perspective because of stratospheric ozone's role in absorbing biologically damaging ultraviolet radiation. It is now well established that for each 1% decrease in atmospheric ozone, penetration of UV radiation to the earth's surface will increase by 2%. As scientific research on potential threats to the ozone layer intensified during the 1970s and early 1980s, concerns mounted regarding the impact such depletion might have on skin cancer incidence. Since more than 90% of nonmelanoma skin cancers are associated with exposure to UV radiation in sunlight, any increase in ultraviolet exposure could be expected to result in more skin malignancies. In 1982 the National Academy of Sciences reported that for every 1% decrease in the concentration of atmospheric ozone, cases of basal cell carcinoma would likely rise by 2–5%, squamous cell carcinomas by 4–10% (Maugh, 1982). In 1992, as efforts to do something about the problem were moving into high gear, the United Nations Environment Programme underscored the urgency of the international effort by releasing estimates forecasting a 26% worldwide increase in nonmelanoma skin cancers if stratospheric ozone levels dropped by 10%.

The "Hole in the Sky"

In the United States, an intense public debate on threats to the ozone layer focused largely on aerosol propellants and resulted in a nationwide ban on such products, effective in 1978. Canada, Sweden, and Norway enacted similar bans in 1980, but aerosol products continued to be used elsewhere. This action lulled the public into assuming the problem had been solved, and for several years little more was heard about the issue. During the early 1980s, both government and many scientists downplayed the ozone depletion threat, asserting that earlier forecasts of ozone loss had been exaggerated and assuring skeptics that CFC production had leveled off and thus presented little cause for concern. This sense of complacency was suddenly shattered in 1985 when members of the British Antarctic Survey announced the existence of a large hole in the ozone layer over the South Pole. Although the gap was temporary, opening in early September (Antarctic spring) and closing by mid-October as the southern atmosphere grew warmer, it had been increasing in size each year since the British researchers first noticed it in 1981; by the time of their startling revelation, the "hole" represented a 40% decline in ozone concentrations. Subsequent confirmation by NASA that the ozone hole was real led to intensified research efforts to learn what was going wrong in the polar skies. U.S. scientists sent to McMurdo Bay in the years following discovery of the "hole in the sky" revealed that the springtime depletion of ozone was steadily getting larger, appearing earlier, and lasting longer. In 1987, ozone losses totaled 50%; by 1991 they reached 70% over an area four times the size of the United States and measurements of UV radiation reaching the ground were the highest ever recorded in Antarctica up to that time. During the 1990s and into the early 21st century the Antarctic "ozone hole" grew ever larger, reaching an all-time record of 11 million square miles (28.4 million km^2) in both 2000 and 2003. It was considerably smaller in 2002 and 2004, a fact scientists attribute to natural variations in atmospheric conditions.

During the late 1980s and early 1990s conflicting theories regarding the cause of this depletion were vigorously debated by researchers. Chemical pollution, cyclical solar flares, and natural atmospheric variation were the main contenders for chief villain. Within a few years the weight of evidence tilted toward the chemical pollution theory with the discovery that concentrations of ozone-destroying chlorine molecules were 400–500 times higher within the ozone hole than outside. The presence of chlorine was widely regarded as a "smoking gun"—evidence establishing a direct cause-and-effect link between CFC emissions and ozone layer destruction.

Throughout the 1990s, evidence continued to mount that the pace of ozone loss was accelerating, not only over the South Pole but also above the more populous regions of the Northern Hemisphere. Since 1979 the U.S. government has been collecting data on atmospheric ozone from ground-based survey stations and the Nimbus-7 satellite. By 1993 NASA scientists were reporting record low concentrations of stratospheric ozone above the middle latitudes of North America and Eurasia—down by as much as 20% from their normal levels. While this dramatic drop in ozone may be blamed, at least in part, on debris hurled into the upper atmosphere by the massive 1991 eruption of the Philippine volcano, Mt. Pinatubo, researchers pointed out that even prior to this event about 3% of the ozone layer above the United States, Europe, Russia, Japan, and China had been lost. Moreover, when the ozone dipped by 3% over the United States, it dropped by 4% over Australia and New Zealand, and 6% in Scandinavia. More ominously, this loss was occurring in the spring and summer when human exposure to sunlight is at peak levels ("Ozone Takes," 1993; WRI, 1992). While winter ozone losses over the Arctic haven't occurred as predictably year after year as they have over the South Pole, the winter of 1997 saw the highest Arctic ozone depletion yet recorded, a reminder that the problem is still very much with us.

Until the 1990s, a major weakness in the claim that observed declines in stratospheric ozone levels represented a serious environmental health threat was the scarcity of data documenting an actual increase in ultraviolet light penetration anywhere except in Antarctica—where the number of exposed humans is negligible. That data gap was essentially closed in November 1993, with the publication of a five-year study conducted in Toronto by two scientists working with Environment Canada (Canadian equivalent of EPA). From 1989 to 1993, the researchers took ground-level measurements of UV radiation every hour from sunrise to sunset during winter and summer (seasons when UV levels are at their highest and lowest, respectively). They found that at wavelengths around 300 nanometers (the portion of the UV spectrum most strongly absorbed by stratospheric ozone), ultraviolet radiation increased by 35% per year in winter, 6–7% per year in summer. Since measurements of stratospheric ozone concentrations above Toronto had documented a 4% annual decrease in winter and a 2% summer decline each year during the study period, skeptics' arguments that air pollution or cloud cover will counteract the effect of ozone loss have been proven wrong (Kerr and McElroy, 1993).

Policy Response—The Montreal Protocol

After years of controversy among scientists, the chemical industry, and government policymakers as to the extent of ozone depletion, the identity of the main culprits, and the most effective approach for halting—or at least slowing down—the process, consensus has emerged that ozone depletion is real, that it presents a major threat to life on this planet, and that global cooperation is required to combat a phenomenon that threatens us all. A major step forward to meet this challenge was taken in September 1987, when diplomats from 29 nations, meeting in Montreal, Canada, signed an international accord aimed at controlling the chemicals most responsible for ozone layer depletion. As originally ratified, the Montreal Protocol called for the freezing of CFC consumption at 1986 levels by 1990, to be followed by a 50% reduction in the production of these chemicals by the end of the century. The treaty went into effect in January 1989, after ratification by nations representing more than two-thirds of the world's CFC production (eventually 184 nations signed the Montreal Protocol). By the early 1990s, scientific evidence that ozone depletion was occurring much more rapidly than anticipated prompted several strengthening amendments to the international treaty. The list of chemicals targeted for controls was expanded to include halons, carbon tetrachloride, methyl chloroform, hydrochlorofluorocarbons (HCFCs), and methyl bromide; in addition, the timetable for phasing out production and use of ozone-depleting substances was advanced. For industrialized nations, the ban on domestic sale and use of CFCs took effect on January 1, 1996, and has met with near-universal compliance; developing countries, whose production and use of these chemicals rose rapidly during the 1990s, were required under the Montreal Protocol to freeze production at their 1995–1997 levels by 1999 and to halt production completely by 2010. Industrialized countries ceased manufacturing halons in 1994, an action developing nations are not required to take until 2010. Phaseout of other ozone-depleters will follow in the early decades of the 21st century.

Unfortunately, even full implementation of the treaty's requirements will not prevent further losses of ozone. Millions of pounds of CFCs already released are gradually drifting up toward the ozone layer and will remain in the atmosphere for many decades. Nevertheless, the cutbacks in CFC production called for in the Montreal Protocol are already having an impact. In August 1993, atmospheric physicists working for the National Oceanic and Atmospheric Administration (NOAA) announced that the unexpectedly rapid drop in industrial production of CFCs even prior to the implementation deadlines set by the treaty had resulted in a substantial slowdown in the rate at which ozone-depleting chemicals were accumulating in the atmosphere. By the early 2000s, depletion of the ozone layer was measured at about 4% per decade, down

Box 11-1 Bumps in the Road to Ozone Recovery

Declining concentrations of ozone-depleting substances (ODS) in the atmosphere, along with encouraging reports that world consumption of CFCs and halons has plummeted by approximately 95% since 1986, have prompted a number of observers to predict complete recovery of the ozone layer by mid-century. Trends indeed seem favorable, but several confounding factors suggest that progress toward this goal could be much slower than anticipated.

The first challenge to ozone recovery efforts was the emergence in 1994–1995 of a lucrative black market in CFCs and other ODS, undermining the intent of the Montreal Protocol. After ratification of the international treaty, the United States and most other industrialized countries launched a commendably rapid transition from CFCs to more ozone-friendly alternatives. Although the changeover cost industry billions of dollars to re-tool manufacturing processes and products, cooperation by CFC producers, industry, and government enabled most developed countries to meet the 1996 deadline date for a halt in production of CFCs and halons for domestic use. By 1994–95, production cuts and excise taxes had driven the retail price of CFCs in the United States from $1/pound to $15/pound—a predictable market response to rapidly dwindling supply and high demand. The excise taxes were intended to encourage recycling of CFCs still in use and to provide a cost incentive for converting equipment to use CFC substitutes. Instead, they substantially increased the cost of U.S.-produced CFCs even before the 1996 ban took effect and led to a sudden explosion in black marketeering.

CFC smuggling to both the United States and European Union countries reached a peak in 1995, when about 20,000 tons were illicitly traded. The primary source of this contraband was Russia, which at that time produced half the world's CFC supply and where the Russian Mafia was deeply involved in Freon trafficking. By 1997, as prohibitions on the manufacture, use, and importation of CFCs took effect in the U.S. and other industrialized countries, increased Customs enforcement and a crackdown on illegal Russian production resulted in a sharp drop in black market CFCs entering the United States. By that time, however, the focus of smuggling had shifted to developing countries, where a freeze on production levels was to take effect in 1999, followed by phaseout of the chemicals by 2010. In Asia, production and use of CFCs and halons had increased rapidly during the 1990s, most notably in China and India. In these countries and elsewhere in the developing world, a great deal of equipment still relies on CFCs and owners are loath to pay the much higher prices charged for CFC alternatives—an ideal situation for smugglers and black marketeers. Surprisingly, a significant portion of the ODS smuggled into Third World nations originates in several European Union (EU) countries that can still legally produce CFCs and halons for export to developing nations.

The Environmental Investigation Agency (EIA), an organization that has been actively tracking the global black market in ODS since the mid-1990s, has conducted undercover operations to describe worldwide smuggling operations. EIA found that although EU production facilities were operating in accordance with the law, the chemicals produced were often sold to unscrupulous dealers who then diverted them to more profitable markets, often using third countries as transit points to divert CFCs onto the black market. By selling their product to brokers rather than directly to a buyer, CFC manufacturers are absolved of the responsibility to verify that the material was delivered to its intended destination or that the amount delivered was not in excess of the country's yearly consumption. Greedy dealers willing to ignore controls, falsify paperwork, conceal smuggled goods behind nonprohibited chemicals, or mislabel products find it relatively easy to evade the lax enforcement of anti-smuggling laws in most developing countries. To deal more effectively with illegal trade in ozone-depleting substances, a new alliance of governments, international agencies, chemical producers, and nongovernmental organizations met in Bangkok in March 2004. There participants agreed to cooperate more effectively, sharing information and intelligence to halt what they all agreed was an environmental crime that could substantially prolong ozone layer recovery. Nevertheless, while international law enforcement efforts to end the illicit trade in CFCs are welcome, some activists are convinced that global smuggling networks are so sophisticated that as long as CFCs and halons continue to be manufactured, black marketeering will persist. The only permanent solution, in their view, is to end all production of ODS.

Although an ODS phaseout would solve one ozone depletion problem, a more difficult issue has recently emerged—a hitherto unrecognized linkage between stratospheric ozone depletion and global warming. It was long assumed that these two phenomena represented two entirely separate issues, with different causes and different solutions. New research, however, has cast doubt on that assumption. Evidence emerged in the late 1990s that the processes associated with global climate change are further aggravating ozone loss. Researchers hypothesize that as greenhouse gas concentrations continue to rise, the stratosphere will become colder as the troposphere and earth's surface heat up. Such cooling of the stratosphere is likely to increase ozone depletion by favoring the formation of the polar stratospheric clouds on whose surfaces the chemical reactions leading to ozone destruction occur. If this scenario proves accurate, an "ozone hole" similar to that over Antarctica could develop over the middle and high latitudes in the Northern Hemisphere. Other scientists examining the linkage suggest that as temperatures in the troposphere above tropical regions rise, more water vapor will enter the stratosphere and raise the threshold temperature below which the chemical reactions resulting in ozone loss occur. As a consequence, these researchers foresee springtime ozone losses above the Arctic increasing from their current 15% to as much as 50% and suggest that global warming trends now underway may explain why total stratospheric ozone continues to decline, even though atmo-

spheric concentrations of chlorine and bromine are beginning to fall.

New awareness of a possible relationship between ozone depletion and climate change has raised a perplexing practical issue related to CFC alternatives. Determined to end use of the most damaging ODS as quickly as possible, negotiators of the Montreal Protocol accepted substitutes (e.g., HCFC) that subsequently proved to be ozone-depleters themselves, albeit somewhat less damaging. Recognizing the problem, deadline dates for phaseout of HCFCs were set, with these products being regarded as transitional to another group of chemicals called hydrofluorocarbons (HFCs). Hydrofluorocarbons play a critical role in the phaseout of CFCs and halons, since they are effective substitutes and are ozone-friendly. HFCs, however, turn out to be powerful greenhouse gases, contributing significantly to global climate change. Their continued use thus presents decision-makers with a paradox: while HFCs are an essential element in solving the ozone depletion problem, they exacerbate the even more serious problem of global warming. Since HFCs are not ozone depleters, the Montreal Protocol is unable to deal with this issue and the dilemma to date remains unresolved.

These uncertainties raise questions regarding when full recovery of the ozone layer will be realized and suggest that there needs to be a more holistic approach to dealing with problems affecting the earth-atmosphere system. As the experts continue to wrestle with these issues, citizens lulled into thinking ozone depletion is no longer a problem might be well advised to hang onto their sunscreen.

References

Environmental Investigation Agency (EIA). http://www.eia-international.org

Parson, Edward A. 2003. *Protecting the Ozone Layer: Science and Strategy.* New York: Oxford Univ. Press.

from 8% in the 1980s. Although concentrations of chlorine in the upper stratosphere continue to increase, they are increasing at a slower rate than previously, an indication that the Montreal Protocol's phaseout of ozone-depleting substances is having a positive impact. These observations have given rise to optimism in many quarters that recovery of the ozone layer is now underway. Although the transition from CFCs and halons to more environmentally benign substitutes is still incomplete, scientists and policymakers are pleased with progress to date, predicting that recovery of the ozone layer to its pre-CFC condition could occur by 2050. The international efforts to protect the ozone layer exemplified by the Montreal Protocol are extremely significant in that they represent the first time in history that the nations of the world have agreed to work together to prevent a disaster of global proportions before it's too late. Initial indications of the success of this approach offer hope for similar cooperation in tackling even more difficult environmental challenges—such as global climate change.

Rising Levels of Atmospheric CO$_2$— Moving toward a Warmer World?

> The inhabitants of Planet Earth are quietly conducting a gigantic environmental experiment. So vast and so sweeping will be the impacts of this experiment that, were it brought before any responsible council for approval, it would be firmly rejected as having potentially dangerous consequences. Yet, the experiment goes on with no significant interference from any jurisdiction or nation. The experiment in question is the release of carbon dioxide and other so-called greenhouse gases to the atmosphere.
> —Wallace S. Broecker, geochemist, Columbia University (Mintzer, 1987)

As mentioned earlier in this chapter, the relative concentrations of the four major atmospheric gases—nitrogen, oxygen, argon, and carbon dioxide—have remained constant for at least several hundred million years. Several decades ago, however, scientists began raising concerns that a decrease in oxygen levels and an increase in the amount of atmospheric carbon dioxide might be occurring due to the sharp rise in fossil fuel combustion (a process that consumes O$_2$ and releases CO$_2$), the worldwide destruction of forest cover, and the poisoning of oceanic phytoplankton by pollution of the seas. (Plants are the source of atmospheric oxygen and also capture and store huge amounts of CO$_2$, thereby removing it from the atmosphere.) Fortunately, studies of the oxygen balance have shown that no oxygen depletion has yet occurred and forces operating at the present time are deemed far too insignificant to constitute a real threat so far as oxygen supply is concerned (Broecker, 1970).

The fears regarding carbon dioxide increase, on the other hand, have proven to be well founded and the prospect of a long-term global warming due to CO$_2$-induced enhancement of the greenhouse effect has become the most pressing and politically charged of all global environmental issues. Levels of atmospheric CO$_2$ have been gradually rising ever since the dawn of the Industrial Revolution as a result of the ever-increasing use of coal, oil, and gas to power the world's factories and vehicles. By 2002, fossil fuel combustion was releasing 6.44 billion tons of carbon to the atmosphere—four times the amount emitted in 1950 (Sheehan, 2003). When fossil fuels are burned, one of the primary combustion products is carbon dioxide; the combustion of one ton of coal, for example, releases three tons of CO$_2$. In past ages, excess carbon dioxide released through volcanic outgassing was gradually absorbed into the oceans and eventually incorporated into carbonate rock or was photosynthetically "fixed" by green plants, particularly rapidly growing young forests (mature forests, by contrast, give off about the same amount of CO$_2$ as they take in). Scientists estimate that perhaps as much as half of the CO$_2$ emitted by human activities each year is currently being absorbed by the oceans and by land plants, with the latter serving as a repository for more carbon than the amount released annually by deforestation.

Table 11-1   Carbon Dioxide Emissions by Top Ten Emitting Countries, 2002

Country	Emissions (Million Metric Tons Carbon Equivalent)	Share of Global Total (%)
United States	1,568.0	23.4
China	908.1	13.6
Russia	415.2	6.2
Japan	321.7	4.8
India	279.9	4.2
Germany	228.6	3.4
Canada	161.4	2.4
United Kingdom	150.8	2.3
South Korea	122.9	1.8
Italy	122.4	1.8
All Other Countries	2,411.9	36.0
Global Total	**6,690.7**	**100.0**

Source: Lila Buckley, "Carbon Emissions Reach Record High," *Eco-Economy Indicators* (Washington, DC: Earth Policy Institute, 2004. www. earth-policy.org). Based on data from U.S. Department of Energy, *International Energy Annual 2002* (Washington, DC: June 2004).

Unfortunately, many researchers believe that the ability of land and water to act as a "carbon sink" is reaching capacity and will decline as concentrations of atmospheric CO_2 continue to rise. As today's young forests mature, they will take up less and less excess CO_2; similarly, after more than a century of absorbing billions of tons of excess carbon, the ocean's buffering capacity is near the point of saturation and as ocean temperatures continue to rise, less carbon dioxide will be absorbed by the world's seas (the warmer the water, the less soluble is CO_2).

While fossil fuel combustion has received most of the attention—and blame—in relation to rising CO_2 concentrations, the wide-scale destruction of natural vegetation, particularly deforestation in the tropics, contributes nearly one-fourth (23%) of all global CO_2 emissions. Both forests and the organic matter in soil humus hold immense quantities of carbon that are oxidized and released as carbon dioxide when vegetation is destroyed. Space satellite monitors have revealed that the impact of forest destruction on CO_2 release may be even greater than previously realized. Data collected over the Amazon basin indicate that the thousands of fires deliberately set every year by settlers and ranchers clearing the Brazilian rain forest are generating such enormous quantities of gases and particles that they alone may account for at least one-tenth of the carbon dioxide released by human activities each year (Watson et al., 1990). The equilibrium that has prevailed for millennia has been disrupted, with the result that atmospheric CO_2 levels are now sharply increasing.

In 1999, a team of Russian, French, and U.S. scientists working at Russia's Vostok research station in Antarctica published data showing that current greenhouse gas levels are higher than any in the past 420,000 years. By chemically analyzing air bubbles trapped in ice cores drilled two miles into the Antarctic ice sheet, the researchers were able to construct a record of past climatic conditions, demonstrating increases and decreases of carbon dioxide and methane as warm interglacial periods alternated with colder glacial epochs. They found that even the highest concentrations of greenhouse gases in past millennia, present during the warm interglacial years, were well below present-day levels, strongly suggesting that humans are influencing today's climatic patterns (Petit et al., 1999). Since the beginning of the Industrial Revolution two centuries ago, concentrations of atmospheric CO_2 have risen by nearly 30%, from 280 ppm to 375 ppm in 2004; throughout the preindustrial portion of the past millennium, atmospheric CO_2 concentrations never varied by more than 5 ppm (Indermühle et al., 1999). Since the early 1980s, CO_2 levels in the atmosphere have been rising at a rate of 0.4% (1.5 ppm) per year and are now 31% higher than they were in 1750, prior to the Industrial Revolution. If current emission rates persist, carbon cycle models project that atmospheric CO_2 concentrations will rise to anywhere from 540 to 970 ppm by 2100—90% to 250% higher than their preindustrial level (IPCC, 2001).

The sense of alarm felt by those monitoring this situation relates not to any adverse effect that CO_2 might exert on human health—the gas is not a toxic pollutant but a natural and necessary constituent of the biosphere—but rather is due to the impact increasing levels of carbon dioxide will have on global climate. As mentioned earlier in this chapter, atmospheric CO_2 plays a vital role in moderating the earth's temperature, a phenomenon known as the **greenhouse effect.** Just as the glass in a greenhouse permits light to enter but prevents the escape of heat, thereby warming the air within, so the absorption of infrared ground radiation by carbon dioxide and its subsequent reradiation back toward the earth helps to maintain an average global temperature of 59°F (15°C). Without CO_2 in the atmosphere, the earth's average surface temperature would fall to about 0°F, making the existence of life as we know it impossible. By way of comparison, the planet Venus, with a dense, CO_2-rich atmosphere, has a surface temperature of 890°F (hot enough to melt lead) while Mars, whose atmosphere consists primarily of CO_2 but is very diffuse and contains but a trace of water vapor, is colder than Antarctica, with an average temperature of –53°F (Revkin, 1992; Houghton, Jenkins, and Ephraums, 1990). However, as carbon dioxide levels increase, more infrared radiation will be absorbed and over time average global temperatures will correspondingly rise.

Comprehensive scientific efforts to determine whether global warming is actually occurring as a result of human activities have been underway since the late 1970s, drawing on evidence derived from such diverse sources as ice core analyses, orbiting satellites, ocean current studies, and computer modeling. The result of these wide-ranging investigations has been an evolving scientific consensus that rising greenhouse gas concentrations have, indeed, altered the global energy balance enough to raise average world temperatures by 1.4 to 5.8°C (2.5 to 10.5°F) over the period spanning 1990–2001. This is in addition to the 0.6°C (1°F) increase in the global average surface temperature during the 20th century. The range in projected future temperature increases reflects the results of computer modeling studies based on 35 different emission scenarios, but all represent a global climate warmer than anything experienced during at least the last 10,000 years (IPCC, 2001). Until the mid-1990s, the international scientific community was hesitant to attribute incipient signs of climate change to human causes, pointing out that natural fluctuations in the past had resulted in alternating cycles of warming and cooling and could be doing so again.

In 1990 the Intergovernmental Panel on Climate Change (IPCC), jointly established by the World Meteorological Organization and the United Nations Environment Programme to assess information related to climate change, issued its First Assessment Report. Based on the limited data available at that time, IPCC concluded that global warming was occurring, but couldn't establish whether human or natural forces were to blame. By the time IPCC published its Second Assessment Report in 1995, its findings were less ambiguous, stating that "the balance of evidence suggests a discernible human influence on global climate," but acknowledging remaining uncertainties. IPCC's most recent Third Assessment Report, released in 2001, cast aside remaining doubts on causation, stating that there is now new and persuasive evidence that human activities are, indeed, to blame for most of the warming observed over the last half-century (IPCC, 2001). Since the IPCC, comprising 2,500 scientists from nearly 100 countries, is regarded by governments around the world as the official advisory body on issues pertaining to global warming, its statements carry considerable weight. Although a small minority of dissident scientists (the so-called "greenhouse skeptics") still argue to the contrary, IPCC's conclusions constitute an important affirmation of the breadth and depth of agreement within the scientific community about the reality of global climate change and the dire consequences of human interference with the earth-atmosphere system.

Turning Up the Heat: Other Greenhouse Gases

As if humanity doesn't have enough to worry about with the rise in carbon dioxide levels, climatologists now warn that increasing atmospheric concentrations of several other gases—specifically, methane, nitrous oxide, and halocarbons—are further enhancing the greenhouse effect by capturing wavelengths of infrared radiation not readily absorbed by CO_2. Although present in concentrations far below that of carbon dioxide, these trace gases are much more efficient than CO_2 in absorbing outgoing heat waves. A molecule of methane, for example, can trap 20–30 times more infrared radiation than does a molecule of CO_2. Equally worrisome is the fact that emissions of trace gases are increasing at a substantially faster rate than CO_2 and originate from sources that may be even more difficult to control. A brief look at the situation regarding the other "greenhouse gases" reveals the following picture.

Methane (CH_4). Although current atmospheric concentrations of this gas are less than 2 ppm, as opposed to CO_2 levels of 375 ppm, methane is far more potent as a greenhouse gas and is increasing at a 0.6% annual rate. Curtailing methane emissions will not be easy, since over half originate from rice cultivation (due to the respiration of anaerobic bacteria in waterlogged paddy fields) and from microbial activity in the intestines of cattle and termites (it is estimated that a cow belches methane approximately twice a minute!). Other significant sources more amenable to controls include landfills, emissions from gas and coal production, flares on oil rigs, and tropical deforestation (when vegetation is burned during clearing activities).

Nitrous oxide (N_2O). With atmospheric concentrations up by 17% (46 ppb) since 1750 and still rising, the so-called "laughing gas" once used as a painkiller by dentists is a more efficient greenhouse gas than CO_2 but because its total atmospheric concentrations are in the parts per billion range, its overall contribution to global warming is still fairly limited. Nitrous oxide is a natural by-product of the metabolism of certain soil microbes, but the generation of this gas has been boosted significantly by the increased worldwide use of nitrogen fertilizers. Combustion of fossil fuels, increased land cultivation, burning of biomass, and the decomposition of agricultural wastes and sewage are additional sources of N_2O.

Halocarbons. A group that includes the ozone-depleting chlorofluorocarbons (CFCs), as well as **perfluorocarbons** (PFCs), **sulfur hexafluoride** (SF_6), and the **hydrofluorocarbons** (HFCs), halocarbons are potent greenhouse gases, each molecule of which has a direct warming effect 12,000–20,000 times greater than that of a CO_2 molecule. It is assumed that the halt in CFC production mandated by the Montreal Protocol will result in a decrease—or slower increase—in atmospheric concentrations of these gases in the years to come. However, concentrations of PFCs, HFCs, and SF_6 continue to rise due to their increasing commercial and industrial use as substitutes for CFCs and other now-banned ozone-depleting chemicals.

It should be noted that water vapor is another important greenhouse gas, but because human activities have negligible impact on its atmospheric concentrations and because the amount of water in the air varies widely from place to place and day to day, levels of this atmospheric constituent are not taken into consideration when discussing global warming scenarios.

While the lion's share of public attention regarding climate change has thus far focused on carbon dioxide emissions, it is now agreed that the cumulative effect of the other greenhouse gases will be nearly equivalent to that of CO_2. Ironically, until now air pollution has helped counteract the heat-capturing potential of greenhouse gases to some extent. Airborne sulfate particles released when fossil fuels and other organic materials are burned reflect solar radiation, thereby exerting a cooling effect on climate. Thanks to increasingly stringent air pollution control laws in many countries, however, the impact of sulfate aerosols in slowing global warming is likely to decline in the years ahead. Indeed, the most recent IPCC projections for global average temperature increase (1.4–5.8°C) are largely due to expectations that sulfur dioxide emissions will continue to decline (IPCC, 2001).

Impacts of Global Warming

To many people, the prospect of temperatures a few degrees higher than they are at present seems little cause for dismay—particularly when they happen to be contemplating such a scenario during a January blizzard. The major impact of a global warming trend, however, would not be felt in terms of human physical discomfort but rather in a possibly drastic alteration of worldwide rainfall and temperature patterns.

While climatologists are unable to make accurate detailed predictions regarding CO_2-induced climatic changes in specific areas of the globe, their computer modeling studies support widespread agreement that while temperatures everywhere are rising to some extent, the global warming trend is not evenly distributed. The high latitude regions of the Northern Hemisphere are expected to experience the greatest temperature increases, perhaps twice as high as the world average. Already parts of Alaska have experienced nearly a 5°F increase in average temperatures since 1900, as opposed to a 1°F global average increase during the same time period. In mid-latitude regions (including the continental United States), greenhouse warming also will exceed the global average, with winter temperatures increasing more than summer temperatures. Regional changes in rainfall patterns are even more difficult to predict, but computer models suggest that our grandchildren's generation may witness heavier precipitation in the already-wet equatorial regions, more winter precipitation in the polar regions, much drier summers in the midwestern United States, and drier winters in California. Along with such widespread regional climatic alteration, localized weather changes such as the frequency and intensity of storms will also be pronounced. More frequent "January thaws" during winter and more unusually hot days during the summer may become commonplace. Whereas Washington, D.C. now averages only one day each year when the mercury tops 100°F, a doubling of CO_2 levels could result in two weeks of triple-digit temperatures in our nation's capital; residents of Dallas, who currently suffer through 100°F heat approximately 19 days each year, can look forward to 78 such days in the warmer world projected by climatologists.

Scientists and policymakers alike are now striving to determine what changes are likely to occur as temperatures climb and to formulate strategies to ameliorate detrimental effects as much as possible. The more significant potential impacts of global warming are discussed in the following sections.

Diminishing Crop Yields

The hotter, drier weather forecast for some of the world's most productive agricultural lands is bad news at a time when global food demand is steadily increasing. For farmers, major climatic change could bring benefits to some regions, severe hardship to others. Climate models predict that greenhouse warming would result in shifting rainfall patterns that could bring substantially heavier monsoon rains to India, but 30–60% less summer precipitation to the American Midwest. Higher temperatures could force a northward shift of agricultural zones, perhaps boosting crop yields in Canada and Russia while turning the American "Breadbasket" into a dustbowl. Although some observers have suggested that rising concentrations of CO_2 might actually enhance food production by increasing photosynthetic rates, recent research indicates that higher atmospheric CO_2 concentrations have a distinctly negative impact on crop production. A report submitted to Congress in August 2004 stated that excess CO_2 boosts the growth of several important species of invasive weeds far more than it stimulates crop growth; it also reduces the nutritional value of certain rangeland grasses. Greenhouse gas-induced warming can reduce harvests, a fact demonstrated by researchers in the Philippines who demonstrated a 10% reduction in rice yields with each 1°C (1.8°F) increase in night temperatures during the growing season (Peng et

Box 11-2   Has Global Warming Begun?

The reality of global climate change has been vigorously debated for years. Although the experts continue to wrangle, a majority of Americans, according to opinion surveys, are convinced that climate has changed already. Such convictions are based on personal observation of less predictable weather patterns and milder winters today than in years gone by. Scientists and policymakers, however, demand more than anecdotal evidence, and one of the serious hindrances in formulating a comprehensive government response to the threat of greenhouse warming has been the lack of conclusive proof that global warming has begun. Nevertheless, an increasing flood of research data from a wide variety of sources around the world is providing ample grounds for concern and suggests the public's "gut reaction" may be correct. A sampling of recent findings includes the following:

1. Spring in the far North is now arriving a week earlier than it did in the 1970s and autumn lasts 2–4 days longer, according to researchers at the Scripps Institution of Oceanography in San Diego. As a result, plant growth has been stimulated over wide areas of Alaska, northern Canada, Siberia, and northern Europe. The increase in plant growth—as great as 10% in some regions—is pointed to as one of the best indicators yet of ecosystem response to a warming climate.

2. Mountain glaciers are melting. Switzerland's Aletsch glacier, the largest in mainland Europe, has retreated more than a mile since the mid-1800s and has shrunk by more than 300 feet in thickness. Alpine glaciers as a group have lost one-third to one-half their ice volume during the past century. On Africa's highest peak, more than 80% of the legendary "snows of Kilimanjaro" have melted since 1912; the remainder is expected to vanish by 2020. In Asia, experts predict that most glaciers in the central and eastern Himalayas will be gone by 2035. Some wags suggest Americans should hold a contest to select a new name for Montana's Glacier National Park, since, at their current rate of melting, all the park's ice sheets could disappear within 30 years.

3. Ocean water temperature is rising. Deep-water temperature increases of about 0.5°C (0.9°F) have been recorded in the southwestern Pacific, the Indian Ocean, and in the North Atlantic. More dramatic increases have occurred in the Arctic Ocean, where a rise of 1°C (1.8°F) since the mid-1980s has been documented. This increase may already be having a detrimental impact on salmon in the North Pacific, where populations of several species of this commercially valuable fish crashed during the exceptionally warm years of 1997 and

1998. When water temperatures rise, salmon need more food just to survive and above a certain threshold they starve. Another valuable marine resource, coral reefs, are similarly devastated when water temperatures increase. The epidemic of coral "bleaching" currently being witnessed in tropical waters around the globe is another suggestive indicator that global warming has already begun.

4. Just as rising CO_2 concentrations are causing the oceans to heat up, they are also altering marine chemistry, reacting with water to form carbonic acid and thereby reducing the ocean's natural alkalinity. Biologists fear that the increasing acidity of seawater will lead to conditions that dissolve calcium carbonate, the main constituent of coral reefs and the shells of mollusks and plankton. Researchers have documented a significant expansion of ocean layers where the water chemistry has shifted from conditions that promote shell and coral growth to those that cause shells to dissolve and say that these changes are occurring far too rapidly to be blamed on natural fluctuations.

5. Air temperatures in the far North are noticeably rising. In Barrow, Alaska, the average temperature is now 4.16°F higher than it was 30 years ago; Juneau is 3.54°F warmer, Anchorage 2.26°F. As a result, permafrost is melting, causing roads and buildings to settle and releasing more CO_2 from decaying plant material into the atmosphere, thereby constituting a "positive feedback mechanism" that stimulates even more climatic warming.

6. Sea ice is melting, thanks to the rise in both air and water temperatures in polar regions. Over the past 30 years, the area permanently covered by Arctic sea ice has decreased by 9% per decade and has become 40% thinner, according to submarine sonar data. Large areas of the Arctic Ocean near Russia, Alaska, and Canada are now ice-free during summer months. Dwindling sea ice has had a devastating impact for such Arctic species as walruses, polar bears, and certain sea birds that rely on ice floes for hunting grounds and breeding sites. Western Antarctica has also experienced warming, as dramatized by the spectacular collapse of a 1,250 square mile section of the Larsen Ice Shelf in 2002. The region's average annual temperature has increased by 4.5°F since 1950; average winter temperatures are up 8.8°F for the same period and sea ice has dwindled by 20% since the mid-1970s. As a result, Adélie penguin numbers have dropped precipitously. Biologists attribute the problem to a decline in the penguins' main food, krill, which normally thrives in plankton-rich areas near sea ice. Melting of the ice has resulted in a crash in krill populations, depriving the Adélies of a food staple. Compounding the penguins' problems, warmer temperatures have increased spring snowfall, and scientists studying the birds worry about reproductive failure as penguin eggs are buried under unaccustomed piles of snow.

7. Distribution patterns of plants and animals are shifting. Scientists have long predicted that if climate changes, the established range of various wildlife species will shift in response. Ecologists are now witnessing the accuracy of that prediction. A researcher at the University of Texas has documented a northward shift of about 60 miles in the population of the Edith's Checkerspot butterfly, with the insect vanishing from the southern extreme of its traditional range and expanding from its northern boundary. Scientists attribute the shift to rising temperatures, which have caused the snapdragon plants on which the checkerspot larvae feed to dry up earlier in the season than usual, depriving the insects of a food source. Plants, too, are on the move. In eastern Switzerland and western Austria, nine species of alpine plants have been moving up mountainsides at a rate of about 12 feet (4 meters) per decade since the early years of the 20th century. More troubling than the migration of butterflies or wildflowers has been the spread of disease-carrying mosquitoes, both northward and to higher altitudes, where temperatures previously were too cool for them to survive. Already yellow fever mosquitoes are appearing in certain mountainous regions of South America where they were previously absent.

All these converging lines of evidence should provide food for thought to those still inclined to debunk the urgency of global climate change in the absence of overwhelming catastrophe.

The retreating Monteratsch glacier in the Swiss Alps is one of many Alpine glaciers that have shrunk during the past century. [*Author's photo*]

al., 2004). U.S. agricultural researchers analyzing the impact of climate on corn and soybean yields came to a similar conclusion, reporting that their studies indicate a 17% drop in yields for those two crops with each degree of warming (Lobell and Asner, 2003).

Global warming could have other less obvious impacts on agricultural productivity. Livestock production will suffer due to heat-induced declines in animal fertility; pastures and rangelands can be expected to sustain heat damage. As temperatures rise, the range of plant pathogens and crop-destroying insects expand considerably; pests currently confined to southern latitudes may spread northward, causing serious agricultural losses. A shift in the balance between pest and predator species, prompted by changing environmental conditions, could also have adverse repercussions for farming by favoring the survival of more resilient pest species over that of their natural enemies. These increased pest infestations may prompt farmers to increase applications of chemical pesticides, raising the probability of more surface and groundwater pollution problems. Crop losses are likely to be further compounded by increasing levels of tropospheric ozone, a pollutant gas that forms most readily on hot, sunny days. Conflicts over access to irrigation water are bound to increase, pitting farmers against city dwellers within nations and heightening international tensions where disputed water supplies cross national borders. In the U.S. this problem may become particularly contentious in California, where EPA predicts that climate change produced by a doubling of CO_2 will result in a 7–16% reduction in annual water supplies to the now highly productive Central Valley—a region already beset by burgeoning water demand.

The extent to which greenhouse warming will affect agricultural production will depend in large measure on the rate at which these climatic changes occur. Most of the world's major food crops are already adapted to a wide range of environmental conditions and if climatic change is gradual, agricultural scientists will have time to develop new, even more tolerant varieties. IPCC scientists are optimistic that on a worldwide basis, harvests can be maintained relative to baseline production levels despite global warming, but warn that regional food production—particularly in the tropics and subtropics—may suffer. A study commissioned by EPA concluded that by 2060, grain production in the developing countries may fall by 9–11% as a result of global climate change. Like so many other environmental problems, global warming is likely to have its greatest impact on those already living a marginal existence.

Loss of Biodiversity

Climate change will impose even greater stresses on natural ecosystems than on domesticated plants and animals, since many nonagricultural species have gradually become adapted to life in a specific habitat and have a rather narrow range of tolerance to changing environmental conditions. Plants and animals, particularly those living in temperate regions, will be forced to move hundreds of miles toward the poles (or thousands of feet up mountainsides) in order to maintain the temperature conditions to which they have become adapted. For many species such migration will be virtually impossible. Plants, for example, can shift location only as far as their seeds are dispersed. A gradual poleward migration might be conceivable if the rate of climate change is very slow, but if warming is so rapid that the present habitat becomes unsuitable before a new area can be colonized, then the species will die out.

One might assume that animals, capable of moving under their own power, would find migration relatively easy. In today's world, however, barriers to migration in the form of cities, highways, dams, and so on make large-scale movements of many species highly problematic (visualize the challenges faced by a group of alligators heading north out of Okefenokee Swamp as they attempt to traverse Atlanta!). While some animal species migrate easily, others are genetically programmed to be highly territorial and wouldn't even try to move as their environment became uninhabitable; others might be capable of migrating, but if the plant species on which they feed don't move also, they would perish of starvation.

Prevalence of infectious diseases among plant and animal populations is likely to increase as the climate warms, presenting another threat to species survival. Pathogens already have been implicated in the rapid die-off of frogs in Australia and Central America, birds in Hawaii, and wild dogs in Africa. Scientists warn that climate change could exacerbate host-pathogen interactions in numerous ways, among them: warmer winters are likely to permit the survival of many pathogens currently killed by low temperatures (more than 99% of pathogens responsible for plant diseases typically die over winter); warmer summers may promote pathogen development, increase rates of disease transmission, and increase the number of generations per year; a pathogen's plant or animal host may become more susceptible to infection as temperatures rise. Researchers report that several plant diseases such as Dutch elm disease and wheat stripe rust are more severe following mild winters. Among wildlife populations, rising incidence of vectorborne disease is expected as their insect carriers respond to higher temperatures by expanding their geographic range and experience increased rates of reproduction, population growth, and biting. Animal parasites also will exhibit faster development rates and increased infectivity as the world grows steadily hotter (Harvell et al., 2002). Biodiversity, already suffering severely from pressures imposed by overhunting, pollution, and habitat destruction, may find greenhouse warming the most devastating blow of all.

Rising Sea Levels

The most dramatic consequence of global warming will be a worldwide rise in sea level due to both the thermal expansion of water as temperatures in the ocean rise and to the melting of the Greenland and Antarctic ice sheets. Although this development could be a boon to navigation in the Arctic (the fabled "Northwest Passage" might become a practical alternative to the Panama Canal!), its impact on densely populated coastal regions worldwide will be devastating. In its 2001 Third Assessment Report, the IPCC estimates a global average rise in sea level of somewhere between 9 and 88 centimeters (3.5 to 34.5 inches) by 2100, depending on the emission scenario employed in the calculations. Looking beyond the current century, some scientists warn that if atmospheric CO_2 levels and temperature continue to rise for hundreds of years into the future, the immense Greenland and Antarctic ice sheets could melt, raising sea levels by more than 30 feet and submerging vast areas of densely inhabited coastal lands worldwide.

Even the relatively modest increases in sea level projected by the IPCC for the near term could be problematic. At particular risk are the inhabitants of low-lying coral atolls. Residents of small island nations such as the Bahamas, Maldives, and Marshall Islands have been the most vociferous proponents of measures to curb greenhouse gas emissions as they confront the prospect of their homelands disappearing beneath the waves. Along the edges of continents, towns and cities built on barrier islands, river deltas, or low-lying shorelines can anticipate a similar scenario unless they soon embark on multi-billion dollar coastal defense construction projects. In many desperately poor, densely populated regions of the world, such expenditures are obviously impossible. It is anticipated that Egypt may lose 15% of its arable land to encroaching seas by the mid-21st century; in Bangladesh, climate models indicate flooding in that country is likely to increase by as much as 40% in the years ahead, due to global warming. If the IPCC's worst-case scenario of a 5.8°C temperature increase by 2100 proves correct, researchers warn that slightly over half of Bangladesh would be covered by nearly 6 feet (1.8 meters) of flood water more than nine months of the year (Mirza, 2003)—a staggering prospect for a nation whose population in 2004 topped 140 million, expected to rise to 280 million by 2050. When one pauses to consider the number of major world cities now located at or near sea level, the impact of such a rise on human settlement patterns becomes clear. Although sea level will advance gradually (no one foresees the likelihood of Boston or Galveston or Miami being submerged overnight!), even a slight increase can have significant consequences; it is estimated that there could be an 8-foot horizontal retreat of sandy beach shorelines due to erosion for every one-inch rise in sea level. Some experts feel that a six-inch rise during the 20th century was responsible for much of the coastal erosion that has occurred, and experts contend that a continuation of present trends will obliterate most beaches along the eastern coast of the U.S. by 2020. Greenhouse warming of ocean waters also will exacerbate coastal problems by provoking more severe hurricanes and storm surges. Over the next hundred years or so, global warming is expected to result in a gradually increasing risk of category-5 hurricanes, featuring storms with higher wind velocity and heavier rainfall than those typical of our present climate. Although there is insufficient evidence at present to predict whether hurricanes will form more frequently in a warming world, their greater intensity increases the likelihood that tropical storms of the future will be much more destructive than past hurricanes and cyclones (Knutson and Tuleya, 2004). Considering that by 2010 three-fourths of the world's people will be living within 36 miles (60 km) of a coastline, such projections are not good news.

Human Illness

Although global warming is primarily an environmental problem rather than a human health issue, the increasing frequency of heat waves will have an impact on morbidity and mortality rates. Extreme heat will result in some excess deaths, mainly due to heart attacks and strokes; 726 Chicagoans died of heat stress during four days of record-high temperatures in July 1995, while an estimated 15,000 deaths in France were attributed to a blistering heat wave affecting much of western Europe in August 2003. Warming temperatures also will promote the formation of additional photochemical smog, worsening air pollution and contributing to higher rates of respiratory disease (Eyles and Consitt, 2004). However, the most significant public health problem associated with global warming is the likely spread of certain vectorborne tropical diseases such as malaria and dengue fever into regions where they are currently unknown. As a possible portent of things to come, unusually hot, humid weather during the mid-1990s sparked a dengue epidemic in Mexico and Central America when virus-carrying mosquitoes moved from endemic coastal areas into the usually cool highlands. An Asian Development Bank survey predicts a similar scenario in Indonesia, projecting a quadrupling of dengue cases in the years ahead as a warming climate facilitates the spread of mosquitoes from the lowlands into Indonesia's mountain regions (O'Meara, 1997).

Rate of Global Warming

As mentioned earlier, the rate at which global temperatures rise will be extremely important in determining how serious the impacts of climate change will be. Humanity may be able to adjust reasonably well to a very gradual warming trend, whereas a more rapid change could be catastrophic. Which of these two scenarios is more likely? Several years ago Columbia University geochemist Wallace Broecker, in testimony submitted to a congressional hearing, remarked that:

> Earth's climate does not respond in a smooth and gradual way; rather it responds in sharp jumps. If this reading of the natural record is correct, then we must con-

Figure 11-3

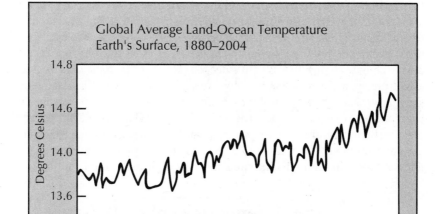

Source: Adapted from NASA Goddard Institute for Space Studies data.

sider the possibility that the major responses of the system to our greenhouse provocation will come in jumps whose timing and magnitude are unpredictable. Coping with this type of change is clearly a far more serious matter than coping with a gradual warming.

In this context, reports from scientists working in Greenland provide considerable cause for alarm. Analysis of air bubbles in layers of ice from cores drilled deep into the island's massive ice cap provides evidence for the rate of climate change in the distant past. University of Rhode Island researchers have found that the end of the last ice age, slightly over 11,000 years ago, occurred much more rapidly than previously thought possible. In just a few decades or less, average temperatures in Greenland suddenly rose 9–18°F. A similarly abrupt, though less extreme, warming trend occurred over much of the Northern Hemisphere at this time (Severinghaus et al., 1998). Another study conducted by researchers from Columbia University's Lamont Doherty Earth Observatory focused on Atlantic Ocean sediments for clues to how quickly climate change might occur. Working off the northwestern coast of Africa, researchers discovered that since the end of the last ice age, ocean temperatures there have experienced wide, abrupt fluctuations roughly every 1,500 years. These changes, and their consequent impact on regional climate, occurred within a period of about 50 years. Converging lines of evidence from these and similar investigations suggest that the relatively stable climate of the past 10,000 years, the period during which human civilizations developed and flourished, is an anomaly—an exception to the rule of frequent and sudden change throughout much of geologic time.

A major concern at present focuses on the possibility of abrupt change in the ocean's **thermohaline circulation**, responsible for carrying heat from the equator to polar regions of the North Atlantic. The warm, salty surface waters of the Gulf Stream gradually cool as they flow northward, becoming more dense and sinking deeper into the ocean as they release heat to the atmosphere. In doing so, they help to keep western Europe nearly 10°F warmer than it would be otherwise. Some scientists worry that as rising temperatures cause increased precipitation and melting of ice in the far North, the increased flow of freshwater into polar seas could shut down this thermal conveyor belt by diluting the salt content of ocean waters, making them less dense and hence too light to sink. If this should happen, Gulf Stream flow could weaken or halt entirely and average temperatures over Europe would drop by as much as 9°F. Scientists are unable to predict how great an influx of freshwater would be necessary to cause a shutdown of the Gulf Stream, but if the tipping point is exceeded, western Europe could experience drastic climate change in less than a decade (an ironic example of how global warming might precipitate a regional mini-Ice Age!). While present IPCC climate models do show a weakening of ocean thermohaline circulation, resulting in some reduction of heat transport to high latitude areas of the Northern Hemisphere, they nevertheless predict a net temperature increase in Europe at least until 2100, due to rising greenhouse gas concentrations. They do not, however, rule out a complete, and possibly irreversible, shutdown in thermohaline circulation if CO_2 levels continue to rise indefinitely.

The Greenhouse Policy Debate

Since the early 1970s, climatologists have been raising increasingly strident warnings about the impending greenhouse warming, urging policymakers to take action to forestall this so-called "doomsday issue." While the general public until recently tended either to ignore such predictions or to regard them as plot material for a science fiction novel, there has been a steadily growing chorus of experts who claim that global climate change has already begun. Testifying before a Senate subcommittee during the torrid summer of 1988, James Hansen of the NASA Goddard Institute for Space Studies told the assembled lawmakers that "the greenhouse effect has been detected and is changing our climate now." Despite Hansen's warning and mounting scientific evidence, most policymakers, acutely aware of the intense opposition by the politically influential fossil fuel industry, have been reluctant to endorse any meaningful policy actions to reduce greenhouse gas emissions. Some refuse to acknowledge a problem even exists; in 2003, Senate Environment and Public Works Committee Chairman James Inhofe (R-OK) went so far as to call global warming "the greatest hoax ever perpetrated on the American people." Nevertheless, as the politicians dithered, temperatures continued to rise. Worldwide, the 1990s was the warmest decade since recordkeeping began in 1860; surface air temperatures in 1998 were the hottest ever, each month breaking every previous record for that date. The years since then have been almost as warm, the second to fifth hottest years yet recorded being 2002, 2003, 2004, and 2001, respectively. Ocean water temperatures also hit new highs during the 1990s. Greenhouse skeptics are thus having an increasingly difficult time arguing that global warming is "an alarmist fantasy." As Howard Ferguson, a meteorologist with the Canadian Atmospheric Environmental Service, remarked: "All the greenhouse scenarios are consistent. These numbers are real. We have to start behaving as if this is going to happen. Those who advocate a program consisting only of additional research are missing the boat."

Calling for action is easier than implementing such changes, however. Delegates to the United Nations' Earth Summit, held in Rio de Janeiro in 1992, took the first substantive steps when they endorsed the **Framework Convention on Climate Control (FCCC)**. Calling for a *voluntary* reduction in signatory nations' greenhouse gas

"Gentlemen, it's time we gave some serious thought to the effects of global warming."

emissions to 1990 levels by 2000, the treaty was quickly ratified by the U.S. Senate and equivalent legislative bodies in Canada and Australia. By 1995, 186 countries had signed on to the FCCC, agreeing in concept with the treaty's ultimate objective—"stabilization of the greenhouse gas concentrations in the atmosphere at a level that would prevent dangerous anthropogenic interference with the climate system." Negotiators at the Rio Conference agreed that the rich developed nations whose greenhouse gas emissions are largely responsible for the present state of affairs must take the lead in emissions reductions and, although it was assumed that at some future time the developing countries would need to curb their emissions as well, no specific timetable for their doing so was established.

When the FCCC was negotiated in 1992, emissions in most participatory nations were only slightly above their 1990 levels and achieving the necessary reductions within the established time frame appeared relatively easy. However, although a few industrialized nations *were* successful in lowering their emissions (most notably the U.K., which rapidly substituted North Sea natural gas for coal, and Russia, whose economic collapse during the early 1990s resulted in the closure of many polluting enterprises), most countries experienced a sharp rise in emissions during this period. Between 1990 and 1996, CO_2 emissions in the U.S. increased by 8.8%, while those in Japan and Australia rose by 12.5% and 9.6%, respectively. By the mid-1990s it was glaringly obvious that voluntary goals were inadequate for achieving the targeted reductions.

Consequently, delegates representing countries that had signed the FCCC met in March 1995 in Berlin and again in July 1996 in Geneva and decided that legally binding goals, rather than optional ones, were necessary if the desired emissions reductions were to be realized. Release of the IPCC's Second Assessment Report, removing any previous scientific uncertainty regarding human involvement in observed warming trends, gave delegates added incentive to finalize a meaningful agreement. A third international meeting, held in Kyoto, Japan, in December 1997 and attended by representatives from 171 nations, concluded with the signing of the **Kyoto Protocol**, a treaty that set *mandatory* emissions reductions for 38 industrial nations. Aimed at reducing emissions of six greenhouse gases (CO_2, CH_4, N_2O, HFCs, PFCs, and SF_6) by the industrialized nations as a group to 5.2% below 1990 levels, the Protocol assigned each individual country its own goal: European Union, 8%; United States, 7%; Canada, 6%; Japan, 6%; Russia, 0% (by contrast, Australia was permitted to peg its emissions at a level 8% *higher* than its 1990 figure; Ireland was assigned a limit 10% above 1990). The agreement calls for these cuts to be made gradually, between 2008 and 2012. The Kyoto Protocol was signed by 84 countries, including the United States (then under the Clinton Administration), but would become legally binding only after ratification by the legislatures of 55 countries representing 55% of the world's 1990 greenhouse gas emissions.

Several important details for achieving the goals of the Kyoto Protocol, enforcement procedures among the most contentious, were left for resolution at future meetings. No progress was made at a gathering at The Hague, Netherlands, in the fall of 2000, intended to establish the criteria by which industrialized nations could meet their Kyoto-mandated emissions targets. Arguments over the extent to which industrialized countries could offset their required emissions reductions by such mitigation activities as planting new forests or how much financial aid should be provided to help developing countries reduce their emissions stymied any agreement and the meeting ended in failure. Nevertheless, discussions at The Hague achieved a virtual consensus that climate change is indeed a serious problem and delegates left with the determination to reach an accord at meetings scheduled for the following year.

Such hopes suffered a severe setback in March 2001, when U.S. President George W. Bush, just two months after assuming office, declared the Kyoto Protocol "dead" and announced that the United States was withdrawing from the treaty because it would hurt the American economy. President Bush's unilateral rejection of Kyoto provoked outrage in the international community (and among U.S. environmentalists) and made prospects for the treaty's eventual implementation highly problematic, since attaining ratification by countries representing 55% of total emissions would be difficult without participation of the biggest emitter of all (U.S. emissions in 1990 represented 36.1% of the world's total). Nevertheless, determined not to concede defeat and galvanized by an added sense of urgency, representatives from over 170 other nations met in Bonn, Germany, in June and again in Marrakech, Morocco, in November of 2001 to hammer out an agreement resolving most of the pending details. Led by the European Union and vowing to move ahead with or without the U.S., the 4,500 delegates to the Marrakech meeting declared their intent to implement a wide range of policies to curtail greenhouse gas emissions (Firor and Jacobsen, 2002). Securing enough ratifications for the treaty to enter into force took longer than anticipated, but success finally was achieved in late autumn 2004, when Russia became the 127th nation and last major emitter (17.4% of world greenhouse gas emissions in 1990) to ratify the Kyoto Protocol. The treaty's provisions took effect in February 2005, 90 days after Russia delivered its signed papers to the United Nations.

While the federal government in the United States continues to sidestep meaningful action, many state and local governments throughout the country have launched a multitude of innovative initiatives to combat greenhouse warming. More than 30 states have adopted climate change mitigation policies, primarily through encouraging the use of alternative fuels. At the forefront of state leadership on climate change initiatives is California, which in June 2004 announced an ambitious plan that would require car manufacturers to reduce automotive emissions of CO_2 30% by 2015. A month earlier, Massachusetts had indicated it planned to require emissions cuts of 10% by 2020. Since the only way to achieve these goals is to reduce fuel consumption, such requirements essentially are mandates to make cars more fuel-efficient. While the auto industry has vowed a court challenge against California's proposed ruling, the initiative is expected to prompt similar actions by other states and raise public awareness of the climate change threat. On the East Coast, New York Gov. George Pataki is spearheading formation of a 10-state regional compact aimed at reducing carbon emissions from power plants and has declared that he intends to follow California's lead on automobiles. At least 13 states, including Texas and Nevada, are forcing electric utilities to diversify their energy sources to include wind and solar power in addition to coal and oil. Renewable, nonpolluting alternative energy sources are rapidly becoming a viable option for reducing greenhouse gas emissions while simultaneously mitigating air quality problems and reducing dependence on imported oil. Although the federal Energy Information Agency reports that alternatives such as solar, wind, geothermal, hydropower, and ocean energy collectively accounted for a mere 6.7% of total U.S. energy consumption in 2004, their share is steadily increasing. Recent improvements in alternative energy technologies, along with the soaring cost of oil and natural gas, have drastically narrowed the price gap between fossil fuels and renewables; with rising political support for government mandates such as those cited above, an imminent takeoff in the use of such technologies is widely predicted.

Local governments as well are becoming active on the climate change front, motivated as much by concerns that global warming could negatively impact local economies in the years immediately ahead as by more general fears of long-term environmental catastrophe. Over 140 U.S. cities and counties representing 16% of the nation's population and a similar percentage of its greenhouse gas emissions have joined the Cities for Climate Protection Campaign. Among them is San Francisco, where voters overwhelmingly approved a measure to make their city the United States' largest producer of solar electricity.

Private industry is similarly moving ahead aggressively, recognizing that even in the absence of federal regulation, emissions reductions typically save companies money and promote the development of innovative technologies. Among the corporate leaders in commitments to greenhouse gas reductions are DuPont (65% cut in emissions between 1990–2010) and Alcoa (25% cut by 2010). Shell, BP Amoco, Alcan, International Paper, and Motorola, among others, have all pledged to reduce emissions below their 1990 level within the next few years. The Green Market Development Group, made up of eleven major companies, is working to develop markets for renewable energy; a General Motors executive whose company is investing millions to develop hydrogen-powered cars with zero CO_2 emissions acknowledges that a low-carbon economy will profoundly change the automobile industry. Even within the utility industry, some far-sighted CEOs are recommending their companies begin planning now for the mandatory reductions they see on the horizon (Carey, 2004; Speth, 2004).

Policy Options

Among those wrestling with the challenge of reducing greenhouse gas emissions, there is now general agreement that a two-pronged approach is needed:

1. Mandatory emissions reductions and/or a "carbon tax." Requiring that specified sectors of the economy meet government-imposed CO_2 emission limitations is an approach already being pushed by some U.S. states and will be a fact of life for greenhouse gas emitters in many countries as the Kyoto Protocol takes effect. The key to achieving these mandatory reductions is improving the efficiency of energy use and breaking modern society's addiction to fossil fuels. Contrary to the belief of most Americans that the best way to prevent global warming is to reduce air pollution (Kempton, 1997), end-of-pipe pollution control technologies do nothing to reduce emissions of CO_2, a gas that is the natural by-product of burning any carbonaceous material. Improvements in energy efficiency, along with related energy conservation measures, result in less fuel combustion and hence fewer CO_2 emissions. Since fully 5% of all the carbon dioxide released worldwide each year comes from U.S. motor vehicles (TRB, 1997), simply improving automobile gas mileage could have an enormous impact on atmospheric carbon levels. It has been calculated that raising the fuel efficiency of the average American car to 45 mpg would result in a 40% drop in vehicle CO_2 emissions. Similarly, mandated efficiency standards for electrical appliances, power tools, and lighting, or tax credits for manufacturers who invest in new, more efficient plants are ways government could promote CO_2 reductions. At the same time, increased funding for research and development of "soft energy path" technologies such as solar, wind, ocean wave, or geothermal power, as well as tax incentives for bringing such sources on-line, could give a major boost to anti-global warming efforts.

Alternatively, a so-called "carbon tax," in which production of gasoline, heating oil, coal, natural gas, and electricity generated from fossil fuels would be taxed incrementally according to the carbon content of those fuels, could also result in a significant drop in emissions. Such a tax scheme recognizes that not all fossil fuels pollute equally; burning coal emits twice as much CO_2 as does natural gas, 1.5 times more than oil. A differential tax would provide financial motivation for energy purchasers to choose less-polluting fuels and would incorporate the environmental costs of energy use into energy prices. A carbon tax also would encourage consumers to shift to alternative energy sources such as solar or wind power, since these emit no carbon and hence would be tax-free.

Box 11-3 *"The Answer, My Friend, Is Blowin' in the Wind . . ."*

Those who question how modern societies can possibly move to a low-carbon economy without "freezing to death in the dark" might well consider the haunting refrain from singer-songwriter Bob Dylan's 1962 hit, *Blowin' in the Wind.*

Worldwide, wind capacity has grown by 30% a year since the early 1990s and is currently the fastest-growing sector of the alternative energy market. In Germany, the world's foremost wind energy producer, wind power provided 6% of the country's electricity in 2004, a share the government promises will rise to 25% by 2025. Denmark, for years the global leader in wind turbine production, has nearly reached Germany's goal, generating more than 20% of its electricity from wind. While about 86% of global wind capacity in megawatts (MW) is now localized in just four countries—Germany (14,609 MW), the United States (6,374 MW), Spain (6,202 MW), and Denmark (3,110 MW)—at least 48 countries are now generating electricity from wind. Carbon dioxide emission reductions mandated by the Kyoto Protocol will undoubtedly motivate many more nations to switch to carbon-free wind power as compliance deadlines approach. Already the United Kingdom has announced plans to construct more than 1,000 wind turbines at 15 offshore sites, pledging that wind will supply 7% of Britain's electricity by 2010 and will catapult the U.K. to world leadership in offshore power generation.

The modern era of wind power dates back to 1981, when commercial generators began to proliferate in California. The United States led the world in wind energy capacity until European countries surged ahead in the late 1990s. The future for wind power in the U.S. remains bright, however; although wind currently contributes less than 1% of the nation's electricity, experts estimate its generating potential at 10,777 billion kilowatts/hour annually—three times the amount generated by all energy sources in the U.S. today. Wind power has become big business; the solitary, picturesque old windmills that dotted Midwestern and Great Plains landscapes years ago, pumping the groundwater that sustained several generations of farm families, are now long gone,

replaced by clusters of sleek metal and fiberglass machines. Wind energy technology has made rapid progress since the early 1980s; by comparison with prototype machines, contemporary models are taller and more powerful, with lighter, more flexible blades, variable speed operation, and direct drive generators. As wind machines become ever more efficient and powerful, the per kilowatt hour (kWh) price of wind-generated electricity is plummeting, from approximately 46¢/kWh in the early 1980s to 3–5¢/kWh at good wind sites today—cheaper than power currently generated by natural gas-fired plants.

Although California has set the pace for wind energy development in the U.S. and remains the leader in domestic wind power, 16 other states have greater future potential for becoming major wind energy producers. The breezy, wide-open expanses of the Great Plains states are currently regarded as the most promising area for U.S. wind development. Experts estimate that the energy potential from North Dakota, Kansas, and Texas alone, if fully exploited, could satisfy the electrical demand of the entire country.

Although the emerging wind power industry has generated considerable interest and enthusiasm in the business community and among many environmentalists, the prospect of "wind farms" sprouting on the horizon doesn't please everyone. Some environmentalists, in fact, have been among the most vocal critics of the new technology, complaining that wind machines are noisy, ugly, a threat to migrating birds, and a deterrent to tourism. Efforts by wind power developers to defuse public opposition by moving wind farms offshore have sometimes backfired, creating even more antagonism. A classic case in point is "Cape Wind," a proposed wind farm off the Massachusetts coast in Nantucket Sound, between Cape Cod and popular vacation spots for the rich and famous on Martha's Vineyard and Nantucket Island. The prospect of 130 huge wind turbines spread over a 24-square-mile area just 5 miles from land galvanized strong opposition from a citizens' group protesting the aesthetic intrusion. Developers counter by pointing out many

economic benefits, including job creation; whether Cape Wind becomes reality remains to be seen, but the likelihood of numerous additional proposals for wind energy development along the populous East Coast ensure continuing controversy.

Citizen complaints related to turbine-generated noise have declined in recent years, thanks to technological improvements resulting in quieter machines, as well as by improved siting procedures. Bird mortality has remained a troublesome issue, however. At one facility—Altamont Pass, 50 miles east of San Francisco—the 7,000-turbine wind farm was associated with nearly 200 bird deaths between 1989–1991, including several endangered California condors and golden eagles. Elsewhere, bird mortality has been generally lower and even many environmental groups admit that, by comparison, wind farms represent but a miniscule percentage of the bird death toll taken by glass windows, house cats, cars and trucks, hunting, and transmission line collisions. While wind turbines do kill some birds, they don't kill very many. The wind power industry is making adjustments to its machines—installing perch guards and replacing old machines with modern turbines on high monopoles—to reduce the toll even further.

Advocates for wind power development argue that the best approach for defusing public opposition to wind farms is simply to avoid choosing sites likely to provoke conflict. While doing so may necessitate foregoing some sites that appear attractive from a wind velocity perspective, the abundance of other locations where residents are eager for wind development projects ensures ample availability of suitable sites. Foremost among these in the United States is the Great Plains, where strong, steady winds, wide expanses of open land, low population density, and a desperate need for new revenue sources create a hospitable attitude toward wind energy development among local citizens. Since wind turbines can coexist with crops or cattle, farmers and ranchers can earn supplemental income by installing and operating wind turbines on their land—extra income that can make the difference between prosperity and bankruptcy. Wind development offers a major boost to 21st century rural economic development, providing well-paid construction jobs, local tax revenues, and yearly royalties to farmers. In some regions of the country, contrary to the early fears of public officials, wind turbines have even boosted tourism, prompting the creation of organized tours and the sale of souvenirs.

U.S. wind power has been enjoying rapid growth in recent years, becoming increasingly competitive as its cost per kilowatt-hour falls while that of natural gas rises. However, to compete with coal, at present the leading conventional fuel for power generation, wind power needs a small subsidy to bridge the price gap. Congress has provided an "on-again, off-again" Production Tax Credit (PTC), most recently set at 1.9¢/kWh, to promote wind development. Whenever the subsidy has been allowed to lapse, as it did at the end of 2003, project development comes to a sudden halt. The uncertainty created by such boom-and-bust cycles, a result of inconsistent government policies, deters the financial investment necessary for wind energy to reach its full potential and explains why European countries, fully committed to a low-carbon future, continue to outpace the U.S. in the transition to renewable fuels. Fortunately, laws now in force in 13 states requiring utilities to include a specified percentage of renewable energy in the total amount of electricity delivered to customers provide a big incentive for wind power development. To comply, producers can either generate the renewable energy themselves, buy it from another party, or purchase credits—"green tags"—from producers who have excess. Such incentives, along with continued technological advances that further drive down costs, are advancing wind energy's progress toward self-sustained profitability. As societies around the world begin the necessary transition from an economy addicted to fossil fuels to the renewable energies essential to avert global warming, we can say that at least a part of the answer is "blowin' in the wind."

References

Pasqualetti, Martin J. 2004. "Wind Power: Obstacles and Opportunities." *Environment* 46, no. 7 (Sept).

Sawin, Janet L. 2004. "Mainstreaming Renewable Energy in the 21st Century." *WorldWatch Paper* 169 (May).

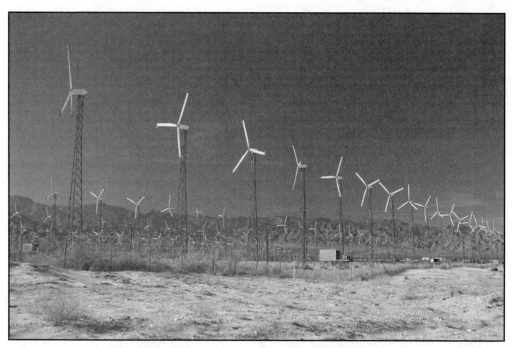

Wind power is the fastest-growing sector of the alternative energy market.

2. Establishment of a global emissions-trading program. Once a country's greenhouse gas emissions ceiling is set, governments will allocate specific reduction levels among targeted segments of that nation's economy—manufacturing plants, utilities, transportation, and so forth. Those industries will then be allowed to achieve the mandated reductions in any way they choose. With the establishment of a worldwide emissions-trading program, innovative, proactive companies whose energy-efficient technologies or adoption of alternative fuels have enabled them to exceed their mandated emissions reduction goals will be able to sell credits for those excess emissions to other companies unable or unwilling to make the changes necessary to meet their assigned targets. These tradable emissions rights ("assigned amount units" in Kyoto Protocol jargon) provide a strong incentive for all parties involved to find the most effective, least-costly route to a low-carbon future.

Under the Kyoto Protocol's Joint Implementation provision, a government or company can earn credits toward its emissions reduction cap by investing in specific emissions-lowering projects in another developed country (usually one of the former Soviet republics) or, under the Protocol's Clean Development Mechanism, can similarly meet a portion of their Kyoto-assigned target by engaging in Third World projects—activities such as tree planting or installing low-emission technologies in factories—that will help developing countries reduce their emissions. Since climate change is a global phenomenon, with greenhouse gases circulating widely throughout the earth's atmosphere regardless of point of origin, an emissions-trading system that allows a company to meet its emissions reduction goal in the most cost-effective manner—even when those reductions are accomplished half a world away—makes environmental sense. This reasoning prompted such initiatives as American Electrical Power Company's investment in Chilean renewable energy projects and a "carbon offset" program in Guatemala where a Connecticut-based utility donated $2 million for the planting of 52 million trees.

Although the U.S. has not yet joined the international community in ratifying the Kyoto Protocol, the Chicago Climate Exchange (CCX®) in December 2003 began a pilot program trading rights to emit greenhouse gases among a group of North American companies committed to reducing their emissions by 4% by 2006. The previously described local and state climate change initiatives proliferating throughout the U.S. are also beginning to spark a response in Congress. In 2003, Senators Lieberman (D-CT) and McCain (R-AZ) cosponsored a bill to establish a market-based "cap-and-trade" system to reduce greenhouse gas emissions from industries, utilities, businesses, and transportation. Although weaker than the Kyoto Protocol, the legislation, if passed, would constitute an important step in the right direction for a meaningful U.S. response to the climate-change challenge. Meanwhile, in January 2005, the European Union initiated its own CO_2 cap-and-trade program for its 25 member countries. This European Union Emissions Trading System represents the first large-scale attempt at greenhouse gas regulation and will be scrutinized closely for the lessons it provides on how market-based policies can best be used to address environmental problems (Carey, 2004; Speth, 2004; Kruger and Pizer, 2004).

Averting Catastrophe

As atmospheric CO_2 levels and temperature continue to rise, the need for effective, immediate action to implement the long-term strategies outlined above becomes increasingly urgent. Many scientists warn of catastrophic consequences if Earth's climate warms by more than 2°C—a temperature increase likely to occur if CO_2 concentrations rise from their current 375 ppm to 550 ppm, a figure roughly double that of pre-industrial levels. In a business-as-usual world with no efforts made to curtail emissions, CO_2 levels could reach 450 ppm by 2030, 800–1000 ppm by the end of the 21st century. Because greenhouse gases persist in the atmosphere for centuries, global average surface temperatures will continue to rise even after their concentrations have stabilized. Nevertheless, they will rise at a much slower rate after stabilization, so the lower their level at the time of stabilization, the less the total temperature change will be. Consequently, time is of the essence—the longer we wait to take effective action, the higher will temperatures ultimately rise and the more drastic will be the impacts of climate change (IPCC, 2001). The modest initiatives just now getting underway are encouraging, but they won't succeed in reversing global warming unless all countries enlist in the effort. Even if the United States eventually joins the other industrialized nations in taking action, rapid economic growth in developing countries such as China and India—currently exempt from Kyoto Protocol-mandated emissions cuts—will result in a further increase in atmospheric CO_2. Although the developing nations today contribute less than one-fifth the greenhouse gas emissions generated by the industrialized world, by the end of the century, as their economies and populations continue to grow, their emissions will soar to 2–3 times the level of those in developed countries. Mustering worldwide cooperation to combat what is perceived by many as a distant threat is extremely difficult, since the basic problem stems from daily energy use decisions of billions of individuals throughout the world. Unfortunately, even if every government were to ratify the Kyoto Protocol and move immediately to fulfill treaty commitments, capping emissions slightly below their 1990 levels as the Protocol requires wouldn't be sufficient to forestall global warming. This is because current rates of CO_2 emissions, stable or not, are so much higher than those of the preindustrial period that natural processes of absorption or sequestration—which formerly maintained a rough equilibrium—cannot keep pace and the atmospheric reservoir of CO_2 continues to increase. Merely stabilizing atmospheric carbon dioxide concentrations at 550 ppm would require a worldwide slashing of emissions by more than 60%.

Even then, there is no assurance that this would be a safe level; what *is* certain is that the longer we postpone sharp emissions reductions, the deeper future cuts will have to be in order to achieve the same ultimate effect (WRI, 1998). Some observers conclude that it is already too late; the degree of worldwide cooperation and coordination necessary to achieve any meaningful reduction in CO_2 releases would, in their view, be impossible to attain in a world "hooked" on fossil fuels. Instead of a crash fuel-switching effort, such voices call for accelerating research on CO_2 and its effects and for a policy to improve society's ability to adapt to changing circumstances, preparing the economy for the consequences of global warming. Perhaps the best summation of the differing assessments of what society's response to greenhouse warming ought to be is that given more than a decade ago by Harvard planetary scientist Michael McElroy:

> If we choose to take on this challenge, it appears we can slow the rate of change substantially, giving us time to develop mechanisms so that the cost to society and the damage to ecosystems can be minimized. We could alternatively close our eyes, hope for the best, and pay the cost when the bill comes due. (Revkin, 1992; EPA, 1992)

References

Broecker, Wallace S. 1970. "Man's Oxygen Reserves." *Science* 168 (June 26).

Budyko, M. I. 1986. *The Evolution of the Biosphere*. D. Reidel Publishing.

Carey, John. 2004. "Global Warming." *Business Week* (Aug. 16):60–69.

Environmental Protection Agency. 1992. *Climate Change Discussion Series: Agriculture*. Office of Policy Planning and Evaluation, May.

———. 1990. *Policy Options for Stabilizing Global Climate: Report to Congress*. Washington, DC: EPA.

Eyles, John, and Nicole Consitt. 2004. "What's At Risk? Environmental Influences on Human Health." *Environment* 46, no. 8 (Oct).

Firor, John, and Judith Jacobsen. 2002. *The Crowded Greenhouse*. New Haven, CT: Yale Univ. Press.

Gribbin, John. 1982. "Carbon Dioxide, Ammonia—and Life." *New Scientist* 94 (May 13):413–416.

Harvell, C. Drew, Charles E. Mitchell, Jessica R. Ward, Sonia Altizer, Andrew P. Dobson, Richard S. Ostfeld, and Michael D. Samuel. 2002. "Climate Warming and Disease Risks for Terrestrial and Marine Biota." *Science* 296, no. 5576 (June 21).

Houghton, J. T., G. J. Jenkins, and J. J. Ephraums, eds. 1990. *Climate Change: The IPCC Scientific Assessment*. Cambridge: Cambridge Univ. Press.

Indermühle, A., T. F. Stocker, F. Joos, H. Fischer, H. J. Smith, M. Wahlen, B. Deck, D. Mastroianni, J. Tschumi, T. Blunier, R. Meyer, and B. Stouffer. 1999. "Holocene Carboncycle Dynamics Based on CO_2 Trapped in Ice at Taylor Dome, Antarctica." *Nature* 398 (March 11):121–126.

Intergovernmental Panel on Climate Change (IPCC). 2001. *Climate Change 2001: The Scientific Basis, Third Assessment Report of the Intergovernmental Panel on Climate Change 2001*, edited by J. T. Houghton et al. Cambridge: Cambridge Univ. Press.

Kasting, James F. 1993. "Earth's Early Atmosphere." *Science* 259, no. 5097 (Feb. 12).

Kempton, Willett. 1997. "How the Public Views Climate Change." *Environment* 39, no. 9 (Nov):12–21.

Kerr, J. B., and C. T. McElroy. 1993. "Evidence for Large Upward Trends of Ultraviolet-B Radiation Linked to Ozone Depletion." *Science* 262 (Nov).

Knutson, Thomas R., and Robert E. Tuleya. 2004. "Impact of CO_2-Induced Warming on Simulated Hurricane Intensity and Precipitation: Sensitivity to the Choice of Climate Model and Convective Parameterization." *Journal of Climate* 17, no. 18 (Sept. 15).

Kruger, Joseph A., and William A. Pizer. 2004. "Greenhouse Gas Trading in Europe." *Environment* 46, no. 8 (Oct).

Lobell, David B., and Gregory P. Asner. 2003. "Climate and Management Contributions to Recent Trends in U.S. Agricultural Yields." *Science* 299, no. 5609 (Feb. 14).

Maugh, Thomas H. 1982. "New Link Between Ozone and Cancer." *Science* 216 (April 23).

Mintzer, Irving M. 1987. "A Matter of Degrees: The Potential for Controlling the Greenhouse Effect." World Resources Institute, Research Report 5, April.

Mirza, M. Monirul Qader, R. A. Warrick, and N. J. Ericksen. 2003. "The Implications of Climate Change on Floods of the Ganges, Brahmaputra, and Meghna Rivers in Bangladesh." *Climatic Change* 57, no. 3 (April).

O'Meara, Molly. 1997. "The Risks of Disrupting Climate." *World•Watch* 10, no. 6 (Nov/Dec):10–24.

"Ozone Takes a Nose Dive after the Eruption of Mt. Pinatubo." 1993. *Science* 260 (April 23).

Panofsky, Hans A. 1978. "Earth's Endangered Ozone." *Environment* 20, no. 3 (April)

Parson, Edward A. 2003. *Protecting the Ozone Layer*. New York: Oxford Univ. Press.

Peng, Shaobing, Jianliang Huang, John E. Sheehy, Rebecca C. Laza, Romeo M. Visperas, Xuhua Zhong, Grace C. Centeno, Gurdev S. Khush, and Kenneth G. Cassman. 2004. "Rice Yields Decline with Higher Night Temperature from Global Warming." *Proceedings of the National Academy of Sciences* 101, no. 27 (July 6).

Petit, J. R, J. Jouzel, D. Raynaud, N. I. Barkov, J. M. Barnola, I. Basile, M. Bender, J. Chappellaz, M. Davis, G. Delaygue, M. Delmotte, V. M. Kotlyakov, M. Legrand, V. Y. Lipenkov, C. Lorius, L. Pépin, C. Ritz, E. Saltzman, and M. Stievenard. 1999. "Climate and Atmospheric History of the Past 420,000 Years from the Vostok Ice Core, Antarctica." *Nature* 399 (June 3):429–436.

Revkin, Andrew. 1992. *Global Warming: Understanding the Forecast*. New York: Abbeville Press.

Severinghaus, J. P., T. Sowers, E. J. Brooke, R. B. Alley, and M. L. Bender. 1998. "Timing of Abrupt Climate Change at the End of the Younger Dryas Interval from Thermally Fractionated Gases in Polar Ice." *Nature* 391 (Jan. 8):141–146.

Sheehan, Molly O. 2003. "Carbon Emissions and Temperature Climb." *Vital Signs 2003: The Trends That Are Shaping Our Future*. New York: Worldwatch Institute/W.W. Norton.

Speth, James Gustave. 2004. *Red Sky At Morning: America and the Crisis of the Global Environment*. New Haven, CT: Yale Univ. Press.

Strahler, Arthur N., and Alan H. Strahler. 1973. *Environmental Geoscience*. Hamilton Publishing.

Transportation Research Board (TRB) and National Research Council (NRC). 1997. *Toward a Sustainable Future: Addressing the Long-Term Effects of Motor Vehicle Transportation on Climate and Ecology*. Washington, DC: National Academy Press.

Watson, R. T., H. Rohde, H. Oeschger, and U. Siegenthaler. 1990. "Greenhouse Gases and Aerosols." *Climate Change: The IPCC Scientific Assessment*, edited by J. T. Houghton, G. J. Jenkins, and J. J. Ephraums. Cambridge: Cambridge Univ. Press.

World Resources Institute (WRI). 1998. *World Resources 1998–99: Environmental Change and Human Health*. New York: Oxford Univ. Press.

———. 1992. *World Resources 1992–93*. New York: Oxford Univ. Press.

12

Air Pollution

> ... why, it appears no other thing to me
> but a foul and pestilent congregation of vapors.
>
> —William Shakespeare (*Hamlet*)

Humans have undoubtedly been coping with a certain amount of polluted air ever since primitive *Homo sapiens* sat crouched by the warmth of a smoky fire in their Paleolithic caves. An inevitable consequence of fuel combustion, air pollution mounted as a source of human discomfort as soon as people began to live in towns and cities. More recently it has become an extremely serious problem on a worldwide basis for two primary reasons: (1) there has been an enormous increase in world population, particularly in urban areas, and (2) since the early 1800s the rapid growth of energy-intensive industries and rising levels of affluence, first in the industrialized nations and recently in several of the large developing countries as well, have led to record levels of fossil fuel combustion.

Prior to the 20th century, problems related to air pollution were primarily associated, in the public mind at least, with the city of London. As early as the 13th century small amounts of coal from Newcastle were being shipped into London for fuel. As the population and manufacturing enterprises grew, wood supplies diminished and coal burning increased, in spite of the protestations of a long series of both monarchs and private citizens who objected to the odor of coal smoke. One petitioner to King Charles II in 1661 complained that due to the greed of manufacturers, inhabitants of London were forced to "breathe nothing but an impure and thick Mist, accompanied by a fuliginous (sooty) and filthy vapour, which renders them obnoxious to a thousand inconveniences, the Lungs, and disordering the entire habit of their Bodies. . . ." (Evelyn, 1661).

In spite of such railings, English coal consumption increased even faster than the rate of population growth and by the 19th century London's thick, "pea-soup" fogs had become a notorious trademark of the city. Numerous well-meaning attempts at smoke abatement were largely ignored during the heyday of laissez-faire capitalism, epitomized by the industrialists' slogan, "Where there's muck, there's money."

The same conditions that had made London the air pollution capital of the world began to prevail in the United States as well during the 19th and early 20th centuries. St. Louis, plagued by smoky conditions, passed an ordinance as early as 1867 mandating that smokestacks be at least 20 feet higher than adjacent buildings. The Chicago City Council in 1881 passed the nation's first smoke abatement ordinance. Pittsburgh, once one of the smokiest cities in the United States, was the site of pioneer work at the Mellon Institute on the harmful impact of smoke both on property and human health.

In spite of gradually increasing public awareness of the problem, levels of air pollution and the geographical extent of the areas affected continued to increase. Although by the late 1950s and 1960s large-scale fuel-switching from coal to natural gas and oil had significantly reduced smoky conditions in many American cities, other newer pollutants—products of the now-ubiquitous automobile—had assumed worrisome levels. Today foul air has become a problem of global proportions; no longer does one have to travel to London or Pittsburgh or Los Angeles to experience the respiratory irritation or the aesthetic distress that a hazy, contaminated atmosphere can provoke. In the early 21st century, virtually every metropolitan area in the world, from Beijing to Bangkok, Delhi, Tokyo, Athens, Moscow, and Mexico City—all are grappling with the problem of how to halt further deterioration of air quality without impeding industrial productivity and development.

Sources of Air Pollution

Where is all this dirty air coming from? Not surprisingly, the sources of air pollution are quite diverse and vary in importance from one region to another. Some air contaminants are of natural origin; volcanic eruptions, forest fires, and dust storms periodically contribute large quantities of pollutant gases and particles to the atmosphere. In June 1991, immense quantities of volcanic ash and an estimated 18 million metric tons of sulfur dioxide (roughly equivalent to U.S. emissions of this pollutant gas during an entire year) were spewed into the atmosphere during a single massive eruption of Mt. Pinatubo in the Philippines. For several months during the fall of 1997, fires deliberately set by farmers and loggers to clear land on the Indonesian island of Sumatra burned out of control, creating a pall of pollution over much of Southeast Asia. Covering an area inhabited by 200 million people, the smoke provoked acute respiratory problems throughout the region, caused transportation accidents that killed hundreds, devastated the tourist trade, and severely damaged the economies of the nations affected. British experts estimate that the burning forests released more greenhouse gases than were emitted in an entire year by all the cars in Europe. Less dramatic but worthy of note, considerable amounts of methane gas are released into the air when organic matter decays in the absence of oxygen, and some plant species produce volatile hydrocarbons that are thought to be responsible for the blue haze observed in the Smoky Mountains and other forest regions. However, most of the pollutants befouling our air today come from emission sources that have proliferated with the development of industries and transportation networks.

At present in the industrialized world the largest sources of air pollution, in order of importance, are (1) transportation, primarily automobiles and trucks; (2) electric power plants that burn coal or oil; and (3) industry, the major offenders being steel mills, metal smelters, oil refineries, and pulp and paper mills. Of less importance now than in past decades is the contribution made from heating homes and buildings and burning refuse. The general trend toward heating with oil, gas, or electricity instead of with coal greatly reduced pollution from space heating. At the same time, increasingly common municipal bans on home refuse burning, along with the utilization of sanitary landfills or incinerators equipped with pollution control devices for community solid waste disposal, have accounted for a marked decline in emissions from trash combustion. Within any one region or community, of course, the relative importance of various emission sources may differ from the overall national rankings noted here. In most metropolitan areas, automobiles contribute by far the largest amount of air pollutants; in small towns, by contrast, significant levels of contamination may be caused by just one polluting factory.

Criteria Air Pollutants

Air pollution, of course, is no single entity; thousands of gaseous, liquid, and solid compounds contribute to the atmospheric mess. The nature of some of these substances is well known while others are only now being studied and their threat to human health assessed. The most common and widespread air pollutants include six that the federal government has designated **criteria pollutants,** requiring the Environmental Protection Agency to gather scientific and medical information on their environmental and human health effects. These are the pollutants for which **National Ambient Air Quality Standards (NAAQS**—familiarly referred to as "nax") have been set, specifying the maximum levels of concentration of these pollutants allowable in the outdoor air. The six criteria air pollutants are discussed in the following sections (it should be noted that most industrialized countries, and some developing nations as well, now have regulations controlling these same air contaminants).

Particulate matter (PM_{10} and $PM_{2.5}$). All airborne pollutants that occur in either liquid or solid form, including pollen, dust, soot, smoke, acid condensates, and sulfate and nitrate particles are referred to as particulate matter. Particulates range in

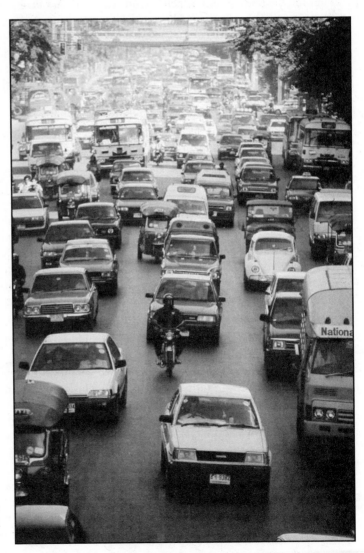

Motor vehicles constitute the largest source of air pollution in the industrialized world.

size from pieces of fly ash as large as a thumbnail to tiny aerosols less than 1 micrometer in diameter—so small that they remain suspended in the air and are transported on wind currents as easily as are gases. To many people, particulate matter and "air pollution" are synonymous, since easily visible dark plumes of smoke and soot or clouds of dust are the only forms of air pollution of which they are aware. Marked reductions in particulate levels in a number of urban areas in recent years have led many citizens to conclude erroneously that air quality is no longer a problem, since most other air pollutants are invisible.

Particulate matter is generated by a wide variety of activities—fuel combustion, road traffic, agricultural activities, certain industrial processes, and natural abrasion. The most visible damage caused by particulate matter is the layer of grime deposited on buildings, streets, clothing, and so on. Prior to pollution-control efforts launched during the 1970s, it was estimated that in the most polluted areas of big cities as much as 50–100 tons of particulate matter per square mile fell each month (Air Pollution Primer, 1969). Particulate matter can obscure visibility and corrode metals; more important is the fact that when inhaled, particulates irritate the respiratory tract. Most dangerous in this regard are the tiny aerosols that, because of their very small size, can evade the body's natural defense mechanisms and penetrate deeply into the lungs (in most cities, these very small particles comprise 50–60% of suspended particulates). In recognition of this fact, the EPA in 1987 replaced the original standard for total particulates with a revised standard that applies to those particles with a diameter of 10 micrometers or less (PM_{10}) that are small enough to penetrate to the highly sensitive alveolar region of the lungs. In 1997, EPA again revised the standards for particulate matter, adding new requirements for particles smaller than 2.5 micrometers in diameter. This action was taken in response to studies indicating that the characteristics, sources, and health effects of these smaller particles are substantially different from those in the PM_{10} category.

Sulfur dioxide (SO_2).   The major source of this colorless pollutant gas is fuel combustion, inasmuch as sulfur is present to a greater or lesser degree as an impurity in coal and fuel oil. When these sulfur-containing fuels are burned, the sulfur is oxidized to form SO_2. By itself sulfur dioxide is not particularly harmful, but it readily reacts with water vapor in the atmosphere to form other sulfur compounds such as sulfuric acid, sulfates, and sulfites that irritate the respiratory system, corrode metals and statuary, harm textiles, impair visibility, and kill or stunt the growth of plants. Sulfur dioxide is also one of the main precursors of acid precipitation, recognized now as an environmental threat of major proportions and a subject that will be dealt with in greater detail later in this chapter.

Carbon monoxide (CO).   No other pollutant gas is found at such high concentrations in the urban atmosphere as is the extremely toxic, odorless, and colorless carbon monoxide. Any type of incomplete combustion produces CO, but the most significant source in terms of urban air pollution is automobile emissions; according to EPA, in the mid-1990s motor vehicles accounted for fully 81% of all CO emissions to the ambient air (in indoor situations, cigarette smoking is a major source of carbon monoxide). When inhaled, CO binds to hemoglobin in the blood, displacing oxygen and thereby reducing the amount of oxygen carried in the bloodstream to the various body tissues. For this reason, carbon monoxide is the air pollutant that provokes the most severe reactions among heart patients. Studies have shown that more deaths among heart attack victims occur during periods of high CO concentrations than at other times. Patients suffering from angina pectoris, a coronary disease in which there is an insufficient supply of oxygen to the heart during exercise, experience a much

Box 12-1   Brown Cloud Over Asia

Little has been heard in Western countries about the "Asian Brown Cloud," but for several billion people in India, Pakistan, Afghanistan, Bangladesh, China, and elsewhere in south and southeast Asia, the two-mile thick haze hovering over cities and countryside alike is an omnipresent reminder that air pollution has become one of the region's most pervasive and serious environmental problems.

First described by an international team of more than 200 scientists from India, the U.S., and Europe working on the Indian Ocean Experiment (INDOEX), the Asian Brown Cloud briefly made headlines in August 2002, with the publication of a United Nations Environmental Programme (UNEP) report, released in time to coincide with the opening of the UN-sponsored World Summit on Sustainable Development in Johannesburg. Following the international conference, both the media and governments moved on to other issues and have scarcely mentioned it since; nevertheless, the situation described in the UNEP document continues to endanger human health and economic progress for societies living under the "brown cloud." Lands thousands of miles away may be affected as well; Japan, Korea, and Taiwan already receive particulate fallout from their Asian neighbors and in April 2002, a cloud of pollutants similar to the Asian Brown Cloud was carried by prevailing winds from the Mongolian-Chinese border across the Pacific to the western United States, with fallout detected in Arizona and Colorado. This incident removed any doubt that pollution can cross oceans to affect regions half a world away.

The blanket of smog so apparent in satellite images of the Indian subcontinent originates from a variety of sources, about 80% of them related to human activities. These include fires deliberately set to clear land or to burn agricultural wastes; industrial emissions; exhaust fumes from the region's burgeoning fleet of cars, trucks, and motorcycles; and smoke from millions of inefficient home cookstoves. Of all these sources, scientists believe that fossil fuel combustion (e.g., coal-fired power plants, gasoline-or diesel-fueled motor vehicles) and the burning of biofuels (e.g., firewood,

cow dung) are most responsible for the witches' brew of ash, black soot, sulfate particles, NO_x, carbon monoxide, acids, and toxic aerosols that comprise the pervasive haze. Confounding the situation, enormous amounts of CO_2 also are being released to the atmosphere, with serious future implications regarding global climate change.

Among the various impacts associated with the pall of pollution, the most direct effect documented by INDOEX scientists is a 10–15% reduction in the sunlight reaching the earth's surface—a result of the reflection and scattering of incoming visible light waves by ambient sulfate aerosols. The result is a cooling of land surfaces in the region. At the same time, black carbon—another component of the Asian haze—absorbs solar radiation and is causing temperatures in the troposphere to rise by 50–100%. The inversion layer formed by a cap of warm air above relatively cooler surface air traps even more pollutants close to the ground, further exacerbating air quality conditions in the region. Researchers fear that the combination of surface cooling and tropospheric warming is also altering winter precipitation patterns, resulting in a 20–40% decrease in rainfall over northwestern India, Pakistan, Afghanistan, and western China while increasing precipitation and flooding in northeastern India, Nepal, Bangladesh, and elsewhere in eastern Asia. Areas beneath the brown cloud may also see a reduction in the frequency of rainfall as a consequence of particulate pollution causing the formation of smaller, more numerous raindrops and longer-lived clouds. If such forecasts prove accurate, the implications for water supply and water quality in the world's most densely populated area are disturbing.

Aside from disrupting the region's hydrologic cycle, the Asian Brown Cloud is already having an impact on human health, reflected in reports of the rising incidence of respiratory diseases and asthma. Research conducted in seven large Indian cities estimated that by the mid-1990s air pollution was responsible for approximately 37,000 premature deaths annually in those cities as a group; further east, in China, Thailand, and Korea, air pollution is provoking similar health problems.

Agricultural productivity in southern Asia is yet another concern. As mentioned previously, airborne particulates block a portion of incoming sunlight, reducing rates of photosynthesis and resulting in a decline in plant productivity. Fly ash and soot settling on leaves likewise reduce the exposure of chloroplasts to solar radiation. Deposition of acidic aerosols or acid precipitation can injure foliage of crop plants or trees and may cause leaching of essential mineral nutrients from the soil; already Asia is the recipient of more acid rain than North America and Europe combined. Research in India indicates that the pollutant-laden haze has caused a 10% decline in the winter rice harvest—an ominous trend for a nation that needs to feed over a billion people. Water stress caused by the haze-induced decrease in winter precipitation in western areas under the brown cloud will be problematic for farmers due to decreased snow melt in the spring. Irrigated agriculture in the region depends heavily on snowmelt to replenish water supplies, so any shortfall in snowfall could have a serious impact on agricultural production.

INDOEX researchers concede that definitive conclusions regarding the climate impacts of haze cannot be drawn from their limited sets of modeling studies Nevertheless, their preliminary findings strongly suggest that the brown cloud forming over the Indian subcontinent each winter may be profoundly affecting the climate, hydrology, and agricultural productivity of the region. Realizing the need for more in-depth research to quantify air pollution's impact on regional climate, scientists have initiated the Asian Brown Cloud Project (ABC Project), aimed at establishing observatories to study the haze and to analyze its impacts on human health, agriculture, and water supplies. It is hoped that a more thorough understanding of the complex physico-chemical reactions occurring within the Asian Brown Cloud can help policymakers devise strategies to reduce haze without derailing the region's impressive economic development. That may be difficult, since the most troublesome pollutants are those emanating from the open fires or inefficient biofuel stoves relied upon by millions of poor families to prepare their meals and provide warmth during the winter. Unable to afford cleaner fuels, such people are unlikely to be persuaded to eat uncooked food or shiver in the cold for the sake of forestalling adverse weather conditions in the years ahead. For policymakers as well, remaining scientific uncertainties and the need for more research provide an excuse for postponing action. Society can only hope that a decade or so from now when all the data have been gathered, the problem has not grown to unmanageable proportions.

References

Hsu, Margaret, and Laura Yee. 2003. "The Asian Brown Cloud (ABC)." San Francisco University High School, Global Environmental Issues, http://www.sfuhs.org/features/globalization/asian_cloud/ Accessed 11/16/04.

United Nations Environment Programme (UNEP). 2002. *The Asian Brown Cloud: Climate and Other Environmental Impacts*, UNEP Assessment Report, Center for Clouds, Chemistry, and Climate.

more rapid onset of pain during periods of increased carbon monoxide pollution. Depending on the concentration of CO in the air and the length of exposure, inhalation of carbon monoxide can result in adverse health effects ranging from mild headaches or dizziness at relatively low levels of exposure to death at high levels. Fortunately, the health effects of short-term carbon monoxide exposure are reversible, but people who work for many hours in areas of heavy traffic (e.g., police officers, toll collectors, parking garage attendants) are obviously receiving substantial doses. Some evidence indicates that blood absorption of CO slows down mental processes and reaction time, raising the suspicion that many rush-hour traffic accidents can be at least partially attributed to low-level carbon monoxide poisoning.

Nitrogen oxides (NO_x). Consisting primarily of nitric oxide (NO) and nitrogen dioxide (NO_2), oxides of nitrogen are formed when combustion occurs at very high temperatures. Nitrogen oxides enter the atmosphere in approximately equal amounts from auto emissions and power plants (in urban areas, cars are generally the predominant source of NO_x emissions). Nitrogen dioxide is the only criteria pollutant gas that is colored. The yellow-brown "smoggy" appearance typical of southern California on bad days is due to the high concentrations of NO_2 in the air. At high levels of pollution, nitrogen dioxide has a pungent, sweetish odor. When present in the high concentrations that sometimes occur indoors in the vicinity of gas stoves or other sources of combustion, NO_2 can provoke shortness of breath or coughing; children living in such environments suffer an enhanced risk of respiratory disease. Nitrogen dioxide also stunts plant growth and visibly damages leaves. It reduces visibility and, like sulfur dioxide, contributes to the formation of acid rain.

Ozone (O_3). The main constituent of a group of chemical compounds known as **photochemical oxidants,** ozone and such fellow travelers as peroxyacetylnitrate (PAN) and various aldehydes are considered to be auto-associated pollutants even though they are not emitted directly from the tailpipe into the atmosphere. Instead, these substances form in a complex series of chemical reactions when nitrogen dioxide and **volatile organic compounds (VOCs),** especially certain hydrocarbons from both auto exhausts and a variety of stationary sources, react with oxygen and sunlight to produce a witch's brew of chemicals dubbed **photochemical smog.** First observed in the Los Angeles area in the 1940s (the bright sunlight, warm temperatures, frequent atmospheric inversions, and heavy traffic make southern California particularly well-suited for photochemical smog formation), photochemical smog is now often observed in other cities as well, especially on bright summer days ("ozone season" is considered to extend from May 1 through September 30). Ground-level ozone, an early and continuing product of the photochemical smog reaction, is the chemical whose presence is used to measure the oxidant level of the atmosphere at any given time. This pungent, colorless gas irritates the mucous membranes of the respiratory system, causing coughing, choking, and reduced lung capacity. Heart patients, asthmatics, and those suffering from bronchitis or emphysema are at special risk during periods of high O_3 levels. Ozone also cracks rubber, deteriorates fabrics, and causes paint to fade. The eye irritation and watery eyes frequently experienced during smog episodes is caused both by ozone and by PAN. Plant growth is severely impacted by ground-level ozone; either alone or in combination with SO_2 and NO_2, ozone accounts for about 90% of annual U.S. crop losses due to air pollution. Symptoms of ozone damage are most visible between the veins on the upper surface of leaves, exemplified by tiny flecks (irregular light tan spots) or small stipples (darkly pigmented areas); alternatively, in some plant species a bronzing or reddening of the leaf surface is characteristic of ozone injury. Among evergreen species such as pine, needle tips turn yellow and die. Premature leaf or needle drop is a typical consequence of such damage. Less visible but equally harmful, ground-level ozone interferes with a plant's ability to photosynthesize, thereby reducing plant biomass and lowering crop yields.

Lead (Pb). The adverse impact of this toxic metal on the intellectual development of children (see chapter 7) caused it to be added to the list of criteria pollutants when the Clean Air Act was reauthorized in 1977. Since most airborne lead can be traced to automobile emissions, the major control strategy for this pollutant was to phase out the use of leaded gasoline, a process completed in the United States by the end of 1995. Approximately 50 other nations have subsequently joined the U.S. in discontinuing the use of leaded gasoline, including Canada, Japan, Sweden, Germany, India, Brazil, Turkey, Egypt, and China.

Hazardous Air Pollutants (HAPs)

In addition to the criteria air pollutants, a large number of less common, but much more hazardous, chemicals are released into the atmosphere from a wide range of industries and manufacturing processes, as well as from motor vehicles. Although the sources of these emissions are more localized than are those of the criteria pollutants, the fact that many of them are either toxic or carcinogenic suggests that they deserve special attention. In 1970 Congress directed the EPA to develop a list of industrial air pollutants that can cause serious health damage even at relatively low concentrations and to establish protective emission standards for those so listed. No deadline date for listing substances as hazardous was mandated, however, and implementation of the congressional directive was exceedingly slow.

By 1990, twenty years after the original congressional mandate, only eight toxic air pollutants had been listed—**asbestos, mercury, beryllium, benzene, vinyl chloride, arsenic, radionuclides, and coke oven emissions**—and standards had been set only for the first seven (a standard for coke oven emissions was finally promulgated in 1993). Frustrated with this snail's pace, environmentalists for years had prodded EPA to speed up the evaluation process, urging the agency to list and set standards for additional toxic air pollutants that pose a special hazard to public health. In 1986, congressional passage of the Emergency Planning and Community Right-to-Know Act (Superfund Amendments and Reauthorization Act, commonly referred to as SARA Title III), prompted by a tragic chemical accident in Bhopal, India two years earlier, led to heightened public awareness of the toxic threats lurking in hundreds of communities across the nation. By requiring that manufacturers disclose information on the kinds and amounts of toxic pollutants they discharge into the local environment each year, this law prompted demands from community activists and the media for tighter controls on health-threatening emissions. In turn, the necessity of revealing data that might alarm previously complacent local residents prompted voluntary emissions reductions by a number of firms eager to maintain a positive corporate image. In 1990 Congress responded to the mounting pressure to "do something" about air toxics by identifying 189 chemicals that it ordered EPA to regulate as hazardous air pollutants and by establishing comprehensive, technology-based controls for dealing with this largely ignored public health threat; two of the original air toxics have now been delisted—caprolactam in 1996 and ethylene glycol mono-butyl ether (EGBE) in 2004—leaving 187 regulated HAPs. The new regulatory approach to controlling air toxics will be discussed in greater detail later in this chapter.

Impact of Air Pollution on Human Health

If dirty skyscrapers or impaired views were the only consequence of polluted air, concern about the phenomenon would undoubtedly be considerably less than it is today. The unfortunate fact is, however, that over the years there has been a steadily growing mass of evidence indicating that the quality of the air we breathe has a measurable impact on human health.

Some of the ill effects of air pollution have, of course, been known for a long time: Los Angelenos knowingly curse the smog as they wipe tears from their burning eyes; motorists hopefully roll up their car windows in heavy traffic, trying to avert a carbon monoxide-induced headache; and asthmatics brace for an attack when the weather forecaster proclaims an ozone alert. For many years discomforts such as these were shrugged off as necessary consequences of economic growth. Only after several air pollution "disasters" made world headlines did the general public begin to realize the extent of the threat posed by dirty air. In each case, already-bad air quality was made much worse by an atmospheric anomaly known as an **inversion**—a condition where a layer of cool surface air is trapped by an overlying layer of warmer air. This situation is a reversal of normal conditions in which the air is in a constant state of flux, with air near the earth's surface rising as it warms, carrying with it and gradually dispersing pollutant particles and gases. During an inversion the cool air, being heavier than the air above, is unable to rise and mix, remaining atypically stable. If the inversion layer remains in place for several days, pollutant emissions within the affected area have nowhere to escape and can accumulate to health-threatening concentrations.

This is precisely what happened in Belgium's heavily industrialized Meuse River Valley in 1934 when 60 people died of the foul air during a 3-day inversion; thousands of others fell seriously ill, coughing and gasping for breath. In the fall of 1948, the small Pennsylvania town of Donora, near Pittsburgh, similarly fell victim to a 5-day inversion. Situated in a valley characterized by smokestack industries, Donora was enveloped in a cold, damp blanket of murky air permeated with the smell of sulfur. During this time, fully 42% of the town's population suffered eye, nose, and throat irritation; chest pains; coughing; difficulty in breathing; headaches; nausea; and vomiting. When the inversion finally lifted, it was found that 20 people had died during the period (Waldbott, 1978). Most notorious of all was London's famous killer smog of 1952. For a period of five days shortly before Christmas, emissions from coal-burning home fireplaces, factories, and motor vehicles accumulated to 10 times their usually smoggy levels. Even at noon the pervading gloom was so thick that car-train collisions were common and cinemas were forced to close because the projector beam from the back of the theater couldn't reach the screen. When the inversion layer finally lifted, officials were shocked to discover the grim health toll of this episode—4,000 excess deaths, most of them among elderly sufferers of heart or respiratory diseases (Goldstein and Goldstein, 2002).

Road and rail traffic were reduced to a crawl during London's infamous killer smog of December 1952. [© *Topham / The Image Works*]

These dramatic examples of pollution-induced death and disease were all associated with levels of air contamination considerably worse than those experienced by most urban residents today, even those living in visibly smoggy cities. For many years researchers have been trying to determine whether air pollution at levels typically encountered in metropolitan areas can, by itself, increase mortality and morbidity rates and, if so, which specific pollutants pose the greatest hazard. Results obtained from a number of studies now confirm fears long suspected—air pollution kills, and at levels of pollutant concentration well within the legally allowable limits established by the NAAQS.

The Air Pollution-Health Connection

Investigations aimed at determining precise cause-and-effect relationships linking given levels of pollution with specific health responses have encountered numerous difficulties. One such problem relates to scientific ethics: it simply isn't acceptable to expose the most vulnerable members of society—children, the elderly, asthmatics, etc.—to high levels of air pollution and then watch to see what happens to them. In addition, because urban air contains so many different pollutants, determining with certainty *which* pollutant at *what level* is causing an observed health effect has been problematic. The likelihood that synergistic effects play a role in determining the response to polluted air is a further complicating factor, as is the possibility of contributory occupational exposure. Particularly vexing to researchers has been the overwhelming influence of cigarette smoking—i.e., how much is due to the pollutants in city air and how much is due to self-inflicted tobacco pollutants? In spite of these challenges, a substantial body of evidence documenting the health effects of air pollutants has been compiled by researchers in many parts of the world. Epidemiological data collected in the United States since the 1970s supports environmentalists' contention that air pollution can be deadly. An estimated 2–3% of all deaths in the U.S. each year are attributed to air pollution-induced respiratory or cardiovascular disease. Similar levels of mortality due to dirty air have been reported in Poland and the Czech Republic (WRI, 1996). According to a World Health Organization (WHO) report released in 2003, urban air pollution reduces life expectancy in Europe more than any other environmental risk factor. WHO estimates that long-term exposure to air contaminants from road traffic alone is responsible for 80,000 European deaths each year. Mortality due to foul air is even higher in cities of the developing world, where soaring rates of urbanization, rapid industrial development, proliferation of motor vehicles, and lack of effective pollution control programs combine to produce far worse air quality than anything experienced by the industrialized nations. Very few developing countries possess the data required to evaluate air pollution's public health impact, but observers have no doubt the toll is significant. As evidence they point to the high rates of acute lower respiratory infection, one of the leading causes of child mortality in the Third World and known to be enhanced by exposure to air pollution. Worldwide, WHO estimates that approximately 5–6% of all deaths each year can be attributed to air contaminants, both indoors and outdoors, providing ample justification for government regulation of air pollution in order to protect human health (Saksena and Smith, 2003).

Major Health Effects

Not surprisingly, air pollution's major impact on health is the result of irritants acting on the respiratory tract. Not all air pollutants are equally harmful, however. Research indicates that the most serious health effects associated with polluted air can be attributed to elevated levels of very fine particulates—those with an aerodynamic diameter of 2.5 micrometers or less—and to sulfate particles. These pollutants have been more directly associated with heightened risk of death and disease than have any other contaminants in the ambient air; the fatalities that occurred during the air pollution disasters previously described have all been attributed to this group of pollutants. Even today, research indicates that airborne particulates cause over 100,000 deaths annually in the United States alone (Schwartz, 2000). These tiniest aerosols have no threshold level below which they don't present a health risk; inhaled deeply into the lungs, they lodge in sensitive pulmonary tissue and constitute a chronic source of irritation. Epidemiologic studies conducted from 1975–1988 in six U.S. cities convincingly demonstrated the link between high levels of particulate air pollution and death due to lung cancer, respiratory disease, and heart ailments—even after controlling for individual risk factors such as smoking, occupational exposure, excessive weight gain, and so on. The correlation was most dramatically evident in Steubenville, Ohio, the most polluted city in the survey group, where adjusted mortality rates were 26% higher than in Portage, Wisconsin, the least polluted of the six communities studied. Interestingly, the link between pollution levels and increased risk of premature death was statistically significant only in relation to concentrations of fine, inhalable particles; varying levels of total suspended particulates, NO_x, SO_2, or ozone appeared to have no measurable impact on death rates—an indication that fine particulates constitute the most dangerous form of air pollution in terms of human health impact (Pope et al., 2002; Dockery et al., 1993). Ground-level ozone can also be a killer. Scientists studying the impact of short-term outdoor ozone exposure in 95 U.S. metropolitan areas, home to 40% of all Americans, found that a 10-ppb increase in the previous week's ozone concentrations resulted in a statistically significant (0.52%) increase in daily mortality rates, primarily involving deaths due to cardiovascular or respiratory disease. The researchers calculated that for the 95 communities studied, ground-level ozone was responsible for an estimated 3,767 excess deaths each year—clear evidence that this common air pollutant is negatively affecting public health (Bell et al., 2004).

When polluted air is inhaled, both the structure and the functioning of the respiratory tract can be altered. Although much remains to be learned about the precise physiologic mechanisms by which exposure to air pollution can kill, some of the ways in which air pollutants can induce illness include the following.

Inhibit or inactivate natural body defenses. The human respiratory system is well constructed to restrict entry of foreign particles and to rid the body of such intruders if they succeed in penetrating the first lines of defense. As a result, the approximately 10,000–20,000 liters of germ-and particle-laden air inhaled by a person each day are effectively cleansed by the time they reach the lungs. Particles are removed both by deposition and by clearance, the precise site at which this occurs depending on particle size. Large particles may be trapped by nasal hairs or are deposited on the walls of the nose or throat, while smaller particulates generally escape these defenses and travel deeper into the respiratory tract. Here the slower air movement causes all but the smallest particles to settle out on the surface of the trachea or bronchi (the conducting airways). Upon settling, the invading particles are trapped by mucus produced by cells lining the airways. They are then swept upward by the constant beating movement of millions of tiny **cilia,** hair-like projections of epithelial cells lining the respiratory tract. This mucociliary action transports dirt and pathogens to the upper respiratory passages from whence they are expelled by nose blowing, coughing, sneezing, or swallowing. The tiniest aerosol particulates that evade removal in this manner are deposited on the lining of the **alveoli** (terminal air sacs), where they may be attacked and devoured by specialized scavenger cells called **macroph-ages,** thus removing them from the lungs.

Although not always successful, these defense mechanisms are extremely impor-tant in shielding the respiratory system from assault. Research has shown that expo-sure to certain air pollutants can induce health problems due to the effect of these contaminants on the body's natural defenses. When pollutant gases are inhaled, espe-cially ozone, NO_2, or SO_2, the action of the cilia lining the airways may be slowed down or halted altogether. At high pollutant concentrations, patches of ciliated cells may be killed and slough off; macrophage cells in the alveoli also may function improperly. Any of these effects greatly reduces the body's ability to withstand inva-sion from pathogenic organisms such as bacteria or viruses. Thus a common health consequence of breathing polluted air is increased susceptibility to infectious airborne diseases such as pneumonia or acute bronchitis.

Cause constriction of the airways ("chronic airway resistance"). Exposure to gases such as O_3 or SO_2 may result in a swelling of the membrane lining the airways, thereby reducing the diameter of the opening and resulting in more labored breathing.

Induce fibrosis and thickening of alveolar walls. Ozone is particularly effec-tive in altering the wall structure of the delicate terminal air sacs. When ozone comes into contact with sensitive alveolar cells, tiny lesions are formed. The breaks subse-quently heal, but in the process scar tissue is formed. Lung tissue becomes thicker and stiffer, making it more difficult for air to penetrate and thereby reducing functional lung capacity ("Health Effects," 1978).

Fortunately, in most of the industrial democracies, the public has recognized the serious health hazards posed by air pollution and has demanded air quality controls that have significantly reduced levels of contamination. Although air quality continues to worsen in many developing nations, today in most parts of the United States, Japan, and western Europe it is very unlikely that another air pollution disaster such as that of Donora in 1948 or London in 1952 could occur again. For this we can thank the persistent efforts of a dedicated coalition of citizens and scientists who wouldn't allow the public to ignore the air pollution-health connection and the legislators, both state and federal, who had the political courage to impose mandatory controls on polluters.

Pollution Control Efforts—The Clean Air Act

As air quality in the United States steadily deteriorated during the 1950s and 1960s, it became increasingly evident that a broad-based, concerted effort was needed to deal with what was increasingly perceived as a problem of national scope. Until 1955 any attempts to regulate pollutant emissions were based solely at the local or state level; in that year the first federal law dealing exclusively with air pollution offered research and technical support to states and municipalities, thereby initiating a policy of federal-state-local partnership in the pollution control effort. By 1963, wors-ening levels of air pollution generated pressure for more effective action and led to passage of the first Clean Air Act, which gave the federal government a modest degree of authority to attack interstate air pollution problems and further increased the flow of federal dollars to state and local pollution control agencies. By 1965 recognition of the automobile's contribution to air quality problems precipitated the first emission standards for automobiles (these standards, set for carbon monoxide and hydrocarbon emissions, took effect with 1968 model year cars). In 1967 the comprehensive Air

Quality Act established a regional approach for establishing and enforcing air quality standards, though the main responsibility for control of emission sources (except for automobiles) remained at the state and local levels of government. This gradual transition from total reliance on state and local authorities to an increasing federal involvement grew out of general recognition that the problems of air pollution were so immense, diverse, and complex that environmental improvement could be achieved only through intergovernmental cooperation at all levels.

Although such laws were well intentioned, they relied on voluntary compliance by states, many of which were reluctant to adopt strict controls for fear of driving away industry, thereby forfeiting jobs and tax revenues. As a result, pollutant levels continued to rise and public outcry mounted. By 1970, spurred by a grassroots demand that something be done about the environmental crisis facing the nation (a public outcry that culminated in the first national observance of "Earth Day" on April 22, 1970), an historic turning point was reached with congressional passage of the **Clean Air Act Amendments of 1970** (henceforth referred to here simply as the Clean Air Act). This landmark piece of environmental legislation provided the first comprehensive program for attacking air pollution on an effective nationwide basis.

The 1970 Clean Air Act established a number of legal precedents that form the basis of U.S. air quality control regulations in effect today—and, coincidentally, served as a model subsequently adopted by many other nations. Some minor modifications to the law, primarily in the form of deadline extensions for meeting stringent new auto emission requirements, were made in 1977. However, by the early 1980s, continuing problems with high levels of certain auto-related pollutants, complaints that portions of the act had not been implemented with sufficient vigor, and the emergence of acid rain as a troublesome new issue not even addressed by the 1970 mandate, gave rise to vociferous demands from the environmental community for changes that would make the Clean Air Act both stronger and more comprehensive. At the same time, the new Reagan Administration viewed its mission as one of dismantling many of the environmental programs enacted during the 1970s. Although Congress refused to approve most of the changes proposed, decisions by the Reagan EPA to waive implementation of certain regulations deemed burdensome to industry resulted in a gradual reversal of air quality improvements. On the most contentious issue of all— what to do about acid rain—the Reagan White House adamantly opposed any new initiatives other than further study, remaining steadfastly unconvinced that the phenomenon posed any real problems.

As a result of this impasse, efforts to reauthorize the Clean Air Act as required by law languished throughout the 1980s, in spite of continued public support for improving air quality. The legislative logjam remained unbroken until 1988 when newly elected President George Bush, citing his desire to be remembered as the "Environmental President," threw his active support behind efforts to resolve the clean air controversy. Within Congress the clash among regional interests and competing ideologies frequently threatened to derail negotiations, but eventually, after months of heated debate, the differences were resolved. Passage of the Clean Air Act Amendments of 1990, signed into law by President Bush in November of that year, marked a significant strengthening of U.S. air quality legislation. The amendments expanded the scope of regulatory requirements, addressed new issues ignored by the 1970 act, and made the law more consistent with other environmental mandates. Although these amendments won't be fully implemented until 2010, they should result in major measurable improvements in U.S. air quality. Some of the most significant provisions of the Clean Air Act are discussed in the following paragraphs.

National Ambient Air Quality Standards (NAAQS)

In setting national ambient air quality standards for the six criteria air pollutants, the EPA reviews the existing medical and scientific literature to establish **primary standards** at levels intended to safeguard human health, allowing a margin of safety to protect more vulnerable segments of the population such as young children, asthmatics, and the elderly. These standards are subject to periodic revision as new data become available. The Clean Air Act differs from other major environmental laws in requiring that primary standards be set solely on the basis of protecting health, without regard for the costs of pollution control.

The primary standards were originally mandated to be attained by 1975, with penalties (e.g., bans on the construction of new sources of pollution, cut-off of federal highway construction funds, etc.) to be imposed on those **nonattainment areas** that failed to bring their pollution levels into conformance with the NAAQS. Twenty years after passage of the original legislation, numerous urban areas were still in violation of the primary standard for ozone, historically the most difficult-to-control pollutant, and many cities also exceeded the standard for carbon monoxide as well. Therefore, with the enactment of the 1990 amendments, Congress revised its approach for dealing with nonattainment areas. Under the current program, regions still in violation of any of the air quality standards are classified according to the seriousness of their pollution problems (categories range from "marginal" to "extreme"), and are given varying amounts of time—anywhere from 3 to 20 years, depending on the severity of nonattainment—to comply with the standards. The higher the pollution levels, the more regulatory steps states must take in dealing with the problem. The 1990 amendments further require specified annual emission reduction goals to ensure steady progress toward full compliance, lest affected areas postpone action until deadlines are imminent.

In addition to the primary standards, EPA was told to set more stringent **secondary standards** that would promote human welfare by protecting agricultural crops, livestock, property, and the environment in general. No timetable for compliance with secondary standards has been set. However, since the secondary standards set by the EPA are, in most cases, identical to the primary standards, the lack of a deadline date is largely irrelevant.

It is difficult to overemphasize the importance of national (as opposed to state or local) air quality standards. As experience prior to 1970 amply demonstrated, drifting air pollutants pay little heed to political boundaries, a fact that largely nullified feeble state attempts to improve air quality within their own borders. States or cities that tried to impose emission controls on polluters within their jurisdictions found that air quality gains were minimal due to airborne pollutants arriving from less concerned—or less courageous— states upwind. Threats by polluting industries to leave a particular state and relocate in a more lenient regulatory environment made many state legislatures extremely reluctant to get tough with polluters. Thus, establishing uniform nationwide standards has been a key element in improving air quality since 1970.

Emission Limitations for New Stationary Sources of Pollution

The intent in establishing **new source performance standards (NSPS)** for factories and power plants is to reduce pollutants at their point of origin by ensuring that pollution controls are built in when factories and plants are newly constructed or substantially modified. Note that this requirement is not retroactive; that is, polluting power plants or factories already in operation at the time the Clean Air Act was passed are not affected by the NSPS guidelines. However, if "grandfathered" facilities are expanded or rebuilt in ways that increase their total output of pollutants, under its **new source review (NSR)** program the Clean Air Act requires they obtain a permit specifying what emission levels must be met and requiring installation of modern pollution controls. The new source performance standards are set on an industry-by-industry basis, taking into account such factors as economic costs, energy requirements, and total environmental impacts such as waste generation and water quality considerations. The 1990 amendments strengthened this provision by adding a requirement for all stationary sources to obtain operating permits from the state regulatory agency, specifying allowable levels of pollutant emissions as well as required control measures.

Strict Emission Standards for Automobiles

Emission standards for automobiles and other mobile sources form an integral part of Clean Air Act requirements, inasmuch as motor vehicles spew more pollutant emissions into the outdoor air than any other single source. In the U.S., on-road vehicles contribute 51% of all CO emissions, 34% of NO_x, and 29% of VOCs in the ambient air; in traffic-congested metropolitan areas, the percentage of these pollutants originating from mobile sources often exceeds 90% (EPA, 2001; WRI, 1996). Detroit eventually settled upon modified engine design plus installation of catalytic converters as the chief means by which American car manufacturers would reduce emissions, and by 1981 new cars for the first time were able to meet Clean Air Act standards. According to the EPA, automobiles coming off the assembly lines today emit 90% less carbon monoxide, 80–90% fewer hydrocarbons, and 70% less nitrogen oxides than did cars manufactured prior to passage of the Clean Air Act. To ensure that in-use vehicles continue to achieve these emission reductions, the 1990 Clean Air Act Amendments require that all nonattainment areas in the U.S. institute auto **inspection and maintenance (I/M)** programs to detect those vehicles whose emissions control systems are malfunctioning and to require that they be repaired. Since surveys have shown that the majority of mobile source emissions come from the worst 10% of vehicles on the road, such programs represent one of the most effective and least costly means of combating urban smog, short of prohibiting driving altogether. EPA estimates that a well-run I/M program can reduce levels of air pollution in a traffic-congested city by as much as 30%. Currently I/M programs are operating in all or parts of 39 states, some requiring annual inspections, others testing every two years.

Improvements in urban air quality resulting from reduced auto emissions since the mid-1970s have been dramatic, but a shift in vehicle preference among American motorists has, at least temporarily, slowed progress toward clean air goals. Sports utility vehicles (SUVs), minivans, and light-duty trucks now comprise almost half of all new vehicle purchases and account for a steadily increasing proportion of vehicle miles traveled. This fact poses serious air quality concerns because a loophole in the 1970 Clean Air Act, enacted when these types of vehicles comprised a small percentage of the nation's fleet, permitted such vehicles to emit 2–3 times as much pollution as ordinary passenger cars. That situation is now being rectified; during the 1990s, emissions requirements for SUVs were gradually tightened and in 2004 the phase-in of even more stringent "Tier 2" standards began. When completely in place by 2009, all passenger cars, SUVs, and light trucks will be subject to the same emissions requirements. Nevertheless, the legacy of past discrepancies in allowable emissions will persist for many years until most of the current SUV fleet is no longer on the road (Plotkin, 2004).

While reducing tailpipe emissions has been a key component of efforts to curb mobile source pollution, other approaches are being pursued as well. Altering the rel-

Inspection/Maintenance program: (top) vehicles await their turn for emissions testing in Chicago; (bottom) a monitor inserted into the tailpipe of an automobile measures emissions of carbon monoxide and hydrocarbons. [*Illinois Environmental Protection Agency*]

ative proportions of the ingredients used in making gasoline can have a major impact in reducing emissions of ozone-forming chemicals and toxic air pollutants such as benzene. Recognizing the pollution-reducing potential of such reconfigured fuels, the 1990 amendments to the Clean Air Act mandated the use of so-called **reformulated gasoline** (see box 12-2) in the major metropolitan areas experiencing the most severe ozone problems. In addition, service stations in such areas were told to install vapor recovery systems on gasoline pumps to capture hydrocarbons that would otherwise be

---

Box 12-2 Fighting Smog with Reformulated Gasoline

All gasoline is not created equal. Hundreds of different formulations are used to make the fuel that powers the spark-ignited engines found in the vast majority of automobiles and small trucks. The composition of these various blends is periodically altered to conform to the power and performance requirements of the vehicles in which the gasoline is burned. However, prior to passage of the 1990 Clean Air Act Amendments, the emissions performance of a particular gasoline formulation was not an issue.

During the congressional debate that preceded enactment of the new law, the petroleum industry advanced the idea that **reformulated gasoline (RFG)** could be a valuable weapon in the war against air pollution. In comparison with conventional gasoline, RFG has lower levels of certain compounds that contribute to air pollution and doesn't evaporate as easily; thus, industry argued, reformulated fuels can have a major impact on the amount of pollutant emissions released by fuel combustion. In pushing RFG, oil industry lobbyists were protecting their own interests, since federal legislators were on the verge of requiring the use of alternative, nonpetroleum fuels as a means of improving air quality. By the late 1980s, oil companies were already marketing a type of RFG in California that reduced emissions from older vehicles no longer able to use leaded gasoline, and they managed to persuade lawmakers that RFG was a more practical alternative than nongasoline fuels. Industrial spokespersons argued that RFG could immediately be used in the nation's existing car fleet, while alternative fuels, by contrast, could only be phased in as new cars engineered to use them rolled off the assembly lines. In the end, they succeeded in convincing Congress to scuttle most of the alternative fuel proposals in favor of RFG.

The reformulated gasoline program went into effect in 1995 and targeted urban areas that were consistently in violation of the national ambient air quality standards for ozone (i.e., smog) and carbon monoxide, developing specific RFG requirements to deal with each of these problems. In the nation's smoggiest cities, the government ruled that RFG must contain a minimum oxygen content of 2% by weight, no more than 1% benzene, and must be free of lead, manganese, and other heavy metals. Although several compounds potentially could be used to meet the oxygen requirement, in most formulations the oxygenate of choice until recently was **methyl tertiary butyl ether (MTBE)**, an additive first introduced in the 1970s as an octane enhancer to replace lead. Numerous major metropolitan areas across the nation are now required by federal law to use RFG as a means of reducing ozone pollution; many others experiencing smog problems have voluntarily opted to use reformulated fuels, with the result that RFG is now being sold in 19 states and the District of Columbia.

In regions of the country where attainment of the NAAQS for carbon monoxide has been problematic, the Clean Air Act Amendments require the *wintertime* use of RFG containing higher oxygenate levels than those required for ozone nonattainment areas—in this case a minimum of 2.7% by weight. To meet this requirement, the fuel of choice has been **ethanol**. Added to RFG, both ethanol and MTBE have the effect of "leaning-out" the air-to-fuel ratio, promoting more complete combustion during cold temperature months when cars need additional fuel to start and when catalytic converters operate less efficiently.

By the late 1990s, several controversies over oxygenates used in RFG raised questions about their safety and effectiveness. In

1999, the California Energy Commission voted unanimously to end the use of MTBE in that state by Dec. 31, 2002, a deadline subsequently postponed until January 1, 2004. Sold in California since the 1970s, MTBE was targeted for phaseout because an estimated 10,000 wells in that state show evidence of MTBE contamination, a result of leaks from underground storage tanks and accidental spills. Several months later MTBE producers got more bad news when an EPA advisory panel recommended that the agency promptly begin reducing MTBE use across the country because of the contamination threat to groundwater supplies. While not calling for an immediate ban, panel members urged that alternatives be brought onto the market as soon as possible. During the next several years, 16 additional states imposed total bans on the use of MTBE and market demand for the additive has sharply declined. As of 2004, Congress had not yet banned MTBE nationwide, but most states where it had once been the oxygenate of choice have now switched to ethanol. The ethanol industry itself is facing a potential problem as the EPA steps up its war on ozone pollution. Although ethanol additives help gasoline burn cleaner during the winter, it also increases vapor pressure during the warmer months of the year—an ozone-enhancing feature that MTBE doesn't share. All gasoline, both RFG and conventional blends, must meet federal requirements limiting the Reid Vapor Pressure (RVP) of gasoline to no more than 9.0 psi during the summer ozone season; an even more stringent 7.8 psi limitation has been set for gasoline sold in ozone nonattainment areas from June 1 to September 15 each year.

While EPA and other proponents contend that the RFG mandate has ushered in significant air quality improvements, other experts are dubious about the overall environmental impact. A 1999 report issued by the National Research Council (NRC) concluded that *neither* ethanol nor MTBE had much impact on reducing emissions that contribute to ozone formation. The real heroes in improving urban air quality, according to the NRC report are (1) better emissions-control equipment on motor vehicles, (2) other nonoxygenate additives to RFG, (3) improved auto engine design, and (4) increasingly stringent air quality regula-

tions. The NRC predicted further improvements in urban air quality in the years ahead, not due to ethanol or MTBE use, but as a result of new technology. Not surprisingly, the Oxygenated Fuels Association takes strong exception to NRC's conclusions, pointing out that the report failed to acknowledge the role oxygenates play in reducing wintertime carbon monoxide levels. EPA also defended the use of oxygenates in reformulated gasoline, stating that they significantly reduce air toxics such as benzene and dilute or displace other fuel components such as sulfur, which then reduces emissions of VOC and NO_X, major precursors of smog formation.

For motorists, the pros and cons of various gasoline additives for enhancing air quality are probably of less immediate interest than the effect of reformulated gasoline on car performance and fuel efficiency. Fortunately, on this score the news is mostly good. Requirements for fuel formulations that burn cleaner have simply been added to long-standing considerations regarding vehicle performance. As a result, RFG has no adverse impact on a car's performance or on the durability of the engine and fuel system components. In terms of fuel efficiency, however, RFG may lower gas mileage in some cars by 1–2% compared to oxygenate-free gasoline, and RFG costs a few cents more per gallon than conventional blends. Residents of RFG marketing areas who travel to parts of the country where the reformulated product is not sold need have no concerns about filling up with conventional gasoline—mixing the two won't have any effect on a car's performance.

Overall, environmental officials regard the reformulated fuels program as a big step forward in clearing the nation's urban air. EPA credits RFG with eliminating over 100,000 tons of smog-forming pollutants each year in RFG areas, as well as 24,000 tons of air toxics annually. For drivers it's a win-win situation: improved, cleaner-burning gasoline, no change in vehicle performance, and more healthful air for everyone to breathe.

Reference

U.S. Environmental Protection Agency. 2004. Office of Transportation and Air Quality.

released during refueling. Cities in violation of carbon monoxide standards were required to use reformulated gasoline containing oxygen additives ("oxygenates") during winter months to increase the combustion efficiency of gasoline, thereby reducing tailpipe emissions of CO.

A major step forward in improving urban air quality was taken in May 2004, with the adoption of tough new regulations on diesel fuel. Prompted by the recognition that emissions from diesel-powered bulldozers, tractors, locomotives, barges, and other off-road vehicles emit more particulates than all the cars, trucks, and buses on American streets and highways, EPA mandated drastic reductions in the sulfur content of diesel fuel, from 3,400 ppm in 2004 to 15 ppm in 2010, for all off-road diesel vehicles except boats and locomotives, which have two additional years to comply with the new standard. Strict regulations for diesel-fueled trucks and buses were adopted in 2000 and are scheduled to take effect in 2007. Health experts, heralding EPA's action, estimate that the new rules curbing diesel emissions will prevent thousands of premature deaths and heart attacks every year.

Looking to the future, many clean air advocates ultimately place their hopes on a transition from the internal combustion engine to nonpolluting "zero emissions vehicles" such as cars powered by efficient hydrogen fuel cells whose only emissions are water vapor. While prestigious authorities such as the National Academy of Sciences contend that hydrogen fuel cell cars remain decades away, some automakers are working on technologies to power conventional engines with hydrogen as well as on dual-fuel hydrogen/gasoline cars they say could be on the market within a few years. In California, the South Coast Air Quality Management District has awarded a $2.3 million contract to Toyota to convert 30 Prius hybrids to run on hydrogen fuel. The State of California also has launched a program requiring auto manufacturers to produce and market millions of low-emission vehicles over the next 15 years (2005–2020). For the immediate future this probably means hybrid electric vehicles, specially modified gas cars, or battery-powered autos, though industry views the latter as a dead-end due to the need for frequent recharging of such vehicles. Currently auto companies are working on a number of different prototypes, striving to meet California's zero emissions mandate—one that several northeastern states are likely to adopt as well.

The success or failure of these initiatives holds important implications for the future because there is little hope of solving auto-related air quality problems solely through reliance on catalytic converters. Even with extremely strict standards for tailpipe emissions, the sheer increase in numbers of cars on the road (by 2002 more than 530 million passenger cars were on the road worldwide, a number that is expected to double by 2030) guarantees a reversal of air quality gains in the years ahead unless a radically different approach to curbing emissions is adopted.

Regulation of Hazardous Air Pollutants through Technology-Based Controls

Under the 1990 Clean Air Act Amendments, EPA was told to adopt a technology-and performance-based approach to reducing air toxics emissions. In response, the agency developed **maximum achievable control technology (MACT)** standards for each group of industrial emitter (source category). These standards are based on levels of control already being accomplished by the best-performing, most proactive industrial plants within that source category. In most cases, MACT standards take the form of a specified percent reduction in emissions or a concentration limit that regulated sources must achieve. Facilities are not mandated to use any specific type of pollution control equipment to achieve the required emissions reductions but rather are allowed to employ whatever methods they find most cost-effective. Such methods might include redesigning industrial processes, installing new pollution control technologies, changing work practices, or capturing and recycling emissions. Once EPA developed MACT standards for the 175 source categories subject to regulation as air toxics emitters, the agency launched the second phase of its program to control HAPs, applying a risk-based approach to determine how successful its technology- and performance-based emissions limitations have been in reducing public health and environmental risks due to air toxics. Depending on the results of this assessment, now in its early stages, EPA will decide whether it is necessary to develop additional regulations to address any significant risks still posed by air toxics.

It should be pointed out that the regulatory program described above pertains solely to stationary sources (e.g., refineries, power plants, factories, gas stations, dry cleaners), which collectively contribute slightly less than half of all human-generated toxic air emissions. The other half comes from mobile sources, including both on-road and off-road vehicles. EPA currently has programs in place that are expected to reduce 1996 levels of mobile source air toxics by more than a million tons by 2010. The new diesel fuel standards, emissions reduction requirements for off-road equipment, reformulated gasoline programs, and further progress in controlling standard tailpipe emissions should all contribute to a further lowering of ambient air toxics concentrations.

Acid Deposition Controls

Perhaps the most bitterly debated issue during the Clean Air Act reauthorization process was acid rain controls. Such controls became a part of federal clean air legislation only after passage of the 1990 amendments. The main focus of the Acid Rain Program has been to reduce 1980 levels of SO_2 emissions from electric power plants by approximately one-half; the current goal is to cap such emissions at 8.95 million tons annually, starting in 2010. NO_x, the other major contributor to acid rain formation, is also a target of emissions reduction efforts. A novel feature of the acid deposition regulations that is attracting widespread interest and attention is a market-oriented system of emissions allowances that utilities can buy, sell, or trade to help finance the costs of pollution controls (see box 12-4).

The Clean Air Act provisions described here represent only the highlights of this extremely complex piece of legislation. Responsibility for implementing and enforcing the federal mandate falls primarily on the environmental agencies of state government, which must develop **State Implementation Plans (SIPs)**, detailing strategies for compliance with Clean Air Act requirements. SIPs must list all the pollution sources within the state, estimating the quantities of each pollutant emitted annually, including both mobile and stationary sources. They must issue operating permits for stationary sources, as well as timetables for compliance, and must include some kind of transportation control strategy for dealing with auto-related pollutants in areas of heavy traffic. States must have their SIPs approved by the federal EPA or be working with the agency to improve a conditionally approved plan before they can issue a construction permit for any new polluting facility.

Enforcement provisions under the Clean Air Act, and the civil and criminal penalties for violation of the law, were significantly strengthened under the 1990 amendments. EPA can levy large financial penalties against facilities in violation of air quality requirements—penalties sufficiently stiff to cancel any economic benefits a firm might derive from delaying compliance. Criminal liability, which may be imposed on people *knowingly* violating the law, can result in fines, imprisonment, or both. The Clean Air Act gives citizens the right to file suit against polluters if the EPA fails to take action. To encourage "whistle-blowing" by people aware of Clean Air Act violations, Congress has authorized EPA to pay informants up to $10,000 for information leading to a civil penalty or criminal conviction (Bryner, 1993; "Easy Guide," 1993; *Environmental Law Handbook,* 1993).

Global Air Quality Trends

Deadline dates have come and gone, hot summers are punctuated with ozone alerts, and a haze of smog still hovers over many of our cities. Nevertheless, 35 years after the Clean Air Act ushered in a "get tough" approach regarding air pollution control, overall trends in American skies are favorable. Elsewhere in the world, progress in cleaning up dirty air varies considerably from one country to another.

A comprehensive assessment of international air quality trends is complicated by the fact that scarcely any routine monitoring has been conducted in the developing nations that comprise the bulk of world population. Anecdotal information suggests that pollution levels in Third World cities are far higher than in most industrialized countries—and getting steadily worse. Many urban areas in the developing world— Beijing, Delhi, Bangkok, Sao Paulo, Hong Kong, Mexico City, to cite just a few—currently experience air pollution levels two to three times higher than those considered "healthy" under World Health Organization guidelines. Some experts fear that air pollution is likely to take a heavier public health toll in the developing countries than it does in the industrialized world, even at similar levels of pollutant concentrations, simply because exposed populations in the Third World include a higher percentage of citizens living in poverty and suffering from malnutrition, both factors that increase the risk of ill health; they also include a much larger proportion of the very young—the most vulnerable age group in any population. As developing nations strive for rapid economic growth, environmental protection may be regarded as a luxury they can't yet afford, while air pollution is but one of many public health issues clamoring for attention (Romieu and Hernandez-Avila, 2003). Air quality problems originate from many sources, but are due primarily to exhaust fumes from the developing world's rapidly growing fleet of motor vehicles, as car ownership becomes synonymous with "the good life" for increasing millions of the newly affluent. In most developing countries, and particularly in Asia, the number of cars on the road is increasing exponentially and the fact that many are old and poorly maintained—and frequently fueled with adulterated gasoline—ensures choking levels of pollutant emissions. Motorcycles and scooters also are proliferating at a record pace, especially in Asia where their highly polluting two-stroke engines further degrade the quality of urban air. Particulate pollution is an especially serious problem in Third World cities, with levels of PM_{10} regularly exceeding WHO guidelines. In Lanzhou, China—ranked among the world's 15 most polluted cities in terms of airborne particulates—the air is so foul that simply breathing is the equivalent of smoking a pack of cigarettes daily. In developing world cities featuring both heavy traffic and bright sunshine, ground-level ozone, a constituent of photochemical smog, is increasingly associated with an upswing in asthma attacks and respiratory problems. Ozone levels in Mexico City exceed WHO air quality guidelines as many as 300 days in a year. Concentrations of sulfur dioxide, another pollutant known as a respiratory irritant and a precursor of acid rain, are increasing in some developing countries, most notably China, as well as in Russia and eastern Europe, where plentiful supplies of high-sulfur coal are burned without pollution controls.

Some positive developments have become evident in recent years, however, as Third World governments begin to take the air pollution/health threat seriously. As

Box 12-3   Air Quality Aloft

Prohibitions on in-flight smoking imposed during the 1980s and now enforced by the vast majority of domestic and international airlines were expected to resolve the most serious concerns voiced by passengers and flight attendants regarding the quality of aircraft cabin air. Certainly such restrictions made air travel more pleasant for the majority of the population who are nonsmokers, but they didn't end complaints, most of them rather broad and specific, about what many travelers and crew members feared were health-threatening levels of airborne contaminants aloft.

While maintenance of good air quality is important in any indoor space, aircraft cabins present a more challenging situation than most, since occupants are in extremely close proximity to one another and are unable to leave if they find conditions oppressive. The steadily increasing number of people traveling by air each year—currently about 1.5 billion worldwide and growing by 6% annually—means that cabin air quality affects a significant portion of the population. In addition, those flying today include an increasing percentage of passengers with preexisting medical conditions such as respiratory or cardiovascular disease, as well as the very young and the elderly, both age groups known to be more vulnerable to environmental stress.

To prevent problems and maintain acceptable cabin air quality, commercial airliners rely on an **environmental control system (ECS)** designed to control cabin pressure, ventilation, temperature, and humidity and to prevent entry of harmful airborne contaminants into the cabin. A typical jetliner uses a mixture of outdoor air, brought in through the engines, and cabin air that is filtered and then recirculated, the portion of recirculated air in the total mix varying from 30% to 55%.

Although the ECS in general does a good job in maintaining safe, comfortable in-flight conditions, the potential exists for a number of airborne contaminants to enter the aircraft cabin. Entry of stratospheric ozone into the cabins of high-flying aircraft could pose a possible health threat to those aboard. At high altitudes, when outside air is drawn into the ventilation system, ozone—a known respiratory irritant—can be present at concentrations that exceed FAA limits on O_3 for cabin air. To avoid this problem, most large commercial airliners now employ O_3 converters which, when new, remove 90–98% of the ozone in the air passing through them. Some concerns have been expressed, however, that there is no process in place to ensure that converters are operating at a high level of efficiency (the useful lifespan of a converter ranges from 10,000–20,000 flight hours); this, plus the fact that some aircraft are still not equipped with O_3 converters, means that on some flights ozone concentrations could exceed existing standards.

Another air quality issue of concern on some international flights involves in-cabin **disinsection**—whereby employees spray insecticides prior to passengers disembarking. Numerous airline passengers have protested this practice, claiming adverse reactions to contact with pesticidal chemicals, but several countries insist it is necessary to rid in-bound flights of any unwelcome insect pests the planes might be harboring. The U.S. Centers for Disease Control and Prevention agrees with those calling for a discontinuation of the practice, asserting that disinsection is both ineffective for its intended purpose and poses a potential health risk for passengers and crew. Nevertheless, India, Uruguay, Grenada, Trinidad, and a few other countries continue to treat all in-bound aircraft while passengers are still on board; the Czech Republic, Switzerland, and the U.K., among others, treat planes arriving from specified areas where malaria is a problem; and Australia, New Zealand, and some Caribbean nations require treatment of aircraft with a residual insecticide when passengers are not on board. The most commonly used pesticides for disinsection are pyrethroid chemicals recommended by WHO for this purpose as effective contact poisons with low human toxicity. Few, if any, studies have been conducted on the amount of pesticide exposure to those on board as a result of disinsection; nevertheless, when on-board spraying is conducted both inhalation and skin (dermal) exposure is inevitable.

The most worrisome in-flight air contaminants are infectious bacteria and viruses, introduced into the aircraft cabin not through the ventilation system but by other passengers or members of the flight crew. Reports regarding transmission of infectious organisms during air travel abound, not surprisingly since such trips involve close contact with a large number of people, in some cases for long periods of time. When such travel involves international flights to tropical destinations, the opportunity for exposure to exotic disease organisms is substantially higher for air travelers than it is for the general public. In addition, with the longer nonstop flights that now characterize much international air travel, passengers are together for more prolonged periods of time than was the case in years past, further increasing opportunities for disease transmission.

Some of the infections known or strongly suspected to have been transmitted in-flight include influenza, measles, and tuberculosis; transmission of acute respiratory infections and meningococcal disease is also considered possible. Contrary to the commonly held belief that germs are spread throughout the aircraft cabin via recirculated air, studies show no difference in infection rates whether or not recirculated air is used. The credit for this is undoubtedly due to the fact that the vast majority of aircraft now employ HEPA filters, capable of removing over 99% of particles and pathogens in the airstream. In-flight sampling studies have shown that concentrations of bacteria are significantly higher near floor vents than in the passenger breathing zone—an indication that airborne microbes are effectively entrained and removed from the cabin with exhaust air. Only in situations where the ventilation system has been shut off, as sometimes happens when ground delays keep a plane sitting on the runway for several hours, are infectious agents likely to spread throughout the cabin. It should be mentioned that air from restrooms is *not* recirculated, in order to avoid the possibility of introducing infectious organisms or odors from sewage disposal systems into the passenger cabin.

The risk of contracting an infectious disease during air travel, therefore, is determined almost entirely by seat assignment; only people sitting (or working, in the case of flight crew) in close proximity to an infected source are exposed to a sufficient number of pathogen-laden droplet nuclei to become infected themselves. The number of source cases and the occupant load of the aircraft are significant factors in determining how many passengers will contract an infection during the flight. Investigations involving suspected cases of disease transmission on aircraft suggest that unless the ventilation system is inoperable, one source case on a plane seldom results in any but adjacent passengers subsequently becoming infected. Clearly, keeping aircraft cabin air free of infectious organisms depends less on equipment (though a properly functioning ventilation system is essential) than it does on common sense and personal responsibility among air travelers. People knowingly suffering from an infectious respiratory disease should postpone flying until they are no longer contagious or, at a minimum, practice good personal hygiene, move around the cabin as little as possible, and cover their mouth and nose while coughing or sneezing. Assuming that many are unlikely to heed such pleas, other travelers are advised to take advantage of immunization against such vaccine-preventable diseases as influenza, measles, and pneumonia (for elderly passengers) as a precautionary measure.

Although current data do not indicate serious air quality-related problems among passengers or cabin crew now that in-flight smoking is no longer permitted, the almost complete lack of detailed studies on contaminant exposure and related health effects, both short-and long-term, make it impossible to state categorically that anecdotal reports of problems are unfounded. Until a systematic effort is launched to collect, analyze, and report health data relating to aircraft cabin air quality, that uncertainty will persist.

References

National Research Council. 2002. *The Airliner Cabin Environment and the Health of Passengers and Crew*. Washington, DC: National Academy Press.

mentioned previously, numerous Asian and Latin American nations have joined the developed countries in outlawing the use of leaded gasoline; Brazil, Thailand, China, India, South Korea, Taiwan, Hong Kong, Singapore, and the Philippines now require all new cars to be equipped with catalytic converters; the entire bus fleet in India's capital city, Delhi, now runs on low-emission compressed natural gas (CNG), as do the city's thousands of 3-wheeled auto-rickshaws. Taiwan has implemented an aggressive program to curb motorcycle emissions, inspiring several of its Asian neighbors to adopt similar programs. Whether such efforts will succeed in reversing the ongoing deterioration of air quality in burgeoning Third World megacities remains to be seen (Walsh, 2003).

In contrast with the downward trends in air quality evident in many developing countries, in parts of the industrialized world emission levels from both stationary sources and motor vehicles have been drastically cut in recent years. While the United States was the pacesetter in air pollution control initiatives until the early 1980s, since then several European nations and Japan have equaled or surpassed the American record. Prompted by international treaty obligations, the European nations reduced sulfur dioxide emissions by 32% between 1980–1990 (McDonald, 1999). Japan requires state-of-the-art controls on automobiles, incinerators, power plants, and steel mills and is the only country in the world that compensates victims of air pollution—deriving monies for those so injured from a tax on SO_2 emissions. The Canadian province of Ontario has an ambient air standard for SO_2 considerably more stringent than that of the United States. Germany, jolted out of complacency in the early 1980s by reports of widespread forest damage due to acid rain, has since implemented one of the world's most vigorous air quality control programs. Unlike the situation in the United States, where power plants in operation prior to promulgation of New Source Performance Standards were exempted from the requirement for the best available technological controls, Germany has mandated the retrofitting of all its medium and large-size power plants, regardless of age, with state-of-the-art pollution control devices. The Swiss and Austrians, similarly concerned about dying forests, have adopted what may be the most stringent air quality regulations in the world, like Taiwan setting emission standards even for motorcycles.

In the United States, air quality in most parts of the country has improved significantly since passage of the Clean Air Act. In 2004 the EPA reported that total emissions of the six criteria air pollutants were at their lowest level since 1970, down 51% (from 301.5 million tons/year in 1970 to 147.8 million in 2003), in spite of population growth, increased traffic volume, rising energy consumption, and continued industrial development during the same time period. Progress in cleaning up the nation's air has not been uniform—concentrations of some pollutants have declined more than others and some regions of the country have experienced air quality trends better or worse than national averages would indicate. Of the criteria air pollutants, since 1970 ambient levels of lead have dropped by a precipitous 98%, while emissions of particulates, SO_2, CO, and the volatile organic compounds that contribute to ozone formation have all declined by 50% or more. Reductions in nitrogen oxides have been somewhat less impressive, down by 25% since 1970. Air toxics emissions have dropped as well, down 30% between 1990 and 1999.

Nevertheless, levels of the criteria pollutants in a number of urban areas still remain high enough to endanger the health of their residents. EPA, which gathers information on air concentrations of the various criteria pollutants from over 4,000 monitoring stations across the United States, reports that in 2003 nearly 126 million people lived in areas that still exceeded the NAAQS for at least one pollutant. In that year more than 100 million resided in areas where ozone levels violated the 8-hour federal standard. It should be noted, however, that smog levels within a region vary considerably from year to year, depending on weather conditions. Since ozone concentrations tend to be highest when daytime temperatures exceed 90°F, increases or decreases in ozone levels for any given year are heavily influenced by how hot a summer the region in question experienced. The fact that ozone levels in 2003 were the lowest since 1980 was due not only to successful emissions control programs, but also to favorable (i.e., cooler) weather during the summer of 2003. Ozone remains by far our most troublesome pollutant in terms of numbers of people affected. $PM_{2.5}$ is problematic as well. In 2004, EPA reported that 225 counties in 20 states and the District of Columbia—home to 95 million people—exceeded the federal standards for fine particulate pollution. It is likely that in the years immediately ahead there will also be much more aggressive efforts to tighten controls for nitrogen oxides, whose emissions appear to be more important contributors to ozone formation than previously realized. Controls are likely to expand over a wide range of formerly unregulated sources of VOCs such as dry cleaning establishments, furniture refinishers, auto body shops—and possibly even consumer items such as charcoal lighter fuel, spray starch, and power lawn mowers! Southern California, a perennial nonattainment area for ozone (partly because the area experiences inversions as often as 340 days of the year), will be most heavily impacted by stricter air quality regulations. There, as well as in several other smog-plagued metropolitan areas (e.g., New York/New Jersey, Chicago/Gary, Houston), EPA anticipates that supplemental local emission control measures will be necessary if the federal air quality standards for ozone are ever to be attained. Accordingly, California has adopted the toughest, most aggressive air quality regulations in the nation—some of which are now being copied by several northeastern states grappling with smog problems of their own.

In spite of these remaining challenges, air quality trends in the United States overall are very encouraging. While declining levels of pollutant emissions are due in some measure to energy conservation, fuel-switching, and the demise of many smokestack industries, a large share of the credit must be given to the regulatory programs that have mandated significant investment in pollution control technologies. Although the battle to control air pollution is by no means over, progress to date proves that the Clean Air Act is working.

Acid Deposition

An air quality problem virtually unrecognized and unmentioned at the time the 1970 Clean Air Act was passed, the issue of acid deposition (commonly referred to as "acid rain," though the phenomenon includes not only rain but also snow, fog, dry SO_2 and NO_2 gas, and sulfate and nitrate aerosols) became political dynamite during the 1980s, pitting region against region, nation against nation. Although the domestic policy battles generated by the debate over acid rain controls were largely resolved by key provisions of the 1990 Clean Air Act Amendments and by the Canada-United States Air Quality Agreement of 1991, the problem itself persists and the damage toll continues to climb. Nor are all the facts concerning acid deposition completely understood even today. To comprehend what the fuss is all about requires a brief look at the nature of acid deposition, how it is formed, and the types of damage it causes.

What Is Acid Deposition?

On a pH scale, distilled water has a pH of 7.0, considered "neutral" because the number of hydrogen (H^+) and hydroxyl (OH^-) ions is equal, making the solution neither acidic nor basic. However, since atmospheric CO_2 tends to dissolve in water, forming a weak solution of carbonic acid, rainfall is slightly acidic by nature. Measurements of the pH of precipitation in many parts of the world have led researchers to conclude that natural, unpolluted rain has a pH around 5.0. Thus, by definition, any precipitation measuring **less than 5.0** on the pH scale is considered acid deposition. Since the pH scale is logarithmic, rainfall with a pH of 4.0 is ten times more acid than precipitation with a pH of 5.0 and 100 times more acid than that of pH 6. A reading below 2.0, such as that recorded during a three-day drizzle in the fall of 1978 at Wheeling, West Virginia, represented a level 10,000 times more acid than unpolluted rainfall.

Extent of the Problem

Acid precipitation had been observed as a local phenomenon in the vicinity of coal-burning facilities since the 19th century. In fact, the term "acid rain" was first coined by an English chemist, Robert Angus Smith, to describe the corrosive brew falling on industrial Manchester more than 100 years ago. In the early 1960s Canadian ecologist Eville Graham, a pioneer of acid rain research in North America, described the acidification of lakes in northern Ontario in the vicinity of the huge Sudbury smelting complex, then the world's largest single source of sulfur emissions (Munton, 1998). Not until the 1970s, however, did acid rain emerge as a regional problem, affecting areas far from the source of pollutant emissions. The alarm was first raised in 1972 by Swedish delegates attending the UN Conference on the Human Environment in Stockholm. After initial disbelief by many national governments, Swedish views about the extent and seriousness of this newly recognized environmental threat became widely accepted. On the basis of measurements taken during the past few decades, scientists have shown that until the late 1990s, when government-mandated controls began to take effect, the pH of rainfall steadily dropped throughout large areas of North America and Europe. Not only did rainfall become more acid in the affected areas, but the geographical extent of the problem widened also. Early measurements of rainfall pH indicated that in the years 1955–1956 only 12 northeastern states were experiencing acid precipitation. By 1972–1973 the number of states experiencing excessive rainfall acidity extended over the entire eastern portion of North America, except for the southern tip of Florida and the far northern regions of Canada. In addition, acid rain was detected in several of the major urban areas of California and in the Rocky Mountain region of Colorado.

Today the pH of rainfall averages 4.4 throughout the United States east of the Mississippi River, with substantially lower readings being obtained during some individual storm episodes. However, encouraging news has been reported by scientists working for the U.S. Geological Survey who documented a steady drop in the concentrations of acid-forming sulfates in precipitation from 1980 to 1991—a decline that has accelerated since the 1990 Clean Air Act imposed strict SO_2 reduction requirements on coal-burning power plants. As a result, in many of the affected regions, the average pH of rainfall has gradually been rising. Such field data are hailed as evidence that pollution control technologies aimed at curbing SO_2 emissions are having the intended impact. Unfortunately, USGS monitoring stations have not seen an equivalent decline in rainfall nitrate concentrations, nor has a nearly 35-year trend toward increasing acidification of waterways been reversed. Indeed, in the streams being monitored, pH levels have continued to fall year after year (Hilchey, 1993).

Beyond North America, acid deposition today also affects most countries of Europe, although on that continent, as in North America, increasingly stringent controls on sulfur dioxide emissions reduced the seriousness of the problem during the decade of the 1990s. By contrast, acid rain has emerged as a growing environmental threat in Asia, particularly in the rapidly industrializing provinces of southeastern

China, a country where acid precipitation now affects more than 40% of the total land area. Japan is reporting acidification problems, and high levels of acid precipitation are now being experienced in northeastern India, northern and central Thailand, and throughout the Korean peninsula (WRI, 1998).

Mystery of the Dying Lakes

During the 1960s and 1970s anglers, campers, and resort owners raised the first alarms concerning what was to become a major environmental tragedy. From the sparkling lakes of the remote Adirondacks, to the popular vacationlands of Ontario and Quebec, to the waterways of Scandinavia, reports of the mysterious disappearance of once-abundant fish, amphibians, and aquatic insects began to generate public concern. The fact that such lakes and streams were far from any of the usual sources of water pollution that have traditionally been associated with fish kills only increased the bewilderment. To a casual observer the water remained blue and clear, uncontaminated by chemical spills or sewage overflows; beneath the surface, however, the affected lakes had become watery deserts, devoid of life. By 2003, surveys showed that in New York's Adirondack Mountains approximately 41% of the lakes had become too acidic for fish and other aquatic life; the same situation applied to 15% of lakes in the New England states (Driscoll et al., 2003). In New Jersey's Pine Barrens, fully 90% of all streams are acidic—the highest percentage in the nation. In eastern Canada the toll is even higher—acidified lakes total 14,000, with approximately 150 now fishless. Such lakes are acid dead, poisoned by pollutants falling from the sky in the form of sulfuric and nitric acid.

Formation of Acid Rain

Acid precipitation forms when its major precursors, sulfur dioxide and nitrogen dioxide, are chemically converted through a complex series of reactions involving certain reactive hydrocarbons and oxidizing agents such as ozone to become sulfuric or nitric acid. The reactions involved can take place either within clouds or rain droplets, in the gas phase, on the surface of fine particulates in the air, or on soil or water surfaces after deposition (Rhodes and Middleton, 1983).

Sulfur dioxide is discharged into the atmosphere in amounts averaging 15 million tons annually in the United States. Of this amount, approximately two-thirds originates from coal-and oil-burning power plants; the remainder is primarily from smelters and industrial boilers. A certain amount of SO_2 enters the atmosphere from natural sources such as volcanoes or mud flats, but such emissions contribute relatively little to the problem of acid rain; it is estimated that in the northeastern U.S., 90% of the sulfur in the air comes from human sources of pollution.

Nitrogen oxides, of which about 20 million tons per year are currently emitted in the United States, come predominantly from auto emissions, power plants, and industry. Until recently, SO_2 emissions have widely been perceived as posing a more serious problem than NO_x in terms of acid rain formation; however, as technological controls are increasingly successful at reducing levels of airborne sulfur compounds, the role of nitrogen oxides as acid rain precursors has grown in importance. Clean Air Act requirements have been far less successful in reducing airborne emissions of NO_x than they have been in controlling SO_2 and most observers agree that additional measures to cut nitrogen emissions will be needed to protect sensitive ecosystems.

Long-Distance Transport

The aspect of acid rainfall that makes it such a politically charged issue is the fact that the pollutant emissions that are the precursors of acid rain formation may be produced hundreds of miles from the regions suffering the effects of acid deposition. Because some pollutants can remain in the air for a relatively long period of time, they can be carried on the prevailing winds across geographical and political boundaries far from their place of origin—a phenomenon known as **long-distance transport**. There are documented examples of acid rain-forming pollutants being carried more than 600 miles before being deposited on the earth's surface.

Ironically, pollution control technologies adopted early in the 1970s to reduce *local* levels of ambient air pollution had the unintended effect of increasing the long-distance transport problem. The approach adopted most often by utilities striving to lower SO_2 concentrations in the vicinity of their plants was to pursue a **tall stack strategy**; that is, to build extremely tall "superstacks" that discharged pollutant gases into the persistent air currents more than 500 feet above the ground. This approach was indeed effective in reducing local pollution levels, but it promoted long-distance transport and thereby increased the range and severity of acid deposition in regions downwind. Until the 1990 Clean Air Act Amendments committed the United States to aggressive acid rain control efforts, relations between Canada and the United States were seriously strained because half of the corrosive rain falling over southeastern Canada originates in the heavily industrialized Ohio River Valley and upper Midwest. New York and the New England states harbored a similar grudge against Illinois, Indiana, and Ohio—the source of fully one-fourth of all U.S. sulfur emissions.

In the same way, much of the acid rain now damaging vegetation and aquatic environments in Japan originated in China, whose sulfur emissions in 1990 were 40–45 times higher than those during Japan's worst air pollution years in the mid-1970s. Japanese authorities estimate that at least 37% of the sulfur deposition over their country is "made in China" and have offered the Chinese low-interest loans to purchase pollution control equipment for reducing SO_2 emissions (Brown, Renner, and Flavin, 1998). Prior to the 1980s, acid rain provoked harsh words among neighboring European countries as well, since the corrosive precipitation wreaking havoc on lakes and forests in Norway and Sweden was produced primarily in central Europe and Great Britain. Such circumstances make the formulation of acid rain control policies politically difficult because those bearing the cost of pollution abatement strategies and those reaping the benefits are not one and the same. Effective action toward resolving this dilemma was taken first in Europe where 35 countries in 1979 signed the **Convention on Long-Range Transboundary Air Pollution,** an agreement requiring the signatory nations to achieve a 30% reduction in SO_2 emissions from 1980 levels by 1993. Targets have subsequently been set for reducing NO_x and VOC emissions as well. In the United States, the acid rain debate raged in Congress for years. Legislators from the Midwest were nearly unanimous in their opposition to proposed federal rules that would impose more stringent sulfur emission controls on coal-burning power plants in their region. Citing the financial burden that would be passed along to electric consumers and the inherent threat controls would pose to coal-mining interests in states like Illinois and West Virginia, midwestern representatives were acutely aware that the environmental gains achieved by tougher regulations would be enjoyed by citizens outside their own constituencies. Conversely, legislators from such states as New Hampshire and Maine, areas that had few large sources of emissions yet were suffering severe economic and ecological damage due to acid rain, were among the most vocal in demanding regulatory action.

Regional Vulnerability to Acid Rain

Although the entire eastern United States is now experiencing acid rainfall, not all areas are suffering adverse ecological effects. An ecosystem's sensitivity to acid precipitation is determined primarily by the chemical composition of the soil and bedrock—an attribute referred to as the **buffering capacity** of that environment.

Buffering capacity refers to an ability to neutralize acids, the buffer acting to maintain the natural pH of an environment by tying up the excess hydrogen ions introduced by acid rain. Regions such as New England, the Mid-Atlantic states, the Southeast, northern Minnesota and Wisconsin, the Rocky Mountain states, and parts of the Pacific Northwest are characterized by soils that are naturally already acidic or underlain by granitic bedrock; these areas are said to have a low buffering capacity and hence are very sensitive to acid rain. By contrast, most parts of the Midwest, the Great Plains, and portions of the Southwest have predominantly alkaline soils and bedrock of limestone, giving them a high buffering capacity. This fact explains why a state such as Illinois, which is currently experiencing rainfall almost as acid as that falling in New York or New England, is not suffering comparable ecological damage. Nevertheless, such apparent invulnerability is not guaranteed to last forever. Over time, a given soil's buffering capacity can be overwhelmed by continual acid inputs, a phenomenon that seems to be occurring already in parts of the upper Midwest. It seems a cruel twist of fate that prevailing wind currents are transporting acid rain-forming pollutants to precisely those regions that are most sensitive to their harmful effects.

Environmental Effects of Acid Rain

Acid precipitation can cause a number of adverse environmental changes, the best-understood of which include the following.

Damage to aquatic ecosystems. That acid rain can decimate the biotic communities inhabiting lakes, ponds, and streams in those regions where natural buffering capacity is low has been well documented in numerous studies. Most freshwater organisms do best in waters that are slightly alkaline—about pH 8. As lakes gradually become acidified due to steady inputs of acid rain, one aquatic species after another disappears. The first affected are the tiny invertebrates that constitute a vital link in aquatic food chains; at pH 6.0 the freshwater shrimp are eliminated; at pH 5.5 the bacterial decomposers at the lake bottom begin to die off, as do the phytoplankton, the producer organisms in aquatic ecosystems. Fish populations, the subject of most human attention, are somewhat more tolerant to increasing acidity; little change in their numbers is noticed until the pH drops below 5.5. Under pH 4.5 all fish species disappear, as do most frogs, salamanders, and aquatic insects ("Acid Rain," 1982).

Interestingly, falling pH levels seldom kill adult fish directly. The primary cause of fish de-population is acid-induced reproductive failure; pH values below 5.5 can prevent female fish from laying their eggs, and those eggs which are laid frequently fail to hatch or result in the production of deformed fry. (Just as the early developmental stages of humans are the most vulnerable to the adverse influence of environmental contaminants, the same holds true for the larval stages of lower organisms.) Interference with hatching is accentuated by the fact that the most critical developmental period usually coincides with the time of the annual snow melt when several months' accumulation of acid suddenly inundates the spawning areas in one massive dose, a situation known as **shock loading** or **episodic acidification**. This sort of periodic drop in pH, due either to snow melt or heavy downpours, is much more common than chronic acidification of lakes and streams. While the abrupt drop in pH levels during such events is generally of short duration, the ecological impact on young fish or fish eggs can be as devastating as chronic exposure. Large-scale reproductive failure leads to a situation in some lakes where the older fish grow larger and larger, thanks to decreased competition for food, and anglers boast of their excellent catches until, with further increases in acidity, all the fish disappear. As a professor at the University of Toronto succinctly states: "There is no muss, there is no fuss, there is no smell. The fish quietly go extinct . . . They simply fail to reproduce and become less and less abundant, and older and older, until they die out" (Weller, 1980).

At one time it was assumed that acid rain's impact on aquatic environments was limited to freshwater ecosystems. It is now recognized, however, that acid precipitation contributes 30–40% of all the nitrates entering Chesapeake Bay. Studies have shown that these airborne nutrients are as important as farmland fertilizer runoff in stimulating the algal blooms that are degrading water quality in that important saltwater estuary.

Mobilization of toxic metals. Contact with acidified water can cause tightly bound toxic metals such as aluminum, manganese, lead, zinc, mercury, and cadmium to dissolve out of bottom sediments or soils and leach into the aquatic environment. Such metals, especially aluminum, can kill fish by damaging their gills, thereby causing asphyxiation. Acid-induced release of aluminum, even at concentrations as low as 0.2 mg/L, has resulted in fish kills at water pH levels that wouldn't have been lethal in the absence of the toxic metal. Toxic metals in the water also can bioaccumulate in fish tissues, making them dangerous for humans to eat.

Mobilization of poisonous metals also presents a direct threat to human health if the acidified lakes are a source of drinking water supplies. A resort owner from the Adirondacks testified before a congressional committee that, in response to his children's complaints about the taste of water piped to their lodge, he had the water tested and found it contained 5 times the safe level for lead and 10 times that for copper. In other communities, acidified water that was originally free of toxic metals became contaminated upon passing through lead or copper plumbing systems—the low pH of the water caused corrosion of the pipes, resulting in leaching of toxic metals into the water. Homeowners who obtain their drinking water from roof catchments in areas affected by acid rain are also at special risk (Boyle and Boyle, 1983).

Deterioration of buildings, statuary, and metals. While it is extremely difficult to assign a precise monetary value to the impact of acid rain on materials, it is nevertheless acknowledged that the scope of the damage is large indeed. Most pronounced are the effects of acid deposition on stone and metal buildings and statues, on textiles, leather, and paint, and to some extent on paper and glass. Many monuments of great historic and cultural significance are today slowly disintegrating under the impact of airborne pollutants, of which various sulfur compounds are by far the most important. Corroding surfaces of the Statue of Liberty, the Washington Monument, the Capitol Building in Washington, D.C., Canada's Parliament buildings in Ottawa, and the Field Museum in Chicago all give evidence of the ravages produced by acid rain. In India, the Supreme Court ordered nearly 300 coal-burning facilities near Agra to close by the end of 1997 because their SO_2 emissions were severely corroding the beautiful marble façade of the Taj Mahal (Brown et al., 1997). On a more mundane level, EPA estimates that acid rain increases the cost of each new car by $5.00 due to the necessity of using more expensive acid-resistant paint on vehicles sold in regions where acid rain is a problem.

Reduction of crop yields. The extent of acid rain damage to field crops is less clear-cut than with other types of acid-induced environmental damage. Yields of some species appear to be diminished by acid rain, some are stimulated, while others show no change as pH levels of rainfall drop (Cohen, Grothaus, and Perrigan, 1982). In Asia, the increasing acidification of rainfall during the 1990s has been blamed for widespread crop damage. Chinese officials report that approximately 40% of their country's agricultural land is affected by acid precipitation, and the World Bank estimates annual crop and forest losses in China at $5 billion (Brown et al., 1998). In northeastern India, steep reductions in wheat yields in fields downwind of a coal-burning power plant are attributed to acid rain damage (WRI, 1998).

Damage to forest productivity. From the wooded slopes of the Adirondacks to the forests of central Europe and Scandinavia, acid-laden rain and fog are contributing to death and reduced growth rates among an ever-increasing number of important tree species. Most affected are conifer forests at high elevations, frequently shrouded in acid fog or mist. At many sites above 850 meters in the White Mountains of New Hampshire or the Green Mountains of Vermont, over half the red spruce have died since the early 1960s. In Germany, the rate at which wide areas of forest have been similarly affected just since the early 1980s has been so dramatic that distraught German scientists have coined a word for the phenomenon—*waldsterben* ("forest death"). By 1989 German scientists were estimating that more than half the trees in the country were suffering some degree of defoliation. Fortunately, the rate of forest decline in Germany now appears to be slackening, possibly in response to the aggressive pollution control policies enacted specifically for that purpose in 1983. The situation looks less hopeful for Germany's central European neighbors, whose forests are dying at an alarming rate. In the Czech Republic and Poland over a third of all forests are moderately or severely affected (75% of Polish trees show some signs of damage); more than 60% of the conifers in Lithuania are ailing—and the situation is worsening annually. One analysis published in 1990 calculated that three-fourths of European commercial forests were experiencing damage caused by sulfur deposition and 60% were receiving more nitrogen than they could assimilate without harm (WRI, 1992).

Acid rain damage is evident in this forest on Mt. Mitchell in western North Carolina. [© *Will & Deni McIntyre/Corbis*]

The extent to which acid rain can be blamed for the decline of forests on two continents is currently a subject of intensive investigation by scientists in Europe and North America. In some cases acid rain causes direct damage to leaves, resulting in the leaching of nutrients such as calcium from foliage. Such loss in certain evergreen species decreases resistance to foliar freezing and is thought to account for the dieback of large expanses of red spruce in mountain areas of the northeast (Driscoll et al., 2003). This phenomenon is particularly associated with the acid fog that commonly occurs on ridgetops and is further enhanced by the presence of ozone. For the most part, however, it appears that acid rain's role in the forest decline drama is less direct. Acid precipitation increases the solubility and migration of soil-bound aluminum ions, which act as a poison to the delicate root hairs responsible for nutrient uptake. Acid rain also causes the loss of essential plant nutrients—calcium, potassium, magnesium—from forest soils. Calcium depletion in particular is emerging as one of the most significant factors explaining forest decline in eastern North America. An essential element for plant growth, calcium is leached out of forest soils into waterways as precipitation becomes increasingly acidic. Research during the 1990s revealed a marked drop in the calcium content of soils in both the northeastern and southeastern United States since the 1960s—a decline linked to acid rain. This trend is worrisome because calcium loss undermines a tree's ability to resist insect attack, disease, and extreme temperatures. Field investigations have documented a distinct correlation between reduced stress tolerance in ailing red spruce and sugar maple forests to soil calcium deficiencies. Unfortunately, calcium that is leached out of soils by acid precipitation is no longer being replaced at the rate it once was. Studies have shown that rainfall today contains approximately 80% less calcium than it did in the 1950s. As a result, even if the problem of acidification were to vanish overnight, forest recovery would require many decades before the damage is repaired. Researchers working at the Hubbard Brook Experimental Forest in New Hampshire's White Mountains have discovered that the acid-impacted forest essentially stopped growing in 1987, with virtually no new biomass added since that time. Such observations may help to explain why natural ecosystems damaged by past acidification fail to show signs of recovery in spite of recent reductions in acid-rain-forming pollutants (Driscoll et al., 2003; Lawrence and Huntington, 1999; Likens, Driscoll, and Buso, 1996).

Acid Rain Controls

Throughout the 1980s a growing awareness of the extent and severity of the acid rain problem led to increasingly vociferous public demands to "Stop Acid Rain!" through regulatory action, primarily in the form of laws requiring stringent pollution controls on coal-burning power plants. Passage of the 1990 Clean Air Act Amendments, containing the strong acid rain control provisions previously discussed, ended nearly a decade of vituperative debate. The innovative market mechanism devised to make the requirements more financially feasible for the affected utilities permits polluters to choose among numerous options for meeting mandated emission limits (see box 12-4).

Observers of the acid rain saga are in unanimous agreement that the control program mandated by the 1990 Clean Air Act Amendments has been resoundingly successful in meeting the Phase I goal of a 10-million-ton reduction in SO_2 emissions. All 110 power plants targeted under this phase of the program met the EPA deadline for both sulfur and nitrogen oxide reduction. By 2003 the electric power industry had cut its SO_2 emissions by 10.6 million tons—a 38% reduction from 1980 levels—while NO_x emissions were down by 4.2 million tons. The biggest surprise was that these reductions were achieved at a far lower financial cost than even the most optimistic

Box 12-4 "Cap-and-Trade": A Market-Based Approach to Clean Air

No longer are the commodities being bought and sold amidst the pandemonium at the Chicago Board of Trade restricted to such mundane items as soybean futures or pork bellies. Thanks to a novel concept known as **allowance trading** created by the 1990 Clean Air Act Amendments, utility companies can now broker government-assigned allowances for SO_2 emissions in an innovative program that makes acid rain controls more effective and affordable. First proposed by the Environmental Defense Fund, the idea of allowance trading was welcomed by legislators as a way to break congressional gridlock over who should pay for rescuing acid-threatened lakes and forests.

Under the strategy devised by Clean Air Act negotiators, EPA has abandoned the traditional regulatory approach that requires polluters to install controls on each piece of equipment. Instead, the agency has set enforceable limits on the amount of sulfur dioxide that power plants can emit each year and has assigned each plant a designated number of emission "allowances." For each allowance granted, the recipient is permitted to discharge one ton of SO_2 annually (the number of allowances assigned to each facility is determined by a complex formula and is specified in the plant's operating permit). The emission limits imposed on individual plants must collectively correspond with the Clean Air Act's mandated nationwide SO_2 reductions. Utilities can subsequently adopt any pollution reduction strategy they wish in order to achieve the mandated reductions. Such strategies might include installing new pollution control equipment, increased reliance on alternative energy sources, switching to low-sulfur fuel, introducing energy conservation measures, or simply reducing usage. Whatever the means chosen, a plant's annual emissions cannot exceed the allowances allocated to it for that calendar year—*unless the utility purchases surplus allowances at market rates from another plant whose emissions were below the designated limit.*

The beauty of allowance trading is that it encourages polluting facilities not merely to reduce emissions to the legal limit, but to cut them as low as possible, thereby accumulating unused emission allowances that can then be traded with another power plant in the same system, sold to another utility on the open market, or "banked" to cover possible excess emissions in future years. Utilities that choose to install newer, cleaner technologies and make efforts to find the most cost-efficient means of reducing pollutant emissions can help cover the cost of their investment by selling surplus allowances to those facilities—usually older, dirtier plants—for which the cost of installing new equipment substantially exceeds that of purchasing another company's pollution credits. The existence of an allowance-trading mechanism also broadens a plant operator's range of choices. For those considering installation of stack gas scrubbers, for example, the availability of emissions credits obviates the necessity of purchasing expensive backup equipment. Under the old system, such equipment was mandatory for use during the inevitable "down-time" of the principal scrubber. With the allowance trading option, plant officials know that in an emergency they can simply buy emission credits to cover pollution released when a scrubber has to be shut down for repairs. The cost of each credit is, of course, determined by market forces. It was initially expected that the value of an allowance would range between $500–$700, while the EPA-imposed penalty for exceeding allowance allocations is $2,000/ton. This cost differential became even more pronounced when trading officially commenced; in 1993 the price for one allowance averaged just $250 and by the late 1990s had fallen to a bargain-basement price of slightly under $100.

Some critics initially opposed the new program on a philosophical basis, complaining that emissions trading promotes the "right to pollute." Advocates point out, however, that on a nationwide basis the same amount of SO_2 will be removed from the air, thus achieving Clean Air Act goals but at a substantially lower cost than under the traditional "command-and-control" regimen.

During Phase I of the program (1995–2000), allowances were allocated to 374 of the largest-emitting units at 110 power plants; the scope of the program expanded considerably in 2000 as allowance trading entered Phase II, encompassing all power units with greater than 25 megawatts generating capacity—a number totaling approximately 3,000 generating units at more than 700 power plants and representing about 99% of all SO_2 emissions from electric utilities. Allowance allocations also have been tightened under Phase II, with a cap of 8.95 million placed on the number of allowances to be issued annually. In effect, this translates into an 8.95 million ton/year limit on SO_2 emissions, ensuring continued progress in efforts to reduce one of our most troublesome air pollutants.

Ten years after its initiation, the SO_2 allowance-trading program is widely acknowledged as a resounding success, responsible for notable emissions reductions at lower-than-anticipated costs and for a significant drop in acid precipitation throughout the eastern U.S. Experience with the program has been so positive that the concept of "**cap-and-trade**" has been expanded to include market-based efforts to reduce NO_x and mercury (see box 7-3) emissions as well. The NO_x Budget Trading Program, initiated in the late 1990s in eight northeastern states, was expanded in 2004 by 11 additional states and the District of Columbia; portions of two more states were added in 2005, for a total of 21. Unlike the SO_2 program, which operates nationwide and is implemented by the EPA, the NO_x trading program constitutes a partnership between the federal government and participating states. Its focus extends beyond the electric utility industry to encompass large industrial emitters such as pulp and paper mills, oil refineries, and steel plants. Under the NO_x program, states have a fixed limit on emissions and allocate allowances to emitters within their jurisdiction by a variety of methods. As with the federal SO_2 trading program, EPA keeps track of the registries that record allowance transfers, verifies emissions data, and ensures that end-of-year emissions correspond with allowances. The NO_x trading program is now almost as large as that for SO_2 and has met with similar success. The first annual Progress and Compliance Report, issued in 2003, reported that NO_x emissions had dropped 30% below 2002 levels in eight northeastern states and the District of Columbia, more than 99% of the targeted emitters were in full compliance, and market trading had been active. EPA anticipates that when the program is fully implemented, NO_x emissions in the trading area will be down by a million tons and the 100 million Americans who live there will breathe cleaner, healthier air.

The promising debut of allowance trading in the United States has sparked interest abroad, where an ambitious cap-and-trade program for greenhouse gas emissions is in its formative stages. The success of a more flexible free-market approach for meeting air quality objectives at surprisingly low cost guarantees that this new problem-solving strategy will be applied to a growing list of environmental challenges in the years ahead.

References

Kerr, Richard A. 1998. "Acid Rain Control: Success on the Cheap." *Science* 282 (Nov. 6):1024–1027.

Kruger, Joseph A., and William A. Pizer. 2004. "Greenhouse Gas Trading in Europe." *Environment* 46, no. 8 (Oct).

analysts had predicted—approximately $1 billion per year as opposed to the $3–7 billion cited by industry lobbyists fighting enactment of the legislation. Although market-based allowance trading is frequently credited for this remarkable accomplishment, several other factors were equally, if not more, instrumental. The unusual degree of flexibility built into the program made it possible for power plant managers to take advantage of unexpected opportunities to cut emissions in the most cost-effective manner. EPA's "just do it" directive—setting limits but not specifying the means for achieving them—prompted most of the affected utilities to meet the designated goal by switching to relatively cheap low-sulfur coal rather than by installing expensive flue gas desulfurization systems ("scrubbers"). The small percentage that did opt for scrubbers were pleasantly surprised to discover that, due to new, more efficient technology and manufacturers' need to keep the purchase price competitive, the equipment was both cheaper and more reliable than originally expected. Finally, as described in box 12-4, the availability of a market-based pollution credit system gave plant operators additional leeway in choosing the most economical way of getting the job done.

Successful as the current approach has been in measurably reducing the acidity of precipitation, however, there is growing doubt that sensitive ecosystems will recover without the imposition of even more stringent controls. Just as particulate pollutants and ozone-laden smog continue to bedevil regulators, so the problem of acid rain promises to remain a challenge for the foreseeable future (Munton, 1998; Kerr, 1998).

Indoor Air Pollution

While the attention of scientists, citizens, and government regulators has until recently been focused almost exclusively on problems of ambient air pollution, recent studies suggest that more serious air quality threats lurk much closer to home. It is now apparent that contaminants within private dwellings may pose a greater risk to human health than do outdoor air pollutants. In fact, with the exception of ozone and sulfur dioxide, all the air pollutants regulated under U.S. laws occur at higher concentrations indoors than out, prompting the EPA to rank indoor air pollution among the top five environmental risks to public health. This is particularly troubling because the majority of people spend more of their time indoors than outside; thus their exposure to indoor air pollutants is nearly continuous. Such pollutants pose a special threat to the very young, the ill, and the elderly—those most susceptible and also the ones most likely to spend long periods of time inside. Justifiable concerns about energy conservation may have worsened the indoor air pollution problem because thick insulation, triple-glazed windows, and magnetically sealed doors greatly reduce air exchange with the outside, effectively retaining and accumulating contaminants inside the home.

While most people tend to equate the risk of harm they might suffer from toxic pollutants to the total amount and toxicity of such substances, in fact the main determinant of danger is the dose actually received by the individual. Thus, large amounts of toxic pollutants such as benzene, formaldehyde, or carbon monoxide, for example, when emitted from a factory smokestack or the tailpipe of a car, pose minimal risk to the average citizen because they break down or are diluted in concentration before individuals are directly exposed to them. By contrast, much smaller amounts of the same chemicals, released in close proximity to people inside their homes or offices, have a quick, direct route into the body and hence pose a much greater overall risk of health damage. Studies demonstrate that personal exposures and concentrations of indoor air pollutants exceed those occurring outdoors for all of the 15 most prevalent chemicals studied (Wallace, 1987). In addition, peak pollutant concentrations, as well as overall averages, are generally higher indoors than in the ambient air.

Some of the more common air pollutants known to be present in the home environment include the following.

Radon Gas

When Stanley Watras started radiation-detection alarms ringing at the Limerick nuclear power plant near Philadelphia one December morning in 1984, he didn't realize that he was about to become a national celebrity, alerting Americans to a hitherto unsuspected menace within their own homes. The radioactive contamination that was detected by Watras when he arrived for work that morning had obviously come from outside the nuclear facility, so Watras requested Philadelphia Electric, the utility company that owned the plant, to check his home in Colebrookdale Township. To everyone's amazement, tests revealed that the Watras home had levels of radon gas approximately 1,000 times higher than normal. Investigators estimated that Watras, his wife, and two young sons were receiving radiation exposure equivalent to 455,000 chest X-rays a year simply by living in their house. As officials of Pennsylvania's Division of Environmental Radiation hastened to determine the extent of the indoor radon threat, it quickly became apparent that the Watras family was not alone in its predicament. Throughout sections of eastern Pennsylvania, New Jersey, and New York, underlain by a uranium-rich geological formation known as the Reading Prong, thousands of homes exhibit elevated levels of radon. Nor is the problem limited to a few mid-Atlantic states. EPA surveys reveal that indoor radon contamination problems span the country and agency officials, as well as the U.S. Surgeon General, urge that all homes be tested for the radioactive gas that is now widely recognized as a serious health hazard.

Radon originates from the natural radioactive decay of uranium. It is present in high concentrations in certain types of soil and rocks (e.g., granite, shale, phosphate, pitchblende), but most soils contain amounts high enough to pose a potential health hazard. Radon dilutes to harmless concentrations in the open air, but when it enters the confined space inside a structure it can accumulate to potentially hazardous levels. Since radon is a gas, it readily moves upward through the soil; small differences in air pressure between indoors and outdoors (very slight negative air pressure inside a heated building results from the "stack effect," created by air's tendency to rise whenever it is warmer than the surrounding atmosphere) cause the gas to seep into homes through dirt floors or crawl spaces, through cracks in cement floors and walls, through floor drains, sump holes, joints, or pores in cinder-block walls. Occasionally, radon gets into well water supplies and enters homes when water is used, particularly for showers or baths. Radon is dangerous because it is radioactive, undergoing decay to produce a series of "radon daughters," the most troublesome of which are alpha-emitters polonium-218 and 214. These can be inhaled and deposited in the lungs where they constitute an internal source of alpha radiation exposure, increasing the risk of lung cancer. Radon's contribution to overall human exposure to ionizing radiation is considerable. The National Council on Radiation Protection and Measurement estimates that the average individual receives fully 55% of his or her yearly dose of ionizing radiation from radon inside homes. The health consequences of such exposure, according to EPA's updated "best estimate," is an annual lung cancer death toll of 21,000—a number that would make radon the second-leading cause of lung cancer deaths in the United States, behind cigarette smoking. In some parts of the country where radon levels are unusually high, hundreds of thousands of Americans are receiving as much radiation exposure from radon in their homes as that received by the Ukrainian citizens who lived near Chernobyl at the time of the nuclear accident there in 1986. An individual's chances of developing radon-induced lung cancer depend on radon concentrations inside the home and the length of time one is exposed. It is thought that long-term exposure to slightly elevated levels of radon poses a greater cancer threat that does short-term exposure to much higher levels. Cigarette smoking has a synergistic effect in enhancing the radon/lung cancer risk by a factor of 10.

Until the 1980s, radon was regarded as a health hazard only to uranium miners, so estimates of risk to residents of radon-contaminated homes have simply been extrapolated from standards set for occupational exposure in the mines. Indoor radon concentrations are measured as the number of picocuries of radiation per liter of air (pCi/L). Outdoors, radon concentrations in the ambient air typically measure about 0.4 pCi/L, while the average indoor level approximates 1.3 pCi/L. Acknowledging

Figure 12-1   EPA Map of Radon Zones

- Zone 1 counties have a predicted average indoor radon screening level greater than 4 pCi/L (picocuries per liter)

- Zone 2 counties have a predicted average indoor radon screening level between 2 and 4 pCi/L

- Zone 3 counties have a predicted average indoor radon screening level less than 2 pCi/L

LEGEND
Zone 1
Zone 2
Zone 3

Guam

Source: EPA, http://www.epa.gov/radon/zonemap.html

that *any* amount of exposure to ionizing radiation entails *some* degree of risk, for practical reasons EPA regards 4 pCi/L as the **action level**—the point at or above which homeowners are advised to take some kind of remedial action. It is estimated that about 6% of homes in the U.S. exceed this action level, the vast majority of them located in geographical regions where the soil and rocks have a high uranium content (Goldstein and Goldstein, 2002). Readings above 20 pCi/L are considered cause for serious concern and may require significant abatement measures (as a basis for comparison, radon levels in the Watras home measured 2,700 pCi/L).

Since it is impossible to predict with certainty which structures are likely to have elevated radon levels (some homes in the Watras neighborhood were essentially radon-free), the need for radon reduction measures can only be determined by actual measurements, which often can be done by the homeowner with relatively inexpensive devices (see box 12-5). If test results indicate the need for some sort of radon remediation efforts, a variety of options are available. Most require the services of a professional contractor, though some can be as simple as covering sump holes or improving ventilation. More extensive—and expensive—possibilities include installing fans or air-to-air heat exchangers to replace radon-contaminated indoor air with outdoor air; covering any exposed earth inside homes with concrete, gas-proof liner, or sheet metal; sealing all cracks and openings with mortar, polyurethane sealants, or other impermeable materials; installing a drain tile suction system around the outer foundation walls of a house; or by installing a series of exhaust pipes inside hollow-block basement walls or baseboard to draw radon out of the voids within such walls before it can enter the living space. In structures with significantly elevated levels of radon, it may be necessary to utilize several methods to achieve sufficient reductions. For people planning to build a new home in areas with known radon problems, use of radon-resistant construction techniques is far more cost-effective than installing a radon reduction system after the fact.

Products of Combustion

Carbon monoxide, nitrogen oxides, and particulates can reach very high levels inside homes where gas stoves or other gas appliances are used, where kerosene heaters or wood-burning stoves are operating, where auto emissions from a garage can enter the house, or where there are cigarette smokers. In homes with gas ranges, for example, nitrogen oxide levels are frequently twice as high as those outdoors. Carbon monoxide emissions from wood, coal, or gas stoves often exceed Clean Air Act standards for outside air. The growing popularity of wood-burning stoves is a particular cause for concern, since wood is a much dirtier fuel than either oil or gas. Wood smoke contains approximately 100 different chemicals, at least 14 of which are the same carcinogens found in cigarette smoke.

Cigarette smoking (the by-product of which is now referred to technically as **ETS** or "Environmental Tobacco Smoke") may constitute the most significant source of indoor air pollution in many homes; particulate levels may go as high as 700 micrograms/m^3, far above the primary ambient air quality standard of 50, when there are smokers in a house. A study conducted by researchers at Harvard University found that household tobacco smoke is the main source of exposure to particulate pollutants for most children. It also demonstrated that whereas typical particulate levels in a home without smokers is 10–20 micrograms/m^3, each smoker contributes an additional 25–30 micrograms/m^3, more than doubling the base level amount (Ware et al., 1984). That parental smoking could be considered another form of child abuse has been amply documented in numerous studies. EPA reports that children exposed to environmental tobacco smoke are at increased risk for lower respiratory tract infec-

Figure 12-2

Points Where Radon Can Enter Homes

Top row of block

Joint between floor and walls

Openings around pipes

Crack in floor

Cracks in wall

Radon Reduction Methods

Outside fan draws radon away from house

Sealant

Sheet metal covers exposed area

Sealant

Sump

Box 12-5   Assessing Home Radon Risk

Radon detection businesses have proliferated rapidly following EPA's announcement advising that homes nationwide be tested for the presence of this apparently ubiquitous indoor air pollutant. Since 1985, millions of homeowners have heeded the agency's advice, but many others have yet to follow through, deterred by the hefty fee charged by many professionals offering radon-monitoring services. Such individuals should be heartened to learn that they can purchase relatively inexpensive devices that will give a reasonably accurate indication of the extent of radon problems in the user's home.

The two most popular do-it-yourself home radon detectors are (1) short-term tests using charcoal canisters—small containers of activated charcoal that should be opened and left in place for three to seven days, then sealed and returned to the manufacturer for analysis and (2) longer-term alpha track detectors that are left in place for several weeks to as long as one year. Since radon levels can fluctuate considerably from day to day and season to season, alpha track detectors are good for determining yearly averages; charcoal canisters are useful for short-term screening tests, but since their results are indicative only of radon levels during the few days when the test was performed, they may over- or under-represent the actual extent of hazard. Both devices, however, can be effectively used by nonprofessionals to give a rough approximation of radon pollution. If laboratory analysis reveals that radon levels are high, consultation with a radon abatement specialist would be advisable, but if the screening test indicates negligible amounts of the gas, the homeowner is saved the expense of contracting for a radon survey that might cost several hundred dollars.

Those interested in doing their own radon monitoring can improve the accuracy and relevance of the results by understanding a few basic concepts about radon. Because radon infiltrates into homes through the ground, basements are likely to exhibit the highest radon levels. For this reason, if residents want to know the peak concentrations to which they may be exposed, a monitoring device should be located in the basement (or lowest level of the dwell-

ing), placed about 3–6 feet above the floor and away from walls, doors, or windows. However, if occupants spend little time in the basement and want a measurement more representative of the exposure they are receiving, monitors can be placed in living areas of the next highest floor. Another likely spot for monitor placement is near suspected sources of radon entry, such as sump holes or crawl spaces (however, don't use charcoal canisters in humid environments such as bathrooms and kitchens; the charcoal absorbs moisture and test results will not be accurate). All windows and outside doors should be closed at least 12 hours before beginning the test; avoid conducting short-term tests during periods of severe storms or strong winds. Since monitoring devices are relatively inexpensive, it may be advisable to use two or three simultaneously in different areas of the house. Radon concentrations in most states tend to be highest in winter, so this is the best time for using short-term monitoring devices.

Home radon detectors are available for purchase online, at hardware stores, supermarkets, or other retail establishments; local public health departments may also be a source of monitoring devices or information on where they can be obtained. Until October 1998, manufacturers could voluntarily submit their products to EPA for evaluation; that program has since been terminated, so any "EPA-Approved" designation on products or services currently on the market is no longer valid.

In situations where preliminary monitoring indicates a need for radon mitigation (i.e., where the radon level measures 4 pCi/L or higher), homeowners would be well advised to consult a remediation professional. Currently two private groups—the National Environmental Health Association (NEHA) and the National Radon Safety Board (NRSB)—offer accreditation/certification for radon testing and mitigation. Anyone planning to contract for radon-related work in a state where licensing of radon professionals is not required by law should first inquire whether the contractor in question has met the certification requirements of one of these organizations.

tions, bronchitis, and pneumonia, with those under 18 months of age more susceptible than older children. Fluid in the middle ear, wheezing, and asthma all occur more frequently among children whose parents smoke. Medical researchers have demonstrated that asthmatic children exposed to significant levels of secondhand smoke suffer 70–80% more attacks than children subjected to little or no such exposure. A significantly greater number of children whose mothers smoke are hospitalized for respiratory conditions than are children of nonsmoking mothers and asthmatic children often experience marked improvement when their parents quit smoking.

Particulates are but one of several indoor air pollutants generated by smokers; carbon monoxide is another, as is benzene, a known carcinogen and a listed toxic air pollutant. Researchers calculate that fully 45% of Americans' total exposure to benzene comes from inhaling tobacco smoke, while a mere 3% is due to industrial emissions (Ott and Roberts, 1998). Such findings have provided scientific justification for the proliferation of smoking bans in restaurants and other public facilities. Even in the absence of enforceable federal standards, ETS has become a socially unacceptable indoor air pollutant.

Formaldehyde

Known to cause skin and respiratory irritation, formaldehyde is now suspected of being carcinogenic as well. A wide variety of household products contain formaldehyde, most notably particleboard, plywood, and some floor coverings and textiles. Levels of formaldehyde are particularly likely to be high in mobile homes, where residents frequently complain of rashes, respiratory irritation, nausea, headaches, dizziness, lethargy, or aggravation of bronchial asthma. Within the same home, formaldehyde levels can fluctuate dramatically, depending on environmental conditions. A 15°F increase in temperature can result in a doubling of formaldehyde levels, while the lowest formaldehyde concentrations have been recorded on cold winter days; similarly, increases in relative humidity cause a corresponding rise in formaldehyde emissions. In terms of its effect as an irritant, there does not appear to be a threshold level for formaldehyde exposure, though few people experience symptoms when concentrations are below 0.1 ppm.

The National Academy of Sciences estimates that as many as 10–20% of the population experiences some form of irritation due to formaldehyde exposure even at very low concentrations. Since formaldehyde is so ubiquitous in the modern environment, avoiding exposure entirely is almost impossible. Nevertheless, sensitive individuals can reduce exposure and thereby minimize symptoms by substituting metal or lumber products for those containing pressed wood or selectively purchasing low formaldehyde-releasing pressed wood construction materials, cabinets, or furniture. Similarly, those allergic to the chemical should always launder permanent-press fabrics prior to use to remove the formaldehyde finish, since a single wash can reduce textile formaldehyde emissions up to 60% (unfortunately, this approach won't work for draperies, which also are large formaldehyde emitters).

Chemical Fumes and Particles

Numerous household products (including furniture polish, hair sprays, air fresheners, oven-cleaners, paints, carpeting, pesticides, disinfectants, solvents, etc.), release chemical fumes and particles that can reach very high levels indoors. While relatively little research has been done on the health impact of inhaling these substances on a regular basis, it is known that several commonly used household chemicals cause cancer in laboratory animals. Paradichlorobenzene, the active ingredient in moth crystals

Box 12-6 Smoky Kitchens = Sick Cooks

Aside from the occasional finger nicked with a paring knife, meal preparation isn't regarded as a particularly hazardous occupation by those of us living in the industrialized world. Nevertheless, in over 100 countries where firewood, animal dung, charcoal, crop residues, or coal constitute the main domestic fuel source, the simple task of cooking dinner is undermining the health of millions of women and their children every year. The World Health Organization (WHO) ranks indoor air pollution as one of the four most critical environmental problems in developing countries, responsible for 1.6 million deaths annually. Stoking fires and stirring pots in the close confines of small, poorly ventilated kitchens, housewives throughout the Third World daily work in a smoke-laden environment with direct exposure to toxic emissions. As a result, they and the small children who spend most of their time close to mother are falling ill and often dying from diseases provoked by indoor air pollution.

Of the various ailments associated with cookstove emissions, acute respiratory infections affect the largest number of people, with infants and toddlers the most frequent victims. Studies of Zulu children in South Africa found that youngsters living in homes with wood cookstoves were five times more likely to be hospitalized with severe respiratory infections. In Nepal, a significant correlation was found between the incidence of moderate to severe respiratory infections among 2-year-olds and the number of hours they spent near a fire. In Gambia, researchers found that babies whose mothers carried them on their backs while cooking over an open wood fire inside a smoky hut were six times more likely to contract acute respiratory infections than were children not exposed to wood smoke. Adult women experiencing long-term smoke exposure are themselves at high risk of developing chronic lung diseases such as emphysema, bronchitis, and asthma. A study conducted in Mexico among women who had been exposed to wood smoke for many years found their risk of lung disease was equivalent to that of heavy smokers and 75 times that of women not exposed. Cancer is another

health threat associated with this form of indoor air pollution, as are reproductive problems such as stillbirths, low-birth-weight babies, and difficulties during delivery for women who inhale cookstove emissions during pregnancy.

The types of pollutants emitted from cookstoves vary, depending on the type of fuel burned. Biomass fuels—wood, charcoal, crop residues, animal dung—are the dirtiest. Used by over two billion of the world's poorest people, wood and other biofuels emit levels of carbon monoxide, benzene, and particulate matter many times higher than WHO limits and significantly add to the haze of pollution blanketing virtually every developing world city today.

Coal, though considered a step up the energy ladder from biofuels in terms of pollutant emissions, is nevertheless a dirty fuel as well, emitting prodigious amounts of $PM_{2.5}$, the most dangerous form of particulate matter. In China, where close to 400 million people rely on coal as their chief domestic fuel, the problem of indoor air pollution has assumed major proportions in both rural and urban areas. The coal used in Chinese cookstoves is, for the most part, mined from deposits containing excessive traces of toxic elements such as arsenic, mercury, fluorine, and antimony. Used directly without washing, these coals release toxic emissions when burned.

The situation is made worse in some parts of China by the practice of drying certain agricultural products, such as chili peppers and corn, directly over coal fires. Doing so results in volatilized toxic metals concentrating in the dried foods. In China's southwestern Guizhou Province, several thousand people suffer from chronic arsenic poisoning due to eating arsenic-contaminated dried chilies (while fresh chili peppers contain less than 1 ppm arsenic, those dried over high-arsenic coal fires have levels that exceed 500 ppm). An estimated 10 million Chinese are experiencing bone deformities and dental fluorosis due to fluoride contamination of foods dried over dirty coal fires. Millions of Chinese homemakers are affected by volatile organic compounds released by coal-burning cookstoves. Polycyclic aromatic hydrocarbons (PAHs) from unvented coal stoves are believed to be the main cause for the high incidence of lung cancer in China. In homes where smoky coal is burned, the lung cancer death rate is five times above the national average. Studies conducted in China by EPA researchers found a strong association between lung cancer incidence in women and the length of time they had spent cooking indoors. Blood samples taken from the women, along with indoor air analyses, demonstrated that indoor coal-burning was to blame for the observed cancers.

The solution to these problems is perfectly straightforward: replace wood and coal-burning stoves with those fueled by solar panels, natural gas, or electricity. Even liquid fuels such as kerosene and liquefied petroleum gas (LPG) would be far preferable to the dirty fuels so widely used today. Unfortunately, a rapid changeover is scarcely conceivable, given the widespread poverty in the countries affected and the sheer numbers of households still dependent on biofuels or coal. In the short term, efforts to improve the health of women and children sickened by poor indoor air quality have focused on designing a better cookstove. Over the past two decades nearly 200 projects have been launched throughout the Third World to develop appropriate cookstove technologies using locally available materials to produce improved stoves at a price poor people can afford. While the main intent has been to enhance the energy efficiency of the stoves rather than improving indoor air quality, many of the newer models that use a flue or chimney to remove smoke from the house have succeeded in substantially reducing pollutants as well (unfortunately, by diverting smoky emissions from inside to outside the house, improved cookstoves have worsened neighborhood air quality problems).

Despite notable progress in some countries to advance the use of cleaner fuels, for many of the world's poorest people, any change in current conditions remains but a distant hope. National governments could, if they desired to do so, help speed up the transition by adopting policies to reduce the cost of new stoves or to subsidize the cost of service connections for electricity. Differen-tial electricity charges could be very beneficial as well; in Thailand, poor urban households that use very little electricity are charged lower rates than better-off consumers who use more. As a result, virtually all urban Thai homes are electrified. Unfortunately, in the developing world, as elsewhere, indoor air pollution—despite its enormous health costs—receives scant attention in comparison with outdoor air quality problems.

In 2002, the Global Partnership for Clean Indoor Air was launched at the UN-sponsored World Summit on Sustainable Development in Johannesburg, inspiring a growing number of individuals and organizations to develop new, affordable technologies for less-polluting cookstoves and fuels. In support of this effort, EPA announced in October 2004 that it had awarded $1.3 million in grants to fund 11 pilot projects in Asia, Africa, and Latin America. Among the activities the agency is funding are the production and sale of 2,000 solar panel ovens in Mexico; the introduction of a methanol stove-fuel cooking system in Nigeria; promotion of more efficient wood-burning stoves in a Honduran city; and the introduction of biogas technology in a rural area of western India. Although the grants are limited in scope, EPA is convinced they will reduce pollution exposure of 160,000 people within the project areas and, equally important, will significantly increase awareness among the wider population regarding the serious health threat posed by indoor air pollution and the benefits of adopting improved cookstove technologies.

References

Finkelman, R. B. et al. 1999. "Health Impacts of Domestic Coal Use in China." *Proceedings of the National Academy of Sciences* 96 (March):3427–3431.

Saksena, Sumeet, and Kirk R. Smith. 2003. "Indoor Air Pollution." In *Air Pollution & Health in Rapidly Developing Countries*, edited by Gordon McGranahan and Frank Murray. Earthscan Publications.

World Resources Institute. 1998. *World Resources 1998–99: Environmental Change and Human Health*. New York: Oxford Univ. Press.

Figure 12-3   Deaths Attributable to Solid Fuel Use

Source: World Health Organization Programme on Indoor Air Pollution.

and many air fresheners and room deodorants, as well as limonene, another odorant, present perhaps the highest cancer risk among indoor organic chemicals. Tetrachloro-ethylene, a solvent used in dry cleaning, is another carcinogen to which household residents may receive significant exposure when wearing freshly dry-cleaned garments or by breathing emissions from closets in which such articles were stored (Smith, 1988).

When used in accordance with instructions, most household chemicals are not known to provoke acute health effects. However, use of pesticides inside homes has occasionally resulted in a wide range of health complaints, including headaches, nausea, vertigo, skin rashes, and emotional disorders. Chlordane, which for almost 40 years was the most widely used insecticide for controlling termites, was taken off the market in 1988 in response to hundreds of complaints about alleged chlordane-induced illnesses among residents following pesticidal applications in homes. Inappropriate pesticide use inside homes can result in long-term exposure to toxic residues and vapors. Chemicals that break down quickly outdoors in the presence of sunlight and bacteria can persist for years in carpets, presenting an ongoing threat to residents (Ott and Roberts, 1998).

Biological Pollutants

A diverse group of living organisms, most of them too small to be seen with the naked eye, also can pose serious indoor air quality problems. Bacteria and fungal spores can enter structures via air-handling systems and occasionally cause disease outbreaks (the Legionnaires' Disease episode in Philadelphia in 1976 is the classic example of this). Many allergies are associated with exposure to household dust that may contain fungal spores, bacteria, animal dander, and feces of roaches or mites.

Perhaps most significant in stimulating allergic reactions are live dust mites, tiny arthropods less than 1 millimeter in size that are found in enormous numbers on bedsheets and blankets where they feed on sloughed-off scales of skin. Humid conditions or the presence of stagnant water seem to favor buildup of large populations of these unwanted guests and their dissemination has sometimes been associated with the use of humidifiers or vaporizers that harbored fungal or bacterial growth. Flooding problems or other water damage to homes can result in an indoor air quality problem that was largely unrecognized until the mid-1990s. Growth of the toxin-producing mold, *Stachybotrys chartarum*, on damp wallpaper, ceiling tiles, carpeting made of natural fibers, cardboard boxes, bundles of newspapers, and, especially, the paper covering sheetrock can cause serious illness among residents of affected structures. Symptoms can include headaches, respiratory distress, recurring colds, heart palpitations, fatigue, skin rashes, and general malaise. Detecting the presence of *S. chartarum* requires careful inspection of areas that may not be readily visible—in wall voids, above false ceilings, in basements—any place where leaks, condensation, or sustained flooding could occur. The fungal mass is black in appearance, slightly shiny when fresh and powdery when dry. Although the mold won't continue to grow once it dries out, spores can be sucked up by the furnace fan and spread throughout a dwelling. If mold growth is found in a structure, the situation requires prompt action, first to correct the water problem and then to clean up the mold. The latter step usually requires professional help, since householders are not advised to tackle any mold-contaminated area larger than two square feet. The surface of small areas can be disinfected using 1 cup of chlorine bleach in a gallon of water (rubber gloves and a dust mask should be worn while working). However, the fungal mycelium within the contaminated material often sur-

Extensive mold growth on the ceiling and walls of this room represents a significant health threat to the home's occupants. [*EPA*]

vives surface disinfection and may subsequently resume growth. Thus most experts advise that while smooth, hard-surface materials such as ceramic tile, glass, or metal can be effectively cleaned and salvaged, it is virtually impossible to remove all fungal contamination from soft porous materials like paper, textiles, cellulose ceiling tiles, or paper-covered gypsum board; if these types of materials sustain water damage, they should, in most cases, be discarded and replaced (Nelson, 1999; IOM, 2004).

Sick Building Syndrome

Some indoor air pollutants can provoke complaints among building occupants of problems such as chest tightness, muscle aches, cough, fever, and chills. These symptoms of what is now termed **building related illness (BRI)** may persist for an extended time period after affected people leave the building, but they have clearly identifiable causes and can be clinically diagnosed. By contrast, a somewhat more mysterious malady reported with increased frequency since the mid-1970s is a condition described as **sick building syndrome (SBS).** SBS refers to situations where building occupants experience various forms of acute discomfort—eye irritation, scratchiness in the throat, dry cough, headache, itchy skin, fatigue, difficulty in concentrating, nausea and dizziness—but no causative agent can be found. Furthermore, these symptoms generally vanish soon after sufferers leave the building (sometimes the complaints are associated with only one part of the building or even with a single room).

This situation has become so widespread in recent years that a committee of the World Health Organization has suggested that as many as 30% of the world's new and remodeled buildings may be generating complaints. While some of the symptoms reported may, in fact, be caused by illnesses contracted somewhere else, by preexisting allergies, or by job-related stress, in many cases poor indoor air quality is the major culprit. Although some of the reported outbreaks of sick building syndrome are eventually traced to specific pollutants—e.g., microorganisms spread through ventilation systems, vehicle exhausts entering intake vents, ozone emissions from photocopying machines, VOCs outgassing from new carpeting—in most cases these contaminants aren't present in concentrations high enough to provoke the reported symptoms. Synthetic mineral fibers released into the air from acoustical ceiling tile and insulating material have been identified by researchers at Cornell University as the prime cause of many SBS situations. Most often, however, SBS has been traced to inadequate ventilation and its rise in frequency parallels efforts since the 1973 Arab oil embargo to incorporate energy conservation features into building design.

Unlike the situation in homes, most new nonresidential structures are equipped with mechanical heating, ventilation, and air conditioning (HVAC) systems and feature windows tightly sealed to restrict air infiltration from outside. These HVAC systems recirculate air throughout the building, with a significant portion of the air being reused several times prior to being exhausted, the purpose of such reuse being to lessen energy costs for heating or cooling incoming fresh air. Building codes require that a specified minimum amount of outside air be provided in order to establish an acceptable balance between oxygen and CO_2 indoors, to dilute odors, and to remove contaminants generated within the structure. Prior to 1973 that specified minimum was approximately 15 cubic feet per minute (cfm) per building occupant; after 1973 the standard was reduced to just 5 cfm, an amount which, in a number of situations, proved inadequate for maintaining healthy, comfortable conditions. In some situations HVAC systems were improperly installed, had defective equipment, or functioned poorly because of improper vent placement. When errors such as these occur, an insufficient amount of ventilation air will be supplied. Once such problems are identified, they can generally be corrected by repairing or adjusting the air-handling system to provide additional outside air; in some cases, however, building design itself may be at fault, requiring much more extensive renovations (Turiel, 1985; Beek, 1994).

In general, the public has been slow to demand action on this problem because access to information about indoor air pollutants has been very limited and possibly because people don't want to believe that pollution problems have invaded the home. Nevertheless, an increasing awareness of the threat posed by indoor air pollutants has stimulated thinking on new ways to deal with this problem. Monitoring and enforcing air quality standards inside millions of American homes is obviously impossible. However, standards could be set to control pollutant emissions by modifying product design or manufacture. For example, the United States and a number of other countries have set standards regulating emissions of formaldehyde from plywood. In the future, updated building codes that incorporate design features and materials which minimize release and retention of indoor air pollutants could ensure that most new structures have acceptable air quality. In the meantime, efforts must be made to educate homeowners and occupants on the impact personal behavior and consumer choices can have on the quality of the indoor environment. Decisions as to which products we buy, how we use certain appliances, our consideration for the health of others as reflected in personal smoking habits—all have a profound impact on indoor air quality.

References

Acid Rain: What It Is. 1982. National Wildlife Federation.

Air Pollution Primer. 1969. National Tuberculosis and Respiratory Disease Association.

Beek, Jim. 1994. "Man-Made Minerals Could Be Key to SBS." *Indoor Air Review* 3, no. 11 (Jan).

Bell, Michelle L., Aidan McDermott, Scott Zeger, Jonathan M. Samet, and Francesca Dominici. 2004. "Ozone and Short-term Mortality in 95 U.S. Urban Communities, 1987–2000." *The Journal of the American Medical Association* 292, no. 19 (Nov 17).

Boyle, Robert, and R. Alexander Boyle. 1983. *Acid Rain.* Schocken Books/Nick Lyons Books.

Brown, Lester R., Michael Renner, and Christopher Flavin. 1998. *Vital Signs 1998.* New York: Worldwatch Institute/W. W. Norton.

———. 1997. *Vital Signs 1997.* New York: Worldwatch Institute/W. W. Norton.

Bryner, Gary C. 1993. *Blue Skies, Green Politics: The Clean Air Act of 1990.* CQ Press.

Cohen, C. J., L. C. Grothaus, and S. C. Perrigan. 1982. "Effects of Simulated Sulfuric and Sulfuric-Nitric Acid Rain on Crop Plants: Results of 1980 Crop Survey." *Special Report* 670, Agricultural Experiment Station, Oregon State University, Corvallis.

Dockery, Douglas W. et al. 1993. "An Association Between Air Pollution and Mortality in Six U.S. Cities." *The New England Journal of Medicine* 329, no. 24 (Dec. 9).

Driscoll, Charles, David Whitall, John Aber, Elizabeth Boyer, Mark Castro, Christopher Cronan, Christine Goodale, Peter Groffman, Charles Hopkinson, Kathleen Lambert, Gregory Lawrence, and Scott Ollinger. 2003. "Nitrogen Pollution: Sources and Consequences in the U.S. Northeast." *Environment* 45, no. 7 (Sept).

"Easy Guide to the Air Toxics Law." 1993. *The Environmental Manager's Compliance Advisor,* no. 344 (Feb. 1).

Environmental Law Handbook. 12th ed. 1993. Government Institutes, Inc.

Environmental Protection Agency (EPA). 2001. *National Air Quality Emissions Trends, 1990–1999.* Office of Air Quality Planning and Standards (March).

Evelyn, John. 1661. *Fumifugium.* London National Society for Clean Air, reprinted 1969.

Goldstein, Inge F., and Martin Goldstein. 2002. *How Much Risk? A Guide to Understanding Environmental Health Hazards.* New York: Oxford Univ. Press.

Health Effects of Air Pollution. 1978. American Thoracic Society.

Hilchey, Tim. 1993. "Government Survey Finds Decline in Building Block of Acid Rain." *New York Times,* Sept. 7.

Institutes of Medicine (IOM) of the National Academies. 2004. *Damp Indoor Spaces and Health.* Washington, DC: National Academy Press.

Kerr, Richard A. 1998. "Acid Rain Control: Success on the Cheap." *Science* 282 (Nov. 6):1024–1027.

Lawrence, Gregory B., and T. G. Huntington. 1999. *Soil Calcium Depletion Linked to Acid Rain and Forest Growth in the Eastern United States.* U.S. Geological Survey, WRIR 98–4267 (Feb).

Likens, G. E., C. T. Driscoll, and D.C. Buso. 1996. "Long-Term Effects of Acid Rain: Response and Recovery of a Forest Ecosystem." *Science* 272, no. 5259 (April 16):244–246.

McDonald, Alan. 1999. "Combating Acid Deposition and Climate Change: Priorities for Asia." *Environment* 41, no. 3 (April): 4–11, 34–41.

Munton, Don. 1998. "Dispelling the Myths of the Acid Rain Story." *Environment* 40, no. 6 (July/Aug):4–7, 27–34.

Nelson, Berlin. 1999. *Stachybotrys chartarum: The Toxic Indoor Mold.* American Phytopathological Society, APSnet Feature (Feb).

Ott, Wayne R., and John W. Roberts. 1998. "Everyday Exposure to Toxic Pollutants." *Scientific American* (Feb):86–91.

Plotkin, Steven. 2004. "Is Bigger Better? Moving Toward a Dispassionate View of SUVs." *Environment* 46, no. 9 (Nov).

Pope, C. A., R. T. Burnett, M. J. Thun, E. Calle, D. Krewski, K. Ito, and G. D. Thurston. 2002. "Lung Cancer, Cardiopulmonary Mortality, and Long-Term Exposure to Fine Particulate Air Pollution." *Journal of the American Medical Association* 287, no. 9 (March 6).

Rhodes, S. L., and P. Middleton. 1983. "The Complex Challenge of Controlling Acid Rain." *Environment* 22, no. 4 (May).

Romieu, Isabelle, and Mauricio Hernandez-Avila. 2003. "Air Pollution and Health in Developing Countries: A Review of Epidemiological Evidence." In *Air Pollution & Health in Rapidly Developing Countries,* edited by Gordon McGranahan and Frank Murray. Earthscan Publications.

Saksena, Sumeet, and Kirk R. Smith. 2003. "Indoor Air Pollution." In *Air Pollution & Health in Rapidly Developing Countries,* edited by Gordon McGranahan and Frank Murray. Earthscan Publications.

Schwartz, J. 2000. "Fine Particulate Air Pollution: Smoke and Mirrors of the '90s or Hazard of the New Millennium?" Presentation at annual meeting of the American Public Health Association, Boston (Nov. 14).

Smith, Kirk R. 1988. "Air Pollution: Assessing Total Exposure in the United States." *Environment* 30, no. 8 (Oct).

Turiel, Isaac. 1985. *Indoor Air Quality and Human Health.* Palo Alto, CA: Stanford Univ. Press.

Waldbott, George L. 1978. *Health Effects of Environmental Pollutants.* St. Louis: C. V. Mosby.

Wallace, L. A. 1987. *Total Exposure Assessment Methodology* (TEAM Study: Summary and Analysis) 1, Washington, DC: Environmental Protection Agency.

Walsh, Michael P. 2003. "Vehicle Emissions and Health in Developing Countries." In *Air Pollution & Health in Rapidly Developing Countries,* edited by Gordon McGranahan and Frank Murray. Earthscan Publications.

Ware, J. H. et al. 1984. "Passive Smoking, Gas Cooking, and Respiratory Health of Children Living in Six Cities." *American Review of Respiratory Disease* 129:366–374.

Weller, Phil. 1980. *Acid Rain: The Silent Crisis.* Between the Lines & the Waterloo Public Interest Research Group.

World Resources Institute (WRI). 1998. *World Resources 1998–99.* New York: Oxford Univ. Press.

———. 1996. *World Resources 1996–97.* New York: Oxford Univ. Press.

———. 1992. *World Resources 1992–93.* New York: Oxford Univ. Press.

NOISE POLLUTION

> **Noise**, *n*. A stench in the ear. . . . The chief product and authenticating sign of civilization.
>
> —Devil's Dictionary (1911)

An ever-increasing cacophony of sound is today grudgingly accepted as an inescapable component of the modern urban environment. From the traffic-clogged streets of New York and Paris to the bustling bazaars of Baghdad and the crowded sidewalks of Hong Kong, the blessings of "the quiet life," extolled by poets of yesteryear, are increasingly difficult to procure. Unfortunately, public and policymakers alike tend to regard noise as an inevitable by-product of modern life, sometimes unpleasant but largely unavoidable. At the same time, polls taken among urban residents in both the United States and Europe reveal that most city dwellers certainly are bothered by noise. According to EPA, every day over 138 million Americans are exposed to noise levels they find annoying and disruptive; among those living in big cities, 87% endure levels of noise that could, over time, impair their hearing ability (Wolkomir and Wolkomir, 2001). In 2004 when Mayor Michael Bloomberg proposed the first complete overhaul of New York City's Noise Code in 30 years, noise ranked as the #1 quality-of-life complaint in that city, prompting nearly 1,000 calls daily to its 311 citizen service hotline. Similarly, a poll conducted by a research group in the United Kingdom found that one out of every three Britons felt their enjoyment of life was diminished by noisy neighbors or the din of traffic (Bond, 1996). In Greece, reputedly the noisiest nation in Europe, a senior member of the Association for the Quality of Life remarked that "noise pollution is becoming the country's greatest health threat. If effective measures are not taken, Greeks will either turn mad or deaf."

Sources of Noise

Most concerns about noise as a pollutant have focused on the occupational environment where high levels of noise associated with machinery, equipment, and general work practices have long been recognized as a serious threat to both the physical and psychological health of workers. However, the sources of noise that torment the general public are far more diverse than those that constitute an occupational hazard. Around the world, rapidly growing numbers of cars, trucks, and motorcycles have been boosting noise levels on crowded streets and highways, while the skies above metropolitan neighborhoods are regularly deafened by the roar of jets taking off or landing at urban airports. Even once-quiet residential areas are losing their tranquility as noise-generating home appliances and motorized yard tools are increasingly regarded as essential components of the good life. Within the last few years a growing avalanche of complaints from communities large and small has been aimed at the cell-phone chatter encountered virtually everywhere, from commuter trains, buses, and planes to restaurants, theaters, and other public places.

While most people perceive community noise as a general din, originating from a multiplicity of sources, vehicular noise—particularly that from motorcycles and large trucks—seems to be regarded as the most annoying by community residents. Unfortunately, overall noise levels are growing steadily worse, in part because modern lifestyles and transportation habits are changing in ways that inevitably result in more noise generation. We also are carrying noise with us to places that formerly were havens of peace and quiet. The advent of snowmobiles, trail bikes, and powerful motorboats have brought noise pollution to once-silent wilderness areas (witness the current controversy regarding curbs on the use of snowmobiles in Yellowstone National Park), as have overflights of helicopters and small planes catering to the tourist trade in places like Arizona's Grand Canyon and Hawaii's Volcanoes National Park. Amplified music now jars city parks when partying crowds forget that not everyone finds loud rock bands pleasurable, and the desert air occasionally reverberates to a similar beat, thanks to "boom car" sound-offs where enthusiasts compete to see whose car stereos are the most ear splitting.

Beyond the technological and lifestyle changes that have made contemporary life noisier than in days gone by, there are simply more of us on the planet, adding to the din. For the most part, levels of outdoor noise are directly related to population density—the more populous the city, the noisier it is likely to be. Predicted trends in noise levels are not particularly encouraging. One of the most important sources of excessive community noise, urban traffic, is expected to increase considerably in the years immediately ahead, with the U.S. Department of Transportation estimating that the number of automobiles on the road will increase by 0.6–0.7% annually. Overseas, a study on noise control strategies revealed that efforts taken to reduce traffic noise in several western European countries (e.g., screens along main highways) helped to offset the increase in traffic noise but didn't result in an overall lowering of noise exposure—simply because of the rapid increase in size of the car fleet. In the Netherlands alone, private car ownership is projected to increase from 4.6 million in 1985 to 7.9 million by 2010, during which time passenger traffic on that nation's highways will have grown by 70%; truck traffic is expected to increase by an even larger percentage. Europeans have been experimenting with rerouting traffic, prohibiting vehicles entirely in certain areas, and constructing noise screens, a combination of which has resulted in some lowering of noise levels in central cities. However, the spread of residential suburbs into rural areas is resulting in a steady expansion of noise exposure into areas formerly undisturbed by such problems (OECD, 1991).

Noise as a Nuisance

More than 2,000 years ago, the Roman Emperor Julius Caesar grappled with the issue of noise as a public nuisance when he attempted to ban chariot racing on the Eternal City's cobblestone streets due to the racket it created. History doesn't record whether or not he was successful, but as the clamor of urban life continued to increase during the ensuing centuries, the irritant value of noise grew apace and has occasionally caused frayed tempers to snap, sometimes with fatal results. An elderly Greek farmer is currently serving two life sentences in a maximum-security prison for shoot-

Box 13-1   The Not-So-Friendly Skies

Motor vehicles still top the public's noise complaint list, but aircraft din is a rapidly growing contender for first place, as millions of people worldwide suffer the environmental impacts of airport construction and expansion. In the United States, air travel is the fastest-growing form of transportation, with the number of annual passenger boardings expected to increase from their current 650 million to one billion by 2011. In Europe, the increase in air passenger loads has been even greater than in the U.S., while total world demand is now approaching two billion passengers each year. Growth in air cargo is also increasing dramatically; by 2001, fully 40% by value of the world's international shipments were transported by air. To meet the burgeoning demand, airports in the U.S. and abroad are expanding operations, building new runways or runway extensions to accommodate a steadily growing number of daily flights.

All of this means a greater noise burden for communities located near these facilities. Of the numerous environmental problems posed by modern airports—air pollution, odorous fumes, toxic releases, contaminated runoff—noise is by far the most frequent complaint voiced by angry airport neighbors. Concerns expressed by affected residents go well beyond mere annoyance and fear of declining property values; studies demonstrate significant health problems among people subjected to the constant roar of planes overhead. Research conducted in the Netherlands near Amsterdam's Schiphol International Airport revealed that incidence of heart disease had doubled and the use of sleeping pills increased 20–50% during a 10-year period after the addition of a new runway. One resident of the area who keeps a decibel meter on his balcony reports regular readings of 100 dB or higher as aircraft roar overhead every 90 seconds during peak hours. Researchers in Sweden found that people living near the Stockholm airport were more likely to have high blood pressure than were those living slightly farther away. The opening of a new international airport in a rural area outside Munich, Germany, provided researchers from Cornell University an opportunity to observe the impact of noise on a group of elementary school children residing within the airport's noise impact zone. By testing the children both before and after operations at the facility commenced, the Cornell scientists demonstrated that exposure to chronic airport noise caused children to exhibit such stress-related responses as increased blood pressure and elevated adrenaline levels. Nor were the children's adverse reactions restricted to physical symptoms; researchers also found that the youngsters' reading skills and long-term memory were impaired as a result of their noisy surroundings. In the United States, similar reports of reading problems among children in a New York school impacted by aircraft noise constitute persuasive evidence of its harmful effects and bolster efforts by groups pressing for stronger noise pollution controls.

Airport authorities, often prodded by citizen complaints or municipal lawsuits, have attempted to alleviate noise problems by altering flight patterns to avoid nighttime jet overflights of residential areas. While providing relief to noise-stressed airport neighbors, however, this practice can pose safety risks to air travelers when weather conditions make landing on the designated runway dangerous. In 1997 a jetliner landing at Schiphol swerved off the assigned runway after being denied use of a safer one due to noise pollution concerns.

In many cases airports can tap federal funds to soundproof nearby homes and schools or even buy out homeowners whose residences are excessively impacted by airport noise. Effective zoning laws also can help forestall citizen complaints about aircraft noise. The FAA strongly urges local governments to prohibit residential development or other noise-sensitive land uses from locating close to airports. However, FAA's admonitions are all-too-frequently ignored and the agency has no authority to overturn local land-use decisions.

The most significant initiative taken to alleviate airport noise, both in the U.S. and abroad, has been the introduction of the quieter planes required by stricter certification standards of the International Civil Aviation Organization (ICAO). This new generation of jet aircraft has had a major impact in reducing aircraft noise. In 1976, before stringent noise-reduction standards were imposed, an estimated 6–7 million Americans were exposed to objectionable levels of aircraft noise. By 2000, when the new Chapter Three standards took effect in the U.S. for all civil turbojet planes heavier than 75,000 pounds, FAA estimated the numbers of Americans exposed to significant aircraft noise levels had dropped to 500,000—in spite of rapid growth in the national aviation system during the intervening quarter-century. Looking to the future, ICAO recently adopted even tougher Chapter Four standards, due to take effect in 2006, which will provide further relief for those living near airports. In addition to these efforts to reduce noise by improving aircraft design, FAA touts other new tools such as Global Positioning Systems (GPS) technology that can help mitigate noise by keeping planes from straying outside designated noise corridors.

The success or failure of these noise abatement initiatives has profound long-term economic, as well as environmental, implications. At a time of rapidly increasing demand for air transportation, numerous aviation construction projects around the world have been delayed or abandoned in recent years due to public opposition to the noise such facilities generate. If aircraft noise problems are not adequately resolved, the ability of the global aviation industry to expand services to meet steadily growing consumer demand will be jeopardized. Further progress in reducing aircraft noise is thus critical not only for human health and quality of life, but for the health of the aviation industry as well.

References

Baliles, Gerald L. 2001. "Aircraft Noise: Addressing a Potential Barrier to Global Growth." *Virginia Lawyer* (June/July).

Evans, Gary W., Monika Bullinger, and Steffan Hygge. 1998. "Chronic Noise Exposure and Physiological Response: A Prospective Study of Children Living Under Environmental Stress." *Psychological Science* 9, no. 1 (Jan):75–77.

"Mad About the Noise." 1998. *Time International* 150, no. 48 (July 27):38.

ing two residents of a neighboring apartment who ignored his repeated complaints about the loud music blasting from their residence. When taken into custody, the old man said that all he wanted was to listen to the evening news in peace ("Mad About," 1998). In Japan a newspaper reported that a woman in densely populated Kawasaki picked up a neighbor's dog and threw it out the window of her apartment, exclaiming that the animal's constant barking was driving her to distraction. The enraged neighbor then retaliated by stabbing the woman to death! Perhaps to avoid just such altercations, more and more Japanese city dwellers are having their canine pets' vocal chords cut or are fitting them with antibarking shock collars to make sure they remain quiet all day in the tiny, yardless living quarters typical of modern Japan (Shapiro, 1989).

Just as beauty is in the eye of the beholder, the perception of a sound as "noise" (arbitrarily defined by one writer as "sound at the wrong time and in the wrong place") depends on the point of view of the individual listener. A case in point is the furor that erupted in Hamtramck, Michigan, near Detroit, in the spring of 2004 when the city council amended its noise ordinance to allow a local mosque to broadcast a call to prayer from outdoor loudspeakers five times daily. Many non-Muslim residents vehemently objected to the council's decision, insisting that one group's right to religious freedom shouldn't impinge on another group's right to peace and quiet. Unfortunately for those attempting to set standards regulating noise exposure, loudness of a noise and the annoyance it causes are not always directly correlated. As any college student partying near a residential neighborhood well knows, people *generating* loud sounds may frequently enjoy them, while those forced to listen usually find the same noise profoundly objectionable. In general, people most easily tolerate noise when (1) they are causing it, (2) they feel it is necessary or useful to them, or (3) they know

Millions of Americans are daily being exposed to levels of noise that could permanently damage their ability to hear. [*Photos top left and right by Nora Byrne*]

where it is coming from. To the extent that other people exposed to the same sounds do not experience equivalent benefits from the noise, conflict between participating and nonparticipating groups is generated (Bugliarello et al., 1976). As the old French proverb aptly puts it, "I do not like noise unless I make it myself."

While most people are well acquainted with the feelings of annoyance and irritation that unwanted sounds can arouse, it is becoming increasingly evident that noise levels commonly encountered in thousands of cities, factories, places of recreation, and even inside homes represent far more than a simple nuisance. Noise today has become a public health hazard; more insidious than easily recognized air and water pollution, noise is invisibly undermining the physical and psychological well-being of millions of people around the world. The remainder of this chapter will describe the ways in which noise affects human health, but first it is necessary to take a brief look at the physical nature of sound and how noise levels are measured.

Nature of Sound

Sound is produced by the compression and expansion of air created when an object vibrates. The positive and negative pressure waves thus formed travel outward longitudinally from the vibrating source. Two basic characteristics of sound, **frequency** (or **pitch**) and **amplitude**, are related to how loud and annoying a sound will be perceived.

Frequency describes the rate of vibration—how fast the object is moving back and forth. The more rapid the movement, the higher the frequency of the sound pressure waves created. The standard unit used today for measuring frequency is the **hertz (Hz),** equivalent to one wave per second passing a given point. Most people can hear sounds within a frequency range of 20–20,000 Hz, though there exists a great deal of individual variation in ability to perceive very low or very high frequency sounds. Because low-frequency sounds (e.g., bass sounds from amplified music, traffic noise) are more penetrating than those of high frequency, they are more difficult to control by shielding and thus are often the main source of irritation related to community noise.

Amplitude refers to the intensity of sound—how much energy is behind the sound wave. Sound waves of the same frequency can be heard as very loud or very soft, depending on the force with which they strike the ear. In technical terms, amplitude measures the maximum displacement of a sound wave from its resting, or equilibrium, position, but it is perceived psychologically as **loudness**, measured with a sound level meter in units called **decibels (dB)**. This system allows comparison of a measured sound's intensity to the level just detectable by normal, healthy ears, with a decibel level of zero representing the threshold of hearing. The decibel scale is logarithmic rather than linear; hence even a small rise in decibel values can make a significant difference in noise intensity. For example, to a pedestrian standing on a subway platform, the noise of the passing train, measured at 90 dB, sounds twice as loud as does street traffic registering 80 dB. It should be noted in passing that this discussion relates to sound measurements in *air*, where the point of reference is the human ear. The decibel scale also is used to measure sound level intensity in water, but a different reference point is employed in making such calculations. For this reason, a sound level intensity of, say, 100 dB in water is not the same as 100 dB in air.

A listener's perception of a sound as loud does not depend entirely on its amplitude, being affected to some extent by its frequency as well. Although hearing ability ranges from 20–20,000 Hz, not all of these frequencies sound equally loud to the human ear. Maximum sensitivity to sound occurs in the 1,000–5,000 Hz range. For reference, normal human speech frequencies can vary from 500–2,000 Hz. However, sounds at the very low or very high ends of the full audible range seem much fainter to our ears than do those in the middle frequencies. Thus, for example, an extremely low-pitched sound must have an amplitude many times greater than a sound of medium pitch in order for both to be heard as equally loud. For this reason, decibel values are sometimes weighted to take into account the frequency response of the human ear. When this is done, the unit measurement designation may be written as dB(A). Table 13-1 indicates approximate decibel values for a number of commonly encountered sounds.

Table 13-1   Sound Levels and Human Response

Common Sounds	Noise Level (dB)	Effect
Air raid siren	140	Painfully loud
Jet takeoff	130	
Discotheque	120	Maximum vocal effort
Pile driver	110	
Garbage truck	100	
City traffic	90	Very annoying, hearing damage
Alarm clock	80	Annoying
Freeway traffic	70	Phone use difficult
Air conditioning	60	Intrusive
Light auto traffic	50	Quiet
Living room	40	
Library	30	Very quiet
Broadcasting studio	20	
	10	Just audible
	0	Hearing begins

Source: Environmental Protection Agency.

Noise and Hearing Loss

... I've shot my hearing; it hurts and it's painful, and it's frustrating when little children talk to you and you can't hear them.

—Pete Townshend

While everyone has experienced irritation due to noise, many people are unaware that the sounds that annoy them may also be affecting their hearing. Pete Townshend's confession during a 1989 press conference that his career as a rock musician had irreversibly damaged his hearing may not have dampened fans' enthusiasm for ear-splitting concerts, but it did serve as a warning to the general public that loud music may produce long-lasting effects. Unfortunately, Townshend is joined by an estimated 10 million Americans who have already suffered full or partial hearing loss due to excessive noise exposure; according to EPA, at least 20 million people in the U.S. are daily being exposed to noise levels that will permanently damage their ability to hear.

Most people are familiar with the temporary deafness and ringing in the ears that occurs after sudden exposure to a very loud noise such as a cap gun or firecracker exploding close to one's head. This type of partial hearing loss generally lasts a few hours at the most and is referred to as **temporary threshold shift (TTS)**. In addition to the obvious impact of sudden, high-intensity sounds, noise research has found that

TTS also can result from longer-term exposure (16–48 hours) to noise and that recovery to normal hearing may take as long as two days, depending on both the intensity and duration of noise exposure (Melrick, 1991). The type of short-term hearing loss typified by TTS is an accepted fact of life among workers in noisy occupations, performers and patrons at rock concerts, wildly cheering spectators at sporting events, and many others. However, most people don't realize that regular, prolonged exposure to noise, even at levels commonly encountered in everyday life, can eventually result in permanent hearing impairment. Because damage to the ear is usually painless and seldom visible, few people recognize the injury they are incurring until it is too late. The Occupational Safety and Health Administration (OSHA) has determined that exposure to daily noise levels averaging just 85 decibels (approximately the loudness of an electric shaver or a food processor) will result in irreversible hearing loss. For this reason, OSHA recommends hearing protection for workers whose 8-hour, time-weighted average noise exposure is at or above 85 decibels; for exposure to noise levels of 90 decibels and above, hearing protection is *required.*

The noise of city traffic, subways, power lawnmowers, motorcycles, certain household appliances, babies screaming, and even people shouting all exceed the decibel level considered "safe." Above 85 dB, progressively higher levels of noise exposure exert ever-increasing risk of damage—and the louder the noise, the shorter the exposure time required to wreak lasting harm. With each additional five decibels of loudness the time required to cause permanent injury is cut in half (Jaret, 1990). For revelers rocking with the beat at a nightclub, where the intensity of sound may hit 120 dB, the damage is done in less than 30 minutes.

Mechanism of Hearing Loss

Noise results in hearing loss through its destructive effect on the delicate hair cells in the Organ of Corti within the cochlea of the inner ear. These hair cells convert fluid vibrations in the inner ear into impulses that are carried by the auditory nerve to the brain, resulting in the sensation of sound. The outer hair cells at the base of the cochlea, primarily associated with high-frequency sounds, are the first to be affected, but continued exposure to loud noise will eventually result in damage to hair cells in other areas of the cochlea. Over a period of time, prolonged exposure to excessive noise levels may result in the complete collapse of individual hair cells, thus affecting the transmission of nerve impulses. The average individual is born with approximately 16,000 sensory receptors within the Organ of Corti; while 30–50% of these hair cells can be destroyed before any measurable degree of hearing loss is detectable, losses above this level result inevitably in an impairment of hearing ability. Unfortunately, there is no method at present by which a doctor can diagnose the beginning stages of noise-induced hearing loss. The earliest warning signs—inability to hear high-frequency sounds—are unlikely to be noticed unless the affected individual has his or her hearing tested for some other reason. By the time enough hair cells have been lost to affect perception of lower-frequency sounds, a process that may require many years of excessive noise exposure, the damage has been done.

This type of hearing loss, categorized as **sensorineural,** is irreversible and cannot be restored by the use of a hearing aid since both the auditory nerve and cochlear structures have been affected. By contrast, hearing loss resulting from infections (e.g., "swimmer's ear," mumps, measles, etc.) or by trauma (e.g., a blow to the head that ruptures the eardrum or puncturing the eardrum with a cotton-tipped swab or toothpick) is referred to as **conductive** hearing loss and can often be corrected by surgery or medication (Thurston and Roberts, 1991). To a limited extent the ear can protect itself against loud continuous noise by a tightening of the membrane at the entrance to the

Figure 13-1   How We Hear

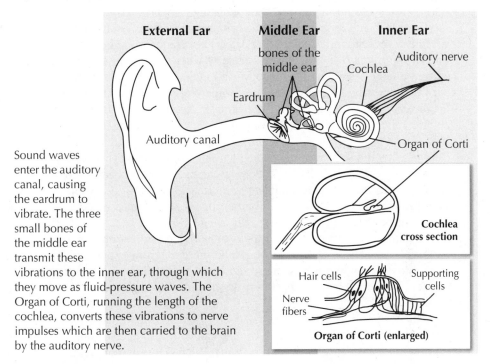

Sound waves enter the auditory canal, causing the eardrum to vibrate. The three small bones of the middle ear transmit these vibrations to the inner ear, through which they move as fluid-pressure waves. The Organ of Corti, running the length of the cochlea, converts these vibrations to nerve impulses which are then carried to the brain by the auditory nerve.

inner ear, thereby dampening sound. However, in situations where noise volume increases very rapidly or instantaneously, as when a military jet makes a low-altitude flyover or someone fires a rifle close to the ear, adaptation processes and reflex protective mechanisms don't have time to function effectively. In such cases, risk of damage to the inner ear is greater than it would be if the volume of noise were increasing more slowly (Ising et al., 1990).

Many people take it for granted that a gradual loss of hearing is one of the inevitable consequences of growing older, a belief bolstered by statistics which report that by the age of 65, one out of four Americans is experiencing hearing loss significant enough to interfere with communication; by the time they reach their 90s, nine out of ten seniors are so afflicted. Many researchers are convinced, however, that the extent of the problem is considerably greater than it need be. Some years ago, an audiologist traveled to a remote African village near the Sudan-Ethiopian border to test the hearing of tribe members who had never heard the blare of amplified music or the din of urban traffic. He found that 70-year-old Africans, unlike their American peers, could easily hear sounds as soft as a murmur from as far as 300 feet away (Jaret, 1990). While some degree of age-related hearing loss (clinically described as **presbycusis)** may be inevitable, the Sudanese experience provides a meaningful lesson—one of the best ways to preserve lifelong sharpness of hearing is to limit as much as possible one's exposure to a noisy environment.

Effects of Hearing Loss

Hearing disability caused by noise can range in severity from difficulty in comprehending normal conversation to total deafness. In general, the ability to hear high-frequency sounds is the first thing to be affected by noise exposure; for this reason, tests for early detection of hearing loss should pay special attention to hearing ability in the 4,000 Hz range. People affected often have difficulty hearing such sounds as a clock ticking or telephone ringing and cannot distinguish certain consonants, particularly *s, sh, ch, p, m, t, f,* and *th.* Individuals suffering hearing loss not only have trouble with the volume of speech, but also with its clarity. They frequently accuse people with whom they are speaking of mumbling, particularly when talking on the telephone or when background noises interfere with conversation; listening to the radio or television may become impossible. The psychological impact of such difficulties—the fear of being laughed at for misunderstanding questions or comments, the frustration of not being able to follow a conversation, the feeling of isolation or alienation experienced as friends unconsciously avoid trying to converse—are frequently as severe as the physical disability. Individuals experiencing hearing loss tend to become suspicious, irritable, and depressed; their careers suffer and their social life becomes severely restricted, sometimes to the point of complete withdrawal (Perham, 1979). Some researchers even suspect that the confusion and unresponsiveness blamed on Alzheimer's disease may actually, in some cases, be due to hearing loss.

In addition to these problems, a person with partial hearing loss may suffer sharp pain in the ears when exposed to very loud noise and may experience repeated bouts of **tinnitus**—a ringing or buzzing sound in the head that can drive the victim to distraction, interfering with sleep, conversation, and normal daily activities. Probably the single most common side effect of noise-induced hearing loss, tinnitus can become a permanent condition, though it is usually only a temporary nuisance. To sufferers, the intensity of the noise in their heads can be maddening, likened by one victim to "holding a vacuum cleaner to your ear" (Murphy, 1989). The pitch of the ringing characterizing tinnitus can sound like a high scream, and volume levels as high as 70 dB have been measured. Among those afflicted with permanent tinnitus, certain medications, diet, or relaxation therapies may ease the symptoms, but the condition at this stage is essentially irreversible (Cohen, 1990).

Other Effects of Noise

Hearing loss is the most obvious health threat posed by noise pollution, but it is by no means the only one. Noise can adversely affect our physical and psychological well-being in a host of other ways.

Stress and Related Health Effects

Exposure to unwanted noise involuntarily induces stress, and stress can lead to a variety of physical ailments including an increase in heart rate, high blood pressure, elevated levels of blood cholesterol, ulcers, headaches, and colitis.

Stressful reaction to loud or sudden noise undoubtedly represents an evolutionary adaptation to warnings signaling approaching danger. Bodily responses to the snarl of a predatory beast or the rumble of a boulder crashing down a mountainside cause a surge of adrenaline, an increase in heart and breathing rates, and the tensing of muscles—all physiological preparations for fight or flight that have important survival value. However, these same metabolic responses are today being triggered repeatedly by the innumerable noises of modern society. As a result, our bodies are subjected to a constant state of stress which, far from being advantageous, is literally making millions of people sick—even though they may not attribute their problems to noise. While many individuals insist that they have "gotten used to noise" and are no longer bothered by it, the truth is that no one can prevent the automatic biological changes that noise provokes.

Box 13-2   The Noisy Seas

Humans aren't the only creatures forced to endure excessive levels of noise pollution. Throughout the world's oceans, whales, dolphins, sea lions, and other marine mammals are under increasing stress from human-generated sounds that threaten their hearing, health, behavior—perhaps even the survival of some species.

The oceans, of course, have never been serenely quiet. Marine life evolved in an environment permeated by underwater noises generated by wind-driven wave action, earthquakes, thunderstorms, cracking ice, and, in time, by the myriad sounds produced by sea animals themselves. Sea-dwelling mammals and fish rely heavily on sound to locate food, to navigate, and to communicate with other members of their species. All aquatic vertebrates have ears and auditory capabilities and they utilize sound as a critical means of learning about and surviving in their watery environment.

In recent years, awareness of the importance of sound to marine mammals has led to growing alarm among scientists and concerned citizens who fear that the steadily increasing underwater din produced by a wide range of human activities may be adversely affecting the lives of these creatures. Ocean noise levels that had remained more or less constant from primordial times until the mid-1800s began to escalate during the past century and a half as the Industrial Revolution accelerated and expanded across the globe. Commercial ship traffic early became, and still remains, the leading anthropogenic component of noise in the marine environment, as sailing ships gave way to mechanically powered vessels and as the number and size of ships steadily increased. In localized areas, high-speed yachts contribute significantly to underwater noise, as do outboard and inboard motor-boats. In recent years the growing popularity of whale-watching has resulted in a documented change in the behavior of killer whales, as the animals increase the duration of their calls to compensate for the noise generated by numerous boatloads of tourists circling near their pods.

Over the past 60 years since the end of World War II, numerous other noise-generated activities have proliferated in or adja-cent to the world's seas, further contributing to the underwater cacophony and raising fears of serious resultant harm to ocean mammals. Among these newer sources are activities related to offshore oil and gas exploration and production—seismic surveying utilizing air guns, drilling, emplacement and removal of drilling platforms, and provision of supplies to these platforms by noisy low-flying helicopters or power boats. Construction and other industrial activity along seacoasts further contribute to human-induced ocean sound levels. Dredging and pile-driving are both very noisy activities, as are power plant operations and certain types of industries; the increasing proliferation of near-shore power-generating windmills are a relatively recent addition to the long list of anthropogenic noise in the marine environment.

Attracting the most attention from environmentalists is the widespread use of sonar systems, employed for both civilian and military purposes, to characterize physical properties of the seabed and to locate underwater objects such as schools of fish, sunken ships, or enemy submarines. Proponents of sonar use correctly point out that, to date, sonar is the most powerful remote-sensing tool available for such tasks, a tool that has produced significant practical benefits and increased our general understanding of marine geology. Sonar also comprises an essential weapon for maintaining national security, providing a means to detect and track missile-carrying submarines, thus providing an early warning of potential danger to naval vessels in the general vicinity.

While the benefits of sonar and other types of underwater acoustical devices are undeniable, such technologies, nevertheless, raise legitimate concerns as to whether they affect the normal activities of marine mammals and their long-term ability to sustain healthy populations. As long ago as 1972, the Marine Mammal Protection Act mandated controls over noise sources that could negatively impact whales and other ocean mammals. However, there was limited public interest in the issue until 1992 when the Office of Naval Research (ONR) launched its Acoustic Thermometry of Ocean Climate project, utilizing high-intensity, low-frequency sound waves from a source deployed deep in the ocean and transmitted over thousands of kilometers to gather basic scientific information on the properties of ocean basins. The controversy generated by this project and the increasing levels of scrutiny it attracted from marine biologists, environmental groups, and other concerned parties have prompted ONR to require that all of its research programs utilizing underwater acoustic transmissions identify and mitigate against any possible harm to the marine environment and adhere strictly to all federal and relevant state environmental laws and regulations.

These safeguards have not silenced critics of such activities, however. In 2002 immediate protests erupted when the Navy was given a permit to deploy its low-frequency active (LFA) sonar system, intended for submarine detection, across three-fourths of the world's oceans. Because the project calls for warships to tow a vertical line of up to 18 loudspeakers emitting an effective noise level of 235 dB through vast areas of the ocean, opponents alleged that whales or dolphins swimming nearby could be injured, deafened, or even killed by the excruciatingly loud noise. Even 300 miles from the source, they charged, noise levels would be high enough to interfere with the animals' normal activities. While research data pertaining to the effects of anthropogenic sound on marine life are scanty, there are valid reasons for such concerns. In 2001 in the Bahamas and 2002 in the Canary Islands, mass strandings of beaked whales (*Ziphius cavirostris*) occurred shortly after the Navy engaged in military exercises testing high-energy, mid-frequency (1–10 kHz) sonar. A team of scientists from London's Institute of Zoology examined the whale carcasses soon after the strandings and concluded the animals died of decompression sickness, their livers and kidneys damaged by gas bubbles that formed in the whales' blood as they shot to the surface to escape the sonar. This study constituted the most direct evidence to date that sonar can be lethal to marine mammals.

When news of the Navy's LFA sonar permit was announced, environmental groups quickly rallied to block commencement of the research project. Leading the opposition, the Natural Resources Defense Council (NRDC) filed a lawsuit against the Navy and the National Marine Fisheries Service (the agency issuing the permit), charging that deployment of the LFA system would violate the Marine Mammal Protection Act. In October 2002, just days before the Navy intended to commence operations across 14 million square miles of the Pacific, NRDC won a preliminary injunction to block such action; in August 2003, a federal judge issued a final ruling barring the Navy from pursuing its project as originally proposed, thereby protecting critical habitat of endangered whales and sparing countless marine mammals and fish from death and injury. However, the injunction permits the Navy to test its sonar system in a limited area off the coast of northeastern Asia and allows use of the system in case of war.

While this most threatening source of oceanic noise has been forestalled at least for the immediate future (as this book goes to press, the Navy is appealing the federal court's 2003 ruling), numerous others continue to proliferate. The extent to which they adversely affect the well-being of marine mammals is as yet little understood and experts agree that far more broad-ranging research is needed to clarify and quantify the impact of human-generated sounds on the health and behavior of these animals.

Reference

Jepson, P. D., et al. 2003. "Gas-Bubble Lesions In Stranded Cetaceans." *Nature* 425, no. 6958 (Oct. 9).

National Research Council. 2003. *Ocean Noise and Marine Mammals*. The National Academies Press.

Teratogenic Effects of Noise

The human uterus is not an inner sanctum of peace and quiet. Research has shown that fetal development proceeds amidst constant internal noise generated by the throbbing of maternal arteries and rumbling of bowels. Background noise levels within the pregnant uterus have been variously estimated as ranging anywhere from 56 to 95 dB (as compared with, for example, a typical office environment where decibel levels average about 50). Although the mother's body tissues to some extent attenuate penetration of external noise into the womb, both experimental and anecdotal evidence indicate that outside noise can provoke a physical response in the developing unborn child.

For over half a century, one method used by physicians for determining fetal viability has been to place a sound source near the mother's abdomen and expose the fetus to noise of 120 Hz frequency. Since a fetus' hearing ability is well developed by the 28th week of pregnancy, such noise exposure causes a noticeable increase in heart rate and kicking among third-trimester fetuses. Less scientific but equally persuasive testimony comes from pregnant women who have reported that they felt considerably more fetal movement while listening to music in a concert hall, the kicking reaching a peak when the audience began to applaud!

While the fact that noise exposure begins well before birth is undisputable, it is less clear whether such exposure presents any risk of hearing impairment to the unborn child. The question is of some concern because approximately 45% of the U.S.

Contemporary American life is much noisier than in days gone by due in part to advanced technology, lifestyle changes, transportation habits, and population density. [*EPA Journal*]

workforce is now female and many of these women will experience one or more pregnancies during their working years. Since occupational noise pollution control frequently is focused on providing ear protection to workers, the question of possible noise-induced hearing damage to the fetuses of pregnant employees is of more than academic interest. While a few epidemiologic studies have reported some degree of hearing impairment among children whose mothers received occupational noise exposures up to 100 dB during pregnancy, most of the limited research done to date indicates that hearing loss induced in a fetus by external noise is highly unlikely. The insulating effect of maternal tissues, which limits the amount of outside sound penetrating the uterine environment, renders noise an unlikely teratogenic agent (Thurston and Roberts, 1991).

Much more research is needed to define the extent of the relationship, if any, between noise and birth defects, as well as to establish how high noise levels must be to cause developmental problems. Lacking definitive information, some doctors recommend that pregnant women try to avoid noise exposure to the greatest extent possible, one such expert offering the tongue-in-cheek advice that "any expectant mother should get out of New York."

Effects of Noise on Learning Ability

It has long been recognized that noisy surroundings at school and in the home can adversely affect children's language development and their ability to read. A classic study in the early 1970s, comparing reading ability among children living on different floors of an apartment building located adjacent to a busy highway, revealed that youngsters living on the higher (i.e., quieter) floors had better reading scores than those living on lower (noisier) floors. It also showed that the longer a child had experienced excessive noise exposure, the poorer was his/her reading ability. Investigators concluded that a noisy home environment has more of an impact on reading skills than do such factors as parents' educational level, number of children in the family, or the child's grade level (Cohen, Glass, and Singer, 1973).

More recently, an important study conducted by a Cornell University researcher on first-and second-grade students whose school is located within the flight contour of a major New York metropolitan airport (overflights during school hours averaged one flight every 6.6 minutes) demonstrated convincingly that children constantly exposed to noise have poorer reading skills than children attending school in quiet areas. Investigators concluded that the children's reading difficulties stem, at least in part, from noise-related impairment of their ability to recognize and understand spoken words. In order to cope with the constant noise to which they are subjected, children living and attending school near the airport unconsciously reduce their noise burden by "filtering out" certain sounds, including human speech (Evans and Maxwell, 1997). Given the large number of schools worldwide located near airports or busy highways, as well as the increase in residential area noise levels in developed and developing countries alike, the link between noise exposure and children's language development should be a serious concern to educators and parents.

Safety Aspects of Noise

Safety, as well as health, can be in jeopardy when noise levels are high. A tragic case in point involved a Bloomington, Illinois, teenager who was killed when struck from behind by an Amtrak train while walking in the middle of the tracks en route to school. Investigators subsequently concluded that the young man failed to hear the approaching train because he was wearing large earphones while listening to a radio set at high volume. As a police officer at the scene remarked, "The engineer blew the horn, then laid on it to get this person off the tracks. It didn't work. We believe he never heard the train because he had his stereo on" (Simpson, 1997). In the occupational environment as well, high noise levels can pose a safety hazard by preventing workers from hearing shouts of warning or cries for help. Many traffic accidents are thought to be caused by drivers' inability to hear emergency sirens. Both by interfering with shouts for help or by masking warning signals, high levels of background noise pose a very real threat to public safety.

Table 13-2   Permissible Noise Exposures Established by OSHA

Duration per day (hours)	Sound level (dB)
8	90
6	92
4	95
3	97
2	100
1½	102
1	105
½	110
¼ or less	115

Source: OSHA

Sleep Disruption

Sleep is a biological necessity. We need sleep to repair the wearing out of bodily tissues and to rejuvenate them; deprivation or disruption of sleep can thus directly threaten both physical health and mental well-being.

Noise can prevent people from going to sleep, can waken them prematurely, or can cause shifts from deeper to lighter stages of sleep. While individual response to noise in relation to its impact on sleep varies widely, in general adults are wakened by noise more easily than are children; the elderly are more sensitive than the middle-aged; sick people are more affected than healthy ones; and women are more easily disturbed than men (Bugliarello, 1976). In 1996 the World Health Organization cited noise as a significant health threat and the following year published guidelines that recommended lowering average nighttime noise levels suitable for undisturbed sleep from 35 to 30 decibels, with a peak nighttime maximum of 45 dB(A). Given such recommendations for healthful sleep, it is troubling to note that millions of people currently are subjected to noise levels well above the WHO guidelines. Indeed, a survey of traffic noise in western Europe estimates that 16% of Europeans are subjected to more than 40 decibels in their bedrooms every night (Bond, 1996). Given this situation, it shouldn't be surprising that results of a German study, discussed at a 2004 conference in Bonn on sleep and health, found that 80 million Europeans—20% of all EU residents—suffer from stress and sleep disorders serious enough to affect their health.

Noise Control Efforts

Historically, noise abatement efforts have consisted primarily of local ordinances directed at specific community nuisances. One of the earliest such laws was a London ordinance that went into effect in 1829, allowing stagecoach horses to be confiscated if they disrupted church services (Lipscomb, 1974). Over the years since then, cities have adopted a wide variety of local restrictions on noise sources. A brief sampling of such regulations include: requirements for mufflers on cars; bans on leaf blowers; prohibitions against construction activity, garbage collection, or lawn mowing during early morning or evening hours; bans on roosters or other noisy animals within city limits; restrictions on auto horn-blowing; bans on truck traffic through residential neighborhoods; and prohibitions on "boom cars" or other forms of amplified music outdoors. Overseas, governments are taking legislative action against nuisance noise

Box 13-3   Play Can Be Deafening!

The association between high noise levels and hearing loss in the occupational environment has been recognized—and regulated—for years. The Occupational Safety and Health Administration (OSHA) has set an eight-hour time-weighted average of 90 dB(A) as the maximum permissible noise exposure for the American worker. In recent years, however, it has become increasingly clear that dangerous levels of noise are found not only in factories but also in the home and in association with a wide range of recreational activities. The same individual whose hearing is protected by regulations while on the job may, during off-work hours, incur irreparable damage by engaging in noisy activities where sound levels are totally unregulated and where those exposed seldom wear ear protection.

Perhaps most at risk of nonoccupational noise-induced hearing loss are millions of children and young adults whose ideas of fun are often inseparable from noise: listening to amplified music, playing electronic arcade games, participating in noisy sports events, playing in the school band. Researchers have been surprised to discover that noise-induced hearing loss can begin at 10–20 years of age, much earlier than they previously had thought possible. In 1990 a group of British researchers reported unexpected frustration in their efforts to study hearing damage among youths aged 15–23. Their project was stymied because they couldn't assemble a sufficient number of young people to serve as "controls"—virtually all the candidates had already been exposed to loud music!

Hearing impairment among rock musicians is legendary, as testimony by such notables as Pete Townshend, Ted Nugent, Joey Kramer, and others bears witness. Employees of nightclubs featuring loud music are also at risk. A survey of noise levels in a sampling of San Francisco dance clubs found that all violated the CAL-OSHA workplace noise regulations; club employees were resigned to hearing loss as an inescapable consequence of working in such a noisy environment. The impact on those whose exposure is limited to *attending* rock concerts or noisy nightclubs is probably less dramatic. Attendees are typically exposed to noise levels of 100 dB or higher (OSHA standards permit no more than 2 hours exposure to noise of this intensity in the workplace). They frequently experience temporary threshold shift (TTS) but generally recover within a few hours to a few days after exposure.

The roar of the crowd at athletic events may be endangering fans' hearing, particularly if the event in question happens to be a Minnesota Twins game at the Metrodome. Perhaps because its dome is smaller than average, with a roof configuration that returns noise to the field, the Metrodome may reverberate with noise levels exceeding 100 dB when the stands are full and the home team is winning. As in the situation with rock concerts, spectators who spend a limited amount of time in these raucous surroundings are at minor risk of long-term harm, but Twins players and the concessionaires who spend most of the season amidst the cheering throngs are at serious risk of permanent hearing impairment.

Many household appliances expose people of all ages to noise levels that frequently exceed the 85 dB "safe" level; fortunately the duration of exposure to such noises as the whir of a food processor or the drone of a vacuum cleaner is generally quite brief. On the other hand, certain power tools such as chainsaws or leaf blowers could present a risk if used for prolonged periods without hearing protection. Similarly, farm equipment such as tractors can be a significant cause of hearing impairment for rural youngsters. A study conducted in Wisconsin revealed that more than half the children involved in farm work experienced some degree of noise-induced hearing loss, double the rate of children *not* working on farms.

Of all the dangerous forms of recreational noise exposure, however, the greatest toll on young ears (and older ears as well!) is wrought by hunting and target shooting, activities regularly enjoyed by an estimated 13% of the U.S. population. With decibel levels frequently exceeding the threshold of pain, the crack of gunfire, or even cap pistols, can instantly destroy receptor cells in the inner ear and irreversibly damage hearing ability. Among a study group of 94 children or teenagers who were victims of noise-induced hearing loss, an analysis of the noise sources revealed that fully 46% suffered because of guns or fireworks; only 12% had been damaged by exposure to live or amplified music, 8% by power tools, and 4% by recreational vehicles.

Since noise-induced hearing loss is cumulative, growing slowly but steadily worse with continued exposure to a wide variety of high-decibel activities, people of all ages, but especially children, need to become more aware of the importance of wearing ear protection when engaged in noisy activities. Natural defenses unfortunately are insufficient; as an 18th century Englishman long ago commented, "I have often lamented that we cannot close our ears with as much ease as we can our eyes."

References

Clark, William W. 1991. "Noise Exposure from Leisure Activities: A Review." *Journal of the Acoustical Society of America* 90, no.1 (July).

Gauthier, Michele M. 1988. "Clamorous Metrodome Hard on Ears and Foes." *The Physician and Sports Medicine* 16, no. 3 (March).

U.S. Congress. 1991. *Turn It Down: Effects of Noise on Hearing Loss in Children and Youth*. Hearing before the Select House Committee on Children, Youth, and Families, July 22. Washington, DC: U.S. Government Printing Office.

as well. In Beijing, China, the municipal government regulates car alarms, requiring that they ring for no more than 35 seconds and then only when the engine catches fire; when a door, trunk, or hood is opened; or when the entire car is moved. These regulations were provoked by a flood of complaints about excessive noise from the city's 300,000 vehicles with anti-theft devices, some of which were so sensitive they began ringing when the car was merely touched or even when exposed to thunder, hail, or rain! New York City's new noise code targets barking dogs and Mr. Softee ice cream trucks as well as jackhammers, overly loud bars and nightclubs, and noisy air conditioning units—just to name a few. In Switzerland, public complaints about truck noise resulted in passage of a nationwide referendum requiring that heavy trucks tran-

A wide range of recreational activities can create noise volumes with the potential to endanger the hearing of fans and participants.

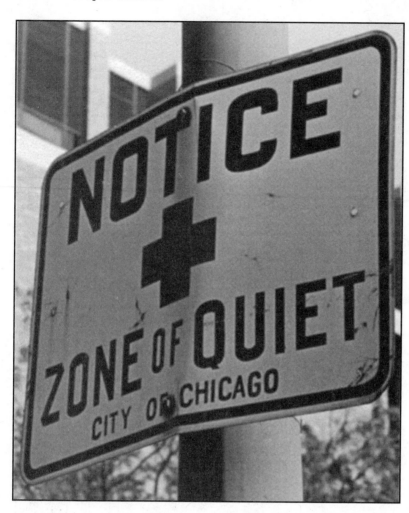

In most urban areas noise-control regulations are nonexistent or are routinely ignored. [*Nora Byrne*]

siting the country will have to be put on trains when they cross the Swiss border to spare that small Alpine country the associated pollution, as well as the thundering noise that occasionally has been known to cause avalanches and landslides.

The federal government entered the noise control arena in 1972 with passage of the Noise Control Act—the first national law aimed at relieving overstimulated American ears by regulating certain commercial products considered to be major noise sources. The law called for noise emission limits to be set for products such as medium- and heavy-weight trucks, buses, motorcycles, power lawnmowers, jackhammers, and rock drills. In addition, the EPA was to draft noise labeling requirements for noisy products as well as conduct studies on the health impact of noise in order to provide an objective basis for the numerical noise standards yet to be promulgated.

In 1978 the Noise Control Act was amended by the Quiet Communities Act, which authorized EPA to work in partnership with state and local governments, helping them to develop antinoise programs appropriate to their own special needs and abilities. Federal funding provided aid in the form of grants, seminars, and training programs to assist lower levels of government. With the EPA serving as a coordinating agency and providing seed money for local initiatives, hundreds of community noise abatement programs were launched during the 1970s. Noise control efforts suffered a serious setback in the 1980s, however, with the advent of a Reagan Administration committed to an antiregulatory agenda on environmental issues. In 1982, to the dismay of noise experts, EPA's Office of Noise Abatement and Control (ONAC) was disbanded and has yet to be restored. Without EPA leadership, technical assistance, or funding, research on the impact of noise on health and hearing has declined sharply since the early 1980s. Most information on noise pollution appearing in current textbooks is still based on studies conducted during the 1970s. The promising proliferation of municipal noise abatement efforts that characterized the late 1970s has suffered a similar reversal. Although the Noise Control Act mandates are still theoretically in effect, they are not being enforced. Regulations that were about to be promulgated at the time ONAC closed were never completed and those that had been finalized have been ignored. Of the wide range of equipment targeted by the Noise Control Act, the only products for which noise emission standards have yet been promulgated are air compressors, motorcycles, trucks, and waste compactors. In 1991 hearing experts testified before a congressional committee, urging restoration of EPA leadership in national noise abatement efforts and calling for renewed noise emission information and warning labels on dangerously noisy equipment. Unfortunately, these initiatives were not followed by legislative action and noise pollution control remains an issue largely neglected by policymakers. Undoubtedly the most serious obstacle to implementing effective programs is the difficulty of convincing both policymakers and the public that noise pollution is really important. As one EPA official remarked, "Noise is something we grow up with, and it is very difficult to believe that such a common pollutant could be doing anything serious to our health or the environment." Until voters insist that excessive noise is a community health hazard that must be controlled, it is unlikely that elected officials will give noise abatement efforts the attention they deserve.

References

Bond, Michael. 1996. "Plagued by Noise." *New Scientist* 152, no. 2056 (Nov. 16):14–15.

Bugliarello, George, Ariel Alexandre, John Barnes, and Charles Wakstein. 1976. *The Impact of Noise Pollution.* Pergamon Press.

Cohen, Peter. 1990. "Drumming: How Risky Is It To Your Hearing?" *Modern Drummer* (Oct).

Cohen, S., D. C. Glass, and J. E. Singer. 1973. "Apartment Noise Auditory Discrimination and Reading Ability in Children." *Journal of Experimental Social Psychology* 9:407–422.

Evans, Gary W., and Lorraine Maxwell. 1997. "Chronic Noise Exposure and Reading Deficits: The Mediating Effects of Language Acquisition." *Environment and Behavior* 29, no. 5 (Sept):638.

Ising, Hartmut, Ekkehard Rebentisch, Fritz Poustka, and Immo Curio. 1990. "Annoyance and Health Risk Caused by Military Low-altitude Flight Noise." *International Archives of Occupational and Environmental Health* 62:357–63.

Jaret, Peter. 1990. "The Rock & Roll Syndrome." *In Health* (July/Aug).

Lipscomb, David M. 1974. *Noise: The Unwanted Sounds.* Nelson-Hall.

"Mad About the Noise." 1998. *Time International* 150, no. 48 (July 27):38.

Melrick, William. 1991. "Human Temporary Threshold Shift (TTS) and Damage Risk." *Journal of the Acoustical Society of America* 90, no. 1 (July).

Murphy, Elliott. 1989. "Townshend, Tinnitus and Rock & Roll." *Rolling Stone,* July 13–27.

OECD. 1991. *Fighting Noise in the 1990s.* Paris: OECD.

Perham, Chris. 1979. "The Sound of Silence." *EPA Journal* 5, no. 9 (Oct).

Shapiro, Margaret. 1989. "Crowds are Made in Japan Too." *Washington Post,* Feb. 13.

Simpson, Kevin. 1997. "Train Kills Teen in B-N." *The Pantagraph,* Bloomington, IL, Oct. 18:A-1.

Thurston, Floyd E., and Stanley L. Roberts. 1991. "Environmental Noise and Fetal Hearing." *Journal of the Tennessee Medical Association* 84, no. 1 (Jan).

Wolkomir, Richard and Joyce Wolkomir. 2001. "Noise Busters." *Smithsonian* 31, no. 12 (March).

WATER RESOURCES

> All the rivers run into the sea, yet the sea is not full; to the place from whence the rivers come, thither they return again.
>
> —Ecclesiastes 1:7

Although the ancient writer of Ecclesiastes expressed his scientific observations in poetic form, his statements relating to the cycling of water through the hydrosphere are basically correct, albeit overly simplified. Water moves in what is essentially a closed system, circulating from one part of the earth to another, changing in form from liquid to solid or gas and back to liquid again, yet remaining relatively constant in total amount. Water occurs as vapor in the atmosphere, as rain or snow falling on the earth or oceans, as ice locked in massive glaciers or ice caps, and as rivers, streams, lakes, seas, and subterranean groundwater. The manner by which water moves from place to place, changing from one form to another, is called the hydrologic cycle.

Hydrologic Cycle

The hydrologic cycle, like virtually all other processes on earth, is powered by energy from the sun that causes water to evaporate from the surface of the oceans, rivers, lakes, and from the soil. The movement of this water vapor in the atmosphere is an important factor in the redistribution of heat around the earth. Because heat is absorbed when water evaporates, the atmosphere becomes a reservoir of heat energy. This heat energy then drives the hydrologic cycle that gives rise to the atmospheric forces involved in weather and climate. The principal processes involved in the hydrologic cycle are:

1. Evaporation of water from surface waters and from the soil.
2. Transportation of water by plants; because both evaporation and transpiration produce the same result (i.e., the addition of water vapor to the atmosphere), the two processes are often collectively called evapotranspiration.
3. Transport of atmospheric water from one place to another as water vapor or as liquid water droplets and ice crystals in clouds.
4. Precipitation when atmospheric water vapor condenses and falls as rain, hail, sleet, or snow.
5. Runoff, whereby water that has fallen finds its way back to the oceans, flowing either on or under the surface of the continents.

Figure 14-1   Hydrologic Cycle

The amount of time required for the completion of the cycle can vary widely from place to place and from one part of the cycle to another. On the average, a water molecule spends nine days in the atmosphere from the time it evaporates until it falls again as rain or snow (Ehrlich, Ehrlich, and Holdren, 1977). However, if it happens to fall as a snowflake on the Antarctic ice sheet, it may remain there for thousands of years before it breaks off as part of an iceberg and melts into the ocean; conversely, if it falls during a desert thunderstorm, it might evaporate in an hour or two.

Approximately 71% of the earth's surface is covered with water, a resource amounting to almost 1.5 billion km^3 in total volume. Of this amount, however, only a very small percentage is readily available for human use. Most of the water on the planet, about 97.4%, is found in the world's seas and oceans—enormously abundant but too salty for drinking or agricultural use; 2% is freshwater locked up in glaciers and polar ice caps; the remainder, less than 1% of the total, consists of freshwater in rivers, lakes, groundwater, and water vapor in the atmosphere (World Resources Institute, 1992; Maurits la Riviere, 1989). Obviously, for humans this is the portion of greatest significance, since it constitutes the water we drink, bathe in, and use for irrigation and industrial purposes. Of this small percentage of water on which human life depends, only a minuscule portion is found in the rivers, streams, and lakes of the world. Likewise, at any given moment only a tiny amount of the world's water occurs as atmospheric water vapor. By far the greatest amount of all available freshwater, approximately 96.5% of the total, is found beneath the surface of the soil in the form of groundwater.

Water Quantity and Health

The human body's absolute dependence on regular intake of water is second only to its need for oxygen. While an individual can, if necessary, survive for a number of

Box 14-1   Desalination—Solution to the Water Crisis?

Answering a reporter's question as to what scientific progress he would like to see during his term of office, President John F. Kennedy in 1961 replied that if we could perfect technology to convert seawater to freshwater at reasonable cost, such an accomplishment "can do more to raise men and women from lives of poverty than any other scientific advance." Like Kennedy and numerous other visionaries, inhabitants of arid coastal regions have long dreamed of transforming seawater into a potable beverage. President Kennedy's aspirations may have sounded far-fetched in the early 1960s when there were only five desalination plants in the entire world. Today, however, such schemes no longer seem unrealistic, as pressures on the world's freshwater resources spur developments that make desalination projects both technologically feasible and increasingly common in water-short areas of the world.

Worldwide desalination capacity has been growing at an annual rate of 11% in recent years. According to the United Nations 2003 World Water Development Report, by 2002 there were about 12,500 desalination plants in operation in more than 120 countries around the globe. Of various sizes and types, these facilities produce, collectively, about 4 billion gallons (14 million cubic meters) of freshwater from the sea each day (an amount which, nevertheless, represents less than 1% of total water use). The leading producer of desalted seawater is the oil-rich desert kingdom of Saudi Arabia, boasting 34 desalination plants that yield over 800 million gallons a day of desalted water. Approximately 70% of the world's desalinated water is produced there and in several neighboring Gulf countries. A distant runner-up is the United States (6.5% of total world capacity), where the largest desalination facility in North America commenced operations in March 2003. Located on Tampa Bay, Florida, production at the facility has been intermittent due to financial and technical problems, but local water authority officials anticipate that the Tampa Bay desalination plant will soon be producing 25 million gallons of high-quality drinking water daily—an amount intended to supply 10% of the drinking water needs of the rapidly growing tri-county Tampa area.

Elsewhere in the U.S., five projects are in the developmental stage in southern California; the San Diego Water Authority hopes by 2008 to open a $270 million desalination facility twice the capacity of the Tampa Bay plant. Located adjacent to the Encina Power Station in Carlsbad where it can utilize the existing infrastructure for intake and discharge of seawater, San Diego authorities expect the output of this plant to meet almost 10% of the region's need for imported water. Plans for other desalination facilities are currently under review by coastal cities in Texas and Florida. Two other large plants, one built at Key West in the 1980s, the second at Santa Barbara in the 1990s, functioned only briefly due to high operational costs and to the fact that both municipalities subsequently found cheaper sources of water elsewhere.

The technologies for desalting seawater are straightforward and relatively simple. The traditional fuel-intensive method, still in use at most desalination plants in the oil-rich Middle East, employs a multistage flash distillation process, in which water is heated under pressure and then injected into a low pressure chamber where it instantly "flashes" into steam which is captured and condensed into pure water. The fact that pressurized hot water from a single source can be flashed into several chambers simultaneously makes it possible to produce large amounts of water quite dependably by this method. The modern, more energy-efficient approach, utilized by the Tampa Bay facility and in the development plans for the San Diego desalination plant, relies on reverse osmosis, a process by which seawater is forced, under high pressure, through semipermeable membranes that permit passage of water molecules but screen out the slightly larger ions of sodium and chlorine.

The problem with both methods—and the main factor limiting desalination—is the enormous amount of energy needed to power both processes, a requirement that translates into a high price per unit of water. Although recent advances in reverse osmosis technology have cut desalination costs by more than half, it is still considerably more expensive than obtaining the same amount from conventional freshwater sources. While the premium price associated with desalinated water may be acceptable to meet the escalating demand for drinking water in arid regions where other supply alternatives are scarce or nonexistent, desalination is still far too expensive for irrigation or industrial purposes—categories that comprise 85% of all water demand. While some skeptics point out that water conservation measures can, in many situations, provide the additional water to meet growing demand at a small fraction of the cost of desalination, in some regions water from the sea may be the only available option. At a time when global warming threatens increased likelihood of prolonged dry spells and worsening of current water shortages,

desalination offers a drought-proof solution to humanity's water supply needs. The fact that many of the regions currently most in need of water border oceans or seas is another reason for aggressive pursuit of the desalination option. Although encouraging progress has been made in recent years, a greater research commitment on the part of both government and the private sector is needed if desalination is to satisfy more than a small fraction of the world's water needs anytime in the foreseeable future.

References

Levin, Ted. 2004. "Turning Oceans Into Tap Water." *On Earth* 26, no. 2 (Summer).

Simon, Paul. 1998. *Tapped Out*. Welcome Rain Publishers.

U.S. Desalination Coalition. 2004.

weeks without food, deprivation of water will result in death within a few days at the most. Water makes up approximately 65% of the adult human's body, a somewhat higher percentage in children. Blood consists of 83% water, while bones contain 25%. Water is essential for the body's digestion of food, transport of nutrients and hormones, and removal of wastes. Depending on a person's size, weight, degree of activity, and the prevailing level of temperature and humidity, an individual requires approximately 1–3 liters of water daily just to maintain bodily functions.

To maintain good health and an adequate standard of living, however, 50 liters of water per day are considered the bare minimum essential for drinking, food preparation, cooking, dish washing, and bathing (Simon, 1998). The use of sewer systems for safe removal of human wastes—wastes that present serious problems when mismanaged—also requires considerable amounts of water. In typical urban residential areas, sewers will not transport wastes efficiently if per capita water use is less than 100 liters a day. In industrialized countries and among the more affluent segments of the urban population in developing nations, water quantity is generally more than ample to meet these basic human needs; average daily water consumption in such situations ranges between 200–400 liters per person per day. However, in developing countries almost 1.5 billion people still lack access to adequate supplies of safe water, in spite of impressive gains made during the United Nations-sponsored 1981–1990 International Drinking Water Supply and Sanitation Decade (WRI, 1998). In many rural areas the problem is not the lack of water per se, but rather that the source of such water is far from the point of use. In some countries, women may spend several hours each day hauling water from a distant river, well, or standpipe to their homes, leaving little time for more economically productive tasks such as gardening or trading in the marketplace. The sheer physical effort involved in carrying water long distances also exerts a toll on the health of rural women who, not infrequently, may be malnourished and overworked. In most urban areas of the Third World, water supply systems are in place, but frequently they are in poor condition or are unreliable, functioning perhaps only a few hours each day. While walking distances for the urban poor are less than for their country cousins, such people nevertheless spend hours waiting in long lines for their turn at the standpipe. Among many poor urban residents in the Third World,

In developing countries like Ethiopia, women must often travel long distances on foot to obtain the daily water supply for their households.

water is obtained by purchasing it from vendors at a cost many times higher than the cost per unit of a piped-in municipal supply. The necessity of buying water imposes a heavy financial burden on family incomes; in Port-au-Prince, Haiti, 20% of a typical slum-dweller's household budget is spent on water.

In situations such as these, where safe water is in short supply, difficult or time-consuming to obtain, or exorbitantly expensive, important aspects of personal hygiene and basic sanitation such as washing hands and eating utensils are frequently neglected. In addition, there is a strong temptation to utilize polluted sources of water if higher-quality supplies are not easily accessible. A study published by the World Health Organization demonstrated that improved access to water reduced the incidence of diarrheal cases by 25%, while improvements in both water quality and access reduced such illnesses by fully 37%. Perhaps the most essential prerequisite for improving the health and living standards among the Third World poor is an increase in readily available safe water (Briscoe, 1993).

Water Supply: Our Next Crisis?

While water is indeed a renewable resource, the rate at which it is renewed within the global hydrologic cycle is both fixed and slow. Water also is a finite resource—although human technologies can devise means for utilizing the existing supply more efficiently, science cannot create additional water nor alter the rate at which water is circulated through the biosphere. Faced with these realities, many water resource experts view current water use trends with alarm, warning that the approaching "water crisis" which they foresee could be the first resource constraint to impose serious limits on future world economic growth. Such fears are based on the fact that over the past 300 years worldwide, withdrawals from freshwater resources have increased more than 35-fold and continue to grow rapidly. Since the beginning of the 20th century, water consumption has risen more than twice as fast as the rate of population growth. A continuation of this trend in the years ahead appears likely, as water demand from growing cities, industry, and irrigated agriculture steadily increases. A recent United Nations assessment of freshwater resources reported that 2.3 billion people live in river basins now experiencing "water stress," defined as those where the amount of renewable freshwater per person is under 1,700 cubic meters annually, a situation that could result in frequent water shortages. Of these people, 1.7 billion reside in regions where yearly per capita water availability is under 1,000 cubic meters, a situation termed "water scarce." In these river basins inadequate water supplies can adversely impact food production, economic development, human health, the provision of sanitary services, and the viability of natural ecosystems. If current water use trends persist, researchers project that the number of people living in water-stressed river basins could rise to 3.5 billion people—48% of world population—by 2025, with 2.4 billion of these enduring high stress water shortages (WRI, 2000).

According to experts, recent water emergencies, precipitated by drought or water mismanagement, are harbingers of more difficult times to come. At first glance, such gloomy predictions seem at variance with the facts. Although the amount of freshwater readily available for human use constitutes less than 0.01% of all the water on earth, it still represents an abundant supply—theoretically sufficient to satisfy the needs of 20 billion people if equally divided (Maurits la Riviere, 1989). Obviously, however, neither the planet's water resources nor its human population are evenly distributed. Depending on local patterns of annual precipitation and evaporative demand (i.e., the maximum amount of moisture the atmosphere is capable of absorbing), water availability varies widely from one region to another. In the United States, for example, average annual rainfall is approximately 30 inches. This amount is distributed quite unevenly, however; whereas the Pacific Northwest receives about 80 inches of precipitation annually and the states east of the Mississippi River average 40–45 inches, the Great Plains and the Southwest are chronically water short. The driest state, Nevada, receives only 9 inches of rainfall in an average year. Viewing the world as a whole, nations lying between 20–30 degrees of latitude both north and south of the equator (the transition zone between temperate and tropical regions) tend to have the lowest annual rates of precipitation and also are most subject to recurrent droughts. Perhaps not by coincidence, these lands are home to some of the world's poorest countries and experience some of the highest population growth rates. Even within regions where water supplies are usually adequate, periodic dry spells and increasing industrial and municipal demands may result in localized shortages. Compounding the problem of regional disparities in water supply is the fact that everywhere—both in water-rich and water-poor areas of the world—pollution is rendering much of the available supply unusable without extensive (and expensive) treatment.

Impact of Population Growth on Water Demand

To some extent, water demand within a society is determined by that society's level of affluence and technological development. On a per capita basis, today's largest water consumers are the rich nations of the industrialized world. Although data issued by the U.S. Geological Survey in 2004 revealed that per capita water consumption in the United States has dropped more than 25% since its peak in the late 1970s, thanks largely to water conservation initiatives, the average American still consumes, directly or indirectly, many times more water each year than the average Third World resident. However, in the years ahead the major factor accounting for increased water demand, especially in urban areas, will be the explosive growth of human populations. Within any region, the amount of available water, determined primarily by precipitation, is finite. Thus, the amount available per capita is directly proportional to population size. While more efficient water management can help ensure more equitable distribution and prevent wastage, unchecked population growth will inevitably result in chronic water shortages. The problem is most acute today for the countries of the Middle East (see box 14-2), a naturally arid, drought-prone region with some of the world's highest birth rates. Of the 15 countries currently designated by the UN as "water scarce," 12 are in the Middle East or North Africa. Among these are Yemen (where per capita water availability is already less than 250 cubic meters per year) and the Palestinian Territory, both of whose populations will double in about 20 years and where the economic and technological ability to deal with the challenges posed by water scarcity is extremely limited (Roudi-Fahimi, Creel, and de Souza, 2002).

The impact of burgeoning population on water supplies promises to be most sorely felt in Third World cities. Even in countries where national averages indicate adequate water resources, runaway rates of urbanization and industrialization are seriously endangering both the quantity and quality of water supplies within many metropolitan areas. In China, where authorities admit that existing water supplies can sustainably support no more than half that country's current population (Hinrichsen, 2003), overpumping of groundwater to meet soaring urban water demand has resulted in drastic lowering of the water table in many areas. Since the 1960s, the water table

Box 14-2 War Over Water?

"Whiskey is for drinking and water is for fighting over." This truism from the 19th century American "Wild West" could be relevant to future struggles simmering just below the surface in many water-short regions of the world today. World population passed the 6 billion mark in 1999 and is expected to increase by another 2.5–3 billion within the next 25 years. Water *demand*, driven by a rising global standard of living, is increasing at twice the rate of population growth, but the world's water *supply* is constant and finite. Today nearly 1.5 billion people lack access to adequate supplies of clean water, a third of all countries are experiencing water stress, and the problem is steadily growing worse. Obviously a crisis looms in the not-too-distant future; neither people nor nations can survive without water and when faced with a dangerously dwindling essential resource, governments typically resort to war. As one international law expert warns, a shortage of freshwater is likely to be *"the* national security issue of the 21st century." Prospects for peaceful resolution are not helped by the fact that 261 large rivers flow between two or more countries, while 80% of the avail-

able freshwater and close to 47% of the world's land area (excluding Antarctica) lies within shared river basins. Yet in spite of the potential for conflict, no enforceable body of international law governs the use or allocation of these waters. As a result, those who pay attention to such matters are bracing for trouble. Klaus Toepfer, Executive Director of the United Nations' Environment Programme, sees future wars over water as a distinct possibility.

A number of potential flashpoints for water wars exist around the world, including the Ganges basin in south Asia, where water diversions to boost Indian crop yields are depriving Bangladeshis of their traditional share of the river's flow, and the River Nile, indispensable to the life and economic survival of 75 million Egyptians, yet controlled by upstream Ethiopia and Uganda who have plans of their own for utilizing its waters. After signing the historic peace accord with Israel, Egyptian President Anwar Sadat remarked that henceforth only water could induce Egypt to go to war again.

Perhaps nowhere is the looming water supply crisis more acute than in the volatile Middle East, where all major rivers are shared and where several nations are over-pumping groundwater from common aquifers. Throughout the region, the nature of each country's water woes is remarkably similar: a naturally arid to semiarid climate, rapidly falling water tables due to over-pumping, and exploding population growth.

In the Jordan Valley, Israelis, Palestinians, and Jordanians compete for shrinking water supplies which, even if equitably shared, are insufficient to meet the demand. In Israel, renewable water supplies are being overdrawn by close to 30% annually. Thanks to rapid population increase spurred by unprecedented levels of Jewish immigration from Russia, as well as high birth rates among Israeli Arabs, water demand in Israel has been soaring. Certainly the current water situation is complicating efforts to conclude a lasting peace agreement with Israel's Arab neighbors, who feel Israel is taking more than its fair share of the region's water. Jordanians protest Israeli diversions from the Sea of Galilee into an aqueduct serving Tel Aviv, thereby diminishing the flow of the Jordan River and rendering it too saline for irrigation. Jordanian attempts to stave off impending water shortages by drilling deeper wells, improving the efficiency of irrigation, and reusing wastewater effluent for irrigation constitute little more than stop-gap solutions. For a nation that is 70% desert, has only one small river entirely within its own territory, and a population of 5.5 million, expected to double within 28 years, Jordan's water supply challenges appear almost insurmountable.

In the occupied West Bank, Palestinians chafe under military orders that cut off their access to irrigation water from the Jordan River while simultaneously setting limits on the amount of water they can withdraw from existing wells and prohibiting the digging of new ones. In the meantime, Palestinians charge, Israeli settlers pumping from the same aquifer are under no such restrictions and have withdrawn so much water that many Arab wells have gone dry. One resentful Palestinian commented to an interviewer that "No one can accept that he does not have water to drink and his neighbor has a swimming pool." In Gaza the water situation is even more critical. Completely dependent on a single heavily polluted aquifer, Gazans are pumping water out of the ground at more than twice the rate of natural recharge. As a consequence, the water table is falling rapidly, and saltwater intrusion into the coastal aquifer, added to the chemical and biological contamination, threatens to render Gaza's groundwater reserves undrinkable within the next few years.

While political tensions over water appear most immediate and serious in the Jordan basin, in the Tigris-Euphrates watershed two other nations with rapidly growing populations—Syria and Iraq— nervously speculate on the water-hoarding intentions of an upstream neighbor. Turkey, one of the few Middle Eastern countries with an adequate supply of water within its borders, is engaged in a major development project in its arid southeastern Anatolia province. Consisting of a series of irrigation and hydroelectric dams on the Tigris and Euphrates Rivers, including the massive Ataturk Dam 340 miles southeast of Ankara, Turkey's Southeast Anatolia Project has neighboring countries seriously worried. While bringing immense benefits to the Turkish people in terms of electrical power and water for irrigation, the project could conceivably reduce the volume of the Euphrates by as much as 50% by the time it reaches Syria. Further downstream, Iraq could experience diminished flows of as much as 90% if water-sharing agreements are not worked out among the three countries. Although Turkey has behaved responsibly thus far, Turkish leaders intend to expand their irrigated acreage, a fact that almost certainly means less, more saline water for nations downstream.

As pressures on water resources mount throughout the world, logic suggests that national leaders would set aside the fear, mistrust, and hostility that have poisoned their relations in recent decades and seek common ground in forging cooperative water management agreements. Unfortunately, there are few indications as yet that either political leaders or the general public are giving the issue of water scarcity the priority it deserves. By the time they do, it may be too late to prevent disaster.

References

Simon, Paul. 1998. *Tapped Out*. Welcome Rain Publishers.

Ward, Diane R. 2002. *Water Wars*. Riverhead Books.

beneath portions of Beijing has dropped more than 110 feet, and by the mid-1990s farmers in the surrounding rural areas were no longer allowed to draw irrigation water from nearby reservoirs because city dwellers' demands for existing water supplies took precedence over the needs of agriculture (Postel, 1996; Brown and Halweil, 1998). Pollution of existing sources further reduces the usable water supply in many cities of the developing world. Bodily wastes generated by soaring numbers of urban poor lacking the most basic sanitation facilities have so polluted many urban water supplies with microbial pathogens that cities from Shanghai to Lima have been forced to divert millions of dollars from other urgently needed projects to finance increased levels of wastewater treatment. Such problems will become even more severe in the years ahead if current population growth trends persist.

Groundwater

Mention "water resources" and most people immediately think of rivers, lakes, and constructed reservoirs—surface water sources that are visible, accessible, and useful not only for direct consumption but for transportation and recreation as well. However, as pointed out earlier, over 96% of all available freshwater supplies occur in the form of groundwater, a resource whose immense importance is often overlooked and little understood by the general public. More than 25% of the U.S. water supply consists of groundwater. Over half of all Americans and 1.5 billion people worldwide rely on underground sources for their drinking water (Glennon, 2002). In Asia, groundwater provides over half the drinking water in most countries, while in Europe the proportion of domestic supplies derived from groundwater is even higher—as much as 98% in Denmark, 96% in Austria, and 88% in Italy (Gleick, 1993). This vast, unseen reservoir flows very slowly toward the sea and is a major source of replenishment for most surface water supplies. Estimates indicate that most rivers receive as much of their flow from groundwater seepage as from surface runoff; such rivers may experience a drastic diminution of flow or dry up entirely if too much water is pumped from nearby wells.

Groundwater supplies constitute an invaluable natural resource—one that has long been regarded as having certain inherent advantages over surface water supplies. Groundwater is usually cleaner and purer than most surface water sources. This is true because the soil through which it percolates filters out most of the bacteria, suspended materials, and other contaminants that find easy access to rivers and lakes. In addition, because evaporation is virtually nil and seasonal fluctuations in supply are small, groundwater supplies are dependable year-round. In terms of cost, groundwater has advantages also. The expense of digging a well is generally less than that of piping surface water to its place of use, and because of its greater purity it is less expensive to treat prior to consumption.

Until recently, communities relying on groundwater for their municipal supplies tended to take this resource largely for granted. Today, however, a sense of alarm is spreading with the realization that the twin evils of pollution and over-use are threatening the integrity of groundwater supplies. To understand how this situation has come about, it is necessary to take a brief look at the physical characteristics of our groundwater resource.

Nature of Groundwater

When rain falls upon the earth, that which is not taken up by plant roots or lost as surface runoff percolates downward through the soil until it reaches the water table.

Contrary to what some people think, the water table is not a vast underground lake or river, but the upper limit of what hydrologists call the **zone of saturation**—an area where the spaces between rock particles are completely filled with water. Such moisture-laden strata are called **aquifers** (Latin for "water carriers"). Above the zone of saturation lies the **zone of aeration,** where some soil moisture may be found as capillary water—useful for plants but incapable of being pumped out by humans. The zone of saturation extends downward until it is limited by an impermeable layer of rock. Sometimes there are successive layers of groundwater separated by impermeable rock layers. Aquifers may range from a few feet to several hundreds of feet in thickness and they may underlie a couple of acres or many square miles. They may occur just below the soil surface or thousands of feet below the earth, though seldom deeper than two miles.

Figure 14-2   Nature of Groundwater

Source: U.S. Geological Survey, *A Primer on Groundwater.*

The amount of water that any given aquifer can hold depends on its **porosity**—the ratio of the spaces between the rock particles to the total volume of rock. Sand and gravel aquifers are examples of rocks with high porosity. Additionally, if water is going to move through an aquifer, its pores must be interconnected. To qualify as a good aquifer, a rock layer must contain many pores, cracks, or both. The rate of water movement through an aquifer varies, not surprisingly, with the type of rock: through gravel it may travel tens or hundreds of feet per day; in fine sand only a few inches or less per day. When hydrologists measure the flow of surface streams, they do so in terms of feet per second; when measuring groundwater flow, figures in feet *per year* are the rule.

Groundwater Pollution

The inherent superiority of groundwater over surface water due to its supposed freedom from contamination can no longer be taken for granted. In recent decades, chemical, biological, and radiological contaminants from a wide variety of sources have been identified in groundwater deposits throughout the world. Although estimates by the National Research Council suggest the total geographic extent of groundwater pollution in the United States remains quite limited, such cases tend to occur in populated areas where the aquifer in question may be the principal or only source of local drinking water. Such findings have raised legitimate concerns among the public regarding both acute and chronic health effects and have resulted in the closure of hundreds of wells, affecting the water supplies of millions of Americans. In numerous cases involving synthetic organic chemicals, levels of contamination have been many times higher than those found in the most heavily polluted surface waters. Within affected communities the discovery that wells are contaminated frequently has come as an unwelcome surprise since, contrary to the situation in lakes and rivers, groundwater pollution is in a sense hidden, out of sight and difficult to detect without sophisticated chemical analyses. Since many pollutants in groundwater are colorless, odorless, and tasteless, citizens may unknowingly consume health-threatening poisons for years. Because routine tests performed to ensure drinking water safety have only recently been expanded to include monitoring for toxic chemicals, well water pollution in the past was often detected only when noticeable numbers of people began to fall ill. Amendments to the Safe Drinking Water Act in 1986 significantly expanded the number of contaminants that public water systems must monitor in both surface and groundwaters. However, these regulations do not cover the approximately 10.5 million private wells, mostly in rural areas, which frequently are shallower and thus even more vulnerable to pollution than municipal wells (Sanford and Oosterhaut, 1991). Since well water traditionally has been regarded as pure enough to drink untreated, not all the public water systems in the U.S. that utilize groundwater sources disinfect the water prior to distribution. Likewise, very few of the noncommunity systems disinfect well water and a negligible number of private well owners chlorinate their supplies. Given the extent of microbial contamination that has been identified in groundwater in recent years and the failure of many suppliers to treat such water, it's not surprising that over half (58%) of the reported waterborne disease outbreaks in the U.S. between 1971–1994 were traced to the consumption of microbially tainted groundwater (NRC, 1999).

Degradation of groundwater supplies by human-generated pollutants occurs largely due to faulty waste disposal practices or poor land management. The most significant sources of contamination include the following.

Waste storage, treatment, or disposal facilities. Unplanned seepage from open dumps, landfills, waste ponds, underground storage tanks, tailings piles—even

Figure 14-3 Sources of Groundwater Contamination

Ground Water Movement
Intentional Input
Unintentional Input

Sewer Leakage

Pumping Well

Factory

Landfill, Dump, or Refuse Pile

Water Table Aquifer

Aquifer (fresh)

Water Table

Pumping Well

Irrigation Pesticide

Septic Tank Cesspool Discharge

Injection Well

Confining Zone

Leakage

Confining Zone

Discharge of Injection

Source: EPA, 1998. "National Water Quality Inventory 1996 Report to Congress." EPA Office of Water, 841-R-97-008 (April).

graveyards!—constitutes a well-recognized and severe groundwater pollution threat if such facilities are improperly sited. In the U.S., petroleum products leaking from underground storage tanks constitute the leading source of groundwater pollution in most states, with landfill seepage close behind (EPA, 1998). Design requirements for the development of new land disposal facilities emphasize incorporation of barriers to prevent leachate migration, thereby protecting groundwater quality.

Septic systems. On-site sewage disposal facilities constitute the third most commonly reported source of groundwater contamination in the United States. Such systems feature the deliberate discharge of wastewater effluent directly into the ground. If such facilities are properly sited, waste discharges pose little hazard, but if located adjacent to or uphill from an aquifer or well, a potential for pollution exists. Contamination from septic systems, which serve approximately 30% of U.S. households, can be either microbial or chemical. A number of outbreaks of waterborne diarrheal diseases such as salmonellosis, hepatitis A, and typhoid fever have been traced to well water contaminated by sewage from septic systems.

Pipes, materials transport, transfer operations. Unintentional leakage from sewers or oil pipelines or accidental spills during transport or transfer of hazardous substances can be another source of groundwater pollution. Studies of well water contamination with agricultural chemicals conducted by the Illinois EPA revealed that the majority of problems—and all those involving high concentrations of pollutants—could be traced to locations where pesticidal formulations were routinely prepared (and routinely spilled on the ground!) prior to field application.

Nonpoint sources of pollution. Many instances of groundwater contamination can be traced to substances discharged as a result of other activities: irrigation practices, mine drainage, field application of farm chemicals or manures, de-icing of highways, and urban street runoff, among the most notable examples. Sources such as these are responsible for a host of water quality problems, among them the elevated nitrate levels found in numerous private wells in farming areas and the high chloride content in wells in some northern states where large quantities of road salts are applied during the winter months.

The most disturbing aspect of groundwater pollution is the fact that by the time the problem is discovered, it is generally too late to do anything about it. Because of the very slow rate of groundwater flow, chemical pollutants will not be flushed out of an aquifer for many years after the source of contamination is cut off (conversely, and for the same reason, contamination of one part of an aquifer does not necessarily affect the use of other parts). Unlike the situation in surface waters, where naturally occurring microbes gradually break down organic pollutants, groundwater is largely devoid of the oxygen needed by the bacteria and other decomposer organisms that endow streams and lakes with their capacity for self-purification. Cleanup of a polluted aquifer, while theoretically possible, is so expensive and time-consuming that it is usually not feasible. The process generally involves drilling numerous wells, pumping out enormous quantities of water, treating the water to remove the contaminants, and then reinjecting the water into the aquifer (Rail, 1989). For all practical purposes, a community that finds its groundwater seriously contaminated has little choice but to close the affected wells and seek a new water supply. Groundwater protection strategies, therefore, logically focus on preventing pollution in the first place rather than on efforts to clean up an aquifer after the damage is done.

Groundwater Depletion

With water demand and per capita water consumption increasing steadily in recent decades, many groundwater-dependent regions of the world have experienced an alarming decline in the water table, a direct result of overpumping. Periodic fluctuations in the level of the water table are normal, with levels rising during wet periods and falling during dry spells (generally the water table is highest in the late spring, sinks in summer, rises somewhat during the fall, and reaches its lowest point just before the spring thaw). However, when the water table lowers persistently it means that more water is being taken out of the groundwater reservoir than is being returned to it through precipitation or stream flow. Such a situation is akin to mining an aquifer, and if continued over an extended time period it can permanently deplete the groundwater supply or render it uneconomical to exploit due to excessive pumping costs. Groundwater depletion problems have assumed major proportions in parts of the Middle East, North Africa, India, China, Thailand, Mexico, and the western United States (Postel, 1992).

Instances of groundwater "mining" can occur even in well-watered areas when demand generated by rapid population growth, along with residential and commercial development, result in a sharp decline in groundwater reserves. In the United States, however, depletion is most acute in arid regions such as the Great Plains and Southwest, where the insatiable demand for irrigation water and the water needs of homes and industries in the booming cities of the Sunbelt have resulted in serious groundwater overdrafts.

A classic case of groundwater depletion in the American West is exemplified by the exploitation of the Ogallala Aquifer, the world's largest underground water reserve. Underlying portions of eight states in the High Plains, the Ogallala supplies almost one-third of all the groundwater used for irrigation in the United States. This enormous sand and gravel formation was deposited millions of years ago as the eastern front of the Rocky Mountains eroded. The plentiful rains of Pleistocene times saturated the formation with water, but due to subsequent changes in the geology and climate of the region, replenishment of the aquifer by natural recharge ceased long ago. Consequently, the Ogallala in a very real sense represents **"fossil" water**—a nonrenewable resource much like coal or oil which, once gone, is gone forever. Thus the heavy rates of groundwater withdrawal which, beginning in the early 1940s, transformed 11 million acres of shortgrass prairie into lush expanses of corn, cotton, and alfalfa raised serious concerns about the region's long-term economic viability as the water table plummeted. Overpumping has been most pronounced in the Texas Panhandle where, by 1990, 24% of that state's portion of the aquifer had been depleted. Rates of extraction during the peak years of the early 1970s led some experts to project that the Ogallala's reserves would last only 40 more years and that production of corn, the crop with the highest water demand, would cease entirely within a few years. In fact, irrigated acreage in the High Plains of West Texas declined by 26% between 1979 and 1989. These cutbacks, along with more efficient irrigation techniques, have substantially reduced the rate of groundwater withdrawal in the region, but depletion is still estimated at 12 billion cubic meters annually (Postel, 1996).

Elsewhere in the world, several governments are repeating the mistakes made on the American High Plains. Both Saudi Arabia and Libya have embarked on short-sighted efforts to irrigate desert fields with prodigious amounts of fossil groundwater reserves. Although food self-sufficiency is the stated objective of these undertakings, many experts question the economic wisdom of depleting a nonrenewable resource for agricultural commodities that could be purchased with petrodollars at a much lower price than they are currently spending to encourage domestic production. At current rates of pumping, experts predict Saudi water reserves could be exhausted by 2007, while Libya's aquifer may be pumped dry sometime around 2050.

The impact of groundwater overdrafts extends well beyond constraints on irrigated agriculture. Aquifer depletion can precipitate serious environmental problems, the most visible of which is the drying up of many surface lakes and streams (recall that many rivers, particularly in dry climates, receive the bulk of their flow from underground sources with which they are in hydrologic contact). In Arizona, approximately 90% of streams that used to flow year-round, including Tucson's Santa Cruz "River," now just a dry wash, have dried up completely or been seriously degraded due to overpumping of groundwater. While rivers in the arid West have suffered most, similar scenarios have played out in recent years in eastern states as well; Massachusetts' Ipswich River and the Flint River in Georgia have both experienced drastic declines in volume due to excessive groundwater withdrawals from the aquifers that supplement their flow (Glennon, 2002).

In coastal areas around the world, excessive pumping of groundwater to meet the demands of growing urban populations has resulted in migration of seawater into depleted aquifers, contaminating existing freshwater supplies. Saltwater intrusion is now a serious problem in such far-flung cities as Jacksonville, Florida; Dakar, Senegal; Jakarta, Indonesia; and Lima, Peru. Along Israel's Mediterranean shoreline, 20% of the important coastal aquifer is now polluted and officials fear that one out of five coastal wells may have to be abandoned within the next few years. In the United States, saltwater intrusion is endangering water supplies in southern California, south Florida, and in portions of Long Island and New Jersey (WRI, 1992; Postel, 1992; Ashworth, 1982). In addition, as groundwater reserves are depleted, land subsidence is occurring, accompanied by the formation of fissures and faults that disrupt irrigation canals and highways, as well as endangering buildings. In Mexico City, where the pumping of groundwater to supply the needs of 18 million people greatly exceeds the rate of natural recharge, the 16th century Metropolitan Cathedral dominating the city's historic plaza is one of many structures now sagging precariously, and a main thoroughfare has assumed a roller-coaster configuration, both victims of land subsidence. Around Orlando and northern Tampa Bay, Florida, overexploitation of groundwater reserves has created huge sinkholes that virtually overnight swallow up chunks of roads, yards, and, occasionally, homes. Falling water tables are also resulting in the abandonment of hundreds of thousands of acres of irrigated lands, as energy costs render pumping too expensive to make such farming economically feasible.

Natural Recharge

Under natural conditions, aquifers are recharged by moisture filtering downward from the surface or by seepage from a lake or stream. The area of land that is the main source of the groundwater inflow is called the **recharge area** of the aquifer, and is characterized by permeable soils. This recharge zone may be many miles from the point at which the water is pumped out of the ground; and because groundwater flows so slowly, the natural refilling of an aquifer may be a very slow process, requiring many centuries in some cases.

In recent years it has become increasingly apparent that a major threat to both the quality and quantity of our groundwater supplies is the growth of industrial, commercial, and residential development within the critical recharge areas of an aquifer. When urban sprawl strips natural areas of most vegetation and covers what once was forest, farms, or pastureland with buildings and asphalt, the amount of precipitation that can penetrate the soil is greatly reduced. Even in rural areas, land degradation due to deforestation or overgrazing can have an adverse impact on groundwater recharge by reducing the absorptive capacity of soils and increasing the rate of surface runoff. Such factors assume heightened significance in regions where most of the annual precipitation falls during a distinct "rainy season." In some parts of India, for example, where 80% of the rainfall occurs during the summer monsoon, degraded soils can no longer capture as much of the deluge as in previous years and hence even high-rainfall areas now find themselves short of water during the nine dry months of the year.

Development within the recharge area can affect the quality as well as the quantity of groundwater. As human activities within such areas intensify, the potential for infiltration of contaminants from waste facilities, leaky sewage pipes, chemical spills, or street runoff increases. A growing realization of the importance of protecting groundwater resources has prompted many state governments in recent years to enact laws regulating the types of development and activities permitted within the critical recharge area of aquifers. In some areas land acquisition plans, funded by either state or local governments, have been instrumental in preserving sensitive recharge areas from potentially harmful development. Often, local citizens' groups have been extremely effective in generating the public support necessary for developing and implementing such programs.

Water Management: Increasing Supply versus Reducing Demand

"When the well's dry, we know the worth of water."

—Benjamin Franklin

In the past, as population increase and industrial development boosted urban water demand, cities typically sought to quench their growing thirst by searching for new sources to augment dwindling local supplies. Frequently their reach extended far beyond municipal borders to exploit previously untapped resources in the rural hinterlands. Doing so seemed an obvious solution for a number of reasons: the potential supply appeared limitless and, therefore, relatively cheap; such water generally was of high quality and required little expenditure for treatment; and legal rights to the watershed lands could usually be obtained easily, especially since rural residents seldom had the political savvy necessary to outmaneuver the urban interests that frequently dominated state legislatures. Thus today in places like southern California, where local sources supply only a third of the demand generated by a burgeoning population, the water that maintains lawns, fills swimming pools, and makes life pleasant in the Golden State is imported from the Colorado River, 170 miles to the east, and from sources in northern California as far as 400 miles distant. Similarly, when New Yorkers turn on the tap in Manhattan, the liquid that flows out could have originated from one of a thousand streams in the Catskills, Hudson, or Delaware River valleys. Hetch Hetchy Valley in Yosemite National Park provides much of the water supply for San Francisco; Denver taps the headwaters of the Colorado on the opposite side of the Rocky Mountains; and Oklahoma City pipes its supplies from reservoirs in the northeastern Oklahoma hill country more than 100 miles away (Ashworth, 1982).

Since the 1970s, however, city planners have tempered their once-automatic response of pursuing supply-side solutions. The scarcity of new untapped sources; the sharply escalating costs of building dams and reduced federal funding for the same; competition between urban and agricultural interests for existing supplies; growing opposition to such projects on environmental grounds; plus organized legal resistance

Box 14-3   Megadam on the Yangtze—Mega-Trouble Ahead?

"I hate all dams, large and small. If you are against a dam, you are for a river."

This sentiment voiced over 30 years ago by the late David Brower, an internationally renowned conservationist and founder of the Earth Island Institute, would probably be echoed today by Chinese environmentalists witnessing the ecological impacts wrought by ongoing work at the world's largest hydroelectric project. Construction of a gigantic dam to tame the mighty Yangtze River has been a dream of Chinese policymakers since the idea was first conceived by Sun Yatsen in 1919. Decades of political and economic upheaval postponed implementation of the grandiose scheme until 1994, when work began to excavate and prepare the dam's foundations. In November 1997, Chinese engineers diverted the Yangtze out of its riverbed and building of the Three Gorges Dam in Hubei province commenced. By the summer of 2003, electricity had begun to flow from the first batch of generators, with the dam scheduled for completion in 2009 when all 26 of its 700-megawatt turbines will be in operation. With a price tag of at least $24 billion (unofficial estimates range as high as $75 billion), Three Gorges may constitute the single most expensive construction project in history; whether it constitutes a wise investment or a catastrophic boondoggle remains a subject of intense controversy in China and abroad among experts debating the benefits and drawbacks of massive water management projects.

The practice of obstructing the flow of rivers with earthen barriers, thereby creating a reservoir of stored water, is at least 5,000 years old. Throughout history, humans have engaged in dam building to ensure an adequate supply of water for irrigating crops or to control flooding. By the 20th century, dam construction was also being promoted as a means of providing cheap, clean power, while the reservoirs created by hydroelectric dams offered opportunities for water-based recreation. Until the early 1900s, all dams were relatively small, but improvements in engineering technology and building skills ushered in a new era of megadam construction. In 2000 the World Commission on Dams counted 47,655 large dams (those 15 meters or more in height) in

more than 140 countries. During the first half of the 20th century, the United States was at the forefront of this trend; by 1945 the five largest dams on earth (Hoover, Bonneville, Fort Peck, Shasta, and Grand Coulee) were all in the western U.S.

In recent decades, however, the allure of megadams has been fading in the United States and other industrialized nations and few, if any, are expected to be built in the years ahead. Lack of suitable sites, high up-front costs, and mounting opposition due to a realization of the serious environmental and social impacts of large dams are constraining future dam construction. In fact, since the 1970s, nearly 300 small dams across the country have been dismantled, allowing waterways to resume normal flow. In 1997, for the first time ever, the U.S. government refused to relicense a small hydroelectric dam on Maine's Kennebec River and ordered its destruction because it was preventing migratory fish from returning to their spawning grounds upstream.

In the developing world, by contrast, the outlook for megadam construction is far different. Third World leaders view large dams as symbols of modernity and a highly visible source of national pride. Opponents of China's Three Gorges Dam are convinced that project is being promoted by government hardliners largely for political reasons—to demonstrate China's technological skills and the superiority of socialism. The current dam construction boom is fueled by rapidly growing demand for irrigation water and electricity, both of which additional dams are expected to provide. Today nearly half (22,000) of the world's large dams are in China; however, India currently has more dams under construction than any other country. Although Nepal's Pancheswar Dam will soon be the world's highest and Lesotho's Highlands Water Project represents the biggest dam-and-tunnel project on earth, nowhere will the impacts of dam construction, both positive and negative, equal those at the Three Gorges Dam.

In spite of the much-touted economic benefits of controlling the flood-prone waters of the Yangtze and harnessing the river's energy to ease electrical shortages in much of eastern and central China, groups opposed to the project are convinced these benefits will be more than offset by the dam's environmental and social costs. Construction at Three Gorges will irreversibly alter the ecology of the Yangtze River basin. Dam-induced changes in water chemistry and temperature are expected to have a seriously adverse effect on the river's now-abundant fish species, some of which are unique to the region where the reservoir will form. Observers fear that many commercial fish stocks are likely to disappear as a result. The dam itself will block upstream migration of at least 172 different fish species, preventing spawning. Periodic releases of water from the reservoir will scour the riverbed downstream, washing away small islands that constitute critical habitat for endangered species. Of most concern to local ecologists is the fate of the Chinese River Dolphin (*Lipotes vexillifer*), a "living fossil" descended from a 30-million-year-old species found only in the middle and lower reaches of the Yangtze. With fewer than a hundred individuals left, the dolphins' survival is severely threatened by loss of habitat, decline in food supply, and the potential for accidental collisions with increasing ship traffic. Efforts to relocate the dolphins to nature reserve areas elsewhere on the Yangtze have proven unsuccessful and Chinese naturalists hold out little hope that these unique aquatic mammals can be saved from extinction. Stressing the importance of the Yangtze as a genetic reservoir of freshwater species, Chinese ecologists are racing against the clock to identify and move to safer territory as many threatened fish and plant species as possible before they vanish forever.

Loss of high-quality agricultural land is another unavoidable consequence. Approximately 14,000 hectares of farmland will be inundated and more than 150 towns and hundreds of small villages will be flooded as well. In addition, extensive tree removal associated with dam construction is likely to result in high rates of erosion throughout the watershed, adding to rates of siltation in the world's muddiest river. While exact amounts are difficult to predict for such a mammoth undertaking, most experts agree that more than 70% of the sediment carried by the river will be trapped behind the dam each year, gradually reducing its hydropower potential and clogging the harbor at Chongqing. With its rate of flow impeded by the dam, the Yangtze's ability to flush human and industrial wastewater downstream will be diminished and pollution of the river is likely to worsen, especially as an increasing number of factories relocate close to the reservoir to take advantage of cheap power.

As the impounded Yangtze waters rise to form a 370-mile long reservoir behind the dam, China will lose approximately 1,300 archaeological sites, as well as some of the world's most spectacular scenery and a prime tourist attraction. More problematic is the resettlement and compensation of an estimated 1.2–1.9 million people living in the areas now or soon to be underwater. Although the Chinese government promised to give these people new homes and land equal to or better than those they were forced to evacuate, such lands simply don't exist in that already overpopulated country. Many of those displaced have been relocated to overcrowded marginal lands where living conditions are poor and job opportunities scarce. Government funds for resettlement have all-too-often been diverted to corrupt local officials and no channels for voicing grievances have been provided.

Within China, opposition to the Three Gorges Dam has been voiced by a number of prominent intellectuals, scientists, and journalists, but their views have not been widely reported within the country. The editor of a collection of essays (*Yangtze! Yangtze!*) critical of the project was imprisoned for a year without trial and threatened with execution, so it's not surprising that outspoken dissenters are few and far between.

Construction work at the dam continues to proceed "full steam ahead" and opponents acknowledge the project is now unstoppable. Whether Three Gorges turns out to be the economic panacea envisioned by China's political leaders or the "Chernobyl of hydropower" remains to be seen.

References

ChinaOnline, *Three Gorges Dam Project*, www.chinaonline.com. Accessed 08–13–04.

Gleick, Peter H. 1998. *The World's Water*. Washington, DC: Island Press.

Postel, Sandra, and Brian Richter. 2003. *Rivers for Life*. Washington, DC: Island Press.

The world's largest hydroelectric project, China's Three Gorges Dam, will harness the power of the Yangtze River when all phases are completed (estimated around 2009), but carries with it enormous social and environmental costs. [© *China Photos/Reuters/Corbis*]

by groups in areas targeted for water development have basically brought to a close the era in which city planners attempted to solve water problems through a supply augmentation approach. Today, in metropolitan areas as diverse as Los Angeles and Boston, the emphasis for ensuring adequate water resources has shifted decisively from increasing *supply* to managing *demand.*

Demand management, more commonly referred to by environmentalists as **water conservation,** can include several components: reducing overall use, reducing waste, and recycling used water so it can be made available for other purposes.

Water Consumption

To understand how demand management strategies can help meet increased water needs, it is necessary to examine current water use patterns. Worldwide, irrigated agriculture accounts for the lion's share of water consumption—almost 69% of the total. (In Asia, farmers account for fully 82% of all water use; in the United States, 41%; and in Europe, just 30%.) Industries are the second largest consumers of water at 23% (more in heavily industrialized areas, less in others), while household use averages about 8% worldwide (obviously, in regions devoid of irrigated agriculture, the percentage of water use attributed to household and industrial use are considerably greater than world averages indicate). Focusing on these three major categories of water consumers, what opportunities do water managers have for reducing demand?

Agriculture. As the largest user—and the largest waster—of water, agriculture also offers the greatest potential for substantial reductions in water demand, in most cases without reducing crop yields. Because irrigation water is almost everywhere priced far below its true value, farmers are given the impression that the supply is plentiful and thus have little incentive to invest in more efficient irrigation technologies. As

Agricultural irrigation is the largest user—and waster—of water. [*U.S. Department of Agriculture*]

a result, in most parts of the world irrigators continue to channel or flood water across their fields in a manner that would have looked entirely familiar to their ancestors thousands of years ago. Such practices waste, on average, more than 60% of the water applied, as evaporation or seepage from unlined channels robs thirsty plant roots of the moisture intended for them. More widespread use of advanced techniques such as the automated "drip irrigation" method developed by Israeli scientists can cut water loss to 5% and reduce energy expenses in the bargain. Since the 1980s, farmers in West Texas have achieved dramatic savings by adopting techniques of "surge irrigation" or by installing low-energy precision application (LEPA) sprinklers that can achieve water-use efficiencies as high as 95%; buried droplines approach 100% efficiency. Experts estimate that if the world's farmers could reduce water losses due to inefficient irrigation practices by as little as 10%, the amount saved would be enough to double current domestic use (Postel, 1992). Unfortunately, even though the use of water-saving irrigation methods has grown impressively since the mid-1970s, it is still used on less than 1% of the world's irrigated croplands (WRI, 1998).

Industry. The huge amount of water needed by factories and power plants for processing, cooling, or generating steam accounts for a sizeable portion of total water use in Europe (55%), North America (47%), and other highly developed areas of the world (WRI, 1998). Since water used by industry is not "consumed" in the traditional sense (i.e., it may become heated or polluted but isn't used up), industrial water use can be substantially reduced by recycling. Within the past decade or so, increasingly stringent federal mandates requiring treatment of industrial wastewater prior to discharge, coupled with the escalating costs of waste treatment and disposal, have given industry a strong incentive to embark on waste minimization strategies that entail recycling and reuse of process waters. Such efforts have resulted in sharp declines in water withdrawals in many industries. Further savings are likely in the years ahead as more and more industries recognize the advantages of climbing aboard the pollution prevention bandwagon.

Households. Although domestic water consumption averages far less than that used for agricultural and industrial purposes, societal norms and public health considerations require that such water be of very high quality, necessitating expensive treatment and distribution systems. In past years, municipal efforts in some areas to restrict residential water consumption were launched as a temporary reaction to drought conditions, largely abandoned when the rains returned or new supplies were tapped. Today urban planners are urging that water conservation become a way of life, even in areas of adequate rainfall, as a means of enhancing water availability and containing rising water costs. Contrary to popular belief, a call for water conservation is not a demand for citizens to change their lifestyle radically, nor does it necessarily imply deprivation. Rather, water conservation means making more efficient use of the resource available.

A number of years ago when a lengthy drought in the Northeast had dangerously lowered the levels of reservoirs supplying water to New York City, officials of the Big Apple sponsored a contest for the best water conservation slogan. One of the catchiest advocated, "Save water: take a bath with a friend!" Those who value their privacy can take heart from the fact that today's options for stretching scarce water supplies are far more sophisticated and entail considerably less personal sacrifice than the old Saturday night frontier practice of everyone bathing in the same progressively dirtier tub!

Water Conservation

Some of the major elements in an effective water conservation program include the following.

Rational water pricing. Pricing water to reflect its true cost is fundamental to the success of all other water conservation efforts. Ironically, in many cities current price structures reward profligate users through a system of declining block rates, whereby the cost of additional water units above a certain point is lower than the cost of the initial units. An opposite approach, now used in some major U.S. metropolitan areas, imposes *higher* unit costs on water use above a specified level, thereby encouraging conservation. Peak demand pricing (e.g., summer/winter price ratio of 3:1) can also help curtail profligate use of water for nonessential purposes. Studies conducted in the United States and elsewhere have shown that when water prices increase by 10%, household water consumption drops 3–7% (Bhatra and Falkenmark, 1992). Of course household water use can't be priced appropriately if it isn't metered. The failure of cities in many parts of the world to meter home water use actively discourages water conservation efforts, since consumers see no connection between the amount of water they use and the price they pay. Cities such as New York, Buffalo, Denver, and Sacramento witnessed declines in water use ranging from 10–30% after they installed residential water meters. Use of rational pricing as a tool for encouraging water conservation can be even more effective in the cost-conscious industrial sector. Faced with water prices substantially higher than those in the U.S., German industries use about half the amount of water consumed by their American counterparts (Ward, 2002).

Leak detection/correction programs. Both at the household and municipal level, leaky plumbing can waste enormous volumes of water. In homes, leakage accounts for 5–10% of all residential water consumption. A faucet that loses 1 drop per second due to a worn out washer is wasting 7 gallons of water each day; that figure rises to 20 gallons per day with a steady drip. A leaky toilet tank can waste fully 200 gallons per day without making a sound. (To check for toilet tank leakage, simply pour a small amount of food coloring into the tank; if color appears in the toilet bowl before it is flushed, leakage is occurring, probably caused by a worn-out or defective flush ball.) Correcting these leaks is the easiest and cheapest way to reduce home water consumption.

Figure 14-4 Major Water Users in a Typical U.S. Home

Source: American Waterworks Association.

Box 14-4 A World Marketplace for Water?

The headlong worldwide rush to open and integrate markets across national boundaries—a process known as "globalization"—has sparked one of today's most controversial water resource debates: should water continue to be regarded, as it has been for millennia, as a God-given "social good" available on an equal basis to all humankind or, in an age of increasing scarcity, should it be viewed as a commodity for international trade, subject to the same marketplace rules as diamonds, steel, or toys? As mounting population pressures boost world water demand at the same time climate change, overexploitation, and pollution reduce supply, will countries experiencing water deficits look to the abundant, "unexploited" reserves of water-rich regions as something they should be free to purchase, regardless of whether the people living in those areas oppose such transactions?

Since the early 1990s, concerns among policymakers over the failure of massive international efforts to ensure that people everywhere have access to clean water have led many to conclude that such needs can never be met without a thorough reordering of water use policies and priorities, as well as improvements in the efficiency of water use. Such thinking led delegates to the 1992 International Conference on Water and Environment, held in Dublin, Ireland, to declare that "Water has an economic value in all its competing uses and should be recognized as an economic good." Such a statement has profound implications and immediately provoked a heated, ongoing debate. The idea that water should be regarded as a product, to be bought and sold like any other commodity, is especially alarming to public interest groups, worried that the world's poor could find themselves unable to afford one of life's most essential resources; some compare the idea of trading water for money with selling air and argue that governments are violating their citizens' human and civil rights if they don't provide everyone with water at the lowest possible cost. Environmentalists also fear that free trade in water would ignore ecosystem protection, failing to take into account the vital role played by freshwater in providing habi-

tat for fish and other aquatic organisms, supporting vegetation and animal life along waterways, meeting the needs of water-based transportation and recreation, and contributing to society's aesthetic enjoyment in ways impossible to quantify in monetary terms.

On the other hand, the near-universal practice by which governments supply water at prices that bear little relationship to the true costs of acquiring and delivering that water all-too-frequently results in overuse and wastage. While water subsidies vary widely from city to city, as a global average residents pay their municipal governments just 35% of what it costs to supply that water. All too often, financially strapped cities compensate for the shortfall by neglecting to maintain water storage and delivery systems or by failing to extend service to the poorest sections of the community. Water subsidies also encourage inefficient use, exemplified by the fact that irrigated agriculture consumes 80% of California's water supply yet represents but 10% of that state's economy. Industrial water in California is valued at 65 times that of agricultural water; regarding water as an "economic good" by taking competing uses into account and maximizing water's value to society would radically alter the current allocation of supplies in the Golden State and many other water-scarce areas where irrational water pricing currently prevails. Since subsidized water encourages wasteful use while a classic free market approach threatens to deprive the poor of sufficient water to meet their basic needs, the challenge facing decision-makers is how to get the most value from available water while guaranteeing adequate supplies to those unable to pay and leaving enough water in place to avoid ecological damage.

One potential solution to water supply dilemmas, out-of-basin bulk water shipments are not a new concept, but in the past they have been limited to transfers within the same country or to short-term emergency situations. Since 1955, St. Thomas and St. John in the U.S. Virgin Islands have received sporadic seaborne shipments of water from Puerto Rico; inhabitants of several of the smaller Fijian islands regularly receive water from their larger neighbors during periods of drought; Turkey sends water to its compatriots on ·the island of Cyprus, utilizing both tankers and gigantic plastic-coated "Medusa bags" towed by ocean-going tugboats; Malaysia's offshore island of Penang gets a portion of its water via submarine pipelines from the mainland; and tiny Nauru, an island nation in the Pacific, receives up to a third of its water from Australia, New Zealand, and Fiji on ships returning to the island to pick up loads of phosphate, Nauru's primary export.

Visionary proposals for future international trade in water are more grandiose—and controversial—than these limited transfers, however. For years local boosters in the American Southwest have proposed schemes to divert vast quantities of water from Alaska and northwestern Canada to Arizona and southern California; Italians talk of building a pipeline under the Adriatic Sea to bring Albanian water to arid southern Italy; and Spain only recently dropped long-discussed plans to pipe water from France's Rhone River to Barcelona. As world water demand continues to mount, such proposals receive increasingly serious scrutiny. In March 2004, perennially water-short Israel signed a first-of-its-kind deal with Turkey, agreeing to purchase 50 million cubic meters of water annually for the next 20 years. This water, to be shipped from Turkey's southwestern Manavgat River to Israeli ports in huge converted oil tankers, will comprise about 3% of Israel's annual freshwater consumption and is expected to lay the foundation for that country's long-term water security.

Overshadowing all discussions about future trans-border trade in bulk freshwater is confusion over the rules pertaining to international water trade. Uncertainty persists as to whether bulk water can be considered a "product" and hence subject to existing international trade requirements (the qualifier "bulk water" is important, since bottled water and other processed, value-added waters have been internationally traded for decades, subject to the same trade rules as any other product) and, if so, whether exceptions under the General Agreement on Tariffs and Trade (GATT) would apply to efforts by a government to block or limit water sales it deems objectionable. GATT currently allows a country to impose trade restrictions on a product if doing so is necessary to protect human, animal, or plant life or health and in situations where such restrictions are related to the conservation of natural resources. There is considerable debate among legal experts, however, as to whether these resource conservation principles could be invoked to halt bulk water sales, and few legal precedents exist to suggest how potential future disputes would be resolved. In 1999 the U.S.-Canadian International Joint Commission, an independent binational organization established to help resolve disputes relating to the use and quality of boundary waters, attempted to safeguard Great Lakes water from future export threats by declaring that the Great Lakes constitute a nonrenewable resource, inasmuch as the overwhelming bulk of water they contain was laid down in the distant geologic past. Whether such a statement ensures a GATT exception from the rules governing international trade remains to be seen.

In the near future, large-scale trans-border commerce in bulk water is unlikely, due primarily to the high expense of moving water long distances. Reallocation of water among end users, improvements in water-use efficiency—even the construction of desalination plants—are usually less costly methods of increasing available supplies than shipping water from place to place by tanker. Nevertheless, over time the economics of water trading could change as demand escalates and new water transport technologies emerge. It is imperative that governments act now to formulate and institute national water policies to prevent the overexploitation and export of nonrenewable water resources and ensure that the water needed to safeguard human health and ecosystem stability is protected from the forces driving globalization.

References

Gleick, Peter H. 2002. *The World's Water: 2002–2003.* Washington, DC: Island Press.

Ward, Diane Raines. 2002. *Water Wars.* Riverhead Books.

Cities as well as households may suffer from leaky plumbing. The problem is particularly acute in many developing world cities. Plagued by chronic water scarcity, Amman, Jordan, loses 59% of the water flowing from its water purification plant to homes and institutions, thanks to leaky distribution pipes; in Manila, capital of the Philippines, the figure is 58%; in Mexico City, about one-third (Simon, 1998). Municipalities in the industrialized world are certainly not immune to such problems; it's estimated that cities in the United Kingdom may waste as much as 25% of all treated water due to leakage. In many older U.S. communities the pipes that carry water from a central treatment plant to thousands of homes, institutions, and businesses were installed during the 1800s or early 1900s and have for decades been in serious need of replacement. The current fiscal plight of many urban areas has resulted in short-sighted postponement of these urgently needed renovations. In those cities that have made the necessary investment, however, results have been striking. Prior to a major leak repair program, Boston was losing an estimated 20% of the water entering its distribution system each day; following completion of that program, officials credited leak repair with saving the city 35 million gallons daily.

Installation of water-saving plumbing devices. Technology now exists to cut household water use by close to one-half, with no loss of comfort or convenience. Since more water is used in the bathroom than any other room in the house, the focus of home water conservation efforts has been the installation of water-efficient toilets, showerheads, and faucet aerators. The prime candidate for replacement is the water-hogging conventional toilet which, at 5–7 gallons per flush (gpf), is the single largest water user in a typical American home. By the early 1980s, new low-flush (3.5 gpf) toilets became available, followed several years later by ultra-low flush (1.6 gpf) models offering significant water savings. Although early versions of the ultra-low flush toilets encountered customer complaints of poor performance (mainly the need to double-flush), re-engineering of the bowl has largely eliminated this problem. Recent surveys indicate the vast majority of purchasers find ultra-low flush toilets as good or better than the replaced models. In 1992 Congress passed the federal **Energy Policy Act**, establishing mandatory nationwide water efficiency standards for all toilets, urinals, faucets, and showerheads installed in the United States since 1997. These standards include the requirement that any new or replacement toilets sold or installed in the U.S. must be the ultra-low flush 1.6-gallon type. Since approximately 8 million new or replacement toilets are installed in the country each year, it is estimated that by 2025 water-conserving toilets will have replaced most of the pre-1994 stock currently in use. When complete, this transition is expected to result in nationwide water savings of 6.5 billion gallons per day.

Some cities plagued by chronic water shortages don't want to wait until 2025 to enjoy the full benefits of water savings offered by the new plumbing fixtures. As a result, they are providing financial inducements for citizens to replace older models now. Santa Monica, California, imposed a $2 per month "conservation incentive" fee for all single-family homes that hadn't installed low-volume toilets and showerheads. As a result, the city has now completed its toilet replacement program and achieved a permanent 15% reduction in average total water demand and a 20% decrease in total wastewater flow. Santa Rosa, California, requires that whenever new toilets are installed, all old showerheads and faucets must be upgraded also. To make the switchover more palatable, the city offers customers free low-flow showerheads and faucet aerators. During a plumbing rebate program that ended in 2002, Santa Rosa replaced over 46,000 toilets and city officials estimate the resultant water savings at 1.6 million gallons of water every day.

Altered landscape practices. Americans' deeply held conviction that a broad, verdant expanse of weed-free, neatly manicured grass is an essential component of any respectable residence constitutes a major obstacle to meeting urban water conservation goals. Across the United States, approximately 25 million acres are covered with cultivated lawns that annually consume prodigious amounts of fertilizers, pesticides, and high-quality treated water. In some communities in the western United States, fully 40–50% of household water use is devoted to maintaining lawns and gardens.

In an effort to discourage water wastage associated with landscaping practices, a number of communities have initiated some innovative programs aimed at changing American attitudes toward yard maintenance and design. In southern California, where a six-year drought (1987–1992) prompted major changes in water supply planning, the Metropolitan Water District has implemented landscape water conservation regulations for commercial, industrial, institutional, and multifamily properties; MWD is also encouraging similar practices for single-family residences and urging homeowners to select plantings that can thrive with minimal watering. Elsewhere, some communities have enacted legislation restricting the amount of yard space property owners can devote to grass. On Long Island, the town of Southampton, concerned about groundwater pollution by lawn chemicals, mandates that no more than 15% of a residential lot be devoted to fertilizer-requiring lawns or vegetables, while a minimum of 80% must be retained in its natural wooded condition; in Tucson, Arizona, an ordinance passed in 1991 prohibits planting grass on more than 10% of the landscaped area in new developments (Dziegielewski and Baumann, 1992).

Methods of managing water demand such as those just described, accompanied by intensive public information and conservation education programs, will play a major role in meeting future water needs. Encouraging results are already evident from recently launched programs in such disparate regions as southern California and metropolitan Boston, providing convincing evidence that water conservation not only will provide our largest single source of additional water within the next 20 years but will become an accepted way of life. Provided with appropriate technologies and a cost incentive, citizens, farmers, and industrialists alike will validate the assertion of water managers that the cheapest, quickest, most environmentally benign way to meet future water needs is to use existing supplies more efficiently.

References

Ashworth, William. 1982. *Nor Any Drop to Drink*. New York: Summit Books.

Bhatra, Ramesh, and Malin Falkenmark. 1992. "Water Resource Policies and the Urban Poor: Innovative Approaches and Policy Imperatives." *International Conference on Water and the Environment: Development Issues for the 21st Century*. Dublin, Ireland, January 26–31.

Briscoe, John. 1993. "When the Cup is Half Full: Improving Water and Sanitation Services in the Developing World." *Environment* 35, no. 4 (May).

Brown, Lester R., and Brian Halweil. 1998. "China's Water Shortage Could Shake World Food Security." *World•Watch* 11, no. 4 (July/Aug):10–21.

Dziegielewski, Benedykt, and Duane D. Baumann. 1992. "The Benefits of Managing Urban Water Demands." *Environment* 34, no. 9 (Nov).

Ehrlich, Paul, Anne Ehrlich, and John Holdren. 1977. *Ecoscience*. W. H. Freeman and Co.

Environmental Protection Agency (EPA). 1998. *National Water Quality Inventory: 1996 Report to Congress*. EPA 841-R-97-008 (April).

Gleick, Peter, ed. 1993. *Water in Crisis: A Guide to the World's Fresh Water Resources*. New York: Oxford Univ. Press.

Glennon, Robert. 2002. *Water Follies: Groundwater Pumping and the Fate of America's Fresh Waters*. Washington, DC: Island Press.

Hinrichsen, Don. 2003. "A Human Thirst." *World•Watch* 16, no. 1 (Jan/Feb).

Maurits la Riviere, J. W. 1989. "Threats to the World's Water." *Scientific American* (Sept).

National Research Council (NRC). 1999. *Setting Priorities for Drinking Water Contaminants.* Washington, DC: National Academy Press.

Postel, Sandra. 1996. "Dividing the Waters: Food Security, Ecosystem Health, and the New Politics of Scarcity." *Worldwatch Paper* 132 (Sept).

———. 1992. *Last Oasis: Facing Water Scarcity.* New York: W. W. Norton & Co.

Rail, Chester D. 1989. *Groundwater Contamination: Sources, Control, and Preventive Measures.* Technomic Publishing.

Roudi-Fahimi, Farzaneh, Liz Creel, and Roger-Mark de Souza. 2002. *Finding the Balance: Population and Water Scarcity in the Middle East and North Africa.* Population Reference Bureau.

Sanford, Cynthia, and Joe Oosterhaut. 1991. "Protecting Groundwater: The Unseen Resource." *The National Voter* 40, no. 5 (June/July).

Simon, Paul. 1998. *Tapped Out.* Welcome Rain Publishers.

Ward, Diane Raines. 2002. *Water Wars: Drought, Flood, Folly, and the Politics of Thirst.* Riverhead Books.

World Bank. *The World Development Report 1992: Development and Environment.* Washington, DC: World Bank

World Resources Institute (WRI). 2000. *World Resources 2000–2001: People and Ecosystems, the Fraying Web of Life.* World Resources Institute.

———. 1998. *World Resources 1998–99.* New York: Oxford Univ. Press.

———. 1992. *World Resources 1992–93.* New York: Oxford Univ. Press.

WATER POLLUTION

> Water, water everywhere
> Nor any drop to drink . . .
>
> —Samuel Taylor Coleridge
> (*The Rime of the Ancient Mariner*)

Back in the days when human settlements were relatively small and far apart, the issue of water contamination seldom occupied much attention on the part of the general public. Prevailing sentiment insisted that "the solution to pollution is dilution," and popular wisdom held that "a stream purifies itself every ten miles." While such statements have a certain amount of validity, they lost their relevance as villages mushroomed into crowded cities and as the expanse of countryside between towns steadily contracted under the impact of urban sprawl. The rapid growth of human population and of industrial output resulted in a corresponding decline in water quality, as both municipalities and industry regarded the nation's waterways as free, convenient dumping grounds for the waste products of civilized society. During the 19th century our careless waste-management practices turned most rivers into open sewers and many once-healthy lakes into algae-covered cesspools. It is estimated that most of the world's water drainage basins are polluted with such contaminants as toxic chemicals, human and animal excrement, heavy metals, pesticides, silt, and fertilizers. These contaminants are carried downstream where they are discharged into coastal estuaries and shoreline waters, effecting long-term changes in water quality. The problems posed by such pollutants involve far more than unpleasant sights and odors. Waterborne disease outbreaks, massive fish kills, long-lasting changes in aquatic ecosystems, and severe economic loss to sports and recreation-based industries are all directly related to degradation of water quality by human activities.

Controlling Water Pollution: The Clean Water Act

Although water pollution had been recognized as a major environmental problem in the United States for many decades, it was not until 1972 that a tough, comprehensive federal program to deal with this issue was enacted by Congress. Known originally as the Federal Water Pollution Control Act Amendments (Public Law 92–500), this landmark piece of legislation underwent some "mid-course corrections" in 1977, at which time its name was changed to the Clean Water Act. Prior to passage of this law, our nation's water pollution control strategy, such as it was, focused on attempts to clean up waterways to the point that they could be used for whatever purpose state governments had determined their function should be (e.g., drinking water, swimming, fishing, navigation, etc.). Thus each stream or portion of a stream might have a different water quality standard, and if that standard was not being met, it was up to the state water pollution control agency to determine which discharger was responsible for the violation and to seek enforcement action. This system was totally ineffective for a number of reasons: designations of desired stream use were frequently modified to retain or attract industrial development; insufficient information was available on how pollutant discharges were affecting water quality; blame for violation was difficult, if not impossible, to assess when more than one source was discharging into a waterway; little attention was paid to the effects of pollution on the aquatic environment as a whole; and only contaminants entering a waterway through pipe discharges were given much attention. Undoubtedly the most serious drawback of the pre-1972 water pollution control strategy was the lack of enforcement power. State agencies had to negotiate with all the polluters along a given waterway, trying to persuade each individual source to reduce its discharges to the point at which water quality standards for the particular river or lake in question could be met. Not uncommonly, when industries disliked what they were being told, they would threaten to close down and move to a less demanding state. Also, due to the nature of river basins, many states discovered that in order to improve their own water quality, they had to persuade states upstream to pollute less.

Passage of the Clean Water Act radically altered this approach to water pollution control and took a new philosophical stance toward the problem, reflected in the 1972 Senate Committee's statement that "no one has the right to pollute . . . and that pollution continues because of technical limits, not because of any inherent right to use the Nation's waterways for the purpose of disposing of wastes." Stressing the need to "restore and maintain the chemical, physical, and biological integrity of the Nation's waters," Congress declared as national goals the attainment, wherever possible, of water quality "that provides for recreation in and on the water" (popularly referred to as the "fishable-swimmable waters" goal) by July 1, 1983, and the elimination of all pollutant discharges into the nation's waterways by 1985 ("zero discharge" goal). These goals are not the same as legal requirements—they cannot be enforced and certainly were not attained by the dates indicated; nevertheless, they have been useful in providing objectives toward which to strive and against which progress in improving water quality can be measured.

Progress in moving toward the goals set forth by Congress is difficult to assess on a comprehensive national basis because budgetary constraints, both at the federal and state levels, preclude the possibility of continuously monitoring the quality of all U.S. waterways. In addition, water quality at any one location changes from season to season and year to year. Even determining long-term trends for specific pollutants is somewhat problematic because of the lack of historical records and inconsistencies in the data that have been collected. Also, since the various states and organizations that survey water quality utilize different monitoring strategies, it is often impossible to combine or compare survey results. Active efforts are currently underway to improve nationwide monitoring efforts and to establish an effective, uniform means of collecting, interpreting, and presenting water quality information. In the meantime, policymakers must rely on the EPA's biennial *National Water Quality Inventory*—a compilation of data submitted to the EPA by individual states, territories, Indian tribes, Interstate Water Commissions, and the District of Columbia. Existing data, while incomplete, indicate commendable improvement in the nation's water quality during the years since passage of the Clean Water Act, when fully 95% of all U.S. watersheds were regarded as polluted. During several decades when both the economy and population size have grown substantially, the fact that overall surface water quality hasn't deteriorated gives evidence that the billions of dollars spent on water cleanup efforts have had a positive impact. Nevertheless, EPA's most recent water quality assessment reported that 39% of U.S. rivers, 45% of lakes, and 51% of coastal estuaries surveyed still suffer levels of pollution that impair their use for one or more designated purposes, indicating we have a long way to go before the goals of the Clean Water Act are fully met. While many of the conventional sources and types of water pollution are now being dealt with fairly adequately, newer problems such as toxic chemical pollutants and difficult-to-control runoff from farms, construction sites, and city streets have stymied pollution abatement efforts (EPA, 2002).

Elsewhere in the world, water quality issues rank high on the list of international environmental concerns. Not surprisingly, progress in controlling water pollution varies widely from one country to another. Most developed nations have imposed controls on industrial dischargers similar to those in the United States and the majority have helped finance the construction of sewage treatment plants. As a result, by the first decade of the 21st century the vast majority of North Americans and Europeans were served by wastewater treatment facilities. Similarly, in Japan and South Korea, notable progress has been made during the past few decades in expanding access to sewage treatment, particularly in urban areas. Unfortunately, in many developing nations and most of the former Soviet republics the situation is bad and getting worse. Rapid industrial growth has given rise to numerous toxic "hotspots" of pollution, as industrial dischargers dump poisonous effluent into nearby waterways, unhindered by nonexistent or seldom-enforced water pollution laws. In China, for example, industrial discharges containing both toxic and carcinogenic compounds are fouling rivers that provide the main source of drinking water. Though many people attempt to protect themselves by boiling water before using it for human consumption, doing so has no effect on most toxic contaminants. Throughout the developing world untreated sewage, as well as salt- and fertilizer-laden irrigation return flows, further contaminate lakes, rivers, and coastal waters. In south Asia, south and southeast Pacific, and in Africa modern sewage treatment is virtually nonexistent; of India's 3,119 towns and cities, only 8 provide full treatment of municipal wastewaters. In developing countries as a whole, 95% of urban sewage is discharged untreated (Pimentel et al., 1998). Even in Latin America, where sanitary standards are generally better than in other developing regions, 24% of the urban population and 53% of those living in rural areas still lack access to adequate sanitary facilities (Nash and DeSouza, 2002).

To understand the worldwide impact of water pollution on the health of both ecosystems and their human inhabitants requires a look at the major sources and types of pollution and the problems posed by each. The remainder of this chapter will examine these issues and will describe the pollution control policies developed by the U.S. Congress and regulatory agencies as they strive to protect public health through improving water quality.

Sources of Water Pollution

Pollutants can enter waterways by a number of different routes. Strategies for preventing water contamination must take into consideration the nature of the pollutant source and must devise appropriate methods of control for each source category. Congress has coined two terms—**point source** and **nonpoint source**—to refer to the two general types of water pollution, and pollution control regulations adopted within recent years have by necessity been tailored according to source.

Point Sources

Pollutants that enter waterways at well-defined locations (e.g., through a pipe, ditch, or sewer outfall) are referred to as point source pollutants. Characterized by discharges that are relatively even and continuous, typical point sources of water pollution include factories, sewage treatment plants, and storm sewer outfalls. Point sources have been the most conspicuous violators of water quality standards, but because effluent from such sources is relatively easy to collect and treat, considerable progress has been made in reducing this type of pollutant discharge. The two major categories of point source pollution are sewage treatment plants and industrial discharges. Each will be discussed in greater detail later in this chapter.

Nonpoint Sources

Until the 1980s, nonpoint source (NPS) pollutants—those which run off or seep into waterways from broad areas of land rather than entering the water through a discreet pipe or conduit—were largely overlooked as significant contributors to water contamination. However, when stringent effluent limitations on point sources failed to result in dramatic improvements in water quality, it became increasingly evident that in many waterways the largest pollutant contribution was coming from nonpoint sources. Today the majority of states identify pollutants coming from nonpoint sources as the main reason they have been unable to attain their water quality goals. Nonpoint source pollution (really just new terminology for old-fashioned runoff and sedimentation) results primarily from a variety of human land-use practices and includes the following.

Agriculture. In the United States as a whole, agriculture is the leading source of water pollution, adversely affecting the quality of 50–70% of the nation's surface waters. Among the various contaminants present in farmland runoff, the single most abundant is soil. While most people tend to think of erosion largely in terms of its adverse impact on agricultural productivity, soil entering streams or lakes can severely damage aquatic habitats as well. By increasing the turbidity of the water, sediment sharply reduces light penetration and thereby decreases photosynthetic rates of producer organisms; it buries bottom-dwelling animals, suffocating fish eggs and aquatic invertebrates. Stormwater runoff from fields and pastures carries more than just sediment into waterways, however. Manures from grazing lands or from large livestock management facilities (i.e., "megahog" farms) located adjacent to streams or lakes can contribute five or six times as many nutrients to waterways as do point sources. Manure spread on fields can cause similar problems unless it is applied at rates moderate enough to permit complete uptake of nutrients by plants (i.e., at agronomic rates of uptake). In the same way, chemical fertilizers and pesticides, when applied immediately prior to a storm or in amounts exceeding the assimilative capacity of the crop in question, can be carried by runoff water from fields into adjacent lakes or streams. Upon entering a waterway, farm chemicals can poison fish or promote algal growth; if runoff seeps through the soil into shallow aquifers, it can contaminate drinking water wells. Since these toxic pollutants generally enter waterways attached to soil particles, they can best be controlled by the same strategies used to prevent soil erosion—conservation tillage, terracing, contour plowing, and so on. Additional management strategies include: applying pesticides when there is little wind and the potential for heavy rain is low; using nonpersistent, low-toxicity pesticides; disposing of containers properly; applying fertilizers or manures only when they can be incorporated into the soil (i.e., not when the ground is frozen); and using chemicals in the proper amount and only when field checks indicate they are needed. Controlling runoff from pasturelands

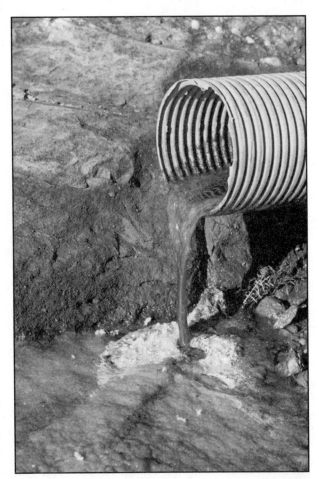

Point source of pollution (*right*): efflu-ents that enter a waterway directly from a factory outfall, pipe, ditch, or sewage treatment plant are the most visible source of water pollution.

Below: Farm runoff (a nonpoint source) is the leading source of water pollution in the U.S. today. [*USDA*]

Box 15-1 Hypoxia in the Gulf of Mexico

Journalists call it the "dead zone"—a huge underwater expanse on Louisiana's continental shelf that each summer becomes so oxygen-deficient that any creatures in the vicinity flee elsewhere or die. Extending over approximately 6,000 square miles (16,000 km^2) from the mouth of the Mississippi River almost to the Texas coast, this **hypoxic zone,** as it is properly termed, is characterized by waters with dissolved oxygen concentrations below 2 parts per million—the minimal amount required for survival of most species of marine organisms. Hypoxia is not a situation unique to the Gulf of Mexico. Several major water bodies—the Black Sea, Baltic Sea, and Chesapeake Bay, to name a few—have always experienced periodic bouts of hypoxia, as do many smaller lakes and ponds. The Gulf "dead zone" is generating unusual concern, however, because of its considerable increase in size during the 1990s and due to its location in the midst of one of the United States' most important commercial and recreational fishing areas. There also is a growing conviction among scientists studying the phenomenon that a better understanding of the "dead zone" will be invaluable for tackling similar problems in many areas around the world.

Gulf hypoxia—to the extent it occurs today—is unquestionably a human-made problem. While a small hypoxic area probably always existed near the mouth of the Mississippi, there is general agreement that today's "dead zone" was gradually created since the 1950s by increasing amounts of nutrients, primarily nitrates and phosphates, discharged into the Gulf by the Mississippi and Atchafalaya rivers. The impact of pollutants draining from the Mississippi watershed into the Gulf was never more dramatic than during the summer of 1993, when record flooding throughout the region caused the hypoxic zone to expand suddenly from 3,500 to nearly 8,000 square miles. To the puzzlement of Gulf ecologists, the area of oxygen depletion has decreased only slightly since 1993, averaging a bit more than 6,000 square miles during the peak months of June-July-August before breaking up in late autumn. In the summer of 2002 it broke all previous records, extending 8,600 square miles (22,000 km^2), an area larger than the state of Massachusetts.

The biological chain of events that gives rise to hypoxic conditions in the Gulf is a phenomenon frequently observed in freshwater lakes and ponds during warm summer months—a process known as **eutrophication.** A term meaning "well fed," eutrophication is initiated when dissolved nutrients enter a body of water where they stimulate the growth and proliferation of algae. These algal "blooms" cause several problems. Because some species produce powerful toxins, their sudden appearance may result in massive fish kills. These so-called "red tides" seem to be increasing in frequency in coastal waters worldwide. Equally important, as algal numbers increase exponentially, large numbers die and drift to the bottom where they constitute an unexpected feast for decomposer organisms, primarily bacteria. As bacterial populations explode in response to the increased food supply, their high rate of metabolic activity causes levels of dissolved oxygen in the water to plummet. The drop in oxygen content is particularly rapid in summer because high temperatures promote more rapid metabolism and because warm water holds less dissolved oxygen than does colder water. The ultimate effect of oxygen depletion is the loss of fish and other organisms requiring high levels of dissolved oxygen and their replacement by species more tolerant of hypoxic conditions.

The source of the nutrients that set this whole process in motion in the Gulf remains the subject of acrimonious debate. Early contentions that Gulf hypoxia simply reflects naturally occurring fluctuations in dissolved oxygen have been put to rest by research results demonstrating a clear association between Mississippi River flow, abundant amounts of riverborne nitrates and phosphates, increased algal growth in the Gulf, and bottom water hypoxia. Although the nutrients discharged to the Mississippi watershed obviously come from a multitude of sources—sewage treatment plant effluent, urban stormwater runoff, atmospheric deposition—the general consensus is that Midwest farmers bear most of the blame for the approximately 1 to 1.5 million tons of nitrogen flowing into the Gulf each year. Using radioisotopes to date animal remains in sediment cores taken from the dead zone, scientists have demonstrated a sharp decline in the numbers of high oxygen-demanding species and a corresponding increase in low-oxygen-tolerant species during the same years that chemical fertilizer applications were soaring in the Corn Belt. As an economist at the University of Minnesota remarked, "The gulf has become the end of the pipe for American agriculture."

Analyzing the cause of the problem is relatively straightforward; reversing the situation promises to be much more difficult, although scientists are optimistic that recovery is possible. A significant reduction (20% or more is regarded as essential) in nitrogen loadings to the Mississippi watershed—a vast area draining over 40% of the land area of the lower 48 states—is key to solving the problem. Phosphorus is usually the limiting nutrient whose overabundance causes eutrophication in freshwater bodies, but in marine environments like the Gulf nitrogen concentrations are more critical. Since industrial and municipal point sources combined are estimated to contribute a mere 3–5% of all the nitrogen carried down the Mississippi, agriculture will bear the brunt of control measures, should they be imposed. Scientists are convinced that only a change in farming practices, particularly in the Corn Belt states of the upper Midwest, can reduce Gulf nitrogen loadings enough to ease hypoxic conditions in the dead zone. Dr. Keith Kelling, a soil scientist at the University of Wisconsin, believes significant reductions are feasible because, he contends, half to three-fourths of the corn acreage in Illinois, Indiana, Iowa, Nebraska, and Minnesota is currently receiving nitrogen fertilizer applications 25% above recommended rates. Dr. Otto Doering, an agricultural economics professor at Purdue, argues that farmers can use a variety of methods, such as not applying fertilizers in the fall, to cut nitrogen runoff by 20–25% without having a detrimental effect on food prices or farm exports. Another proposed approach is the restoration of major wetlands along the Mississippi watershed—an undertaking that would provide significant flood control benefits as well. Suggestions that farmers be paid to create wetlands reserves along riverbanks to capture and contain farmland runoff are now receiving serious consideration by federal and state agencies.

As policymakers discuss the thorny issue of how the burden of resurrecting the dead zone should be shared, researchers continue efforts to expand their understanding of the diverse factors controlling algal blooms and hypoxia. A cooperative venture linking government agencies, private industry, and citizens' groups—The Gulf of Mexico Program—has been studying all the aspects of the hypoxia problem. Meanwhile, as the talk and investigations continue, Gulf Coast fishers and shrimpers bypass the dead zone, knowing any nets or lines cast into the bright blue waters will come up empty.

References

National Oceanic and Atmospheric Administration. 1998. *Gulf of Mexico Hypoxia Assessment Plan.* Committee on Environment and Natural Resources Hypoxia Work Group (March).

Rabalais, N. N. et al. 1996. "Nutrient Changes in the Mississippi River and System Responses on the Adjacent Continental Shelf." *Estuaries* 19:286–407.

Warrick, Joby. 1999. "Death in the Gulf of Mexico." *National Wildlife* 37, no. 4 (June/July):48–52.

can be managed relatively easily by maintaining a buffer zone of vegetation along waterways and using fences to prevent livestock from walking into streams.

Construction activities. Acre for acre, runoff from sites where homes, shopping centers, factories, or highways are under construction can contribute more sediment to waterways than any other activity—typically 10–20 times more than the amounts from agricultural lands. More than 500 tons of sediment per acre per year can wash off such sites into streams during the construction period, frequently carrying with them cement wash, asphalt, paint and cleaning solvents, oil and tar, and pes-

Figure 15-1 Mississippi Watershed and Resultant Hypoxic Zone

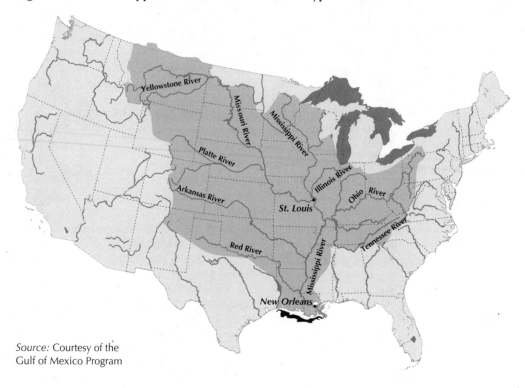

Source: Courtesy of the
Gulf of Mexico Program

July 21–25, 2004 – Area of Bottom Hypoxia

Source: N. N. Rabalais, Louisiana Universities Marine Consortium

ticides. These contaminants from construction sites have impaired an estimated 5% of U.S. surface waters. Fortunately the actual construction time during which land surfaces are unprotected is relatively short and the amount of land exposed is small in comparison with farm acreage. Nevertheless, damage to water quality due to construction site runoff can be severe and long-lasting. Many municipalities are now mandating the use of readily available erosion control techniques on construction sites, the basic approach being to expose the smallest area of land possible for the shortest period of time and scheduling construction activities so that the minimum amount of land is disturbed during the peak runoff period in the spring. Using mulches and fast-growing cover vegetation, retaining as many existing trees and

Nonpoint source of water pollution: construction site runoff. [*Gary Fak, Soil Conservation Service*]

shrubs on the site as possible, roughening the soil surface or constructing berms to slow the velocity of runoff, and building retention basins to detain runoff water long enough to promote settling out of suspended sediment are all well-established management practices for reducing pollutant runoff from construction sites.

Urban street runoff. Although people seldom consider city streets and sidewalks as important sources of water pollution, studies have shown that during storm episodes, particularly storms that terminate a long dry spell, very large amounts of sediment and other pollutants are carried by runoff water into adjacent rivers, streams, or lakes. In many cities, the total pollutant load from urban runoff exceeds that from industrial discharges. Contaminants commonly found in urban runoff include sand, dirt, road salt, oil, grease, and heavy metal particles (lead, zinc, copper, chromium, etc.) from paved surfaces; pesticides and fertilizers from lawns; leaves, seeds, bark, and grass clippings; animal and bird droppings; and other substances too numerous to mention. The EPA has documented discharge of suspended solids from storm sewers in amounts far exceeding those entering waterways from sewage treatment plants. EPA also cited urban runoff as a major contributor of oil to surface waters and a significant source of the pollutants that impair the nation's estuaries (EPA, 2002).

Reducing pollution from this source requires broad-based cooperation and effort on the part of both municipal officials and citizens: more frequent street-sweeping to prevent sediment accumulation on streets; proper disposal of pet wastes; careful and limited application of lawn and garden fertilizers and pesticides; litter control on both public and private property; judicious use of road salt and sand; application of organic mulches to reduce erosion on bare ground; incorporating more green space within urban areas and along waterways to allow runoff to filter into the ground; use of surface ponds, holding tanks, rooftop catchments, subsurface tunnels, or similar structures to hold, retain, and gradually release stormwater.

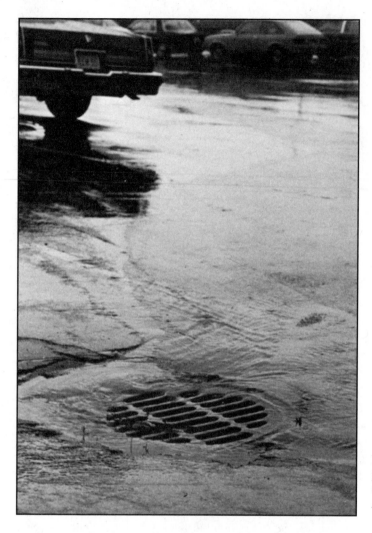

Nonpoint source of water pollution: urban street run-off. [*Illinois Environmental Protection Agency*]

Acid mine drainage. When the iron pyrite found in association with coal deposits is exposed to air and water during mining operations, a series of chemical reactions is initiated, culminating in the formation of a copper-colored precipitate (iron hydroxide) and sulfuric acid. The precipitate frequently covers the bottom of streams in mining regions, smothering bottom life and giving such streams a characteristic rusty appearance. The sulfuric acid lowers the pH of the water, eliminating many aquatic species that cannot survive or reproduce in the acidified water. Both operating and abandoned coal mines of either the underground or surface type are characterized by acid drainage, although only *abandoned* mines are termed nonpoint sources (*active* mines are classified as point source polluters). In West Virginia, the third largest coal-producing state in the United States and home to thousands of inactive mines, acid mine drainage constitutes the leading nonpoint pollution source—a problem shared by many other mining areas as well. Acids, however, are not the only water quality problem posed by abandoned mines. Under the low pH conditions prevailing in such regions, metals such as iron, aluminum, copper, zinc, manganese, magnesium, and calcium are leached from soil and rock, contaminating streams. Large amounts of silt and sediment from slag heaps or refuse piles erode into waterways, clogging streams and burying bottom-dwellers under a thick layer of silt. Legislatively

Figure 15-2 How Excess Nutrients Degrade Water Quality

Source: EPA, *National Water Quality Inventory 1996 Report to Congress,* April 1998.

mandated regrading and revegetation of abandoned strip mines have been helpful in reducing runoff of sediment from abandoned mine sites, but have had minimal impact on acid drainage. Sealing openings to abandoned underground mines, thereby cutting off the supply of oxygen and water that permit acid formation, has been the chief means of combating acid mine drainage. Although this practice significantly reduces acid loadings, it doesn't eliminate them and efforts to find better ways of dealing with the problem continue. In recent years, the use of engineered wetlands to remove toxic chemicals from mine leachate has yielded promising results. More advanced artificial wetlands have incorporated alkaline recharge zones designed to neutralize acids. These and other innovative approaches are undergoing active investigation and offer hope that a solution to acid mine drainage will eventually be found (Bennett, 1991).

Fallout of airborne pollutants. The situation represented by acid rainfall (see chapter 12) is but one example of pollution from the sky causing water quality problems. A great many of the particles released into the atmosphere through human activities eventually return to earth and enter rivers, lakes, or oceans either directly or in runoff. These airborne particles include many hazardous chemicals such as lead, asbestos, PCBs, mercury, fluorides, and various pesticides. The contribution to water pollution by synthetic chemical fallout is surprisingly large—the major portion of PCBs and other toxic chemicals in the Great Lakes and a substantial amount of the hydrocarbons found in the oceans entered these waters through airborne deposition.

As point source pollutants decline in importance, thanks to improved pollution control technology and enforcement of effluent limitations, nonpoint sources such as those just described present the greatest single challenge to attaining our nation's clean water goals. The "top down" strategy, whereby federal and state governments promulgate regulations with which individual polluters must comply under threat of civil or criminal penalties, has served us well in reducing pollution from point sources but is entirely inappropriate for controlling poison runoff from broad land areas. Recognizing the near-impossibility of requiring discharge permits for every farm field or parking lot, regulators striving to control NPS pollution thus far have focused their efforts on altering harmful land-use practices. In 1987 Congress required states to conduct surveys and develop "assessment reports" describing the nature and extent of NPS pollution within their jurisdictions. Subsequently they were to implement management programs to combat the problems identified. Control strategies to deal with NPS pollution fall into one of two possible categories:

1. increasing the land's capacity to retain water, thereby reducing runoff (e.g., a wide variety of erosion control measures), or

2. minimizing the amount of pollutants available for runoff during storms (e.g., keeping manure piles away from streams, judicious application of farm chemicals, regular street sweeping, capturing potential air pollutants before they become airborne and subject to fallout).

Controlling nonpoint pollution unfortunately demands more than just a technological "fix"; it requires instead the cooperation of farmers, ranchers, municipal officials, developers, homeowners, and others in implementing better land management practices to prevent these diverse pollutants from running off the land and into the water.

Past regulatory efforts to deal with NPS pollution were not very successful. State runoff control programs varied widely in their focus, but few emphasized the watershed protection approach so critical to an effective program. Most even today continue to rely on *voluntary* compliance with recommended land management practices—a politically popular stance but not a particularly effective one. Insufficient monitoring data and a perennial lack of adequate funding to implement needed programs have further hindered progress to deal with NPS pollution in a meaningful way.

In an effort to rectify this situation and to improve national water quality management strategies, the federal government in 1998 launched a new initiative, the **Clean Water Action Plan**. Encompassing a wide range of water quality issues, the Action Plan addresses the problem of polluted runoff by encouraging states and tribes to adopt enforceable controls on nonpoint sources. It also has increased incentives and provided new funding to help farmers control polluted runoff from agricultural lands. Most significant for the long term, however, is that the Clean Water Action Plan finally emphasizes the importance of a watershed approach as the most effective means for further improving the quality of our rivers, lakes, and estuaries.

Municipal Sewage Treatment

In 1854 the city of London was reeling under a severe epidemic of Asiatic cholera, a disease characterized by the sudden onset of profuse watery diarrhea and vomiting, resulting in rapid dehydration and death of approximately half of those afflicted. Not all parts of the city were equally affected, however. Within a district called St. James Parish, the cholera death rate hit 200 per 10,000 population, while in neighboring Charing Cross and Hanover Square districts fatalities were considerably lower. Dr. John Snow, a member of the commission of inquiry appointed to investigate the outbreak, noted that the vast majority of individuals who had died of cholera obtained their drinking water from a well on Broad Street; in other respects there seemed to be no fundamental difference between conditions in St. James Parish and nearby districts where cholera rates were low. Although the cholera bacillus and its method of transmission had not yet been discovered, Snow recommended that the handle of the Broad Street pump be removed to prevent further consumption of water from the well.

Shortly thereafter, the cholera epidemic subsided. Subsequent investigations disclosed that prior to the outbreak, residents of one house on Broad Street had been ill with an unidentified disease. Their fecal wastes had been dumped into an open cesspool near the well, a common method for disposing of human wastewater in those years. Unfortunately, the brick lining of the cesspool had deteriorated to the point that the liquid wastes could readily seep through the ground and contaminate the well water with still viable pathogenic organisms. The connection between poorly managed human wastes and serious human disease was clearly demonstrated (Cholera Inquiry Committee, 1855).

London's use of open cesspools as a method of sewage disposal was a well-established practice in many parts of the world until the late 19th and early 20th centuries. These pits in the ground simply collect wastes that are then stabilized by bacterial action. Seepage of liquids into the soil from such holes was common, and since no disinfection was used, contamination of wells and aquifers with human fecal pathogens frequently occurred. During the 19th century the growing popularity of flush toilets in urban areas resulted in greatly increased volumes of wastewater requiring disposal. This additional influx produced frequent overflowing of public cesspools and caused a further spread of filth and waterborne disease, particularly cholera and typhoid fever. Installation of sewer systems that carried wastes directly from homes into nearby rivers helped to alleviate problems of well contamination but caused severe degradation of surface water quality, eliminating many forms of aquatic life and enhancing the risk of waterborne disease in communities downstream that used surface water supplies for drinking.

By the end of the 19th century rapid urban growth convinced city planners that sewage treatment facilities were needed to alleviate the health and aesthetic problems created by dumping raw sewage into waterways. Today in the United States approximately 70% of the population live in areas where domestic wastes pass through a sewage treatment plant before being discharged. The remainder, for the most part, rely on on-site wastewater disposal systems—usually a septic tank and soil absorption field or sand filter. Provision of adequate methods of sewage treatment, along with the chlorination of drinking water, has done far more to reduce the incidence of epidemic disease and to upgrade standards of public health than has the more widely acclaimed introduction of modern medicines and vaccines.

The aim of sewage treatment is to improve the quality of wastewater to the point that it can be discharged into a waterway without seriously disrupting the aquatic environment or causing human health problems. Achieving these goals requires kill-

---

Box 15-2 Water, People, Snails, and Disease: How to Break the Link?

Schistosomiasis, also known as bilharzia or snail fever, has been the target of eradication efforts by public health agencies throughout the developing world for decades, yet infection rates have remained relatively constant for the past 50 years. Today nearly 250 million people—about 3 to 4% of the total world population—are infected with the schistosome parasite, with another 600 million considered at risk. Although an estimated 80% of victims live in sub-Saharan Africa, schistosomiasis is endemic to 74 Asian, African, and Latin American countries where it provokes recurrent fever, chills, muscle pains, and chronic weakness, undermining physical fitness, the ability to work, and intellectual capacity. While few North Americans or Europeans have ever even heard of the ailment, schistosomiasis has been plaguing residents of the Third World tropics for thousands of years and remains today one of the world's most widespread serious infectious diseases.

Unfortunately, development projects in tropical countries, particularly the construction of large dams and expanded irrigation networks, have greatly increased the number of people afflicted and have introduced the disease into areas formerly unaffected. Chances of contracting the illness are further enhanced by lack of awareness among populations most at risk, their extreme poverty, lack of medical facilities, and the unsanitary conditions of daily life. In recent years, mass movements of refugees and those fleeing wars and civil disturbances have facilitated transmission of the disease, as has the rapid growth of urban shantytowns. The Centers for Disease Control and Prevention (CDC) has also reported sporadic cases among tourists and Peace Corps volunteers in Africa who contracted their infections after engaging in recreational swimming and river rafting. As a result, CDC now recommends that any travelers returning to the U.S. from areas where schistosomiasis is endemic and who have had direct freshwater contact while there should be serologically tested to determine whether they harbor the parasite and, if so, should seek treatment.

Schistosomiasis is caused by several species of parasitic flatworms, or blood flukes, which pass different stages of their life cycle alternately inside snail and human hosts. Schistosome eggs enter waterways via the feces or urine of infected humans. Upon contact with water, the eggs open, releasing first-stage motile larvae (miracidiae) that seek out an appropriate species of freshwater snail, which they then penetrate. Multiplying asexually inside its snail host, each larva produces thousands of second-stage larvae (cercariae), which are excreted by the snail into the surrounding water. These free-swimming cercariae have approximately two days in which to locate a human host, through whose skin they penetrate within a few seconds. Making their way to the victim's blood vessels, cercariae travel through the circulatory system to the liver where, within 30–45 days, they mature and mate. Subsequently they migrate to the bladder or the intestines, depending on the species, and there the female worms commence laying 200–2,000 eggs daily for a period of 3–5 years. About half of these eggs are excreted with urine or feces, while the remainder are carried in the bloodstream to other parts of the body where they eventually die. It is these eggs, rather than the worms themselves, that damage the human host, producing inflammation and lesions in the intestines, bladder, and other vital organs. Since there is no multiplication of worms inside the human body, the seriousness of the infection depends on the number of cercariae that penetrate the victim's skin. If the eggs that are excreted reach a body of slow-moving fresh water within a month, they hatch almost immediately and the cycle is repeated.

Although schistosomiasis is seldom fatal—many victims living in affected areas are asymptomatic—20 million people are reported to be suffering severe consequences of the infection while another 120 million experience milder symptoms (blood in the urine is a common indication of urinary schistosomiasis). Because the debilitating nature of the disease gravely impairs the productivity of infected individuals, the majority of whom are farmers or freshwater fishers living in rural areas, its impact on local economic conditions and the general health status of the population can be considerable. In parts of Egypt, Sudan, and northeastern Brazil schistosomiasis has seriously impaired labor productivity among infected farm workers. In some countries there appears to be an association between urinary schistosomiasis and subsequent development of bladder cancer. In rural Egypt where schistosomiasis is widespread, bladder cancer linked to schistosomiasis is the leading cause of death among men in the 20–44 age group, a rate 32 times higher than that in the United States. Schistosomiasis also has a significant impact on the growth rate of children and their performance in school, a worrisome fact inasmuch as the World Health Organization estimates that 66 million children in 54 countries are infected with urinary schistosomiasis, including over 90% of children living in villages around Ghana's Lake Volta.

Reducing the prevalence of schistosomiasis is being tackled via a broad-based public health and education effort to break the link in disease transmission—something that sounds simple enough in theory, but is difficult in practice, given existing conditions of life in the developing world. Attempts to eradicate the snail hosts of the parasite have proven largely ineffective because even a few snails can produce enough schistosome larvae to infect a large number of people. Therefore, snail-killing pesticides would have to be 100% effective in order to break the disease cycle—a near-impossible situation, since many snails could burrow into the mud to survive. Even in the unlikely event that the entire snail population in a given section of waterway is eradicated, there is nothing to prevent the influx of new snails from neighboring areas. In addition, the use of large quantities of pesticides incurs the risk of undesired environmental side effects, while the cost of the chemicals often precludes their use. Increasing the velocity of water flow in canals and irrigation ditches, fluctuating water levels, lining the edges of such waterways with concrete, and removing aquatic weeds along stream banks help reduce snail numbers by altering their preferred habitat, but here again complete eradication is seldom possible.

An alternative approach to controlling schistosomiasis focuses on treating victims of the disease. Although there is no vaccine effective against the parasite, several orally administered drugs, most notably praziquantel, produce a high cure rate after a single dose, have virtually no side effects, can be safely administered by primary health care teams, and are relatively inexpensive. Although subsequent reinfection may occur, serious organ damage is greatly reduced among patients who have received the drug and a noticeable regression of lesions has been noted among children after treatment for schistosome infection. A tribute to the effectiveness of drug therapy is the significant reduction in cases of schistosomiasis within a year or two following community-wide treatment efforts. Nevertheless, praziquantel does not represent a permanent solution to the problem; it is almost always necessary to repeat the treatment, though in areas where transmission rates are low, the interval may be as much as five years. Unfortunately, worrisome evidence has surfaced that the parasite may be developing resistance to the drug, since schistosomiasis cure rates using praziquantel are lower now than they were in the past.

The most promising long-term approach to control of schistosomiasis is an integrated program that includes drug therapy, public health education, improved methods of sanitary waste disposal, provision of safe drinking water, and modifying snail habitat, as described above. If human body contact with water could be avoided, parasites couldn't penetrate the victim's skin; if infected individuals could be persuaded to use latrines instead of urinating and defecating in or near the water, schistosome eggs would be unable to hatch. Unfortunately, avoiding contact with water is virtually impossible in Third World village society, where shallow waterways are used for bathing, swimming, fishing, doing laundry, planting rice, and washing livestock. Altering toilet customs would appear a more feasible option, but centuries-old habits are hard to change, particularly among children and teenage boys accustomed to urinating in the water while swimming and bathing. Efforts by civil authorities to reduce water contact by building bridges over canals and constructing public facilities for laundering, bathing, and recreation offer some promise if the necessary funding can be obtained. Health education efforts, both in the public schools and the mass media, have had a significant impact in raising awareness about disease prevention and the need for diagnosis and treatment. Perhaps most critical to the success of anti-schistosomiasis efforts is the urgent need to expand the provision of clean drinking water. Since field experience has shown that the beneficial results of praziquantel are most pronounced in communities with treated water, governments should give high priority to areas with a high prevalence of schistosomiasis infection when trying to decide where to invest scarce funds for upgrading drinking water treatment. Policymakers, environmental health specialists, and educators, as well as international lending agencies, must increase their efforts to break the cycle of disease that continues to condemn a large portion of the developing world's population to life-long disability.

References

Tucker, Jonathan B., 1983. "Schistosomiasis and Water Projects." *Environment* 25, no. 7 (Sept).

Water for People, Water for Life: The United Nations World Water Development Report. 2003. UNESCO Publishing, Berghahn Books.

ing pathogenic organisms present in human wastes (within any human population there will always be some individuals suffering from various gastrointestinal diseases and releasing the causative bacteria, protozoans, etc., in their excreta; it is assumed, therefore, that domestic sewage entering the treatment facility is contaminated with pathogens capable of causing disease outbreaks) and, to the greatest possible extent, removing organic wastes or converting them to inorganic forms so that after discharge they will not deplete the oxygen content of the receiving waters as they decompose. To accomplish these ends, several levels of sewage treatment are necessary.

Primary Treatment

The used water supply of a community, averaging about 100 gallons/person/day in cities having separate storm and sanitary sewers, flows from homes and institutions into the municipal sewer system, which carries the wastes to a treatment plant (in regulatory jargon a "**POTW**"—publicly owned treatment works). At this point sewage consists not only of human feces and urine, but also of wastes from laundry, bathing, garbage grinding, and dishwashing, as well as all the miscellaneous articles that find their way into the sewer system—sand, gravel, rubber balls, leaves, sticks, dead rats, etc. Primary sewage treatment consists of several mechanical processes designed to remove the larger suspended solids through screening and sedimentation. Though there may be minor variations in the methods used by different treatment plants, in general the incoming flow first passes through one or more screens to remove large floating objects. After the waste-laden water has passed the screens, it enters a grit chamber where the reduced velocity of flow permits sand, gravel, and other inorganic material to settle out. Air is sometimes injected into the tank to maintain aerobic conditions and to remove trapped gases. Following several hours in an additional sedimentation tank (a *primary clarifier*), the wastewater enters the secondary treatment system or, in those POTWs having only a primary level of treatment, is chlorinated and discharged into the receiving waters. The solid material (sludge) that settles out in the sedimentation tank is regularly removed, dried, and disposed of by one of several methods.

While primary treatment is unquestionably better than no treatment at all, it does not result in an effluent of sufficiently high quality to prevent degradation of the receiving waters. During primary treatment approximately 50–65% of suspended solids are removed. In addition, the amount of pollutant organic material in the water, a measurement referred to as **biochemical oxygen demand,** or **BOD,** is reduced by about 25–40%. (When organic matter in wastewater discharged into streams or lakes is acted upon by bacteria, dissolved oxygen is rapidly depleted, resulting in fish kills and drastic alterations in the aquatic environment. Biochemical oxygen demand basically is an indication of how much putrescible organic material is present, with a low BOD indicating good water quality and a high BOD reflecting polluted conditions.) Because the pollution potential of wastewater following primary treatment is still quite high, the Environmental Protection Agency does not consider primary treatment by itself an adequate level of sewage treatment.

Secondary Treatment

Whereas primary treatment is based upon physical and mechanical methods of removing suspended solids from wastewater, secondary treatment depends on biological processes, similar to naturally occurring decomposition but greatly accelerated, to digest organic wastes. Microorganisms, predominantly aerobic bacteria, are utilized in the presence of an abundant oxygen supply to break down organic materials into inorganic carbon dioxide, water, and minerals. This can be accomplished by means of **trick-**

Figure 15-3 Schematic Municipal Wastewater Treatment Process

ling filters—beds of crushed stone whose surfaces are covered with a microbial slime consisting of bacteria, protozoans, nematodes, etc. that absorb the organic material as the wastewater is sprayed over the surface of the rocks—or by the more modern **activated sludge process.** This involves "seeding" a tank of sewage with bacteria-laden sludge, pumping compressed air into the mixture and agitating it for 4–10 hours. During this time the microbes adsorb most of the colloidal and suspended solids onto the surfaces of the sludge particles and oxidize the organic material. After the process is complete, the sludge is separated from the remaining liquid by settling (*secondary clarification*). Most of this sludge, consisting primarily of masses of bacteria, is removed, but some must be retained and fed back into the incoming sewage to perpetuate the process.

After wastewater has passed through both primary and secondary treatment, the level of suspended solids and of BOD has been reduced by about 90–95% (however, cold weather can reduce the efficiency of pollutant reduction because it slows the metabolic rate of the microorganisms on which secondary treatment depends). Secondary treatment is not effective in removing viruses, heavy metals, dissolved minerals, or nutrients (Koren, 1980). In the United States, a federally imposed mandate requiring that all POTWs provide at least secondary wastewater treatment took effect in July 1988.

Advanced Wastewater Treatment (Tertiary Treatment)

A third level of sewage treatment may be required in situations (1) where effluent from the secondary treatment process still contains substances that are causing water

Table 15-1   Tertiary Treatment Processes

Tertiary Treatment Method	Pollutant Removed
Chemical coagulation, followed by filtration or sedimentation	phosphates, tertiary suspended solids, and BOD
Activated carbon adsorption	synthetic organic chemicals, tastes, odors
Nitrifying towers	ammonia
Air stripping	ammonia
Oxidation ponds and aerated lagoons	BOD, phosphates
Reverse osmosis	BOD, nitrates, phosphates, dissolved solids
Electrodialysis	dissolved minerals
Oxidation	organic material
Foam separation	organic chemicals
Land application	phosphates, nitrates, BOD, suspended solids

quality problems; (2) when the sheer volume of effluent is large enough that the remaining 10% of suspended solids and BOD are sufficient to initiate eutrophication; (3) or if the treated wastewater is to be used for purposes of drinking, irrigation, or recreation. Advanced wastewater treatment involves either one or a combination of several biological, chemical, or physical processes designed to remove such pollutants as phosphates, nitrates, ammonia, and organic chemicals. It also further reduces the concentration of remaining suspended solids and BOD to about 1% of that present in raw sewage. Recognition of a growing nitrogen pollution problem in many U.S. waterways and coastal estuaries has prompted requirements for many POTWs to install advanced technologies to remove nitrogen from their wastewater effluent—something that conventional secondary treatment fails to accomplish. The option most commonly chosen uses naturally occurring bacteria in a 3-step process called **biological nitrogen removal (BNR)**. BNR involves the microbial transformation of dissolved organic nitrogen through a series of steps to unreactive elemental nitrogen (N_2), which is released into the atmosphere and no longer poses any water quality threat. The technology to accomplish this is expensive, but treatment plants using BNR have substantially reduced their nitrogen loadings to receiving waterways (Driscoll et al., 2003).

Disinfection

Since the most common waterborne diseases are caused by pathogenic bacteria, viruses, or protozoans present in human excrement, one of the primary purposes of sewage treatment is to kill such organisms before they can infect new victims. Simple exposure to the hostile environment outside the human intestine is sufficient to reduce the number of bacteria appreciably as they pass through the treatment process. However, because a substantial number of live organisms still remain in the wastewater after primary and secondary treatment are complete, it was standard procedure for many years to disinfect treated effluent by adding chlorine prior to discharge in order to eliminate any remaining disease-causing organisms. More recently, the policy of chlorinating all sewage treatment plant discharges has met with increasing resistance and today more than half of all states no longer require that all sanitary wastewaters be disinfected. There are several reasons for this change in accepted practice.

    1. Chlorine is effective in killing bacteria, but less so in relation to viruses and parasites (e.g., *Giardia, Cryptosporidium*), many of which survive this treatment.

Box 15-3 For Want of a Toilet . . .

A clean, properly functioning toilet inside one's own home is an assumed fact of life among the vast majority of industrialized world citizens, living in relatively affluent societies where indoor plumbing and municipal sewers (or on-site septic systems) are near-universal. Not so among the urban poor in most Third World cities. The lack of adequate sanitation in such areas is even more acute than the dearth of safe drinking water and its impact on human health and well-being is equally profound. In Latin America as a whole, only 66% of the population lives in areas where toilets are connected to a sewer system; in Asia and Africa that percentage is much lower, standing at 18% and 13%, respectively. Dismayed by these statistics, delegates to the United Nations-sponsored 2002 World Summit for Sustainable Development set 2015 as their target date for reducing by half the number of people currently lacking access to basic sanitation. Doing so constitutes a monumental task, especially since projected world population growth during the intervening years means that an additional 1.9 billion people will require services in order to meet the goal.

The challenge is particularly acute in the squatter settlements that surround most Third World cities. Largely unplanned and overcrowded, these slum areas frequently lack even the most basic infrastructure found in more affluent neighborhoods. In Nairobi, Kenya, for example, 55% of the population in the mid-1990s lived in informal settlements where only a small minority of homes had toilets and a large percentage of residents had no access to showers or baths. Within the largest slum area, home to almost half a million people, traditional pit latrines provide the only method of excrement disposal. Frequently as many as 200 people are forced to use the same pit latrine; as a result, the pits fill up quickly, presenting a serious excrement disposal problem because the narrow streets are difficult for removal vehicles to access. To make matters worse, little space exists for installing new pits. The situation is even worse in Tanzania's capital, Dar-es-Salaam, where 83% of households rely on pit latrines. Only 12% of the squatter camps in Karachi, Pakistan's largest city, are provided with sanitary facilities. While the situation is bad in the megacities just cited, access to safe, convenient sanitation is even worse in the Third World's smaller urban centers.

Although it may be unrealistic to expect the governments of low-income nations to provide all their citizens with indoor plumbing and a flush toilet anytime in the near future, international development agencies are urging them to ensure, at a minimum, "safe, convenient sanitation" as soon as possible. Doing so would require that human waste be disposed of in such a manner that it doesn't contaminate human hands, clothing, food, or water and that it not be accessible to disease-carrying houseflies. In this context, the current situation in many developing world cities is discouraging. Reliance on public toilets or pit latrines is commonplace. Frequently such shared facilities are so filthy and poorly maintained that they constitute a genuine health hazard to the people they are intended to serve; because of this, they may be shunned and lapse into disuse. In addition, people living at a considerable distance from communal toilets may find them simply too inconvenient to access. Such facilities also are quite impractical to meet the needs of children, few of whom are able to walk the long distance to a public toilet once they decide they "have to go!" Similarly, small children are seldom able to wait their turn in the long lines that often form outside shared facilities. Reflecting such difficulties, a survey conducted in India found that only 1% of children under the age of 6 use public latrines; stools from an additional 5% are deposited in the latrines by their parents. Wastes from the remaining 94% ultimately end up in roadside ditches, streets, or open areas. Another deterrent to the use of public toilets by the urban poor is their cost. In one Ghanaian city, it costs 10–15% of the main breadwinner's daily wage for each member of the family to use the public latrine one time!

For a half-billion or so urban dwellers in developing nations, provision of sanitary facilities—even simple pit latrines—is so poor that people have no choice but to defecate outside on the ground or into a container such as waste paper or a plastic bag which they then throw away. In the Philippines the latter option is jokingly referred to as "wrap and throw"; in Ghana as "flying toilets"! Humor aside, the necessity of defecating in the open presents a humiliating dilemma for millions of women and girls who often feel that in order to avoid being seen and jeered at by men, they must wait until after dark to relieve themselves.

Unsanitary human waste disposal practices also have profoundly negative health consequences. Exposed feces attract flies that then carry human disease organisms to exposed foods. Excrement-saturated soil harbors parasites such as hookworms, the larvae of which burrow through the skin of bare feet, or several species of roundworms, whose eggs can be accidentally ingested with soil when children put dirty hands or objects in their mouths. Such helminthic infections afflict a billion or more people throughout the tropics and can be quite debilitating. Mosquito larvae thrive where sewage-polluted water pools due to inadequate drainage, facilitating transmission of malaria and filariasis. When human wastes contaminate wells or streams used for drinking water, outbreaks of microbial waterborne diseases such as dysentery, typhoid fever, and cholera may occur. Such problems are particularly common after periods of heavy rainfall in unsewered areas, when sewage-laden stormwaters fill streets, courtyards, and adjacent waterways.

Although the United Nations and numerous governmental and private organizations are actively striving to upgrade the provision of sanitation in Third World cities, some of the most successful projects have been carried out at the grassroots level by the residents most directly affected. In Pune, a city of nearly 3 million inhabitants in western India, 40% of the people live in shantytowns lacking plumbing and sewerage. The number of public toilets provided by the municipality is grossly inadequate and those that do exist are often poorly designed and constructed, provided with inadequate supplies of water for washing, and seldom cleaned. In 1999, a local nongovernmental organization allied with the slum dwellers signed an agreement with the municipality to construct and maintain new sanitary facil-

ities. With capital costs provided by the city and local residents closely involved with management of the project, 114 toilet blocks were constructed, containing 2000 adult seats and 500 sized for children. In contrast to the older facilities, the new toilet blocks are well ventilated, bright, and feature better-quality construction. Large water storage tanks ensure that users have enough water to wash after defecation (toilet paper is an unknown commodity in most Indian households) and to clean the toilet after use (fecal material in nonflush toilets is washed into an underlying pit or septic tank by pouring a containerful of water into the toilet bowl). Additional improvements include separate sections of each toilet block for men and women, one block specially designed for children, and toilets designed for elderly or handicapped residents. Maintenance costs were reduced and the quality of service enhanced by including the construction of living quarters for caretakers and their families. Throughout the course of the project, ongoing communication between the government and residents, along with complete transparency in regards to costing and financing the project, established a high level of trust and cooperation between the parties involved. The end result was a major improvement in sanitation that both government and local users could afford.

Pune's example may not be widely transferable, however. In places where good governance is in short supply, it may take years before local residents can afford to invest in household toilets or communities install an adequate number of safe, accessible public facilities. Given the rapidly increasing number of Third World urban residents living in poverty and the enormous health cost of improper management of human wastes, more effective action needs to be taken now to ensure that all the world's people are guaranteed access to the sanitary facilities most of us take for granted.

Reference

Water for People, Water for Life: The United Nations World Water Development Report. 2003. UNESCO Publishing, Berghahn Books.

2. Chlorine is very destructive of fish and other forms of aquatic life, many of which are eliminated for a considerable distance downstream from sewage treatment plants due to the presence of this chemical in the water. For this reason, many wastewater treatment plants that use chlorine as a disinfectant are now required to dechlorinate their wastewater prior to discharge in order to remove potentially harmful residual chlorine.

3. Chlorine treatment poses safety problems at the treatment plant in the eventuality of cylinder leaks or system disruption.

4. Chlorine disinfects only a fraction of the wastes in streams because bacteria-laden runoff from farmland and urban areas enters waterways untreated.

Proponents of chlorinating POTW discharges correctly point out, however, that this practice helps reduce outbreaks of disease that have been associated with swimming in sewage-polluted water or with consuming shellfish taken from contaminated waterways. Although disinfecting such effluent with chlorine does not sterilize the water, in the sense of killing every last microbe, it reduces their numbers significantly and thereby enhances the self-purifying capacity of natural waterways. As the controversy between wastewater chlorination opponents and proponents continues to rage, a compromise solution has been reached in some states where disinfection of discharge waters is required only during the summer bathing season, with the practice being discontinued during the winter when recreational contact with water is unlikely (Shertzer, 1986). In certain states, requirements for disinfecting POTW effluent have been dropped altogether, except in those situations where a drinking water intake point or a bathing beach is located a short distance downstream.

Unfortunately, as population density increases and the distance between POTW effluent discharge points and public drinking water intake pipes shrinks, fewer treatment plants may have the option of bypassing disinfection. This is especially relevant in states like Texas and California, where serious consideration is being given to proposals for discharging treated effluent directly into drinking water reservoirs as a means of augmenting water supplies. As a result, interest in nonchlorine methods of killing microbes is growing rapidly. While some POTWs now employ membrane filtration or ozonation as their method of disinfection, the most popular nontraditional disinfectant is ultraviolet (UV) light. UV kills microbes by disrupting their genetic material, preventing reproduction. Since the technology relies on radiation rather than chemicals, no harmful residual remains in the water post-treatment, eliminating any need to remove disinfectant from the effluent to protect aquatic life downstream. Industry surveys reveal that 25% of all U.S. and Canadian municipal wastewater treatment plants built or upgraded in 2000 opted to install UV systems as their primary disinfectant. UV disinfection technologies are rapidly being adopted in Europe as well, spurred by a European Union regulation that all significant wastewater discharges must be pathogen-free by 2005. Since most European wastewater treatment plants, except for those in the U.K., currently don't disinfect their effluent at all, it is likely that the new mandate will prompt a large percentage to choose UV systems (Ultraguard Water Systems, 2004).

Biosolids Management

Ironically, the high degree of pollutant removal achieved at modern sewage treatment plants has created a new challenge for POTW operators—how to manage the steadily growing volumes of sludge (the term applied to untreated biosolids) that our increasingly efficient sewage treatment technologies are producing. The quantity of biosolids produced annually by U.S. municipal treatment plants has approximately doubled since passage of the Clean Water Act, thanks to continued population growth, further gains in the efficiency of wastewater treatment, and more widespread compliance with Clean Water Act requirements. Because sewage sludge itself can be a pollutant if improperly managed, its treatment, ultimate disposal, and potential use must be handled in ways that will not endanger public health or the environment.

Routinely removed at each step in the sewage treatment process, the watery sludge (before treatment, sludge consists of 93–99% water) generally is first thickened through the use of coagulant chemicals or dissolved air flotation. It is then stabilized through a two-step anaerobic digestion process in order to reduce problems associated with odors and the presence of pathogenic organisms—a process that takes approximately 60 days to complete. To reduce its volume for ease in handling, the sludge is then dewatered, either by mechanical processes or by drying on sand beds. At this point sludge has the appearance of rich black dirt and is largely odor free. A number of POTWs subsequently compost, heat-dry, or otherwise treat their sludge to kill remaining pathogens. Contrary to the negative public image of anything pertaining to sewage, the treated biosolids at this point represent a valuable resource rather than an objectionable waste. Indeed, the nitrates, phosphates, and organic matter present in sludge make it useful as a fertilizer and as a soil conditioner. Biosolids have a long history of use for improving marginal lands, increasing forest productivity (studies have shown that the rate of tree growth doubles on sludge-enriched soil), boosting home garden yields, and reclaiming lands devastated by strip-mining.

Since sewage treatment plants, particularly those in the larger metropolitan areas, generate enormous amounts of sludge during their normal course of operations, finding a place in which to dispose of this material poses major dilemmas for many such facilities. Incineration can present problems of air pollution, and in many communities where landfill space is at a premium, burying sludge is increasingly controversial—and increasingly expensive. In fact, biosolids management has become so expensive that, whatever the disposal option chosen, treatment and disposal of biosolids now account for over 50% of the operating costs of a typical POTW providing secondary sewage treatment.

Since the mid-1990s, EPA regulations have encouraged a marked trend toward **"beneficial reuse"** of biosolids; as a result, 54% of the 6 million tons of dry sludge produced annually by U.S. sewage treatment plants are being recycled, spread on the land as fertilizer. The 1987 Clean Water Act amendments established a comprehensive program for reducing potential environmental risks posed by sludge through requirements that EPA (1) identify toxic substances that may be present in sludge at potentially dangerous levels, and (2) promulgate regulations that specify acceptable management practices and numerical limitations for sludge containing those pollutants. These regulations, referred to as the **Part 503** standards, were issued in February of 1993 and have now been implemented nationwide.

The main concern that has limited beneficial reuse of biosolids in the past is the fact that sewage sludge often contains toxic chemicals and pathogens as well as desirable nutrients such as phosphates and nitrates. In particular, sludge from POTWs receiving industrial wastewater discharges in addition to residential sewage may contain potentially dangerous concentrations of heavy metals and other toxics—cadmium and lead are of special concern, but copper, zinc, nickel, PCBs, and a number of other contaminants also may be present. EPA addressed this issue by setting maximum loading rates on soils for biosolids containing these contaminants, advising POTWs to police industrial discharges in their communities in an effort to eliminate toxic pollutants at the source. Regulatory standards for chemicals in biosolids were painstakingly developed through a risk assessment process that involved identifying those contaminants deemed likely to pose the greatest hazard, characterizing the most likely ways in which a person might be exposed, and then making science-based calculations on the maximum concentrations permissible in biosolids intended for land application and the amount of biosolids that could be applied to a given land area (i.e., loading rate).

EPA took a different approach to ensuring that pathogen levels in biosolids wouldn't present a health risk. Rather than setting risk-based concentration limits for individual microbes, regulators established sludge treatment requirements, such as composting or heat drying, to reduce even further the already relatively low number of organisms present in digested sludge. Depending on the number of pathogens present following treatment, resulting biosolids are characterized as Class A or Class B. The former, characterized by pathogen densities below specified detection limits, can be applied to any lands, including home lawns and gardens, without restriction. Class B biosolids have a somewhat higher pathogen content and, to ensure public safety, Part 503 restricts their use to croplands, pastureland, and forests. Rules also specify the amount of time that must elapse between biosolids application and subsequent crop harvesting, animal grazing, or public access. During this interval it is assumed that environmental factors such as heat and sunlight will further reduce pathogen concentrations (though no on-site measurements are required to verify this assumption).

More than 30 years of research and practical experience have shown that food crops grown on lands fertilized with biosolids are safe for human consumption and the National Research Council (NRC) reports no documented scientific evidence to suggest that current biosolids regulations fail to protect public health. Nevertheless, some environmental groups cite anecdotal, though unsubstantiated, reports of people or animals sickened by exposure to land-applied biosolids, problems ranging from mild allergic reactions to severe and chronic health problems. Recognizing these concerns, the NRC has recommended that EPA reassess the existing Part 503 chemical standards using improved, up-to-date risk assessment practices and review whether additional chemicals should be added to the list of those currently regulated. They also suggest that although a direct link between biosolids exposure and human illness has never been scientifically proven, the EPA should conduct epidemiological studies focused on biosolids applicators, farmers using biosolids, and people living near land application sites in order to lay such fears to rest. Ensuring that existing rules pertaining to such management practices as loading rates and setback distances from waterways are rigorously enforced is another NRC recommendation to agency regulators, reflecting the fact that many complaints are related to excessive rates of biosolids application or to runoff contamination of streams when required setbacks were ignored (NRC, 2002). Responding to these recommendations, EPA is sponsoring scientific research and public health studies on the safety of biosolids use as a fertilizer. In the meantime, many municipal water reclamation districts continue to view land application as the most environmentally acceptable, cost-efficient method for disposing of their sludge. New York City eagerly seized upon this option in 1992 when, ordered to cease ocean dumping, it began shipping its biosolids 2,065 miles across country to the Sierra Blanca Ranch in Hudspeth County, Texas. There the anaerobically digested biosolids are spread over native desert grasslands at a rate of 3 dry tons/ acre/year. Scientists from Texas Tech and Texas A&M Universities monitoring the site report an increase in the density and biomass of grasses and in the number of desirable species. They also report decreased rates of erosion and no buildup of heavy metals (Carlile, 1995).

Although agricultural lands are currently the destination for most of the biosolids being land applied, farmers are not the only ones interested in taking advantage of this "black gold." While some municipalities are giving biosolids away to anyone who will take it, the majority are selling the stuff to home gardeners, nurseries, or landscaping firms at prices ranging from $1–$22 per cubic foot! Milwaukee and Madison, Wisconsin, and Austin, Texas, have employed imaginative marketing skills in promoting their products, selling biosolids under such catchy trade names as *Milorganite, Metrogro,* or *Dillo Dirt* (EPA, 1993; Tenenbaum, 1992).

New Approaches to Wastewater Treatment

Financing the improvements in municipal sewage treatment required by the 1972 Clean Water Act would have been impossible had Congress not included, in that same piece of legislation, the creation of a massive **Construction Grant Program.** This fund provided federal monetary assistance to communities that could not otherwise have afforded the multimillion-dollar expenditures necessary to construct new or upgraded POTWs capable of providing the mandatory secondary level of sewage treatment. Under the Construction Grant Program, the second-largest public works project in U.S. history (exceeded only by construction of the interstate highway system), the federal government agreed to provide fully 75% of the cost of such projects, an amount that was subsequently reduced to 55% by the Reagan Administration in 1981. Over nearly two decades Washington contributed $57 *billion* for sewage treatment plant construction (state and local expenditures during the same period exceeded an additional $70 billion); as a result, by the late 1980s, 58% of the U.S. population was served by POTWs providing either secondary or secondary and advanced wastewater treatment. Since POTWs cumulatively serve about 70% of the American population (most of the remainder utilizing on-site wastewater disposal systems), it is obvious that domestic wastewaters in the majority of sewered communities now receive a commendably high level of treatment prior to discharge.

Nevertheless, remaining sewage treatment needs are considerable. In the late 1980s, approximately one out of every ten Americans lived in communities providing less than secondary treatment—and some small towns still had no sewage treatment at all, discharging raw wastewaters directly into streams. In 1990, EPA estimated the total cost of bringing all municipal dischargers into compliance with CWA water quality requirements could exceed $110 billion—yet by 1990 the federal well had run dry (Adler et al., 1993). Amendments to the Clean Water Act passed by Congress in 1987 called for a phaseout of the federal Construction Grant Program by 1994, replacing it with a **State Revolving Fund** providing low-interest *loans* (no more free gifts from Uncle Sam!) to municipalities with unmet sewage treatment needs. Unfortunately, the demand for such loans exceeds the supply—but federal deadline dates for compliance with CWA requirements remain unchanged and potential penalties can be severe. Thus the fiscal and legal realities of the 1990s provided a major incentive to develop new, less costly, yet equally effective methods of treating sewage—alternatives to the highly engineered, energy-consuming, sludge-producing, exorbitantly expensive POTWs that offered a convenient "technological fix" during the era of free-flowing federal dollars but are an unrealistic option for communities of limited means.

Fortunately, the old adage, "Necessity is the mother of invention," is as valid in relation to emerging wastewater management technologies as it is in other spheres of life. In recent decades a variety of innovative approaches to solving wastewater problems have attracted considerable interest and a number are now in the pilot-project stage, undergoing extensive field studies; several are in full-scale use, having proven their ability to produce good quality effluent at a fraction of the cost of conventional sewage treatment. The majority of new systems are based on the concept that wastewater effluent, like biosolids, should be viewed as a nutrient-laden resource to be utilized rather than as a pollutant to be discarded.

One of the earliest and most widely adopted approaches to alternative treatment was land application of wastewater. This method involves spraying effluent from secondary treatment onto forest, pastures, or croplands. Land application not only helps prevent stream pollution by keeping nutrients out of the water, it also utilizes those same nutrients as fertilizer for the plants on which it is applied. A further advantage of this method is that the wastewater is largely purified as it percolates through the soil to recharge the groundwater supply. Early health concerns that dissolved metals or pathogens in the effluent might contaminate soils or vegetation have been dispelled by many years of problem-free experience with land application at Pennsylvania State University; in communities in Texas, Michigan, California, and New York; and in Germany, France, Israel, and Australia.

In the 1980s, emphasis shifted to the potential for artificial wetlands ("designer swamps"), duckweed systems *(Lemna spp.)*, and water-purifying hydroponics-type systems inside greenhouses. In the United States, the Tennessee Valley Authority (TVA) has been at the forefront of research and development efforts focused on wetlands treatment. TVA views such systems as a viable wastewater treatment option for small communities that lack the expertise, as well as the financial resources, to operate highly sophisticated mechanical plants. Since the mid-1980s, TVA has designed and constructed engineered wetlands for a number of small towns in southern Appalachia, enabling such communities to comply with federal water quality standards at a fraction of the cost of conventional facilities. Although the sizeable land requirements for engineered wetlands have deterred many communities from giving such systems serious consideration, some larger cities such as Orlando, Florida, and Columbia, Missouri, have opted to utilize wetlands as one element in their treatment process.

Of the municipalities nationwide currently employing wetlands systems to treat sewage, the most renowned is Arcata, California, a community of 16,000 located on the north shore of Humboldt Bay. In the early 1980s, Arcata faced a serious fiscal dilemma: effluent from the town's POTW consistently violated discharge permit limitations and Arcata was being pressured by the state environmental agency to close the plant and join with neighboring municipalities in constructing a large regional facility. Wary of the exorbitant costs such an undertaking would entail, Arcata opted for a radically different solution to its problem. Assisted by faculty at Humboldt State University, the town proceeded to develop a series of ponds and marshes to remove the troublesome pollutants remaining in its effluent following primary treatment at the POTW. Today Arcata's wastewater receives secondary treatment in a 50-acre stabilization pond where suspended solids settle to the bottom, while dissolved organic materials are broken down through a symbiotic association between bacteria and algae. From here the effluent flows into a three-celled, five-acre "treatment marsh" where rooted aquatic plants such as cattails *(Typha latifolia)* and bulrushes *(Scirpus acutis)* flourish. The submerged stems of these plants harbor countless numbers of microorganisms that further metabolize dissolved organic nitrates and phosphates. Passage through the marsh also effectively breaks down pesticides, industrial solvents, and most of the heavy metals in wastewater. After passing through the treatment marsh, the effluent is pumped to a chlorine contact tank for disinfection and is subsequently discharged into an "enhancement marsh" for additional wetlands treatment. This enhancement marsh, open to the public, is interlaced with jogging and hiking trails, picnic areas, and a nature center; it also serves as a wildlife sanctuary, annually attracting more than 150,000 visitors and 160 species of birds and other wildlife—living proof that the imperatives of providing for society's urgent wastewater management needs and restoring valuable ecosystems are mutually compatible.

After treatment in the enhancement marsh, the effluent is chlorinated once again and finally discharged into Humboldt Bay (source of 60–70% of California's oyster crop), its levels of suspended solids and BOD by now well below the NPDES limits of 30 mg/L. Completed in 1986, Arcata's wetland system has been both an environmental and financial success. Once a polluter of Humboldt Bay, Arcata's wastewater treatment process produces an effluent that not only exceeds water quality standards but is even cleaner than the seawater into which it flows—and it does so at a cost far lower than that of a standard treatment facility. By the late 1990s, the obvious advantages of Arcata's natural approach to wastewater treatment had persuaded city officials in Davis and Pacifica, California, to construct their own wetlands treatment systems.

Why haven't more communities followed Arcata's example? The major limitation to such systems is the amount of land they require—about 20 acres for a town of 10,000 people. Unless a community already owns land on its outskirts, being able to afford, or even find, this much land may present serious difficulties. Perhaps the biggest obstacle is sheer ignorance and inertia. Only recently have adequate design guidelines become available for engineers and regulators; municipal officials frequently are unaware of the advantages such systems offer; conventionally trained engineers are frequently reluctant to embark on new, little-tried technologies and often lack the understanding of environmental conditions needed to factor these into their designs. Cynics might also wonder if engineers' general lack of enthusiasm might stem from the fact that cheaper artificial marshes translate into lower fees for engineering firms, since payment is typically calculated as a percentage of total project cost ("Small Community," 1993). Despite these obstacles, the idea is gradually winning converts, and not only in small towns. The city of Phoenix, Arizona, is in the process of creating a wetlands system to treat a portion of its wastewater flow because doing so is a much more economical way of meeting effluent standards than upgrading its conventional treatment plant (Brown, Flavin, and French, 1999).

A more futuristic approach to meeting community wastewater treatment needs in an economical and environmentally benign manner is "The Living Machine," marketed by Living Machines, Inc., in Taos, New Mexico. Designed to treat both human wastewaters and high-strength industrial organic wastes, the Living Machine relies on a series of tanks and biofilters containing a wide spectrum of microorganisms, algae, snails, plants, and fish inside a greenhouse-like structure. After passing through this natural treatment system, the resulting effluent is clean enough to be discharged directly into a waterway or to be recycled (Riggle and Gray, 1999). By 2004, over 30 commercial-scale facilities and pilot plants were in operation throughout the U.S. and in seven other countries, providing a low-cost, sustainable alternative to high-tech conventional wastewater treatment. As communities struggle to avoid stringent penalties for noncompliance with mandated effluent requirements in the absence of federal funding, it's likely that alternative natural systems will receive much wider and more serious attention in the years ahead.

Elsewhere in the world, a variant on wetlands treatment is the use of fishponds for treating sewage while simultaneously supporting aquaculture. In Lima, Peru, a portion of the city's sewage is directed to stabilization ponds where solids settle out and bacteria decompose the organic wastes. After three or four weeks the water is sufficiently cleansed of pollutants to use for irrigation and for fish culture. Similar systems are currently in operation in Hungary, Germany, Israel, and a number of countries in South and Southeast Asia. The largest of these can be found in Calcutta, India, where human wastewaters nourish algae in two large lakes. Herbivorous fish such as carp and tilapia feed upon these algae and are subsequently harvested to provide Calcutta markets with approximately 7,000 metric tons of fish each year. Obvious concerns about the potential for contamination of fish with human gastrointestinal pathogens can be allayed by retaining sewage in the stabilization lagoons for at least 20 days before allowing it to enter the fishponds or by transferring the fish to clean waters for a period of time prior to harvesting (World Resources Institute, 1992).

Septic Systems

Approximately 30% of all Americans live in unsewered areas where they must utilize on-site septic systems for the disposal of wastewaters from bathrooms, kitchens, and laundries. Most on-site wastewater disposal systems consist of two basic parts: (1) a septic tank, buried in the ground at some distance from the house, to which it is connected by a pipe, and (2) a soil absorption field or sand filter.

The septic tank itself is a watertight container made of concrete or fiberglass with a minimum capacity of 750 gallons. Sewage entering the septic tank is partially decomposed by bacteria under anaerobic conditions. During this process, sludge settles to the bottom of the tank, while lighter solids and grease, as well as gases from the decomposing sludge, rise to the top to form a floating scum. The partially clarified liquid then passes through an outlet and the effluent is evenly dispersed among several perforated pipes in a carefully designed absorption field, which must be of adequate size and proper soil porosity to ensure that the effluent seeping out of the perforated pipe moves quickly enough to prevent ponding, but not so rapidly as to infiltrate aquifers, wells, or surface water supplies before contaminants in the effluent have been filtered out or oxidized.

Since more than half of the solids in the wastewater settle out during the retention period in the septic tank, the accumulation of sludge at the bottom, as well as the scum layer at the top, must be removed periodically (usually every 3–5 years). If this is not done, the sludge build-up reaches the point that solids are discharged into the absorption field, resulting in clogging and ponding. This accumulation of particulates and scum in the pores of the soil prevents proper drainage of the effluent and eventually results in failure of the system. In addition to improper maintenance of the septic tank, other reasons for septic system failure may be: use of a septic tank that is too small for the householders' needs, excessive household water use (large parties in homes on septic systems can be disastrous; repair men jokingly comment that they routinely notice garbage containers overflowing with beer cans when on a call to deal with sewage backups!), insufficient size of the absorption field, soil too impervious to receive effluent, or tree roots clogging the effluent distribution lines.

Although a well-located, carefully constructed, and properly maintained septic system can be a perfectly adequate method of sanitary wastewater disposal (and is the only feasible option in most rural areas), malfunctioning septic systems frequently give rise to serious nonpoint source water pollution, as leachates containing pathogenic organisms and nutrients seep from absorption fields into water supplies. The rapid growth of rural subdivisions, many of which rely on septic systems installed on lots too small to provide adequate waste dispersal, ensures that pollution problems related to septic systems will continue to plague public health officials.

Industrial Discharges

Effluent discharges from industry comprise the second major category of point source water pollution and consist of a wide range of pollutants which, for regulatory purposes, have been subdivided into three major groups:

1. *Conventional Pollutants*—These include organic wastes high in BOD, suspended solids, acids, oil and grease, etc. Such pollutants originate from food processing plants, pulp and paper mills, steel mills, oil tanker spills and cleaning operations, accidents involving offshore oil drilling, and so forth.

2. *Toxic Pollutants*—A list of 129 priority toxic pollutants was developed by EPA in 1976 (three subsequently have been de-listed); substances listed include heavy metals such as cadmium, mercury, and lead, PCBs, benzene, chloroform, cyanide, arsenic, 2,4-D, and a number of other pesticides. The electroplating and metal-processing industries, plastics manufacturers, and chemical companies are but a few of the industries discharging toxic effluents.

3. *Nonconventional Pollutants*—All the other pollutants not classified by EPA as either conventional or toxic are grouped into this third category—substances such as nitrogen and phosphorus, iron, tin, aluminum, chloride, and ammonia. As in the preceding categories, the sources of such pollutants can be traced to a wide variety of industrial processes.

The Clean Water Act requires EPA to develop technology-based national treatment standards for each category of industrial discharger (e.g., petroleum refiners, textile mills, iron and steel, leather tanning, etc.), directing that standards be reviewed periodically and made increasingly stringent as pollution control technologies advance. Industries discharging directly into the nation's waterways must obtain an NPDES permit, specifying the allowable amounts and constituents of pollutants in their effluent. Dischargers are required to monitor their effluent on a routine basis and violations of permit limitations can result in serious civil or criminal penalties.

For the most part, industry has a better record of compliance with existing water pollution control regulations than do municipal dischargers (i.e., POTWs); EPA estimates that the use of best available pollution control technologies in 22 targeted industrial categories has reduced releases of certain toxic organic chemicals by 99% and heavy metals by 98% since passage of the Clean Water Act in 1972. Altogether, controls imposed on toxic industrial discharges have, according to EPA estimates, prevented the release of more than a billion pounds of toxics yearly into U.S. surface waters; even larger amounts of conventional pollutants have been controlled. Overall, stream monitoring data and self-reporting by industry both indicate a steady downward trend for industrial discharges in recent years—slow but encouraging progress toward the elusive goal of "zero discharge."

Direct Versus Indirect Discharges

Current water pollution laws distinguish two categories of industrial waste discharges: **direct discharges** that flow directly into a receiving stream or lake and **indirect discharges** that go into the sewer system, where they first pass through the municipal sewage treatment plant before entering a waterway along with sanitary wastewater effluent. When citizens think about industrial pollutant discharges, they generally envision the direct type—pipes from a factory leading straight to the water's edge, pouring a poisonous brew onto the back of some hapless fish. In point of fact, however, the majority of industrial discharges are of the indirect type, released by approximately 27,000 industrial users (IUs) who discharge huge volumes of industrial wastewaters into sewer systems every year. In cases where indirect industrial discharges consist primarily of biodegradable organic wastes, sending them to the sewage treatment plant is appropriate, since the same processes that decompose human excreta are effective on other organic materials as well. In situations involving toxic substances, however, indirect discharges via the sewer system have caused a number of very serious problems.

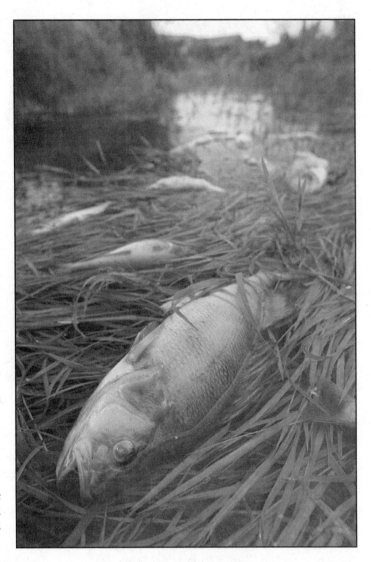

Fish kills provide dramatic evidence of the degradation of water quality by human activities.

Structural damage to sewer system and treatment plant. Industrial discharges of strong acids or alkalis can corrode both sewer pipes and equipment at the POTW. Some chemicals react to produce toxic fumes that can present a serious health threat to workers at the treatment plant, and certain volatile substances can generate a build-up of gas in the sewers, occasionally resulting in explosions.

Interference with biological treatment processes. When toxic chemicals like synthetic organic pesticides pass through a sewage treatment plant, they have the same effect on the microbes responsible for secondary treatment as they do on the target pests—they kill them, and in so doing render the sewage treatment plant ineffective.

Biosolids contamination. Certain toxics such as cadmium, mercury, lead, and arsenic may pass through the sewage treatment plant without damaging equipment or interfering with biological treatment. Nevertheless, they pose major problems because they can be assimilated by the bacteria that provide secondary treatment and subsequently accumulate in the sludge, seriously limiting disposal options for biosolids. Sludge containing excessive concentrations of heavy metals cannot be land-applied

Discharges of hexane from an industry into Louisville, Kentucky's sewer system caused an explosion in 1981 that destroyed two miles of city streets. [© *The Courier-Journal*]

due to concerns that toxics may be taken up by plants or leach into groundwater. Similarly, there are restrictions on incineration of metals-contaminated sludge (Banks and Dubrowski, 1982).

Violation of POTW effluent limitations. Because sewage treatment plants, like industries, must comply with the terms of their NPDES permit, toxic chemicals that pass through the treatment plant and pollute the receiving waters make it necessary for the POTW to install methods of advanced wastewater treatment to prevent such violations from occurring. This, of course, is a costly undertaking, the expense of which is borne by the tax-paying public.

Need for Pretreatment of Indirect Discharges

Problems such as those just described led Congress to legislate a national **pretreatment program** that requires industrial users to detoxify their effluent before discharging it into the sewer. EPA was charged with setting standards for specifically prohibited pollutant discharges as well as categorical pretreatment standards for groups of industries, comparable to the effluent limitations requiring best available technology for controlling pollution from direct dischargers. The work of developing, implementing, and enforcing the program has been assigned to approximately 1,600 local POTWs (those treating five million gallons of wastewater or more on a daily basis) that also have authority to set additional discharge requirements above and beyond the federal standards if such action is deemed necessary. Although originally mandated in 1972, the pretreatment program was extremely slow in getting started, in part because EPA did not formulate basic rules for the program until 1980. Implementation of the program by local sanitary districts moved into high gear by the mid-1980s and today most industries discharging wastewaters to municipal sewers have some form of pretreatment program in place. EPA reports that as a result of the national pretreatment program, industrial users have reduced the amount of pollutants they discharge to POTWs, a fact reflected most dramatically in the sharp reduction in metals present in sludge. A survey of biosolids carried out by the Association of Metropolitan Sewerage Agencies revealed that the concentrations of metals regulated by federal pretreatment rules dropped by 59% between 1986 and 1997. Restrictions on industrial users can't solve every problem related to chemical discharges, however, since not all of the hazardous materials flowing into sewage treatment plants are of industrial origin. Of the regulated toxics entering POTWs, about 15% come from residences—all those bleaches, toilet bowl cleaners, paint thinners, outdated medications, etc., that we flush down the drain don't simply disappear but merge with the myriad of other substances moving through the sewers and eventually arrive at a sewage treatment plant. We all contribute to the problem.

Industrial Accidents, Spills, and Stormwater Runoff

In addition to direct and indirect effluent discharges, some industrial pollutants enter waterways due to transportation accidents, leaks in chemical containers, tanker spills or oilrig blowouts, or chemical runoff from industrial waste sites during storm episodes. Of these various events, the dramatic visual impact of oil spills at sea attract the most public attention. Fortunately, experience from numerous such events indicates their long-term ecological impact is frequently less serious than many fear. Studies of past marine spills show that while petroleum is toxic to many organisms, there is no strong evidence that oil spills have done any permanent damage to the world's ocean resources. Such spills, in fact, comprise a relatively small portion of the oil entering the seas each year. Routine tanker operations such as tank cleaning and ballasting contribute almost twice as many petro-pollutants to the ocean on an annual basis as do spills, even though they attract much less attention. While tanker accidents or offshore rig blowouts can have a catastrophic short-term impact on biotic communities, recovery begins within a matter of months and many such communities have returned to their pre-spill appearance within a year or two.

In 1987 mounting concerns about the adverse environmental impact of urban stormwater runoff prompted Congress to mandate a far-reaching new program to control stormwater discharges. Implementation of the first phase of the program began in 1995, with regulations imposed on more than 170 cities (those with populations of 100,000 or more), 47 counties, approximately 100,000 industrial facilities, and sites of construction activity disturbing five or more acres of land. Affected parties must identify the sources and types of pollutants that could be present in stormwater runoff from their premises and subsequently implement controls to prevent potential contaminants from washing into storm sewers. For municipalities, required preventive measures will include programs to detect and remove illegal connections, ending the improper dumping of used oil and other wastes into storm sewers, preventing and controlling spills, and adopting street de-icing methods less environmentally damaging than the use of road salt. Affected industries, which include those engaged in activities as diverse as manufacturing, airport operations, recycling, mining, wood treating, landfilling—virtually any facility where stormwater could come into contact with raw materials or wastes—must devise improved methods for handling and storing materials and for preventing spills. All potential contributors to stormwater contamination, municipalities and industries alike, are required to obtain discharge permits stipulating exactly how they intend to minimize polluted runoff by developing

Box 15-4 Watch Where You Swim— Recreational Water Illnesses May Be Lurking

A refreshing dip in the pool on a hot summer day, an afternoon at the beach, or a relaxing interlude in a hot tub are pleasures enjoyed by millions of people, totally oblivious to any disease hazard posed by such activities. In recent years, however, many are learning the hard way that microbes and parasites in both treated and natural recreational waters can make them sick. Since the CDC began compiling reports in 1978, the confirmed number of recreational water illnesses (RWI) has been steadily increasing and health authorities assume many more go unreported. In its 2002 surveillance report, covering 25 states during 1999–2000, CDC reported 59 outbreaks, the largest number yet, affecting almost 2,100 people, 25 of whom were hospitalized and four died.

The most frequent outbreaks involved cases of gastroenteritis (diarrhea), acquired while bathing in pools or interactive fountains. Although such facilities are required to comply with state and local regulations regarding maintenance and disinfection, follow-up investigations showed that the majority of pools implicated in waterborne disease outbreaks were poorly maintained and inadequately treated, characterized by disrupted chlorine disinfection. In one situation involving a private pool, not only was disinfection noncontinuous, but there also were ducks swimming in the water! It should be noted that even when pool operators follow proper disinfection procedures, the protective chlorine residual can be depleted more rapidly than usual if the pool is overcrowded with swimmers, if organic material enters the water, or when the weather is particularly hot and sunny. Inadequate chlorine residual permits the survival of waterborne bacteria, which may then be ingested when swimmers accidentally swallow pool water.

In most of the reported outbreaks involving pools, however, bacteria were not the culprits. The vast majority of illnesses were caused, instead, by the protozoan parasite, *Cryptosporidium parvum*, a pathogen not even recognized as a cause of human disease until 1976 but now regarded as a major threat to water safety. Cysts of *Cryptosporid-*

ium, entering the water in fecal material, are highly resistant to chlorination and can remain viable in pools for several days, even when chlorine concentrations in the water meet the standards set by public health authorities. Victims of cryptosporidiosis experience profuse diarrhea that can persist for as long as three weeks. If they go back into the water during that time, they can recontaminate the pool and further spread the disease. This seems to have been the situation in a large outbreak in 2000 at a private swim club in Nebraska, where 225 swimmers contracted cryptosporidiosis over a period of many weeks. Subsequent interviews with victims revealed that 37 of them continued to use the pool while they were still experiencing diarrhea.

While infections associated with swimming pools and interactive fountains most frequently involve gastrointestinal problems, those contracted in hot tubs are more likely to be a form of dermatitis called "hot tub rash." Caused by the bacterium *Pseudomonas aeruginosa*, this itchy skin condition often develops into a bumpy red rash, sensitive to the touch and sometimes featuring pus-filled blisters surrounding the hair follicles. The rash is often worse on areas of the skin covered by the victim's swimsuit, since wet fabric keeps contaminated water in contact with skin for some time after other parts of the body have dried off—a good reason for showering and changing into dry clothes as soon as possible after leaving the water. The causative pathogen, *P. aeruginosa*, is a common organism in soil and water but is effectively controlled through disinfection with chlorine or bromine and by maintaining proper pH levels in the water. To ensure water safety, chlorine/bromine and pH levels should be tested frequently because the warm temperatures typical of hot tub and spa water cause disinfectants to evaporate faster than is the case in swimming pools. Investigations of hot tub-related dermatitis outbreaks almost always identify treatment deficiencies as the causative factor.

Recreational water illnesses are certainly not restricted to treated pools or hot tubs. Swimming in fecally polluted lakes, marine waters, or untreated children's wading pools has led to a number of RWI outbreaks. The pathogen in most reported cases involving freshwater is *E. coli 0157:H7*, the culprit in many serious food-poisoning outbreaks as well. In some situations, just as in the pool incidents previously described, water contamination occurred as a result of infected children, usually toddlers, defecating in or near the water. In other cases, droppings of water birds or mammals introduce fecal bacteria into recreational waters. Point sources of pollution such as POTWs and storm sewers, if located near bathing beaches, may discharge pathogen-laden wastewaters that pose a health risk to swimmers. Malfunctioning septic systems, likewise, can be a source of water contamination. Nonpoint sources can degrade recreational waters when heavy rainfall washes animal wastes, soil, fertilizers, pesticides, and other pollutants off the land and into waterways. For this reason, beach water generally experiences much higher levels of pollution during and immediately after rainstorms, making swimming at such times inadvisable.

In addition to the risk of *E. coli 0157:H7* and other bacterial infections, swimming or playing in contaminated water may result in a parasitic infection properly termed cercarial dermatitis but more commonly known as "swimmer's itch." Caused by a species of flatworm related to the pathogen responsible for schistosomiasis in tropical regions, this temperate-zone pathogen alternates between a snail host and several species of warm-blooded animals, including ducks, geese, swans, gulls, beavers, and muskrats. The feces of infected animals contain worm eggs that hatch into free-swimming larvae when they come into contact with water. The larvae then parasitize snails, which subsequently release second-stage larvae called cercariae. These swim off in search of a host animal, one of those listed above, but sometimes encounter a human bather instead and burrow into the skin. Since humans are not the parasite's natural host, they soon die; before doing so, however, they provoke a tingling, burning, or itching sensation which may persist for as long as a week. Frequently, small reddish pimples appear, often developing into small blisters. Medical attention is seldom required, as the rash gradually fades away; however, since swimmer's itch is essentially an allergic reaction to the parasite, repeated exposures result in increasingly severe symptoms of discomfort. Because the cercariae are most likely to occur in shallow water near the shoreline where snails are common, small children tend to be the most frequent victims of swimmer's itch. Avoidance is the best approach for dealing with this recreational water illness: don't swim in areas where swimmer's itch is a known problem, shower or towel off immediately after leaving the water, and try to prevent the problem in the first place by not feeding (and thus attracting) waterfowl close to areas where people swim.

Growing awareness of the health issues posed by RWIs has prompted greater scrutiny of beach conditions by federal, state, and local health and environmental agencies. Every year hundreds, even thousands, of beaches in the U.S. are posted with warnings or closed for a day or more due to known water contamination. EPA has established federal guidelines to assist states in setting standards for microbial water quality in lakes, ponds, and marine waters, but regulation remains the prerogative of state and local governments. As a result, these vary widely from one jurisdiction to another. Because many beaches are still not monitored at all, or monitored only sporadically, those who swim there have no way of knowing whether or not a hazard exists. To help rectify this problem, the EPA has instituted its BEACH Program (Beaches Environmental Assessment, Closure and Health Program), one feature of which is the agency's Beach Watch Web site (www.epa.gov/waterscience/beacon/) where those interested can access information regarding water quality and local protection programs at specific U.S. beaches.

Common-sense precautions and good personal hygiene on the part of bathers (particularly parents of toddlers and young children), combined with governmental public health efforts, can help ensure that fun in the water won't make you sick.

Reference

CDC. 2002. "Surveillance for Waterborne-Disease Outbreaks—United States, 1999–2000. *Morbidity & Mortality Weekly Report* 51 (SS08):1–28 (Nov 22).

and implementing comprehensive management programs. The second phase of the program, now underway, extends the requirement for stormwater discharge permits to small, municipal storm sewer systems located in urban areas and to construction activities disturbing 1–5 acres of land. Due to the protracted schedule for filing permit applications and extended timetables for achieving compliance, it will likely be years before all sources of urban stormwater are regulated. Nevertheless, after years of handwringing over urban water quality problems caused by stormwater runoff, meaningful steps to tackle this problem are finally underway (EPA, 1999; Goldberg, 1993).

Water Pollution and Health

If a pollster were to conduct sidewalk interviews on what major concerns the average man or woman might have regarding water pollution, it's a safe bet that eutrophication of Chesapeake Bay, fish kills in the Mississippi, or New York City's sludge disposal headaches would rank far down on the list. Among the vast majority of respondents, the number one water quality priority undoubtedly would be assurance that the water flowing from their kitchen or bathroom faucet was safe to drink. Such public concerns stem from the recognition that human health is directly threatened by impure drinking water. There exists today a growing realization that the quality of drinking water is inextricably linked to the quality of our environment as a whole, inasmuch as air pollutants, agricultural chemicals, leachates from landfills, sewage, and industrial effluents all can invade public water supplies. While the nature of drinking water contamination problems differs somewhat in the developing nations versus more industrialized societies, the extent to which polluted water adversely affects health and well-being is a worldwide source of concern.

Microbial Waterborne Disease

Prior to the late 19th century, outbreaks of epidemic waterborne disease in every part of the world claimed a heavy toll in human lives and suffering. As late as the 1880s, typhoid killed 75–100 people per 100,000 population in the United States each year. A major outbreak of the disease in Chicago in 1885 claimed 90,000 victims and persuaded city officials to divert the flow of Chicago's sewage from Lake Michigan, also the source of municipal drinking water supplies, into the Sanitary and Ship Canal (completed in 1900) and ultimately to the Illinois River and the Mississippi—a policy decision that had the unintended side effect of seriously degrading the quality and attractiveness of the Illinois River. Cholera also was a feared disease in 19th century America; a major outbreak in the Mississippi Valley during the 1870s claimed many lives and large numbers of westward-bound settlers died of cholera along the wagon trails.

In the Third World, contamination of waterways with a wide range of microbial pathogens found in human body wastes constitutes the most pressing environmental health problem. The World Health Organization estimates that almost 5,500 people, most of them children, die every day due to fecally contaminated drinking water. The global toll due to infectious diarrhea among all age groups in 2001 was approximately 2 million, 1.4 million of whom were children under 5 years old (United Nations, 2003). The gastrointestinal infections that occur when such pathogens are ingested are the leading cause of illness and death in most developing countries. Reducing the incidence of such disease requires not only the installation of water purification technologies, but also provision of sanitary wastewater disposal and public education regarding personal and household hygiene. During the 1980s, designated by the UN as the "International Drinking Water Supply and Sanitation Decade," significant gains were

Box 15-5 Water and Terrorism: How Vulnerable is America's Drinking Water?

It sounds like the plot for a B-grade movie: foreign terrorists sneak across U.S. borders and kill millions of Americans by surreptitiously poisoning public drinking water supplies. Prior to 9/11, few of us would have spent much time worrying about such a scenario, but following the tragic events of September 2001, efforts to improve national security include a reevaluation of how best to safeguard U.S. water security.

Attempts to use contaminated water as a weapon against enemies are age-old. Examples range from the malevolent dumping of dead bodies into wells to the deliberate lacing of drinking water supplies with pure cultures of the bacterial pathogens that cause cholera and dysentery—a tactic used by the Japanese military against several Chinese cities during World War II.

Despite the fearsome mental images such acts provoke, however, actual instances of the successful use of biological or chemical agents to poison a municipal water supply are few and far between. As the EPA points out, because of rapid dilution, it would take extremely large amounts of an introduced contaminant to threaten large water supply reservoirs. In addition, some of the bacterial species and biotoxins considered likely biological warfare agents are rendered inactive by standard disinfection processes; others could be removed by such advanced treatment technologies as micro- and ultra-filtration and reverse osmosis filtration (technologies which, however, are not currently in place at most municipal water treatment plants). Until now, the need to worry about such eventualities has seemed remote; over the past 100 years, medical records reveal only one death in the entire United States caused by intentionally contaminated water.

Unfortunately, the events of 9/11 and heightened awareness of an international terrorist threat have removed any sense of complacency regarding U.S. water security. Concerns increased in 2002 with the discovery of documents in Afghanistan indicating that al Qaeda operatives were considering various methods for massive disruption of American water supplies and water treatment plants. By then, preparations to increase security at such facilities had already been underway for several years. In 1998 President Clinton signed Presidential Decision Directive 63, identifying drinking water as one of America's critical infrastructures and directing EPA to take the lead in improving water system security. The pace of such activities accelerated significantly following passage of the 2002 Bioterrorism Act, legislation prompted by fears of more post-9/11 terrorist attacks within the U.S. The new law forced water utilities, whose existing emergency preparedness plans dealt solely with natural disasters or acts of vandalism, to focus instead on deliberate attempts by terrorists to disrupt or contaminate water supplies.

Such attacks, if successfully carried out, would have a devastating impact on public health, as well as on sanitation and fire-fighting capability, and could create widespread panic within affected communities. Under the Bioterrorism Act, EPA was required to prepare a baseline threat report, detailing likely threats that utilities should consider when assessing their own vulnerability to terrorism or other deliberate acts to disrupt water supplies. The utilities were then required to conduct vulnerability assessments, examining risks and identifying countermeasures for terrorist attacks against a wide range of water system components. After completing and submitting their vulnerability assessment to EPA, a process now accomplished, utilities must prepare an emergency response plan, based on the results of that assessment.

These new emergency response plans are, by necessity, fundamentally different from previous plans that focused primarily on major water main ruptures or potential tornado, hurricane, or earthquake damage, all of which are immediately recognizable problems. Although some types of terrorist attack, such as the use of explosives to inactivate a treatment plant or to blow up distribution lines, would be apparent within a matter of minutes, other equally devastating forms of sabotage might not be recognized for days. For example, if chemical or biological agents were somehow introduced into the post-treatment water distribution system (considered by experts a much more likely avenue of attack than dumping them into large reservoirs), it is unlikely this would be noticed until the utility started receiving customer complaints about the strange taste, odor, or color of water flowing from their taps—or until hospitals began to report a mysterious surge in emergency room visits. Even telling the public what to do in such a situation would be problematic. The standard "boil order" that typically accompanies a water main break might not be appropriate in a situation where the nature of the problem is still in question. Boiling water intended for drinking or cooking is generally effective in killing bacterial contaminants but does nothing to remove chemical pollutants—indeed, it simply increases their concentration. Similarly, as long as microbially contaminated water is used only for bathing it presents little danger, but the same may not be true for water containing chemical toxins. Until the identity of a presumed contaminant is definitive, the affected utility may have to advise the public not to use the water for any purpose. Currently, information on these and related water security topics is being exchanged among utilities nationwide via Water Information Sharing and Analysis Centers, which serve as an important link between service providers and government agencies dealing with homeland security, public and environmental health, intelligence, and law enforcement.

In addition to performing mandated vulnerability assessments and developing response plans, utilities have been altering many long-established policies and procedures to enhance the security of the water supply infrastructure. Examples of such changes include requirements that those delivering chemical supplies provide advance notification and undergo rigorous identity checks; strict procedures regarding access and parking for contractors and service providers; background checks on new employees; and coordination with local law enforcement agencies for increased surveillance and patrolling of utility grounds. Levels of vigilance have been particularly high in several cities thought to be at special risk. In Chicago, the local Coast Guard conducts regular patrols near that city's water intake site in Lake Michigan. New York City has increased the number of water samples it takes for testing each day and has blocked off some roads near its upstate reservoirs while stationing armed guards at some sites.

Whether all the precautions will be sufficiently protective if terrorists are determined to attack water supply facilities is open to question. Some observers contend that water treatment plants are too large to protect against intrusion, given existing financial resources, and that water distribution pipelines, with hundreds of thousands of access points, are nearly impossible to protect everywhere. Pointing out that the nation's water infrastructure was never intended to withstand terrorism, such critics suggest de-centralizing water treatment, perhaps establishing neighborhood package plants for drinking water treatment or even "point-of-use" treatment, utilizing under-the-faucet filters featuring advanced technologies that could reduce both biological and chemical hazards.

A final, and critical, element in protecting America's water supply is the active involvement of ordinary citizens. A number of utilities have already organized neighborhood watch programs, enlisting the help of residents living near pumping stations, storage tanks, or reservoirs to act as an extra set of eyes, contacting police or the utility if they notice any suspicious activity.

Although most experts regard a successful terrorist attack against America's water supply as unlikely, it is only prudent to establish proactive policies and procedures against intentional destruction or contamination in order to ensure that this country continues to enjoy, as it has for many years, the safest drinking water in the world.

References

American Water Works Association. 2003. *Protecting the Water: Drinking Water Security in America After 9/11.*

Christopher, George W. et al. 1997. "Biological Warfare: A Historical Perspective." *Journal of the American Medical Association* 275, no. 5 (Aug. 6).

Isenberg, David. 2002. *CDI Terrorism Project: Securing U.S. Water Supplies.* Centers for Defense Information. www.cdi.org/terrorism/water-pr.cfm. Accessed 08/22/04.

made in expanding access to safe water supplies, particularly in rural areas where the number of people served increased by 240% worldwide (150% increase among city dwellers). Access to sanitation facilities improved as well, but these gains were largely offset by the continued rapid rate of population growth and urbanization in nations throughout the developing world. In spite of these Herculean efforts, 1.1 billion people today still lack safe drinking water and 2.6 billion remain without adequate sanitary facilities—a reflection of the inability of public works projects in developing nations to keep pace with the needs of rapidly growing populations, as well as the low priority given to such efforts by many Third World governments. In industrialized countries, disease caused by fecal pollution of waterways is much less common now than it was several generations ago. Nevertheless, outbreaks of gastroenteritis traced to microbial contamination of drinking water do occur from time to time, occasionally in headline-provoking magnitude. In the United States, despite the impression that waterborne disease is a thing of the past, periodic surveillance reports issued by the Centers for Disease Control and Prevention (CDC) document numerous outbreaks, thousands of cases of illness, and occasional deaths caused by contaminated drinking water. Although most such occurrences in recent years have been associated with unregulated private wells or small water systems where financial resources preclude the sophisticated equipment and highly trained personnel generally found in larger communities, a 1993 outbreak in Milwaukee, Wisconsin, sickened almost 400,000 people. These numbers, of course, represent only those illnesses that are reported to public health authorities. EPA estimates that for every case of waterborne disease identified, 25 more never appear in the statistics because of haphazard reporting.

Diarrheal illness may be caused by any of a large number of microbial species associated with sewage-tainted drinking water and fall roughly into one of the following groups.

Bacteria. Typhoid fever and cholera are the most notorious of the bacterial enteric diseases and over the centuries have been responsible for millions of human deaths and illnesses worldwide. Other bacterial waterborne ailments include dysentery *(Shigella),* paratyphoid, salmonellosis, *Campylobacter,* and some forms of *E. coli*—ailments which, like typhoid and cholera, can also be contracted by eating food har-

Milwaukee residents stand in line to obtain fresh water after protozoa in the public water supply caused a massive disease outbreak in 1993. [*Milwaukee Sentinel photo*]

boring pathogens of fecal origin. Whereas typhoid and paratyphoid are characterized by headache, muscle pains, high fever, and constipation alternating with diarrhea (all symptoms being less severe in paratyphoid), cholera, dysentery, and salmonellosis are all typified by severe diarrhea (bloody in the case of dysentery) and vomiting.

Viruses. Noroviruses, hepatitis A, poliomyelitis, and rotavirus are among the most common of the several hundred species of enteric viruses associated with waterborne diarrheal illness. Many health authorities suspect that most waterborne ailments caused by unidentified pathogens are, in fact, viral diseases. Viruses are much more resistant to disinfection with chlorine than are bacteria, a fact which explains why outbreaks of hepatitis A have occasionally occurred in communities where drinking water was chlorinated and presumably was safe. While it was once thought that viral pathogens present a concern only in surface waters, it is now known that viruses also contaminate 20–30% of U.S. groundwaters, where they can survive for many months (NRC, 1999).

Protozoans. While more than 30 species of parasites may infect the human gut, only a few present a serious disease threat. Of these, the most common is giardiasis, caused by the flagellated protozoan *Giardia lamblia,* an inhabitant of the intestines of a wide variety of vertebrate animals. Over the past 30-odd years *Giardia* has been blamed for numerous reported outbreaks in the United States, some of them in remote areas where the source of the problem was traced to infected beavers or deer that were polluting the water with feces containing protozoan cysts. Since *Giardia* is largely resistant to chlorination, filtration of drinking water supplies is important in forestalling outbreaks of giardiasis. Another chlorine-resistant protozoan parasite causing serious concern is *Cryptosporidium*, the culprit responsible for the massive disease outbreak in Milwaukee in April 1993, as well as for two other major outbreaks a few years earlier in Georgia and Oregon. Finally, amoebiasis (amoebic dysentery) is another widespread parasitic infection afflicting an estimated half billion people worldwide. Amoebic dysentery constitutes a major health problem in Mexico, eastern South America, western and southern Africa, China, and throughout Southeast Asia (Nash, 1993).

Water Purification

At the beginning of the 20th century, a growing awareness of the link between waterborne pathogens and disease outbreaks prompted municipal officials in North America and Europe to institute various methods of drinking water treatment that largely succeeded in eliminating the serious water-related epidemic diseases of the past. The most important new treatment method introduced at this time was chlorination, first used as a water disinfectant in Belgium in 1903. Introduced to the United States five years later, chlorine disinfection made its American debut in Chicago in 1908 and was swiftly adopted by larger communities nationwide. Such advances in water treatment quickly effected a precipitous decline in deaths due to gastrointestinal waterborne disease and immeasurably improved public health. Nevertheless, the organisms that cause typhoid, cholera, dysentery, and other gastrointestinal ailments are still in our midst, ready to make their presence known whenever a breakdown in water treatment processes affords opportunity for such pathogens to penetrate our technological lines of defense.

Unlike sewage treatment, which is intended to reduce levels of wastewater contamination to the point where the effluent can be returned to a stream without provoking serious health or ecological damage, drinking water treatment theoretically should entirely remove all contaminants in the water, or at least reduce them to acceptable levels. All drinking water, regardless of its source, should be treated prior to consumption, since it can never be safely assumed that such water is totally free from contamination.

Although the precise details of drinking water treatment vary from plant to plant, depending largely on the quality of the local raw water supply (i.e., water from polluted surface sources will require more extensive treatment than does well water drawn from a high quality uncontaminated aquifer), the basic steps in the process can be described as follows:

1. *Sedimentation*—Incoming raw water is detained in a quiet pond or tank for at least 24 hours to allow heavy suspended material to settle out.

2. *Coagulation*—Alum (hydrated aluminum sulfate) is added to the water to cause smaller suspended solids to form flocs, which then precipitate to the bottom of the tank.

3. *Filtration*—Filtration through beds of sand, crushed anthracite coal, or diatomaceous earth further reduces the concentration of remaining suspended solids, including many bacterial cells and protozoans.

4. *Disinfection*—Most commonly accomplished with chlorine (ozone, bromine, iodine, or ultraviolet light also can be used for disinfection), disinfection is the most important method utilized for killing pathogens in water. An important advantage enjoyed by chlorine over other disinfectants is that it leaves a residual in the water that continues to provide germ-killing potential as the water travels through the distribution system to its point of use. Thus in the event of cross-contamination due to faulty plumbing or a break in water lines, some disinfectant is still present to kill intruding bacteria. However, disinfection in the absence of the preceding steps is not highly effective because organic materials and suspended solids in the water interfere with the germicidal action of the chlorine. In addition, occasional outbreaks of hepatitis, giardiasis, and cryptosporidiosis in cities where water has been disinfected indicate that chlorine is not as effective in killing viruses and protozoa as it is against other disease organisms.

In many water treatment plants, particularly those utilizing well water, preliminary treatment also includes aerating the water to remove iron and dissolved gases such as hydrogen sulfide, which impart objectionable tastes and odor to the water. In parts of the country where water contains excess amounts of dissolved calcium or magnesium (i.e., where the water is "hard"), lime and soda ash are added to precipitate these minerals out of solution, thereby "softening" the water. Ion exchange is an alternative method that can be used for this purpose. Finally, many treatment plants today add fluoride to the finished water to reduce the incidence of tooth decay (Koren, 1980).

To ensure that the water treatment process is working efficiently, laboratory tests of finished water samples are carried out on a regular basis. Historically, the presence of appreciable numbers of coliform bacteria in a water sample has been used as an indication that the water is unsafe to drink. In fact, coliforms themselves rarely cause disease; however, because they are common inhabitants of the intestines of warm-blooded animals, present in greater numbers than the pathogenic bacteria, and because they can survive for longer periods of time in water than do the latter, coliforms serve as indicators that the water is contaminated with fecal material and hence potentially hazardous. In other words, the presence of fecal coliform bacteria in a water sample warns health officials that less abundant, but more harmful organisms such as the dysentery bacillus or hepatitis virus might also be present, since all of these organisms live in the intestinal tract and are expelled with fecal material. The predictive value of the coliform test for establishing the safety of a given water supply is not absolute, however. As outbreaks of hepatitis A and cryptosporidiosis have demonstrated, disinfection that kills coliform bacteria may not always eliminate pathogenic viruses and protozoa.

Chemical Contaminants in Drinking Water

Standard water treatment processes, designed primarily to remove bacteria, hardness, and odors from water supplies, have been outstandingly successful in reducing the incidence of acute waterborne disease throughout the industrialized world. However, in spite of the considerable improvement in drinking water quality from a bacteriological perspective, the public today is justifiably alarmed about the safety of water supplies due to recent revelations of toxic chemicals in drinking water. With purification processes aimed at preventing the microbial diseases of the past, few water treatment plants are equipped to remove—or even to detect—the 100,000 or more synthetic organic chemicals now in use, many of which are known to be present in drinking water supplies across the country. Although these substances may be present in concentrations measured in parts per million (ppm) or even parts per billion (ppb), the fact that many of them are known to be mutagenic or carcinogenic raises unanswered questions concerning the long-term health effects of ingesting small amounts of poison on a daily basis. Indeed, the fact that some organic chemicals can be harmful to human health and to aquatic organisms at levels well below those currently detectable by standard analytical methods makes the issue particularly worrisome. A direct cause-and-effect relationship between toxic chemicals in drinking water and human health damage has not yet been conclusively demonstrated, but circumstantial evidence and the testimony of people who, unknowingly, consumed high levels of toxic chemicals with their water for a number of years are alarming.

Synthetic organic pollutants. The kinds of synthetic organic chemicals (SOCs, as they are now called) contaminating surface waters and aquifers worldwide consist of a vast array of pesticides, industrial solvents and cleaning fluids, polychlorinated biphenyls, and disinfection by-products. They originate from a wide range of activities such as chemical manufacturing, petroleum refining, iron and steel production, coal mining, wood pulp processing, textile manufacturing, and agriculture. They enter surface waters through direct and indirect discharges, by surface runoff, or by volatilization and subsequent fallout during precipitation episodes. Well waters can concentrate high levels of SOCs as a result of poor waste disposal practices or downward percolation of farm chemicals after heavy rains. The presence of SOCs in drinking water supplies has been a steadily growing source of public concern since the mid-1970s when several epidemiologic studies suggestively, though not conclusively, linked the presence of these chemicals with an elevated incidence of various types of cancer among exposed populations. Certain disinfection by-products called **trihalomethanes (THMs)** attracted the most attention and initiated a controversy over drinking water disinfection that persists in muted form even today. THMs, which include the carcinogen chloroform, are formed at the water treatment plant itself when chlorine is added to water containing the naturally occurring humic substances found in virtually any lake or river. The fact that traces of chloroform have been detected in almost every water system tested for this chemical led some people to call for the discontinuation of drinking water chlorination. However, since THMs usually are present only in minute amounts, many water experts argue that they pose a minimal health risk. More importantly, they contend that abandoning chlorination would result in a return of the microbial waterborne diseases that pose a much more immediate health threat than

Box 15-6   Good Intentions—Tragic Results

The World Health Organization (WHO) calls it "the worst mass poisoning in history." In the South Asian nation of Bangladesh and the neighboring Indian state of West Bengal, more than 100,000 people are slowly dying of arsenic poisoning and experts predict that millions of Bangladeshis could be similarly afflicted in the years immediately ahead. Ironically, the tragedy unfolding is the unintended outcome of a well-meaning development effort launched years ago by the United Nations' Children's Fund (UNICEF), working with the enthusiastic support of the government of Bangladesh.

For centuries, waterborne diarrheal infections had been the leading cause of death and disease in the lush delta lands adjacent to the Bay of Bengal. Rural villagers who comprise the bulk of the population traditionally drew their drinking water from hand-dug wells or ponds polluted with both human and animal wastes. In the 1970s, UNICEF embarked on an ambitious effort to improve the deplorable health conditions by drilling tubewells into the aquifers underlying the region. The intent was to provide an abundant, pathogen-free supply of water for drinking and irrigation. Over the following 25 years, an estimated 3.5 to 4 million tubewells with hand-operated pumps were sunk throughout Bangladesh, about one million of these drilled by the UNICEF-Bangladeshi government partnership, the remainder by private groups or individuals, often financed by loans from aid agencies. Laboratory analysis of groundwater samples for possible contamination was regarded as unnecessary, since the water was being drawn from supposedly pollution-free deep aquifers. A similar tubewell project was launched in West Bengal by the Indian government in the 1950s, again with the aim of improving access to safe drinking water and providing a reliable water supply for irrigated agriculture. Extensive educational efforts were undertaken to persuade initially hesitant villagers to abandon traditional surface water sources for the new tubewell supplies. The success of these programs was soon evident from health data showing a dramatic decline in deaths due to cholera and other water-related illness, and UNICEF could boast that 97% of Bangladeshis were at last within a short walking distance of safe water. This self-congratulation unfortunately proved premature, as what initially appeared to be a resoundingly successful international development project turned out to be an unmitigated human disaster.

The first reports of arsenic poisoning surfaced in India during the 1980s, but attracted little notice. By the mid-1990s, however, as thousands of villagers in both Bangladesh and the Indian state of West Bengal began exhibiting symptoms of chronic arsenicosis, the problem could no longer be ignored. Studies launched by a number of both national and international groups in Bangladesh and India subsequently revealed that in many localities where groundwater reserves were assumed to be clean enough to drink without treatment, well water contains levels of naturally occurring arsenic far above the World Health Organization standard of 10 ppb. A nationwide survey of about 3,500 wells estimated that at least 1.5 million of the 6–11 million shallow tubewells in Bangladesh are heavily contaminated. In many of those sampled, arsenic levels ranged from 500–1000 ppb, while one topped out at 2,400 ppb. Similar surveys in West Bengal and several other states in northeastern India reveal that a large number of tubewells there also contain arsenic levels 5–50 times greater than WHO permissible limits. Wherever sampling showed well water contamination, signs of chronic arsenic poisoning among unsuspecting villagers were apparent, with many individuals already seriously ill. As a rule, chronic arsenic poisoning takes ten to twenty years to be manifested as outward symptoms of disease; thus people drinking from tubewells drilled in the late 1970s or 1980s are only now beginning to show evidence of arsenicosis. The poison accumulates in the hair, nails, skin, and urine, from which it slowly passes out of the body. As arsenic body burdens gradually increase, affected people begin to experience a variety of health problems, including liver and kidney damage, nervous system disorders, hair loss, and general weakness. Most characteristic, however, is a mottling of the skin and, in more advanced cases, the development of warts and open sores on the palms of the hands and soles of feet. These symptoms constitute a sure sign of the arsenic-induced skin cancers that health authorities fear will become a leading cause of death in the years ahead.

By the time the extent of groundwater contamination was recognized, the number of victims seeking medical care was already in the thousands and climbing; undoubtedly thousands more are ill but not sufficiently aware of the nature of their problems to seek help. The social implications of the situation are nearly as tragic as the health consequences. All over Bangladesh young women disfigured with skin lesions and blotchy appearance are unable to attract husbands, and young men find it impossible to obtain employment. Health experts say that, if caught early, arsenic poisoning can be reversed by removing the source of exposure and eating a nutritious diet, but in the poverty-ridden villages of Bangladesh and West Bengal, neither of these requirements is easily achievable.

Attempts to alleviate the mass catastrophe now unfolding have focused on several pressing needs. One of the most urgent is the need to sample all of the millions of wells in the region to ascertain which are polluted and to prevent their use. Due to quirks in the area's geology, a dangerously polluted well might lie but a short distance from one whose water is uncontaminated. Thus, if informed, villagers theoretically could restrict pumping to safe wells only. In an effort to make the risk readily apparent, in many villages wells that tested positive for arsenic contamination had their pumps painted red—an indication that their use should be avoided. Unfortunately, a general lack of awareness as to the seriousness of the problem, plus a universal human proclivity to take "the easy way out" has undermined the effectiveness of this program. Reports abound of villagers continuing to draw their water from a "red" well because the nearest "green" (i.e., uncontaminated) well is located several houses further away. Similarly, if they need water at night, during a heavy rain, or simply when they're feeling tired, people often ignore any danger and drink from the nearby "red" well.

Once the full extent of tubewell contamination is determined, an even greater challenge is that of finding alternative sources of safe water. Some have suggested reserving one pond in each of Bangladesh's 68,000 villages to use exclusively for drinking water and providing purification facilities for those surface supplies. However, local treatment requires a certain level of expertise in operation and maintenance practices that may not always be available. An abortive attempt to supply villagers with chlorine tablets to disinfect surface waters was terminated by the discovery that the chlorine concentrations used were too high, rendering them more of a health hazard than the arsenic. Suggestions that villagers could remove pathogens from pond water simply by boiling it before drinking foundered on the reality that the cost of fuel for doing so was unaffordable for most families. Rooftop rainwater harvesting is another proposed alternative, though its adequacy during dry spells might be problematic. Arsenic filtration devices offer some promise, but gradually become less effective as the filter becomes saturated with the captured arsenic; safe disposal of the latter also presents potential problems. Recent findings by U.K.-based researchers that anaerobic bacteria within the contaminated aquifers play a key role in releasing arsenic into groundwater may lead to yet more novel approaches for tackling the problem at its source, deep within the affected sediments.

In the meantime, among Bangladeshis impatience and anger are mounting against international aid agencies and visiting researchers. Government officials in Bangladesh are becoming resentful as well. Citing numerous international meetings and seminars on the problem, but little concrete action, a Health Ministry official quipped, "The only beneficiaries in the whole issue have been the national and international consultants."

References

Islam, FS et al. 2004. "Role of Metal-Reducing Bacteria in Arsenic Release from Bengal Delta Sediments." *Nature* 430, no. 6995 (July 1).

Kinley, David H., and Zabed Hossain. 2003. "Poisoned Waters." *World•Watch* 16, no. 1 (Jan/Feb).

West Bengal, India and Bangladesh Arsenic Crisis Information Centre.

do THMs. Nevertheless, the controversy has prompted EPA to lower the maximum allowable level of THMs from 100 ppb to 80 ppb and the agency is considering lowering it even further. Concerns about THMs and the costs associated with their control have also caused a growing number of water treatment plant operators to switch from chlorine to UV radiation for drinking water disinfection.

While a number of the more than 100,000 SOCs currently in use (e.g., chloroform, benzene) are known or suspected carcinogens, establishing a direct causal relationship between polluted drinking water and cancer has been problematic. At present, the human health impact of exposure to organic chemicals in water supplies is thought to be relatively minor. Results of a U.S. Geological Survey study of 20 major U.S. river basins revealed that two or more pesticides were present in every stream sample taken and in half the well water samples. Fortunately, the amounts detected were almost always well below EPA's maximum contaminant levels for drinking water. However, over half the stream samples from both urban and agricultural areas contained at least one pesticide at concentrations that exceeded guidelines for the protection of aquatic life (some of the pesticides most frequently detected are suspected endocrine disruptors). Although public health does not appear to be seriously at risk from the low concentrations of pesticides detected, the survey raises some concerns. Health criteria and guidelines are still lacking for a number of the chemicals detected, nor do standards exist for their breakdown products—some of which are more toxic than the original pesticide. In addition, established guidelines fail to consider possible synergistic effects among the various chemicals present in the waterways sampled nor do they take seasonal pulses of higher-than-average concentrations into account. While not a cause for panic, the USGS report highlights some major challenges for improving protection of our nation's water resources (USGS, 1999).

Lead. That ingestion or inhalation of lead can cause human poisoning resulting in a wide range of health problems has been known for many years (see chapter 7). Government initiatives to lower the lead content of housepaint and to phase out the use of leaded gasoline were prompted specifically by the desire to reduce human exposure to this toxic metal. However, in some areas of the country household drinking water may constitute a significant source of lead exposure. This situation does not mean that municipal water treatment plants are doing a poor job, for in almost all cases lead enters drinking water after it leaves the purification plant or private well. The problem arises either from lead service pipes leading from the water main to the house or from within the home plumbing system as a result of corrosion when water passes through lead pipes or through pipes soldered with lead, when brass fixtures are used, or in situations where the water itself is corrosive (i.e., low pH). This type of reaction is particularly likely with "soft" water; corrosion is also increased by the common practice of using water pipes for the grounding of electrical equipment, since electrical current traveling through the ground wire hastens the corrosion of lead in the pipes.

The age of a home's plumbing system is a major determinant of whether or not a lead problem exists. In older structures—those built prior to the 1930s—lead was commonly used for interior piping as well as for the service connections that joined the house to a public water supply. Obviously if a home has lead plumbing, a potential problem exists. After 1930, copper piping largely replaced lead for residential plumbing, but such pipes were typically joined with lead solder; it is this solder that many authorities consider the main contributor to drinking water contamination with lead. Over time, the amount of lead leaching into water from plumbing decreases because mineral deposits gradually form a deposit on the inside of the pipes, preventing water from coming into direct contact with the solder. For this reason, homes with the greatest likelihood of having high lead levels are those less than five years old (unless the plumbing is made of plastic, in which case there's no problem).

Although telltale signs of corrosion (rust-colored water, stained dishwasher or laundry, frequent leaks) or recognition that the house falls into one of the high-risk age categories mentioned above can alert residents to a potential problem, the only way to make a definite determination of excess lead levels is to have the water tested at a certified laboratory (unfortunately, this is not a cheap procedure).

If lab analysis confirms high lead levels, abatement options short of total replacement of the plumbing system are somewhat limited. Reverse osmosis devices, cartridge filters, and distillation units can be installed at the faucet but are quite expensive and of variable effectiveness. Lead exposure can be minimized by two simple actions that should be taken by anyone who has, or suspects, a lead problem:

1. Don't drink water that has been in contact with pipes for more than six hours. The longer water has been standing, the greater the amount of lead likely to be present. Before using such water for drinking or cooking, flush out the pipes by allowing water to run for several minutes or until it is as cold as it will get (this water can be used for washing, watering plants, etc.).

2. Don't consume or cook with hot tap water, since lead dissolves more readily in hot water than in cold. If you need hot water, draw it cold from the tap and use the stove to heat it.

In response to this health hazard, Congress has prohibited the use of solder containing more than 0.2% lead (formerly, solder was 50% lead) and has banned any pipe or fittings containing more than 8% lead in new installations or for repair of public water systems. In addition, a number of states have now banned all use of lead materials in drinking water systems (EPA, 1987).

The realization that lead in drinking water presents a health hazard in many homes has prompted regulators to take a look at the school environment as well. In 1988, under the Lead Contamination Control Act, Congress urged both schools and day-care centers to test water from electric water coolers (some models of which were believed to have lead-lined tanks or other components made of lead) to ensure that children attending those facilities were not receiving excessive lead exposure. While the recommendations for testing and remediation were purely advisory and thus not legally enforceable, many schools complied with the government's request. Unfortunately, other potential sources of lead-contaminated water such as ice machines, non-cooled water fountains, and classroom and kitchen sinks were not mentioned in the advisory.

Continuing concerns about lead in drinking water have led to further EPA actions to reduce this hazard. In May of 1991 the agency promulgated the Lead and Copper Rule, setting an "action level" (not the same as an enforceable standard) of *15 ppb* lead at the water's point of use. Although EPA does not consider any level of lead in water as "safe," the agency believes that 15 ppb is the lowest level of control achievable by water systems, given current technology and financial resources. In cases where that level is exceeded, the rule calls for the water treatment plant to take steps to reduce the corrosivity of the water—an action designed to reduce the leachability of lead within the plumbing system (Gnaedinger, 1993). New alarms were sounded in the spring of 1994 when EPA issued a warning to millions of private well owners, advising them to have their drinking water tested for possible high levels of lead contamination after research carried out by environmental groups at the University of North Carolina-Asheville revealed that the toxic metal was leaching into well water from lead-based brass and bronze alloys in submersible pumps, particularly from those recently installed (of the 11.8 million U.S. homes with private wells, approximately half feature submersible pumps, though not all such pumps have brass components). Environmental groups promptly urged pump manufacturers to recall all pumps containing lead components and replace them with safe, readily available lead-free models made of stainless steel.

Nitrates

Contamination of drinking water supplies with inorganic nitrates from fertilizer or feedlot runoff, seepage from septic systems, or airborne fallout of nitrogen compounds emitted by industry or motor vehicles has been a concern since the 1940s. At that time a mysterious ailment called "blue baby disease" caused 39 deaths and several hundred illnesses among infants in rural areas. By 1945 the condition, more accurately referred to as **methemoglobinemia**, had been linked to the use of nitrate-polluted water from shallow farm wells to prepare infant formula. Bacteria in the babies' intestinal tract convert nitrates to toxic nitrites which bind to hemoglobin, displacing oxygen and producing a bluish discoloration of the skin; in extreme cases, death by asphyxiation can result. Although all members of a household typically drink from the same contaminated water supply, only infants under six months of age are at risk of developing methemoglobinemia because their stomach juices are less acid than those of older children and adults, and hence support a larger bacterial population. Better understanding of the disease and regular monitoring of public drinking water supplies for nitrate content have greatly reduced the incidence of methemoglobinemia in recent decades. Nevertheless, risk of the disease still persists, particularly in agricultural areas of the Midwest where heavy use of nitrogen fertilizers is standard practice and where shallow aquifers supply much of the drinking water used by rural families (surface waters seldom contain concentrations of nitrates high enough to pose serious concerns). Monitoring of private wells for water quality is not a routine practice, but a 1994 national survey revealed that 22% of private farm wells contain nitrate levels in excess of the 10 mg/L EPA standard for public water supplies (unpol-

Nutrient runoff from manure piles in large cattle feedlots pose water challenges in California's Central Valley.

luted water supplies contain an average of 2 mg/L nitrogen). Because nitrates can persist in aquifers for many years, becoming increasingly concentrated as more nitrogen is applied to the land surface season after season, nitrates in drinking water will remain an ongoing health concern (EPA, 1995).

Safe Drinking Water Act

The federal program to protect drinking water quality in the United States is governed by the provisions of the Safe Drinking Water Act (SDWA), first passed by Congress in 1974 and subsequently amended in 1986 and again in 1996. Prior to 1974, regulation of drinking water supplies was the prerogative of the individual states, with federal involvement limited to developing advisory standards (which the states, for the most part, ignored) and to ensuring that interstate carriers such as railroads and airlines provided safe water to their passengers. Even the latter authority was limited to a focus on microbial pathogens only; not until passage of the SDWA were any enforceable provisions dealing with hazardous chemicals in drinking water incorporated into law. Today the situation is quite different. The SDWA has established a federal-state partnership to ensure compliance with federal standards aimed at protecting U.S. residents from a wide range of contaminants potentially present in drinking water supplies. Under the act, EPA establishes **maximum contaminant levels (MCLs)** for more than 80 biological, chemical, and radioactive pollutants. These MCLs must be met by water supplied by every community water system (defined as one having at least 15 service connections used by year-round residents or regularly serving 25 or more people). Concerns about the hundreds of additional unregulated pollutants known to be present in various water supplies around the country prompted Congress to amend the SDWA in 1996. These most recent provisions require EPA to compile a list every five years of currently unregulated drinking water contaminants that may pose health risks. The agency must then decide whether to develop standards for at least five of those contaminants, ensuring that the list of regulated drinking water pollutants will continue to expand in the decades ahead. In addition to its requirements for setting MCLs, the Safe Drinking Water Act sets uniform guidelines for drinking water treatment and mandates that public water systems follow a prescribed schedule for monitoring and testing the quality of their treated water and report the results to the appropriate state agency. For regulation of some types of drinking water contaminants, specifically microbes, stipulating treatment techniques rather than focusing on maximum allowable concentrations has been the traditional basis for control. Demands that more be done to protect the public from such waterborne pathogens as *Giardia* and *Cryptosporidium* have resulted in amendments to SDWA requiring water suppliers to employ filtration in addition to the standard practice of disinfection. Permission to forego the enormous expense of installing filtration technologies can be obtained only when suppliers can prove that effective watershed protection programs are in place to prevent pathogen-contaminated runoff from entering drinking water reservoirs (NRC, 1999). They also must be able to demonstrate that their disinfection controls are stringent enough to remove 99.9% of all viruses and *Giardia* cysts. These are difficult parameters to meet; EPA estimates that only 12% of the approximately 125,000 unfiltered public water systems serving populations over 10,000 will be able to meet these criteria.

The gradually evolving framework of state and federal drinking water legislation—beginning with simple disinfection requirements and culminating in the highly complex mandates embodied in the SDWA—has given Americans a high degree of assurance that the water they drink won't make them sick. Indeed, the provision of safe water supplies to the vast majority of the U.S. population was one of the great

Box 15-7   Safer from the Bottle?—Not Really

Worried about tap water quality, or simply wanting to make a fashion statement, Americans by the millions have been turning to bottled water to quench their thirst. Surveys reveal that 54% of U.S. residents use bottled water at least occasionally, while over one-third drink it more than once a week. By 2003, according to the New York-based Beverage Marketing Corp., average yearly consumption in the U.S. had reached 22.6 gallons per person, approximately double that of ten years earlier. With over 700 brands from which to choose, American consumers collectively spent $8.3 billion that year for a beverage whose labels evoke such back-to-the wild imagery as "natural alpine spring water," "glacier water," "pristine," or "prepared by Nature." Demand is even greater overseas, as bottled water becomes one of the world's most popular beverages of choice. Western Europeans, in fact, consume nearly half of all the world's bottled water, with Italians winning the prize for quaffing the largest volume per person.

Why the rush to the supermarket for a product much more cheaply available from public water supplies? Primarily because many consumers perceive bottled water as safer and tastier than tap water—and because skillful marketing, particularly of expensive imported brands, has made consumption of bottled water fashionable. The bottled water industry has been quick to take advantage of public fears raised by well-publicized events such as the 1993 outbreak of *Cryptosporidium* in Milwaukee. Advertisements promote their product as 100% contaminant-free and hence a safer, healthier alternative to tap water—well worth its premium price. Whereas a gallon of tap water costs, on average, about one-tenth of a cent, a half-liter bottle of imported "designer water" may carry a price tag of $1.50—a 10,000-fold differential. Ironically, the actual cost of the water itself in bottled brands ranges from a fraction of a cent to a few cents; buyers are paying mostly for bottling, packaging, shipping, advertising, retailing, and profits as high as 25–30% in some cases.

That health and aesthetic factors are important determinants of bottled water's appeal is obvious from the fact that demand is highest in those localities where taste and odor problems are prevalent or where reports of water contamination have prompted consumer worries about waterborne disease. Industry surveys have shown that the more health-conscious people become, the more likely they are to drink bottled water. Concerns about weight and physical appearance come into play also—among the largest consumers of bottled water are women aged 14–32. But can health-conscious buyers really be sure that the bottled water they're purchasing is any safer than the tap water they spurn? In 2002, CDC reported that bottled water appeared to be the culprit in a 10-state outbreak of *Salmonella* Bareilly gastroenteritis—the first time that bottled water had been implicated in a widespread waterborne disease outbreak.

Results from a four-year study published in 1999 by the Natural Resources Defense Council (NRDC), a prominent environmental advocacy group, demonstrated that industry claims of bottled water's superiority are simply untrue. NRDC found that nearly one-fourth of the 103 bottled water brands tested for the presence of chemical or biological contaminants had at least one sample that violated California's water quality regulations, with arsenic or synthetic organic compounds being the contaminants most frequently detected. (*Note:* California has standards considerably more protective than federal EPA maximum contaminant levels for drinking water.) Seventeen percent of the brands tested contained, in one or more samples, bacterial contamination and many contained traces of nitrates or other inorganic contaminants. While the concentrations of these pollutants were not high enough, in most cases, to render the water unsafe, advertising claims of absolute purity are obviously misleading. From a taste standpoint, many municipal supplies are as good or better than bottled water. The public water supply in cities such as New York and Los Angeles, for example, consistently rank among the best-tasting waters in the nation, commercial brands included. However, it is true that bottled waters are free of the taint of chlorine detectable in some publicly supplied waters. This is because most bottling companies disinfect their product with ozone, a chemical that leaves no residual.

The bottling industry emphasizes that its product, like publicly supplied water, is heavily regulated by the federal government, in this case by the Food and Drug Administration (FDA), which classifies bottled water as a "food." FDA regulations require that water be bottled in facilities that follow food plant regulations, that they be processed under federally approved manufacturing processes, and that they be delivered to customers in sanitized containers. In addition to FDA imposed requirements, domestic bottled water must meet EPA's drinking water standards and must comply with any state-imposed regulations. Like any food-processing facility, all U.S. bottled water plants are required to be inspected by federal officials at least once a year. Inspection of foreign bottling plants is beyond FDA jurisdiction, though imported brands are supposed to meet the same regulations as domestically produced water. While these requirements at first glance appear to be sufficiently protective, NRDC points out that the 60–70% of bottled water brands that are packaged and sold within one state are not subject to FDA regulation. While the states in which they operate may regulate them (about 40 states do so), about one out of five do not. In addition, FDA has exempted seltzer water and carbonated water from meeting bottled water standards, and less than half the states require that they do so. Regulatory programs for bottled water at both the federal and state level are seriously underfunded and understaffed, raising concerns about the quality of enforcement and oversight activities to ensure that bottled water complies with mandated standards.

A "truth in advertising" issue raised in recent years concerns the source of bottled water. Brand names and logos alike suggest that water on the supermarket shelves arrived direct from a wilderness mountain stream or Elysian spring. Many consumers are thus shocked to discover that an estimated 25–30% of the bottled water sold in the United States is obtained directly from municipal sources, sometimes given additional treatment, sometimes not. Bottling companies selling these brands simply fill their containers with public tap water, apply a fancy label, boost the price, and put them on the supermarket shelf. PepsiCo's *Aquafina*® brand is a case in point, drawn from eleven different municipal supplies across the country. While such water is perfectly safe, it's not the specialty product its purchasers were led to believe. A more egregious example of misleading labeling was a product being sold in Massachusetts as "spring water," featuring a picturesque lake and towering mountains on the label. Investigators discovered that the contents were actually being pumped from a well located at an industrial warehouse facility next to a hazardous waste site! When the State of Massachusetts petitioned the FDA to take action against the company for misuse of the term "spring water," FDA dismissed the complaint. The agency argued that, under their definition of the term the source could legally be called a "spring" because water sometimes rose to the ground surface in an unpaved area of the industrial parking lot where the well was located. Although the FDA had issued new labeling rules in 1995 in an effort to prohibit misleading claims by less-than-honest bottlers, it's obvious from the example just cited that, while an improvement, the new rules haven't totally eliminated the problem.

Public water supplies provide American consumers with a bargain product—inexpensive and in most communities of such good quality as to make bottled water a nonessential status symbol. Nevertheless, the industry fills an important role as a provider of an alternative source of safe drinking water when emergency situations render a public supply unsafe, when special health or dietary requirements necessitate low sodium or low nitrate water, or when consumers' demands that water taste good and look clean are not met by their municipal source of supply.

References

Natural Resources Defense Council. 1999. *Bottled Water: Pure Drink or Pure Hype?* NRDC, New York (March).

public health success stories of the 20th century. Nevertheless, continued sporadic outbreaks of waterborne disease remind us that vigilance can never be relaxed. Not surprisingly, conditions are most worrisome in impoverished rural areas where the U.S. Department of Agriculture (USDA) estimates that at least 2 million people are experiencing critical problems of drinking water quality and availability. Types of rural water-related difficulties include lack of running water, water contaminated by animal wastes running into streams, chemicals leaching into water supplies from waste disposal sites, inadequate sewage treatment, and water sources that are unprotected or inadequate to meet demand. Because a number of states exempt operators of water purification plants serving fewer than 500 people from certification requirements, employees in these small treatment plants frequently have minimal training and qualifications. This fact, plus local financial constraints that limit the ability to upgrade facilities and equipment, may explain why a disproportionate share of U.S. waterborne disease outbreaks are associated with small public water systems.

Looking Ahead

At the beginning of the 21st century, enormous water quality challenges confront societies worldwide. In the United States, despite significant improvement over the past 30 years, 40% of our rivers, lakes, and estuaries have yet to attain the "fishable, swimmable" goal set forth in the Clean Water Act. Policymakers increasingly acknowledge the need to do far more to reduce the contaminated runoff largely responsible for the degradation of American waterways. The need to address nutrient reduction more effectively is particularly urgent. A consensus is emerging among researchers, policymakers, and the general public that discharges of persistent toxics that bioaccumulate in aquatic organisms must be prohibited altogether; that more federal dollars must be allocated for State Revolving Funds; that enforcement actions be strengthened; that technological innovation and market-based approaches to pollution control should be encouraged; and that our regulatory emphasis must shift from its past focus on "end-of-pipe" controls to a broad-based comprehensive watershed approach, using in-stream biological indicators as a yardstick for measuring progress in cleaning up the nation's surface waters.

In Europe, Japan, Canada, and most other industrialized regions of the world, water quality challenges parallel those in the United States. All have relied heavily in the past on expensive treatment technologies which deal with pollution problems after the fact and all need to refocus efforts on pollution prevention strategies and regional watershed management.

In the developing world the problems are far more daunting. Water quality is steadily deteriorating under the combined assault of human population increase, rapid urbanization, and growing volumes of toxic pollutant discharges. Simply quantifying water quality problems in Third World countries is difficult, since monitoring is virtually nonexistent and few data have been collected even on such basic concerns as sewage contamination and the frequency of microbial waterborne disease. Virtually nothing is known about the extent of toxic chemical pollution beyond anecdotal accounts of sickness and death wherever Third World residents are forced to utilize waters tainted with industrial effluents. For the immediate future, data collection and interpretation will be high on the priority list. At the same time, however, existing knowledge must be used to protect as-yet undegraded waters since wide-scale construction of expensive treatment facilities to deal with pollution problems after damage has occurred is beyond the means of most Third World nations (Nash, 1993).

Around the globe, in developed and developing countries alike, unrelenting human pressures on the environment have created unprecedented water quality challenges. Confronting these challenges will be expensive and will require some fundamental changes in our traditional approach to environmental protection. Nevertheless, the importance of clean water to human well-being—indeed, to our very survival—is so great that we have no choice but to make the effort. A generation ago the U.S. Senate's leading environmentalist, Senator Ed Muskie of Maine, urged his legislative colleagues to override then-President Nixon's veto of the Clean Water Act. His stirring appeal rings as prophetic today as it did in the autumn of 1972:

> Our planet is beset with a cancer which threatens our very existence and which will not respond to the kind of treatment that has been prescribed for it in the past. The cancer of water pollution was engendered by our abuse of our lakes, streams, rivers, and oceans; it has thrived on our half-hearted attempts to control it; and like any other disease, it can kill us.

References

Adler, Robert W., Jessica Landman, and Diane Cameron. 1993. *The Clean Water Act: 20 Years Later.* Natural Resources Defense Council.

Banks, James T., and Frances Dubrowski. 1982. "Pretreat or Retreat"? *The Amicus Journal* (Spring). Natural Resources Defense Council.

Bennett, Lyle. 1991. "Abandoned Mines: Report from West Virginia." *EPA Journal* 17, no. 5 (Nov/Dec).

Brown, Lester R., Christopher Flavin, and Hillary French. *State of the World 1999.* New York: Worldwatch Institute/W. W. Norton.

Carlile, B. L. 1995. "Yankee Biosolids Benefit West Texas Rangeland." *Water Environment & Technology* 7, no. 5 (May):37–38.

Cholera Inquiry Committee. 1855. *Report on the Cholera Outbreak in the Parish of St. James, Westminster, During the Autumn of 1854.* London: J. Churchill.

Driscoll, Charles, David Whitall, John Aber, Elizabeth Boyer, Mark Castro, Christopher Cronan, Christine Goodale, Peter Groffman, Charles Hopkinson, Kathleen Lambert, Gregory Lawrence, and Scott Ollinger. 2003. "Nitrogen Pollution: Sources and Consequences in the U.S. Northeast." *Environment* 45, no. 7 (Sept).

Environmental Protection Agency (EPA). 2002. *National Water Quality Inventory: 2000 Report.* EPA-841-R-02-001 (Aug). Washington, DC: Office of Water.

———. 1999. *Proposed NPDES Storm Water Regulations for Phase II and the "No Exposure" Incentive of Phase I.* Washington, DC: Office of Wastewater Management.

———. 1995. *National Water Quality Inventory: 1994 Report to Congress.* EPA 841-R-95-005. Washington, DC: Office of Water.

———. 1993. "Standards for the Use or Disposal of Sewage Sludge; Final Rules." *Federal Register 40 CFR Part 25 7 et al.* (Feb. 19).

———. 1987. *Lead and Your Drinking Water.* OPA-87-006 (April).

Gnaedinger, Richard H. 1993. "Lead in School Drinking Water." *Journal of Environmental Health* 55, no. 6 (April).

Goldberg, Rob. 1993. "EPA Expands Stormwater Control Permitting." *Water Environment & Technology* 5, no. 7 (July).

Koren, Herman. 1980. *Handbook of Environmental Health and Safety: Principles and Practices.* Pergamon Press.

Nash, Jonathan G., and Roger-Mark DeSouza. 2002. *Making the Link: Population, Health, Environment.* Population Reference Bureau, Measure Communication.

Nash, Linda. 1993. "Water Quality and Health." In *Water in Crisis: A Guide to the World's Fresh Water Resources,* edited by Peter H. Gleick. New York: Oxford Univ. Press.

National Research Council (NRC). 2002. *Biosolids Applied to Land: Advancing Standards and Practices.* Washington, DC: National Academy Press.

———. 1999. *Setting Priorities for Drinking Water Contaminants.* National Academy Press.

Pimentel, David et al. 1998. "Ecology of Increasing Disease: Population Growth and Environmental Degradation." *Bioscience* 48, no. 10 (Oct):817–826.

Riggle, David, and Kevin Gray. 1999. "Using Plants to Purify Wastewater." *Biocycle* 40, no. 1 (Jan):40–41.

Shertzer, Richard H. 1986. "Wastewater Disinfection—Time for a Change?" *Journal of the Water Pollution Control Federation* 58, no. 3 (March).

"Small Community Benefits from Constructed Wetlands." 1993. *Water Environment & Technology* 5, no. 8 (Aug).

Tenenbaum, David. 1992. "Sludge." *Garbage* 4, no. 5 (Oct/Nov).

United States Geological Survey (USGS). 1999. *Many Contaminants Found in Nation's Streams, But Few Drinking Water Standards Exceeded, USGS Report Shows*. News release, USGS Water Resources Division.

United Nations (UN). 2003. *Water for People, Water for Life: The United Nations World Water Development Report*. UNESCO Publishing, Berghahn Books.

Ultraguard Water Systems Corporation. 2004. *Industry Overview*. www.ultraguard.com/technology/IndustryOverview. Accessed 08/27/04.

World Resources Institute. 1992. *World Resources 1992–93*. New York: Oxford Univ. Press.

SOLID AND HAZARDOUS WASTES

> Everyone wants you to pick up the garbage and no one wants you to put it down!
> —William Ruckleshaus (1990)

Throughout the modern world, the "waste not, want not" ethic of past generations has long since been replaced by the consumerist lifestyle of a "throwaway society." The inevitable result of our proclivity to "use once and throw away" has been an ever-increasing volume of refuse which, for both sanitary and aesthetic reasons, must be regularly collected and disposed of in a manner that will not degrade the environment or threaten public health. As pointed out by former EPA Administrator William Ruckleshaus in the statement quoted above, doing so presents major challenges to waste managers because of public opposition to the siting of waste management facilities. The sometimes explosive "politics of garbage" will only be resolved through a deeper public understanding of the issues involved in waste management, and by a societal shift in attitudes and behavior regarding the materials we use and discard.

Waste Disposal—A Brief History

Human generation of wastes is, of course, as old as humanity itself. Anthropologists and archaeologists have gleaned illuminating information about the everyday lives of our primitive ancestors by excavating the rubbish heaps outside early cave dwellings and other ancient settlements. Among rural or nomadic peoples, however, discarded wastes seldom accumulated to an extent great enough to threaten human well-being. The advent of the first cities after the Agricultural Revolution of approximately 10,000 years ago presented humankind with its first serious problems of refuse disposal. The poor sanitary conditions and frequent epidemics that characterized city life from ancient times until the late 19th century derived primarily from the perpetuation of country habits in a crowded urban environment. Human body wastes, garbage, and discarded material items were typically left on the floors of homes or thrown into the streets. A rudimentary awareness of the link between refuse and disease led to the establishment in Athens, Greece, of what was perhaps the first "city dump" in the Western world around 500 BC; this innovation was accompanied by what is believed to be the world's first ban against throwing garbage into the streets, as well as by a regulation requiring scavengers to dump wastes no closer than a mile from the city walls. The Athenian example regarding waste management was not widely emulated, however. Throughout the Roman period and the Middle Ages in Europe, open dumping of wastes in streets or ditches remained the prevailing method of urban waste disposal. An ancient Roman signpost warning citizens to "Take your refuse elsewhere or you will be fined" suggests that governmental anti-littering efforts in those days had a very limited focus!

Attempts by municipal authorities to cope with their citizens' slovenly habits were limited and sporadic. In 1388 the English Parliament prohibited dumping of wastes in public waterways; after the 13th century Parisians were no longer permitted to throw garbage out their windows (they obviously pitched it elsewhere, however, for by AD 1400 the mounds of garbage outside the city gates of Paris were so high that they obstructed efforts by the military to defend the city). As medieval towns gradually developed into modern cities, and particularly after the onset of the Industrial Revolution in Europe at the end of the 18th century, the solid waste problem became even more acute. Urban areas became grossly overcrowded, polluted, noisy, and dirtier than ever. Rising levels of affluence among some segments of society, as well as sheer growth in population size, resulted in the generation of increasing amounts of waste. It gradually became apparent to civic leaders that the accumulation of filth and refuse in urban centers was directly related to disease outbreaks. Thus by the late 19th century, city-sponsored efforts at improving urban sanitation were launched both in Europe and North America. Refuse, previously regarded simply as a nuisance, was finally perceived as a serious threat to human health—a problem so massive that it could be effectively tackled only by municipal governments, not simply by private individuals acting on their own initiative (Melosi, 1981).

Throughout the 20th century and into the 21st, the "garbage problem" has continued to mount at a rate several times higher than the rate of population growth. In contrast to the situation in centuries past, the major forces determining waste output since the 1950s have been an affluent lifestyle and changes in marketing techniques (e.g., multiple packaging), which result in more waste materials. While tossing garbage into the streets is no longer considered socially acceptable, modern methods of waste disposal, for the most part, are not a great deal more advanced than they were at the end of the 19th century. Today the enormous volume of refuse generated by homes, businesses, and industry, coupled with the realization that many of these wastes are of a toxic or otherwise hazardous nature, has prompted a concerted effort on the part of both government and the private sector to develop safer, more effective methods for managing the unwanted by-products of modern society.

Municipal Solid Wastes (MSW)

Every sector of the national economy—farms, mines, and factories as well as businesses, institutions, and households—contributes to the mounting mass of unwanted materials requiring disposal. Nevertheless, municipal wastes, although proportionally far smaller in amount than agricultural and mining wastes, arguably represent our greatest waste management challenge (with the possible exception of industrial hazardous wastes). This is because urban wastes are generated where people live and must be quickly removed and properly disposed of in order to prevent serious environmental health problems. Municipal wastes are also much more heterogeneous than are the wastes produced by agriculture, mining, or specific industries. Paper and paper products constitute the single largest portion of household rejects, but an examination of a typical garbage container would also reveal glass, metal, and plastic containers; rubber, leather, and cloth items; food wastes; discarded furniture, electronic equipment, and numerous other items.

The quantity of these discards steadily increased from 1960 until the peak year of 1994, after which volumes declined slightly. The Biocycle/Earth Engineering Center's

Figure 16-1 What's in Our Trash?

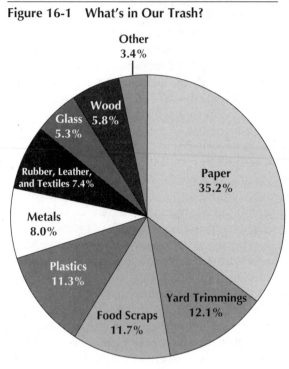

Source: EPA, "Municipal Solid Waste—Basic Facts."
www.epa.gov

2003 State of Garbage in America report indicates the United States generated more than 483 million tons of nonhazardous solid waste in 2002, including construction and demolition debris. Wastes from households and businesses alone, technically referred to as **municipal solid waste (MSW)**, accounted for 376 million tons that year, equivalent to 1.3 tons of refuse tossed away by every man, woman, and child in the United States (Themelis and Kaufman, 2004). EPA estimates that by 2010, each American will generate 4.8 pounds of solid waste daily. Since the late 19th century, Americans have regarded the collection and disposal of urban wastes as a primary responsibility of municipal governments. Today many cities rely on private haulers to collect wastes, and the majority of disposal facilities are privately owned and operated. Nevertheless, municipal officials bear the ultimate responsibility for seeing that waste management services are provided to the satisfaction of their constituents and in compliance with increasingly stringent state and federal environmental regulations.

Municipal Waste Collection and Disposal

The piles of refuse and unsightly, unsanitary conditions that quickly accumulate during the garbage workers' strikes that occasionally plague some cities provide a dramatic illustration of the importance to public health of regular, frequent urban refuse collection. Any breakdown in this essential service, particularly during the warmer months of the year, can result in odor and litter problems or in the rapid growth of fly and rat populations. To prevent such problems, the Public Health Service recommends that refuse be collected twice weekly in residential areas and daily from restaurants, hotels, and large apartment complexes. This is particularly important during the peak of the summer fly-breeding season when eggs may hatch in less than a day and larval stages can be completed in three to four days. Historically, because the public has been far more concerned that refuse be regularly removed than with what happens to it once the garbage truck rounds the nearest corner (the "out of sight, out of mind" philosophy), municipal solid waste budgets traditionally allocated a significantly greater proportion of their resources to refuse collection than to disposal.

From a public health and environmental quality standpoint, proper disposal of urban refuse is just as important as regular collection. Until the 1970s this aspect of solid waste management was given scant attention, resulting in cities utilizing the cheapest method available, with little or no consideration given to the often severe pollution problems thereby created. A new ecological awareness on the part of both the public and policymakers gradually led to the legal prohibition of many long-established practices, such as feeding municipal refuse to hogs or dumping it into waterways. Recognition that garbage-fed hogs frequently were infected with the parasite that causes trichinosis in people who consume undercooked pork diminished the popularity of this waste disposal option. Outbreaks of such diseases as hog cholera among herds of swine fed on raw garbage also provoked second thoughts. By the late 1950s, the U.S. Public Health Service and a number of state health departments passed regulations prohibiting the feeding of uncooked garbage to hogs. Since cooking the wastes made the practice uneconomical, this method of urban refuse disposal has now virtually disappeared. Dumping of municipal wastes into the nearest body of water—a disposal method relied upon for many years by cities such as New York, Chicago, and New Orleans—was halted many decades ago. In 1934 the U.S. Supreme Court banned the dumping of municipal wastes at sea, though certain industrial and commercial wastes were exempted from this ruling. The Marine Protection, Research, and Sanctuaries Act, passed in 1972 and subsequently strengthened by a series of amendments, gradually imposed increasingly strict limitations and now prohibits ocean dumping of industrial waste, sewage sludge, radioactive wastes, and all radiological, chemical, and biological warfare agents.

Until the 1970s, the most common method of urban refuse disposal was **open dumping**, a practice that simply involved hauling collected garbage to a location at the edge of town (usually on "the wrong side of the tracks") and dumping it on the ground. Regarded today as environmentally unacceptable, open dumping epitomizes the problems that can arise when solid wastes are mismanaged. Employed primarily because they are cheap and convenient, open dumps support large populations of rats, flies, and cockroaches that frequently invade nearby dwellings. They contaminate adjacent surface or groundwater supplies when **leachates** (liquids resulting from the interaction of water with wastes) containing dissolved pollutants run off or seep downward through the soil from the dumpsite. If burned over to prevent litter from blowing about or to reduce the volume of wastes, open dumps can pose air quality problems. They are odorous, unsightly, and have a negative impact on property values of adjacent lands. Open dumping as a method for disposing of municipal refuse was outlawed by the federal government in 1976 (earlier by some state governments), and there has been a concerted effort, largely successful, to phase out all open dumping in the United States. In many less-developed areas of the world, however, open dumping remains the most prevalent form of urban waste disposal.

Current Waste Disposal Alternatives

Sanitary Landfilling

In recent decades, most municipalities seeking an economically feasible yet environmentally acceptable alternative to open dumping have opted for sanitary landfills. A sanitary landfill differs from an open dump in that collected refuse is spread in thin layers and compacted by bulldozers. When the compacted layers are 8–10 feet deep, they are covered with about 6 inches of dirt, which is again compacted. At the end of each working day another thin layer of soil is placed over the fill to prevent litter from blowing about, to keep away insect and rodent pests, and to minimize odor problems. When the landfill has reached its ultimate capacity, a final earth cover two feet deep is placed over the entire area and the land can then be used for a park, golf course, or other kinds of recreational facilities.

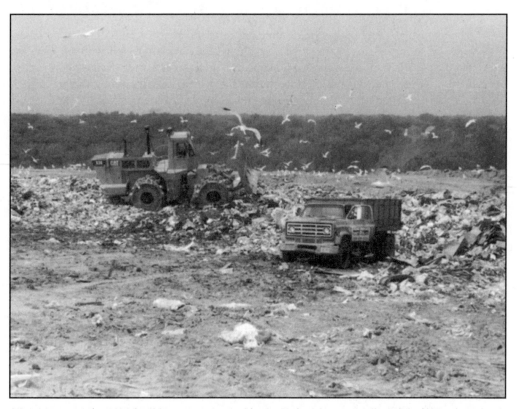

Slightly more than 65% of solid wastes generated in the United States are disposed of in sanitary landfills. [*Author's photo*]

When properly sited, well designed, and efficiently operated, a sanitary landfill can be a perfectly adequate means of urban refuse disposal, free from offensive odors, vermin, or pollution problems. Unfortunately, in the past most so-called "sanitary" landfills were not well sited, properly designed, or well run. As a result, many landfills caused environmental contamination problems little different from those of open dumps and made sanitary landfills unwelcome neighbors wherever they were located. In the mid-1970s it was reported that of 17,000 land disposal sites surveyed, 94% failed to meet the minimum requirements of a sanitary landfill—requirements that in the 1970s were far less stringent than those prevailing today.

Nevertheless, landfills became the overwhelming waste disposal method of choice nationwide, largely because they were (and still are in most places) the most economical of the legal options. In 2002 the average cost for landfilling one ton of MSW (the **"tipping fee"**) ranged from a low of $13.63 in California to a high of $80 in Vermont, with the majority of states featuring tipping fees under $35 per ton. In northeastern states such as Vermont, Massachusetts, New Jersey, New Hampshire, and Connecticut, significantly higher-than-average landfill tipping fees make other alternatives economically attractive. Landfills also appealed to municipal officials because they were capable of receiving any type of waste and could, after completion, be used for facilities popular with the public such as parks, ski slopes, or golf courses. Landfills, of course, are not trouble-free: uneven settling of the land may occur, making them unsuitable as sites for constructing buildings after operations have ceased; anaerobic decomposition of landfilled materials may result in the accumulation of dangerous amounts of methane, which can cause explosions or fires if the gas migrates into

Figure 16-2 Groundwater Contamination as a Result of Unlined Landfill Disposal

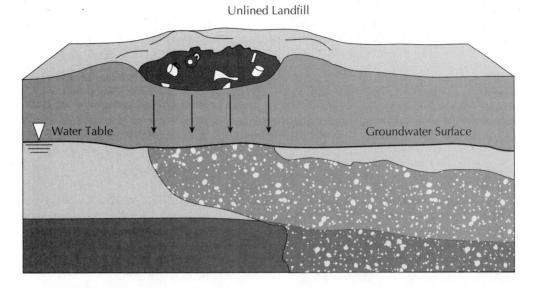

nearby structures; perhaps the most serious environmental impact associated with landfills is their potential for polluting nearby surface streams or underlying aquifers with leachates. This problem can be minimized by careful site selection, choosing locations underlaid by impervious clay formations and far removed from any bodies of surface water. In the past such considerations were frequently neglected, with siting decisions typically based on the price of the land. Unfortunately, in many communities wetland areas, once considered "worthless" because of the cost of developing them for residential or commercial purposes, have been utilized as cheap landfill sites. Aside from the fact that wetlands have intrinsic value for their biologic productivity and flood control attributes, the fact that they are usually in hydrologic contact with groundwater makes wetland areas the *least* appropriate siting choice for a sanitary landfill.

Although landfills have been regarded with increasing public disfavor in recent years, largely due to the long-term environmental liability they represent (approximately 20% of the federal "Superfund" sites slated for multimillion dollar cleanup efforts are former municipal landfills), sanitary landfilling remains the most prevalent method of MSW disposal in the United States. According to the most recent estimates published by *BioCycle* magazine, based on surveys of state waste management programs, 65.6% of the solid waste generated in this country is landfilled (Kaufman et al., 2004).

In the mid-1980s, anxious talk about a so-called national "garbage crisis" dominated discussion of MSW issues in the United States. The tragi-comic voyage of the Islip, New York "garbage barge" during the spring and summer of 1987 focused media attention on the problem of where to deposit society's refuse. Loaded with over 3,000 tons of commercial trash banned from a local landfill reserved for residential refuse, the barge *Mobro* cruised the Atlantic and Gulf coasts for five months, searching in vain for a disposal facility that would accept its increasingly odorous cargo. Eventually the *Mobro* returned to New York, festooned with an enormous Greenpeace banner advising, "Next Time Try Recycling," and its cargo was ultimately burned in a Brooklyn incinerator. Commentators at the time cited worrisome statistics indicating a rapidly dwindling number of landfills in many states and sharply escalating tipping fees at those facilities still in operation. Pointing to still-rising rates of waste generation, they warned that half of all American cities would soon have no place to send their garbage. Compounding the problem—indeed, the essence of the dilemma in a country where open spaces still abound—was the political reality of intense public opposition to landfill siting, a situation which time and again has stymied efforts by local government officials or private waste management firms to develop needed replacement facilities.

The new public focus on MSW concerns sparked intensive efforts by local and state officials to develop new, more sustainable waste management strategies for the decades ahead—and to insist that new and existing landfills be better designed and operated than earlier facilities. A major step toward the latter objective was EPA's promulgation of its new **RCRA Subtitle D** landfill requirements, now in effect nationwide. Mandating that all landfills install groundwater monitoring wells and methane detection systems, Subtitle D has sharply increased the cost of landfill operations but has also ensured that leachates or potentially explosive gases migrating from the fill don't go unnoticed and neglected. Requirements that new cells within a landfill be constructed with double liners and a leachate collection system to remove standing water means that new MSW landfills will be virtually indistinguishable in design from land disposal facilities licensed to accept hazardous wastes. The design features of such landfills render them essentially "dry tombs" where, in the near-absence of moisture and sufficient oxygen, organic wastes degrade very slowly, if at all.

Recently, a new concept in landfill design—**bioreactors**—has attracted attention and several pilot experiments are currently underway to assess their performance. Bioreactors differ from conventional landfills in that the leachate removed from the bottom layer is not discarded but recirculated into the landfill to promote microbial activity. In aerobic bioreactors (an anaerobic version is currently being tested as well), air is injected into the waste mass via wells. This greatly accelerates the decomposition and biological stabilization of landfilled wastes compared to that occurring in conventional landfills. Bioreactors also are expected to generate greater volumes of methane, which can be recovered and sold; leachate disposal costs and post-closure care should be less than for conventional landfills, another economic advantage. Since waste decomposition in a bioreactor decreases its volume, the resulting increase in airspace may permit landfill operators to extend the useful lifespan of the facility. Because bioreactors will be more expensive to build and operate than conventional landfills, it remains to be seen whether the aforementioned cost savings outweigh the increased capital expense of such facilities. By 2005 EPA expects to begin reviewing experimental data regarding the design and operation of bioreactors to assess both their advantages and potential concerns; any agency decision to alter current landfill regulations in light of bioreactor research is, at a minimum, several years away (Dufficy, 2004).

Compliance with Subtitle D requirements, of course, is expensive and owners of many smaller landfills opted to go out of business rather than invest the sums necessary to continue operations under the new regulations. As a result, after the federal rules went into effect in October 1993, the number of operating U.S. landfills dropped from 5,386 to just 2,142 in 2000 (compared to approximately 8,000 in 1988). The sharp decline is much less of a problem than the statistics might suggest, however, for while the *number* of landfills has fallen, remaining landfill *capacity* has not taken a similar nosedive. Although remaining landfill space varies widely across the U.S., many states (Texas, California, Pennsylvania, Illinois, Virginia, etc.) now have adequate capacity to accommodate their needs for the foreseeable future; Wyoming reports its landfills won't be full for at least 100 years! Overall, landfill capacity in the United States is now at its highest level in two decades, and with over 40 states reporting that they are currently in the process of expanding existing landfill space, earlier apocalyptic predictions of garbage piling up in the streets have now largely been discredited. Current trends indicate that for the foreseeable future, MSW will be transported longer distances to fewer, large regional facilities designed and operated in a manner that provides a considerably higher level of environmental protection than the leaky landfills of the past (Kaufman et al., 2004).

In the meantime, waste planners are broadening their perspective, searching for more environmentally friendly MSW management approaches and striving to bring about a paradigm shift in societal attitudes toward the materials we use and throw away. Rather than focusing on one "technological fix" or single disposal alternative to solve every community's problems, most waste management experts view the solution as a combination of approaches, tailored to the specific needs and realities of individual municipalities. The EPA has formulated a recommended three-tiered hierarchy of methods for managing wastes, ranking **waste reduction and reuse** as the most desirable option, **recycling and composting** second, and **waste combustion** and **landfilling** as methods of last resort, to be replaced to the greatest extent possible by the first two alternatives.

Source Reduction

The best—and cheapest—way of managing wastes is not to produce them in the first place. Accordingly, policies of reducing wastes at their source are top-ranked in every priority listing of waste management options. First raised as a possible approach for dealing with U.S. solid waste problems at a 1975 EPA-sponsored Conference on Waste Reduction, the goal of conserving materials and energy through waste prevention or by reducing the volume or toxicity of wastes generated was given little more than lip service until recently. The present sense of urgency to relieve pressures on existing disposal facilities has prompted a more serious look at the potential for source reduction strategies, which most advocates estimate could cut present urban waste streams by about 5%. Approaches to source reduction variously target consumers, manufacturers, or government and can include either voluntary or mandatory components.

Appealing to consumers to use their considerable purchasing power in a more environmentally aware manner has been a key component of source reduction efforts for years. By shopping selectively—buying only the amount of a product that will be used, choosing items without excessive amounts of packaging, buying products that have fewer toxic ingredients than comparable items used for the same purpose, avoiding single-serve disposable packages, or participating in waste exchanges (yard- or garage-sales might be regarded as an effective source reduction strategy!) are all ways of reducing the garbage we throw away. Another approach involves substituting reusable consumer items for single-use throwaway products—cloth napkins and terry towels instead of paper ones; china or plastic dishes instead of paper plates; handkerchiefs instead of Kleenex. Backyard composting of kitchen scraps and garden debris, as well as "grasscycling"—allowing grass clippings to fall and decompose on the lawn or using them for mulch—are other examples of waste reduction that can easily be practiced by individuals.

Opportunities for source reduction of wastes in business or institutional settings are similarly plentiful. Simply asking employees to use their own coffee mugs rather than the ubiquitous Styrofoam cup can noticeably reduce daily waste volume. Copymachines designed to print on both sides of a sheet of paper can save thousands of dollars in business expenditures on paper supplies—as well as on reduced waste disposal fees. Using e-mail rather than paper for interoffice memos, or simply circulating one document rather than making multiple copies, are practices being adopted by thousands of waste-conscious firms.

Manufacturers must play a pivotal role in any national source reduction effort, since their decisions regarding product composition, design, packaging, and durability have such far-reaching implications. Already industry's efforts to reduce packaging and transportation costs through "lightweighting" have had a positive impact on waste reduction trends. When General Mills reduced the thickness of the plastic liners in its cereal boxes, it simultaneously cut the amount of plastic used—and thrown away—each year by half a million pounds. Similarly, since the early 1970s, lightweighting has reduced the weight of a steel can by 43% and decreased that of a one-gallon plastic milk container from 95 grams to under 60 grams today. Many observers feel that manufacturers could do much more, however, by substituting less hazardous components for toxic ones (e.g., Apple Computer several years ago began using brown cardboard packaging containers to replace chlorine-bleached white boxes) and by designing products for easier repair and increased durability, thereby moving away from a corporate policy of "planned obsolescence."

Finally, there are a number of options government could pursue, should it choose to do so, to advance source reduction goals. Aside from efforts at public education—providing citizens with the information they need to make wise purchasing decisions—governments could employ a mix of economic incentives and disincentives, fees, taxes, subsidies, or outright bans to influence consumer choice or manufacturers' behavior. For example, thousands of U.S. municipalities have adopted unit-based pricing (commonly known as "pay-as-you-throw") rather than the traditional flat fee for residential garbage pickup. Essentially a user fee based on the amount of waste discarded, this approach to funding waste management services provides a financial incentive to householders to reduce waste generation and simultaneously encourages recycling and composting. EPA reports an average 14–27% drop in the amounts of MSW discarded in communities that have adopted pay-as-you-throw programs, as well as a 32–59% increase in recycling. Although most unit-based pricing schemes are volume-based (i.e., per-container fees), a few communities have adopted weight-based systems. While a number of municipalities have hesitated to opt for unit-based pricing for fear it would encourage illicit dumping, experience in the communities that have chosen this approach indicates minimal or short-lived problems in this regard. Taxes at the time of purchase on certain hard-to-dispose-of items may not deter their purchase, but can at least provide funds to help offset recycling or disposal costs. A number of states now impose such a tax on tires; motor oil, automobiles, lead-acid batteries, antifreeze, and major appliances are additional products upon which certain states levy taxes that reflect their environmental impact. Outright bans on the use of certain troublesome items have been more difficult to impose due to possible conflict of such mandates with laws governing regional or interstate commerce. Nevertheless, a few have been successfully implemented, most notably the nationwide prohibition against flip-top openers on beverage containers.

The ultimate success of source reduction efforts hinges upon a fundamental shift in society's basic approach to waste management—a refocusing of attention toward ways to *prevent* wastes from being generated in the first place rather than trying to deal with our discards after-the-fact. Source reduction, if wholeheartedly pursued, would also necessitate a different national lifestyle, though not necessarily a less satisfying one. While the concept has yet to capture the hearts and minds of most Americans and has encountered resistance from certain industries that would be directly affected by such policies, the benefits of source reduction programs in reducing waste management costs, saving natural resources, and easing humanity's impact on the environment guarantee a growing commitment in the years ahead to the *practice,* not just the *promise,* of source reduction (League of Women Voters, 1993).

Recycling

More broadly referred to as **resource recovery**—any productive use of what would otherwise be a waste material requiring disposal—recycling and composting are ranked in second place, after source reduction and reuse, on the EPA's list of most environmentally desirable strategies for municipal solid waste management. Perceived by many environmentally aware citizens as "the right thing to do" and by local officials as a way of extending the remaining lifespan of existing land disposal facilities (thereby postponing politically prickly decisions regarding the siting of new landfills or incinerators), recycling of MSW has made impressive gains since the late 1980s. In its 2004 report on "The State of Garbage in America," *BioCycle* magazine reported that, across the nation, 26.7% of MSW was either recycled or composted. In some states the recycling rate is considerably higher than the national average, with Maine (49%), Oregon (48.8%), Minnesota (45.6%), Iowa (41.7%), and California (40.2%) leading the nation in resource recovery efforts (Kaufman et al., 2004). The morale of recycling advocates got a major boost in September 2004 when New York City Mayor Michael Bloomberg announced the resumption of a comprehensive municipal recycling program discontinued two years earlier for financial reasons. A recent escalation in landfill tipping fees altered the equation, making resource recovery far more economical than land disposal—and more politically popular as well. New York City now has a 20-year contract with a highly regarded recycling company that will operate a $25 million state-of-the-art materials recovery facility in Brooklyn. Recyclers across the country are encouraged and excited by New York's change of heart, hopeful that numerous municipalities coast-to-coast will now be inspired to emulate the example of our nation's largest city.

Recycling, of course, is not a new phenomenon. An earlier generation of Americans diligently recycled during World War II, when saving valuable resources to aid in the war effort was widely regarded as a patriotic duty. However, interest in resource conservation waned during the prosperous 1950s and 1960s and only revived with the emergence of the ecology movement and the energy "crisis" of the 1970s. At that time increased emphasis on recycling was promoted primarily for its very real ecological benefits:

1. *Resource conservation*—recycling reduces pressure on forest resources and extends the nation's supply of nonrenewable mineral ores.

2. *Energy conservation*—recycling consumes 50–90% less energy than manufacturing the same item from virgin materials.

3. *Pollution abatement*—manufacturing products from secondary rather than virgin materials significantly reduces levels of pollutant emissions. For example, recycling scrap metal, as opposed to processing iron ore in a coke oven, reduces particulate emissions by 11 kg/metric ton and eliminates the mining wastes generated in extracting iron ore and coal. Recycling aluminum has an even greater environmental impact—both air pollution and energy use are thereby cut by 95%.

In recent years, while acknowledging the environmental advantages of resource recovery, advocates point to a more direct impact municipal recycling efforts could have in their own communities. Not only do such programs have the potential to reduce dependence on landfills and incinerators, they also promote individual responsibility for waste-generating behavior and may eventually help to forge a new public ethic regarding consumerism and sustainable lifestyles.

To encourage more aggressive development and implementation of municipal recycling programs, 42 states, plus the District of Columbia, have set recycling goals

Box 16-1   eCycling

Back in the mid-1990s, observers of national waste generation trends were surprised to discover that the millions of old, outdated personal computers supposedly destined for landfill disposal were nowhere to be seen, raising the inevitable question of "Where are they going?" Those in the know replied, only half in jest, that they were piling up in home basements across the country, sharing shelf space with back issues of *The National Geographic*, the one other consumer item that no one ever wants to throw away! Fortunately, today there are other options besides long-term storage for those who wish to dispose of unwanted electronic equipment such as computer monitors, TVs, and cell phones—and to do so in an environmentally responsible manner.

Electronics recycling, commonly referred to as **eCycling**, was born of the realization that potential dumping of such materials in municipal landfills represents a colossal waste of resources as well as a serious environmental hazard. On average, computer monitors and older TV picture tubes contain four pounds of lead as well as other toxic metals, necessitating responsible e-waste management.

In spite of media reports conveying the impression that North American landfills are awash in obsolete electronics equipment (perhaps prompted by a National Safety Council report that by 2005 Americans were discarding 130 million cell phones a year), e-waste currently comprises only about 1% of all municipal solid waste. Surveys indicate that institutions, businesses, and household residents continue to stockpile old computers and other scrap electronics long after they cease using them. Nevertheless, with National Safety Council projections indicating that nearly 250 million computers will become obsolete before the end of the decade, some recently launched programs are encouraging indications that society has begun responding to the e-waste challenge.

The familiar waste management mantra—"reduce, reuse, recycle"—has been slightly modified in the context of scrap electronics, with **reuse and donation** the #1 e-waste goal. If outdated equipment remains in working order, donating it to those who couldn't otherwise afford it benefits society and protects the environment by diverting such materials from the waste stream. Currently several hundred nonprofit organizations in the U.S. and Canada accept donations of unwanted computers which they then refurbish and send to schools, low-income residents, or organizations in developing countries. Federal legislation such as the 21st Century Classrooms Act has made such donations increasingly attractive to large corporations by granting tax incentives for donations of computer equipment to schools.

For nonworking, nonrepairable e-waste, recycling opportunities are expanding rapidly; indeed, by mid-decade the processing of electronic scrap had become the fastest-growing segment of the North American recycling industry, with at least 850 commercial e-scrap processors and brokers operating in the U.S. and Canada. According to EPA, by 2004 recycling firms were recovering more than 100 million pounds of materials annually from e-scrap (50% of the material inside a personal computer is recyclable).

The logistics of establishing and financing a system for collecting the millions of unwanted computer systems, old TV sets, and other electronic wastes remain challenging, however. In over 1,000 North American communities, local governments have taken the initiative, sponsoring periodic e-waste collection events (often as part of a household hazardous waste collection day) or, in some cases, by establishing permanent e-scrap drop-off centers; some cities have added electronic waste to the list of recyclables eligible for curbside collection.

Hoping to promote ongoing local government programs, in 2003 the EPA launched its **Plug-In to eCycling** campaign, a nationwide effort to increase the amount of e-scrap collected and safely recycled. The campaign is striving to provide the public with information on where they can recycle old computers, TVs, and cell phones, as well as to expand opportunities for safe recycling of e-waste. The agency is currently working to establish partnerships between electronics manufacturers, local and state governments, and retailers to promote shared responsibility for safe electronics recycling. EPA also hopes to advance a life-cycle approach to electronics product stewardship, including environmentally conscious design, manufacturing processes, and the reduction of toxic components in new electronic products. By working with all affected stakeholders, EPA is trying to make it easier and more cost-effective for all involved to divert e-scrap to reuse or environmentally sound recycling while reducing the

Plug-In To eCycling
with U.S. EPA

"environmental footprint" of electronic product use. To achieve its goal, EPA has established a number of targeted programs such as **Design for the Environment**, working with electronics manufacturers to incorporate environmental considerations into project design, and **Waste Wise**, urging campaign partners to set goals for reducing electronics waste. To demonstrate the federal government's commitment to shouldering its own share of responsibility for environmentally responsible e-waste management, in December 2004 EPA awarded its first-ever contracts to assist all federal agencies in the environmentally responsible management of the approximately 10,000 computers disposed of by the government every week (7% of all the world's computers are purchased by the U.S. government!). Under terms of the contracts issued, contractors must maintain an audit trail to the obsolete equipments' final destination to ensure documentation of reclamation and recycling efforts.

Obsolete electronics are not the only wastes associated with the modern world's computer-based culture. In North America more than 350 million plastic printer cartridges are incinerated or discarded in landfills each year—approximately 80–90% of all empty cartridges. In the U.S. alone, it's estimated that 8 cartridges are thrown away every second (unlike old computers or *National Geographic* magazines, empty printer cartridges are not generally considered collector's items!). Since it takes hundreds of years for a landfilled cartridge to decompose and requires approximately a gallon of oil to manufacture a new one, there are obvious environmental and resource advantages to recycling cartridges rather than discarding them. Responding to pressure from environmentally concerned consumers, printer manufacturers like Hewlett-Packard (HP) now offer customers the option of shipping used laser toner cartridges back to the company for recycling, providing a pre-paid, pre-addressed shipping label for returns in every new toner cartridge box. HP claims to have diverted millions of pounds of plastic from landfills since the program's inception and assures participants that all returned cartridges are converted into materials used to manufacture a variety of new products.

However, while recycling is preferable to disposal, waste reduction through reuse is even better—especially when cost savings are included as an added benefit. Within the past few years, entrepreneurial franchisers such as Australia-based Cartridge World have begun to challenge the corporate giants' near-monopoly on the multibillion dollar ink and toner business by establishing retail outlets to refill and refurbish printer cartridges. Today such businesses are diverting thousands of empty cartridges from disposal facilities in communities where franchisees are located. Cartridge World, an EPA *Waste Wise* partner and the world's largest retailer of cartridge refilling services, predicts that for users of printers, photocopiers, or fax machines, refilling cartridges will soon be as routine as separation of recyclables for collection. The concept of refillable cartridges appeals to environmentally conscious customers (an average ink jet cartridge can be refilled 3–8 times, while laser toner cartridges can be remanufactured indefinitely, in both cases without sacrificing quality), as does the price—typically 30–50% less than the cost of a new cartridge. Although by mid-2004 franchise stores that refill and refurbish cartridges accounted for just 20% of the national cartridge market, business was booming and expectations for future growth was high—a win-win situation both for consumers and for the environment.

References

Powell, Jerry. 2004. "Electronics Recycling." *Resource Recycling* 23, no. 8 (Aug).

Tam, Pui-Wing. 2004. "Fill 'er Up, With Color." *The Wall Street Journal*, Aug. 3.

U.S. Environmental Protection Agency. "Plug-In To eCycling." http://www.epa.gov/epaoswer/osw/ conserve/plugin/index.htm.

that local governments within those states are required to meet, specifying deadline dates for achievement (so-called **"rates and dates").** Many have also enacted legislation requiring that local governments develop long-range comprehensive waste management plans, detailing how they intend to comply with state-mandated recycling goals. These planning requirements have forced local officials and citizen advisory groups to look much more closely at waste management problems and solutions in their own communities, leading to a number of innovative approaches for reducing the amount of refuse destined for landfill burial or incineration. Seeking to emulate these state initiatives, the EPA in late 2002 launched its **Resource Conservation Challenge (RCC)**, one goal of which was to boost the national recycling rate to 35%.

To attain these admittedly ambitious goals, waste managers must devise innovative strategies for eliciting greater participation in recycling efforts by householders, businesses, and institutions. One of the most successful approaches to increasing rates of residential recycling in recent years has been the introduction of curbside collection programs that make household recycling as easy as setting out the weekly garbage. From just 1,000 programs nationwide in 1988, curbside collection was provided by 8,875 U.S. municipalities in 2002, serving over 139 million people—almost half of all Americans. Requirements regarding co-mingling or separation of recyclables into one or several containers vary from program to program, as does the range of materials accepted for curbside pickup. While newspapers, glass, and aluminum cans are among

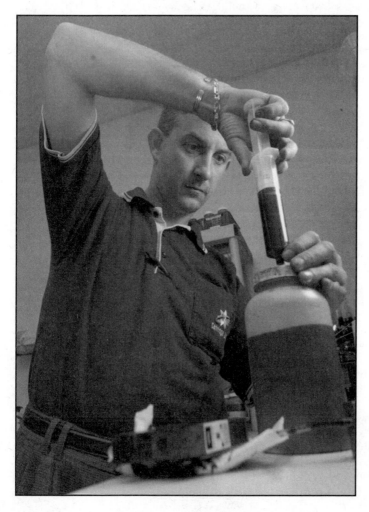

Entrepreneurial franchisers are now opening retail outlets that refill and refurbish printer cartridges at a fraction of the cost of buying a new cartridge. [*The News & Observer*]

the items most commonly included, Santa Clarita, California, made news in 2002 when it became the first—and only—city in the country to collect dirty disposable diapers for recycling. Concerned about statistics showing that approximately 20 billion used diapers ("absorbent hygiene products") from households and elder care facilities are discarded in North America each year and comprise 1.4% of the total MSW stream, civic leaders in Santa Clarita decided to make recycling diapers an environmental priority. During a 10-month pilot project that terminated in 2003, soiled diapers collected from specially designed containers placed at curbside were recycled through a technology patented by Knowaste, a company whose innovative process is currently being used in the Netherlands and Australia. Although Santa Clarita's initiative was popular with participants, the program was discontinued for financial reasons: city staff estimated that the cost of landfilling 40,000 diapers would be approximately $700, in contrast to the $500,000 in state and local funds spent on the pilot recycling program (Whyte, 2003).

Once materials are collected through **source separation** programs (which can include curbside collection, neighborhood recycling centers, community drop-boxes, or periodic recycling drives), they must be sorted and baled prior to being shipped to

Figure 16-3   Recycling Rates of Selected Materials, 2003

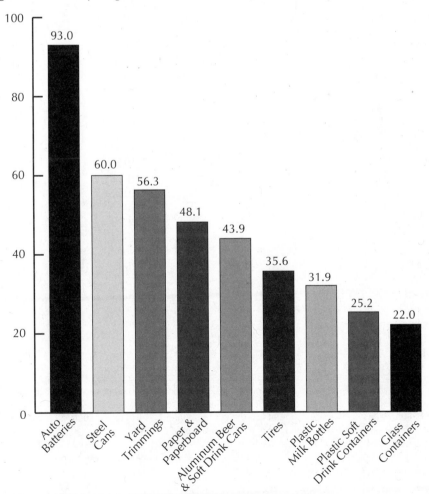

Source: EPA, "Municipal Solid Waste—Basic Facts." www. epa.gov

buyers for reprocessing. These tasks are carried out by **materials recovery facilities (MRFs—referred to in recycling jargon as "murfs")** where mixed recyclables are prepared for marketing.

Table 16-1   State Diversion Goals and Recycling Rates

State	Goal (%)	Rate (%)	Deadline	Is Goal Mandatory?
Alabama	25	23	None	No
California	50	42	2000	Yes
Connecticut	40	23	2000	Yes
Delaware	30[1]	59	None	No
District of Columbia	45	16	2000	Yes
Florida	30	28	1994	Yes
Hawaii	50	24	2000	No
Indiana	50	35	2001	No
Iowa	50	35	2000	No
Kentucky	30[2]	30	2010	No
Louisiana	25	17	1992	No
Maine	55[3]	40	2003	No
Maryland[4]	40	37	2005	No
Massachusetts	70	38	2010	No
Michigan[5]	25	18	2005	No
Minnesota	35/50[6]	42	1996	No
Mississippi	25	16	1996	No
Missouri	40	38	1998	No
Nebraska	50	23	2002	No
Nevada	25	14	None	No
New Hampshire	40	21	2000	No
New Jersey	65	38	2000	Yes
New Mexico	50	9	2000	No
New York	50[7]	42	1997	No
North Carolina	40[1]	26	2001	No
North Dakota	40	11	2000	No
Ohio	50[8]	21	2005	No
Oregon	50	39	2009	Yes
Pennsylvania	35	33	2003	No
Rhode Island	70	24	None	Yes
South Carolina	35[9]	31	2005	Yes
South Dakota	50	n/a	2001	No
Tennessee	25[1]	34	2003	Yes
Texas	40	35	1994	No
Vermont	50	33	2005	No
Virginia	25	29	Annual	Yes
Washington	50	35	1995	No
West Virginia	50	25	2010	No

[1]Waste reduction goal (vs. recyling goal); [2]Goal of 30% reduction by 2010 proposed for 2002 legislative session; [3]50% recycling plus 5% waste reduction; [4]Separate mandated recycling goal of 15–20% for each county and city of Baltimore based on a population of less than or more than 1,511,000. For 2000, all jurisdictions have achieved that goal; [5]Waste reduction goal of 8–12%, reuse goal of 4–6%, composting goal of 8–12% and recycling goal of 20–30%; [6]35% for greater Minnesota counties, 50% for metro area counties; [7]40–42% recycling goal plus 8–10% waste reduction goal; [8]For both MSW and industrial waste; [9]Also an MSW reduction goal of 3.5 lbs/person/day of MSW generated by 6/30/05.

Source: "13th Annual BioCycle Survey: The State of Garbage in America," December 2001. BioCycle, Emmaus, PA. www.biocycle.net. Used with permission.

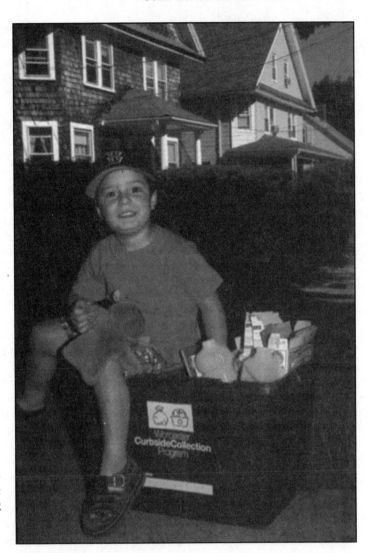

Curbside collection programs have increased the rates of residential recycling in many communities. [*Author's photo*]

In some regions of the country, municipal leaders have opted for an alternative approach to source separation as a means of complying with state-mandated recycling goals. Since even curbside programs, convenient though they are, almost never achieve 100% public participation, some cities don't even make an attempt to involve citizens in recycling efforts. Instead, they simply collect the mixed residential wastes jumbled together in the garbage can— food scraps, old newspapers, dirty diapers, junk mail, empty milk cartons, and so on—and truck them off to a mixed waste processing facility (not-so-affectionately known in recycling circles as a **"dirty MRF"**). There the recyclable components are pulled out of the waste stream and diverted for processing, while the remainder is either landfilled or made into pellets for burning in an incinerator. Proponents of "dirty MRFs" admit that the facilities are expensive to construct and operate, but point out that, in comparison with source separation programs (i.e., separation by the person who generates the waste), mixed waste recovery facilities are theoretically capable of diverting a much higher percentage of recyclables from the waste stream. Some local officials favor such facilities because they don't require any public education efforts to persuade or coerce residents into altering long-established waste-generating behavior. Conversely, opponents contend that, aside from their high cost, "dirty MRFs" are environmentally unsound because the *quality* of potentially recyclable materials pulled from the mixed waste stream is so poor as to have little or no value to a secondary materials industry that demands as clean and homogeneous a waste stream as possible (i.e., who would want to buy paper for recycling once it's smeared with tomato sauce from discarded pizza? How could glass be recovered for shipment to a processor when scattered in small fragments among banana peels, dirty facial tissue, and used tea bags?). As a case in point, Chicago's "Blue Bag" program, launched with much fanfare in 1995, achieved the abysmally low recycling rate of just 6%, largely due to the fact that the blue bags containing source-separated recyclables were intermixed in the garbage trucks with nonrecyclable refuse (Pellow, 2002). These realities have sharply limited the appeal of "dirty MRFs," which comprise less than 15% of all recycling processing facilities nationwide (Berenyi, 1999).

In an effort to promote recycling, governments at the federal, state, and local levels are pursuing a number of options to boost the supply of high-quality recyclables or to stimulate market demand. Among the legislative approaches to increase the amounts of material diverted through source separation efforts are the setting of "rates and dates" as previously described, as well as the passage of **"Bottle Bills,"** laws currently in effect in 11 states (Oregon, Vermont, Maine, Michigan, Iowa, Connecticut, Massachusetts, Delaware, California, New York, and Hawaii) which require consumers to pay a refundable deposit on beer and soft drink containers (California and Maine recently added noncarbonated beverage containers to their deposit laws and other states are considering similar action). Similar mandates are in effect throughout Canada, except for the provinces of Ontario and Manitoba. First adopted by the province of British Columbia in 1970 and the state of Oregon in 1972, bottle bills were originally intended to combat littering. Surveys performed a few years after bottle bills took effect documented a 75–86% drop in the number of beverage containers discarded along roadsides in comparison with predeposit days (although some slovenly individuals persist in tossing cans and bottles away even in bottle bill states, there is now financial motivation for others to retrieve them). Bottle bills have subsequently proven themselves equally effective at boosting recycling rates for aluminum, glass, and PET plastic. Data from bottle bill states indicate that, on average, over 70% of the beverage containers sold in these states are ultimately recycled (95% in Michigan where the deposit is 10¢, as opposed to 5¢ or less in the other ten states). By contrast, in nondeposit states the aggregate rate of beverage container recycling is just 27.9% (Gitlitz, 2004).

Another popular legislative move in recent years has been prohibiting landfill disposal of such materials as yard wastes, lead-acid batteries, whole tires, white goods (large appliances), electronics, and used motor oil. While the main purpose of these bans has been to conserve landfill space or to prevent the formation of toxic leachates, their enactment has greatly enhanced the amount of these materials diverted to recycling centers or composting facilities since there's now nowhere else for them to go.

Minimum recycled content mandates have become an increasingly popular method of creating market demand for old newspaper, glass, and plastic—even telephone directories! Such laws require that targeted products contain a certain percentage of recycled material. For example, by 1998 twenty-seven states had enacted voluntary or mandatory requirements that newspapers sold in those states contain specified percentages of recycled fiber (Miller, 1998).

Government procurement policies that require government agencies, state universities, and public schools to purchase supplies that are recyclable or contain recycled material have long been advocated as a way to promote market demand for recyclables. Since the purchases of goods and services by federal, state, and local governments in the United States cumulatively amount to 20% of the GNP, use of government purchasing power in favor of secondary materials could provide an important boost to the recycling industry.

Take-back programs. The dramatic increase in MSW recycling witnessed during the late 1980s and early 1990s, spurred by programs such as those just described and by the public's perceptions of a national "garbage crisis," has begun to wane in recent years. Municipal recycling rates rose from just 10% in 1980 to 26% in 1995, but then leveled off and have remained relatively stable for the past decade. More discouraging is the realization that increases in recycling have been offset by the ever-growing volume of waste generated by the nation's consumers. It has also become obvious that municipal governments are incapable of managing certain waste streams effectively, since the design of many products—appliances, furniture, and electronic equipment being notable examples—render resource recovery of their various components difficult or impossible. This realization has led to a growing conviction that the *manufacturers* of these products—not local taxpayers, government officials, or waste reprocessors—should bear most of the responsibility for their end-of-life management. Such thinking has given rise to a concept known as **Extended Producer Responsibility (EPR)**. EPR policies, in essence, force manufacturers to consider the environmental impact of products throughout their lifecycle, a process which, ideally, will result in the elimination of unnecessary parts and excessive packaging, as well as promote product design that facilitates repair, recycling, or reuse. In Europe, where the EPR concept was first introduced with Germany's 1991 "Ordinance on the Avoidance of Packaging Waste" and complimentary "Green Dot" (Grüne Punkt) system, many countries now have legislation requiring producers to take back and recycle packaging waste free of charge—a mandate credited with dramatic reductions in manufacturers' use of unnecessary packaging materials. EPR laws in a number of European nations have expanded their initial focus on packaging to include producer **take-back requirements** for discarded electric and electronic equipment, batteries, and automobiles. In most cases, European EPR legislation prohibits the landfilling or incineration of products targeted under the take-back laws and establishes minimum recycling and reuse requirements. As intended, mandatory EPR requirements have motivated European manufacturers to develop new materials or products that can easily be reused or which break down readily once discarded. Examples include a new, infinitely recyclable nylon-6 fiber, produced by the German chemical firm BASF, and a Swiss-manufactured upholstery fabric that naturally decomposes after being removed from a chair at the end of its useful life (Renner, 2004).

In the U.S., proposed federal EPR legislation has made little headway due to strong opposition by manufacturing interests. Nevertheless, the threat of regulation has prompted several voluntary programs by producers, involving product redesign or limited take-backs of certain products (Canada, like the U.S., has a number of voluntary initiatives at the national level, but all ten provinces have various mandatory EPR programs in operation). Except for the 11 state bottle bills, laws enacted by a number of U.S. states assign waste management responsibility for specified products not to the producers of those items, as in Europe, but to government, consumers, or retailers. Examples include used motor oil recycling programs financed by consumer fees or state money, government-managed scrap tire collections funded by fees collected from customers by tire dealers, and retailer take-back programs for used lead-acid batteries, now in effect in 37 states. Thanks to effective lobbying, producer trade organizations—unlike their European counterparts—have successfully avoided any significant take-back responsibility. An industry-wide voluntary take-back program for recovery and recycling of nickel-cadmium rechargeable batteries, launched with considerable

Under a concept known as Extended Producer Responsibility (EPR), manufacturers would be subject to take-back requirements on such products as electronic equipment.

fanfare in the mid-1990s by the Rechargeable Battery Recycling Corporation (RBRC) has been a dismal failure, with a recovery rate hovering around 10%, as opposed to RBRC's 70% stated goal.

The unimpressive results of voluntary initiatives by American industry and the unlikelihood of mandatory federal requirements in the foreseeable future have prompted legislative activity in a number of states. In 2001 Maine became the first to enact a manufacturer take-back law for mercury-containing waste products and to require that car manufacturers pay a bounty to auto salvagers who recover mercury-containing switches. By 2004, approximately a dozen states had passed, and many more were considering, laws either banning mercury in consumer products or requiring that such products bear warning labels. That same year Maine once again set a national precedent, becoming the first state to require that industry take back and recycle discarded television sets and computer monitors. Whether other states decide to emulate Maine's example remains to be seen; if so, industry may decide it prefers a uniform national mandate to a variable patchwork of state laws. Such producer responsibility requirements could give a major boost to U.S. recycling efforts. In the absence of such legislation, the prevailing voluntary approach is unlikely to effect substantial change and the European Union will continue to set the pace for innovative resource recovery and reuse policies (Sheehan and Spiegelman, 2005).

Composting

Since the late 1980s, proliferation of state mandates prohibiting the landfilling of yard wastes has led to an explosive increase in municipal composting facilities in the

Table 16-2 MSW Landfill Disposal Bans for Selected Materials

State	Yard Trimmings	Whole Tires	Used Oil	Lead-Acid Batteries	Batteries (General)	White Goods	Electronics	Others
Arizona		x	x	x				
Arkansas	x[1]				x			
California		x					x	
Connecticut	x[2]			x				
Delaware		x						
Florida	x		x			x		
Georgia	x	x		x				
Hawaii		x						
Idaho					x			
Illinois	x	x	x	x		x		
Indiana	x[3]	x		x				
Iowa	x	x	x	x				
Kansas		x						
Kentucky		x		x				x[4]
Louisiana		x	x	x		x		
Maine		x		x		x		
Maryland	x[5]	x	x		x			
Massachusetts	x	x		x		x	x[6]	x[7]
Michigan	x		x	x		x[8]		
Minnesota	x	x	x	x		x	x[6]	x[9]
Missouri	x	x		x		x		
Nebraska	x[1]	x	x	x		x		
New Hampshire	x		x	x				x[10]
New Jersey	x[11]							x[12]
New Mexico					x			
New York			x	x				
North Carolina	x	x	x	x		x		x[13]
North Dakota			x	x		x		
Ohio		x		x				x[14]
Oregon		x	x	x		x		x[15]
Pennsylvania	x[16]	x		x				
Rhode Island		x				x		
S. Carolina	x[17]	x	x	x		x		
S. Dakota	x		x	x		x		
Tennessee		x	x	x			x	x[18]
Texas		x	x	x				
Utah		x	x		x			
Vermont		x	x	x	x	x		x[19]
Virginia		x		x				
W. Virginia	x	x			x			
Wisconsin	x	x	x	x		x		x[12]
Wyoming				x				

[1]Leaves and grass; [2]Grass clippings; [3]Leaves, brush and woody vegetative matter >3 feet; [4]Yard trimmings are banned from a few landfills; [5]Separately collected loads of yard trimmings are banned from disposal; [6]Cathode ray tubes, [7]Glass, metal and plastic containers and recyclable paper; [8]Containing refrigerants; [9]Source separated recyclables; [10]Ni-Cad batteries; [11]Leaves only; [12]All recyclables in MSW stream; [13]Aluminum cans; [14]Yard trimmings are not banned but disposal is restricted; [15]Cars and other vehicles; [16]Truckloads comprised primarily of leaves; [17]Includes landclearing debris; [18]Oil-based paints and mercury bulbs; [19]Oil-based paint.

Source: "14th Annual BioCycle Survey of Solid Waste Management in the U.S.: The State of Garbage in America," January 2004. BioCycle, Emmaus, PA. www.biocycle.net. Used with permission.

United States. Currently 21 states have enacted such bans and more than 3,200 yard waste composting facilities are operating in the United States (bans on the landfilling of yard wastes have also contributed to booming sales of mulching mowers; results from a four-year demonstration project conducted by the Rodale Institute concluded that use of mulching mowers produces healthier lawns with fewer weeds and no thatch buildup). While a number of European countries have long recognized that composting of organic household waste can reduce the amount of refuse requiring disposal, consideration of composting as a viable waste management alternative in the United States is a much more recent phenomenon. Even though readily decomposable food and yard wastes make up 23% of the U.S. urban waste stream (considerably more during the warmer months of the year, less during the winter), perceived lack of demand for the finished product, plus the ease and low cost of landfilling, led city officials to dismiss composting as an impractical venture. That attitude has now been transformed by the realization that it makes little sense to devote valuable landfill space to grass clippings and autumn leaves when such materials could be converted into a useful and environmentally beneficial product. Nor are yard wastes the only potentially compostable materials in MSW. By 1999, nineteen cities hosted mixed waste composting plants that process the entire organic portion of residential and commercial wastes—food scraps, soiled paper, etc.—removing only noncompostable (but still recyclable) glass, metal, and plastics, as well as any hazardous materials. Though questions have been raised about the quality of mixed waste compost and thus its acceptability to end-users, efforts to educate citizens on the importance of source separation have helped to prevent contamination of the final product and to avoid the loss of potentially compostable materials.

A form of resource recovery, composting utilizes natural biochemical decay processes to convert organic wastes into a humus-like material, suitable for use as a soil conditioner. Although its nutrient content is too low to consider it a fertilizer, compost greatly improves soil structure and porosity, aids in water infiltration and retention, increases soil aeration, and slows erosion. Co-composting of yard wastes with municipal sewage sludge (another increasingly difficult-to-dispose-of waste product), now being practiced in a number of communities, enhances the nitrogen content of the finished product and makes it more valuable for agricultural uses.

A variety of methods for converting wastes to compost are currently in use, ranging from the low-tech, relatively inexpensive **windrow** technique, where long rows of wastes are piled outdoors and mechanically turned periodically to aerate the mass, to highly sophisticated, expensive **in-vessel** operations or processes in which pumps mechanically aerate windrows **(aerated static pile)**, hastening decay and eliminating the need for frequent turning. Choice of the most appropriate composting method depends on the needs and resources of the community in question: if land is abundant and funding scarce, the windrow method may be the best option—though it often requires two or three years for complete breakdown of wastes to occur if the piles are turned only once or twice annually. If available space is at a premium and rapid turnover of wastes desirable, a community might be wise to choose a more high-tech method, provided it can afford the considerably higher price tag associated with such facilities. Whatever the technology, the composting process consists of four basic steps:

1. *Preparation*—incoming wastes are shredded to a relatively uniform size; in most composting operations, nonbiodegradable materials such as glass, metal, plastics, tires, and so on are separated from the compostable wastes. In some composting operations, sewage sludge or animal manures are added to the refuse at this point.

Windrow technique: long rows of composting wastes are piled outdoors and periodically aerated. [*Illinois Department of Energy and Natural Resources*]

2. *Digestion*—microbes naturally present in the waste materials or special bacterial inoculants sprayed on the refuse are utilized to break down organic waste materials. While digestion may be either aerobic or anaerobic, aerobic systems are generally preferred due to shorter time periods required and fewer odor problems. In aerobic decomposition, heat given off by microbial respiration raises the temperature in the windrows well above the 140°F necessary to kill fly eggs, weed seeds, or pathogenic organisms.

3. *Curing*—after digestion of simpler carbonaceous materials is complete, additional curing time is allowed to permit microbes to break down cellulose and lignin in the waste.

4. *Finishing*—to produce an acceptable finished product, compost may be put through screens and grinders to remove nondigested materials and create a uniform appearance. Some composting facilities bag or package the finished product to facilitate marketing or distribution.

While the public rightly regards composting as an environmentally desirable method of organic waste management, composting facilities do not always make good neighbors. Some have been forced to close due to problems with objectionable odors—problems that are gradually being solved as operators compare notes and learn techniques for managing trouble-free facilities. Another public health issue related to composting operations is their potential to emit **bioaerosols**, tiny airborne particles of microorganisms whose inhalation has been blamed for ailments ranging from a runny nose and watery eyes to flu-like symptoms. Bioaerosols, such as spores of the ubiquitous fungus *Aspergillus fumigatus*, were first cited as a potential environmental health concern in 1992 when a New Jersey epidemiologist testified before Congress about potential health risks to people living within a two-mile radius of composting sites. Since that time bioaerosols have attracted intensive scrutiny and have prompted organized community opposition to siting of compost facilities in several localities. Representatives of the composting industry argue that any fears are vastly exaggerated, stating that public exposure to *Aspergillus* emissions from composting are negligible when the process is performed correctly. A report jointly sponsored

Box 16-2 Waste-Eating Worms

While many components of the municipal solid waste stream are now effectively targeted by recycling programs, management of the enormous quantities of food waste discarded daily by households and the food service industry continues to rely heavily on landfill disposal or discharge to municipal sewer systems via home garbage grinders. Recently, however, a somewhat unconventional method of food waste management has been winning enthusiastic converts—a practice known as **vermicomposting**. Derived from the Latin word *vermis* (worm), the term describes a method by which certain species of redworms, most commonly *Eisenia foetida*, feed on organic wastes, converting them into worm castings that are now widely regarded as the best soil amendment available.

Redworms are amazingly voracious little creatures, eating over half their body weight in organic matter daily and creating high-quality compost in the process. Not surprisingly, home gardeners, horticulturists, and organic growers have been leading the vermicomposting bandwagon, but soil scientists and agricultural researchers now support the practice, citing studies that demonstrate a significant increase in seed germination, plant growth, and crop yields when vermicompost is added to growth media or soils. Why worm castings produce such observably beneficial results is now the subject of scientific investigation at a number of universities; researchers hypothesize that plant growth enhancement by vermicompost is due to a worm-stimulated increase in the populations of hormone-producing fungi and bacteria. The water-soluble hormones present in vermicompost stimulate plant growth much more effectively than do the mineral nutrients present in conventional finished compost. Preliminary experiments indicate that vermicompost also markedly suppresses certain soil-based plant diseases and pests such as nematodes, mites, and several species of insects. As a result, use of vermicompost by commercial growers is expanding rapidly—a trend that is giving a major boost to organic waste recycling efforts by the food service industry, feedlot managers, wood pulp producers, and large-scale agricultural operations. For such waste generators, utilizing worms to eat their garbage is a win-win situation, converting troublesome wastes into a saleable product.

Fortunately, vermiculture offers the same rewards at the household level as it does on an industrial scale, giving individuals and families an opportunity to turn kitchen scraps into "brown gold" to nourish houseplants and gardens (it can also provide a fun classroom project for school children and an ecologically beneficial way to dispose of lunch box leftovers!). Unlike the standard outdoor compost pile where decomposition slows to a halt during winter, worm bins for vermicomposting are best kept indoors and hence function year-round—a definite advantage since kitchen waste generation proceeds at a steady pace regardless of the weather.

For those wishing to launch a home vermicomposting project, only a few basic ingredients are needed.

1. **A worm bin**, either purchased or home-made. Numerous types of containers suitable for home vermicomposting are available on the Internet, but bins also can be constructed at home using large plastic or wooden containers (detailed instructions for building a simple worm bin are available on-line or in numerous publications such as *Worms Eat My Garbage* by Mary Appelhof). In general, containers should be relatively shallow (about 8–12'' deep) with holes in the bottom for aeration and drainage; they also need a lid to maintain high humidity and exclude light from the bin. Bricks or wooden blocks should be placed underneath to permit air circulation and drainage. If kept indoors, a tray placed beneath the bin is useful to collect any liquids leaking from the container; these can then be used to fertilize plants.

2. **Bedding** composed of shredded corrugated cardboard or shredded paper (ink poses no problems). To prepare it for use, the dry bedding should be thoroughly soaked with water (it may take several hours to become well saturated), then drained and as much of the excess water as possible squeezed out. The moist bedding should then be fluffed up and placed in the bin to 2/3 its depth.

3. **Redworms**, favored for their rapid reproduction rate and tolerance of high population densities, are available on the Internet, in garden catalogs, or bait shops. Don't try to economize by using night-crawlers or other garden worms—they won't survive in the confines of a worm bin. The amount needed depends on how much food waste is generated daily; for a typical family, one pound of worms is usually sufficient. When starting a new worm bin, simply scatter the worms on top of the bedding; they quickly move down into the shredded material to avoid light. Redworms prefer temperatures in the 55°–77°F (13°–25°C) range; they are likely to die if temperatures fall below freezing or exceed 84°F (29°C).

4. **Kitchen scraps**, including vegetable and fruit peelings, coffee grounds, tea leaves, and non-greasy table scraps. Avoid fat, meat, and bones; citrus peels also may be problematic, since they contain a chemical toxic to redworms. A small amount of gritty material such as cornmeal, coffee grounds, or finely crushed eggshells should be added occasionally to help the worms digest the food. These food scraps can either be spread in a thin layer on top of the bedding or the bedding can be pulled back at one location, the food scraps dumped in, and the bedding pulled back over them (if the latter method is used, vary the location each time more food is added). If odors develop, reduce the amount of food being added or cut it up into smaller pieces.

Assuming that proper environmental conditions have been maintained, the redworms go to work rapidly. Within 3–4 months nearly all of the food scraps and bedding material will be converted to a dark brown material the consistency of coffee grounds. At this point the vermicompost should be harvested, before it becomes odorous and sludge-like. Harvesting essentially means separating the compost from the worms, a process than can be accomplished in one of several ways. One method involves dumping the contents of the bin onto a tarp in bright light, causing the worms to wriggle downward toward the bottom of the pile; the castings at the top can then be scraped away, a process repeated several times until all that is left is a pile of worms which can then be placed in a newly prepared bin. Alternatively, new bedding can be placed on one side of the existing bin, the other side being left undisturbed. Over a period of several weeks, most of the worms will move into the new bedding, allowing the castings on the other side to be removed.

To use the finished compost for container plants, either add it directly to potting mix prior to planting or, for already established plants, spread it thinly on the surface of the soil. When setting out seedlings in the garden, a small amount of vermicompost can be placed in each hole at the time of planting; more can subsequently be worked into the soil around the base of individual plants and watered in. Whatever the application method, the result is beneficial, since worm compost contains 5 times more nitrogen, 7 times more phosphorus, and 11 times more potassium than average soil. Giving a boost to home gardening while simultaneously diverting food waste from landfills, vermicomposting is an idea whose time has come. Give it a try!

References

Cochran, Soni. 2003. *Vermicomposting—Composting with Worms!* Educational Resource Guide #107, University of Nebraska, Lincoln.

Edwards, Clive A., and Norman Q. Arancon. 2004. "Vermicomposts Suppress Plant Pest and Disease Attacks." *BioCycle* 45, no. 3 (March).

by the EPA, USDA, NIOSH, and the Composting Council tends to support industry's contention. Conceding that exposure to bioaerosols could be life-threatening if inhaled by individuals with suppressed immune systems, the report nevertheless points out that the level of such particles is no higher in the vicinity of composting operations than in the general environment. A person is just as likely to inhale *A. fumigatus* spores while mowing the lawn, raking leaves, or cleaning the attic as by living near a composting facility. Experts report that *Aspergillus* at composting sites originates primarily from the storage of bulking agents such as wood chips, with airborne spores being released at the time of initial mixing (the steam rising off the top of wind-rows does *not* appear to be a major source). Operational considerations such as moisture and dust control and minimization of handling can significantly mitigate bioaerosol emissions. While authorities agree that more research is needed, the general consensus at present is that bioaerosols *do not* present concerns serious enough to warrant a reconsideration of municipal composting operations (Greczyn, 1994).

In the past, the difficulty of finding outlets for municipal compost was a major stumbling block in convincing local officials to consider composting as a waste management strategy. In recent years, however, cities' marketing efforts and increased public awareness of compost's desirability as a soil conditioner have created sufficient demand among landscaping firms, nurseries, parks departments, and home gardeners. Public willingness to use compost was threatened in the Pacific Northwest a few years ago when users' crops were damaged by a broadleaf herbicide, chlorpyralid ("Confront"), present as a contaminant in the finished compost. While most herbicides break down during the composting process, chlorpyralid does not and even at very low concentrations it is extremely toxic to many horticultural plants. Fearing that their considerable investment in composting facilities could be jeopardized by public reluctance to use a product that could wipe out their gardens, several local governments in Washington State asked chlorpyralid's manufacturer, Dow Chemical, to cease distributing the herbicide in their area. Subsequently, California, Washington, and Oregon have prohibited use of the chemical on residential and commercial lawns and by 2004 average levels of chlorpyralid in finished compost had significantly declined in those states. Elsewhere, chlorpyralid contamination continues to occur sporadically at composting operations accepting residential lawn clippings. Dow has responded to the problem by amending label information to warn users that grass clippings from lawns treated with chlorpyralid should not be composted or used as mulch (Musick, 2004).

Waste Combustion

Prior to passage of the 1970 Clean Air Act, many communities chose to burn urban refuse at large municipal incinerators because the high cost of land, unavailability of suitable sites, or neighborhood opposition to siting made landfilling unfeasible. By the 1960s, almost 300 municipal incinerators were operating in the United States. As the decade of the 1970s ushered in an era of strict air quality control regulations, however, most of these incinerators closed down, unable to comply with the new emission standards. Studies indicated that in some large cities, close to 20% of all particulate pollutants were coming from municipal incinerators (Melosi, 1981).

By the first decade of the 21st century, incineration was the management option for only 7.7% of U.S. municipal solid wastes, a figure considerably lower than predicted just a few years earlier. During the 1980s, as the nation's mounting garbage woes assumed center stage in the environmental policy debate, interest in burning as an attractive waste management option was revived by the advent of a new generation of incinerators: **waste-to-energy (WTE)** plants. These facilities not only burn refuse, thereby reducing its volume by 80–90%, but also capture the heat of combustion in the form of salable electricity or process steam. Many communities, particularly in the northeastern U.S. where landfill tipping fees were skyrocketing, committed themselves to this new technology as the most feasible alternative to disappearing landfill space. By the mid-1990s, however, increasing landfill capacity and a drop in tipping fees shifted the economics in favor of landfilling. As a result, some municipalities that had been considering construction of combustion incinerators decided to forego that option; elsewhere small, economically marginal incinerators were shut down. By

States are making significant strides in recycling the millions of discarded tires that are piling up throughout the U.S. Some states impose taxes on the sale of tires to help offset recycling costs. [*AP photo/Mike Elicson*]

2004, just 98 municipal solid waste incinerators were operating nationwide, most of them in New England, the Middle Atlantic states, and Florida. Among states, Connecticut is the most reliant on incineration for MSW disposal, burning 45% of wastes generated (Kaufman et al., 2004).

From an environmental standpoint, the euphoria that in the 1980s welcomed WTE incinerators as the ideal solution to our disposal dilemmas is now giving way to a more cautious appraisal, as concerns are raised about possible toxic air emissions, especially dioxins, furans, and heavy metals (e.g., lead, cadmium, and mercury). Proponents of the technology insist such problems can be minimized through good emission controls and proper plant operation; in 1991 tighter emissions limitations required by Clean Air Act Amendments for municipal incinerators were approved by EPA, requiring that facilities install state-of-the-art equipment to control acid gases, metal particulates, and organic products of incomplete combustion, such as dioxin. Smokestacks are now being fitted with acid gas scrubbers, baghouse filters for trapping metal particulates, and activated carbon injection systems for capturing mercury vapors. By utilizing advanced combustion controls, plant operators can maintain furnace temperatures high enough to prevent dioxin formation and to ensure a more complete burn.

Disposal of the considerable volumes of incinerator ash generated by large WTE facilities has been another contentious issue. Incineration is not a complete waste management method; in general, for every three tons of refuse burned, a ton of ash remains, requiring disposal. Until recently the most prevalent method for managing incinerator ash was to bury it in ordinary sanitary landfills or in "monofills"—facilities that accepted only incinerator ash for disposal. However, concerns that this material frequently contains dangerous levels of heavy metals (particularly the fly ash captured by pollution control equipment), have led to demands that incinerator ash be classified as "hazardous waste," thereby necessitating its disposal at a hazardous waste landfill—at an anticipated 10-fold rise in tipping fees. In May 1994, the U.S. Supreme Court settled the dispute by ruling that ash from municipal incinerators must be tested, using specified laboratory procedures, and if results indicate that the waste is indeed toxic, it must be managed as hazardous waste. This ruling, while greeted initially with dismay by municipalities currently relying on incinerators, should give a major impetus to resource recovery programs aimed at removing toxics-containing components of the MSW stream—items such as batteries, paint cans, and electrical equipment. Also, by halting the standard practice of combining the often-toxic fly ash with the far more voluminous but much less dangerous bottom ash, incinerator operators can greatly reduce the amount of ash requiring disposal as "hazardous" (Greenhouse, 1994).

Nevertheless, opponents remain wary, fearing that cities opting for incineration are going to find they've simply traded one set of environmental problems for another. Perhaps the major question regarding the future of WTE incineration, however, is financing their construction and operation. To remain economically viable, incinerators need a steady supply of trash and a dependable market for the energy they produce—but recent developments make both difficult to guarantee. Competing demands from recycling programs for high-BTU trash and recent court invalidation of local **"flow-control" ordinances (**which communities have imposed to ensure incinerators a predictable daily volume of waste) have resulted in a number of municipal incinerators operating considerably below their design capacity—a money-losing proposition. WTE incinerators are exorbitantly expensive to construct and operate (as a rough rule-of-thumb, WTE projects average $100,000–$125,000 per ton of daily waste capacity; a city contemplating construction of a typical 1,000 ton-per-day facility can thus count on investing well over $100 million). Costs are recovered (hopefully!) through tipping fees (which a *BioCycle* survey of 15 states found averaged $62 per ton in 2002) paid by haulers bringing wastes to the facility and through sales of electricity or process steam produced by the plant. Since prevailing regional rates for electricity determine what this amount will be, low power demand reflected in falling prices has caused some communities to cancel plans for incinerator construction, since anticipated revenues from energy sales turned out to be less than originally projected.

The future role of WTE incineration in a comprehensive waste management strategy thus depends on a number of economic and political considerations, including trends in landfill tipping fees (increases make incineration more cost-competitive and vice-versa); demand for energy (high demand equals brighter future for WTE combustion); congressional initiatives (will Congress impose a legislative moratorium on incinerator construction?); and EPA decisions (will the agency further tighten emissions requirements or mandate that communities achieve specified recycling goals before building new incinerators?). WTE combustion remains the most important MSW management method in Japan and a number of European countries. However, given the current abundance of landfill capacity in the U.S. and the large discrepancy between per unit disposal charges at landfills versus incinerators, it is unlikely that the percentage of MSW managed by combustion will increase significantly in the years immediately ahead.

Hazardous Wastes

Late in the summer of 1978 the name of a small residential subdivision in the city of Niagara Falls, New York, entered the American vocabulary and became a household word almost overnight, symbolizing the dangers of our chemical age. The tragic

Box 16-3   Environmental Justice

In 1982 when civil rights demonstrators in predominantly African-American Warren County, North Carolina, rallied to protest the siting of a PCB landfill in their midst, they may not have realized they were leading the vanguard of a new social movement in the United States. They *did* know they were angry that, once again, a small, poor, politically powerless community of color was being targeted as the location for a locally unwanted waste disposal facility.

While the protesters were unsuccessful in forcing closure of the landfill, their cries of outrage reverberated all the way to the halls of Congress where Delegate Walter Fauntroy (D.C.) asked the General Accounting Office (GAO) to look into allegations of racial discrimination in the siting of waste facilities in the South. A year later GAO issued its report, concluding that 75% of the region's hazardous waste was being dumped in predominantly African-American communities. GAO's statement confirmed the existence of what has come to be known as **environmental racism**—the unequal exposure of the poor and people of color to pollution, toxics, and other hazards. It launched the ongoing quest for **environmental justice (EJ)**, an effort to improve the overall quality of life for those same groups, and prompted demands for **environmental equity**, the fair distribution of environmental risks across all population groups.

A major contribution to the struggle against environmental racism was the publication in 1987 of a seminal study by the United Church of Christ Commission for Racial Justice, *Toxic Waste and Race in the United States*, detailing for the first time interrelating issues of race, class, and environment across the nation. This work contended that pollution is anything but an "equal opportunity" affliction, blighting and shortening the lives of African Americans, Latinos, and Native Americans to a far greater extent than white Americans. The Commission for Racial Justice study, as well as subsequent reports on the same topic by several other authors, cited statistics showing that the majority of U.S. landfills and incinerators are located in predominantly African-American or Hispanic communities. Furthermore, 60% of all African-Americans live in communities with

one or more abandoned toxic waste sites (highly segregated southeast Chicago, pock-marked by over 100 such abandoned dumps, is a classic example). To environmental justice advocates, these facts suggest deliberate discrimination, "dumping on the poor" by locating a disproportionate number of undesirable facilities in minority communities.

Federal agencies themselves have been accused of perpetuating environmental injustices. Staff writers at the *National Law Journal* in 1992 charged that EPA was guilty of environmental racism in its implementation of Superfund cleanups, citing evidence of faster action, more thorough remediation, and stricter enforcement of hazwaste regulations in white communities than in minority communities. These inequities prevailed, they asserted, regardless of community income levels—race, and race alone, was the determining factor.

Issues of environmental justice provided the impetus for a "Conference on Race and the Incidence of Environmental Hazards" held at the University of Michigan in 1990. Following that event, a group of participants wrote to then-EPA Administrator William Reilly, requesting that the agency take action to deal with environmental risks in minority and low-income communities. Reilly responded by forming an Environmental Equity Workgroup, and the agency began investigating environmental discrimination charges under the 1964 Civil Rights Act.

Proponents of environmental justice gained an important ally in President Clinton who, on February 11, 1994, signed Executive Order 12898 prohibiting discriminatory practices in any programs receiving federal financial assistance. For the first time, federal agencies were required to consider the racial and socioeconomic characteristics of a community prior to launching a new project or issuing new environmental rules. EPA now has a program in place to guarantee that its rulings don't unfairly impact the poor and powerless, though some groups complain that the agency has not been actively implementing the executive order. On the 6th anniversary of President Clinton's initiative, a group of EJ activists told a Washington press conference that minority groups continued to suffer from the "toxic terrorism" of polluting chemical industries and federal facilities.

During the mid- to late-1990s, EJ groups scored several notable victories, indicating that even the least advantaged segments of society, with little or no official support, could successfully combat the forces of environmental racism. In 1996 a local coalition of environmental, faith-based, and social justice organizations in Chicago calling themselves the West Side Alliance for a Safe and Toxic-Free Environment (WASTE) reaped the rewards of three years of public meetings, marches, and petitions when the city announced plans to close its Northwest Incinerator, a facility that had operated for 26 years, burning over 1,000 tons of refuse daily in a neighborhood largely populated by poor, working class African-Americans. Accusing Chicago officials of environmental racism, one community leader representing the coalition remarked to a reporter, "We know they aren't building these things in rich white neighborhoods. . . . They wouldn't stand for it. This is genocide against poor people and all people of color . . ." An even more significant win came in 1998 when local EJ activists, assisted by the Tulane Environmental Law Clinic (subsequently de-funded by Louisiana's governor for its pivotal role in the struggle), Greenpeace, and several other national environmental organizations, prevented the Shintech chemical company from building a large polyvinylchloride plant in the predominantly African-American town of Convent, located in Louisiana's notorious "Cancer Alley."

Other EJ struggles during the 1990s were less clear cut as to the identity of the "bad guys." A case in point was the raging controversy in Robbins, a Chicago suburb and the oldest city in the northern U.S. governed entirely by African-Americans. One of the poorest suburbs in the country and desperately in need of a steady source of revenue, the town had been actively seeking waste management facilities interested in locating in Robbins. In the late 1980s, local officials struck a deal with an energy company to build a WTE incinerator that would add $2 million in rent to the city coffers each year. This action quickly polarized the community, pitting neighbor against neighbor as opponents protested the negative health impact an incinerator would have on the town while others argued with equal vehe-

mence that the facility would be state-of-the-art and an economic boon for Robbins. Charging that the conflict was provoked by "outside agitators," the mayor argued that "There's always been environmental racism. We're just making it work for us for once!" Supporters of the project prevailed; the state environmental agency approved permits for the facility and the incinerator opened in 1997, processing wastes from 12 Chicago-area communities. Financial problems and accidents plagued the incinerator, however, as did permit violations. The State of Illinois eventually filed suit against the company for exceeding emissions limitations and in 1999 the Robbins facility closed.

Ironically, while the environmental justice movement has been successful in fighting locally unwanted land uses in a number of communities, the recycling facilities that many environmental groups have supported as a "clean alternative" frequently have proven to be as dirty, noisy, and detrimental to the quality of life of nearby residents as the landfills or incinerators they replaced. Most often located, like the latter, in low-income or minority neighborhoods, recycling facilities—particularly "dirty MRFs"—present numerous health and safety threats to workers. As a result, some EJ activists contend that, despite its "green" image, recycling is but the latest example of environmental inequality and charge that the main-line environmental organizations ignore the plight of minority communities.

Whatever the ultimate outcome of the continuing struggle for environmental justice, it has already had the positive effect of heightening awareness and sensitivity to the unequal burden of pollution and poor health suffered by minority and low-income communities. It has also sparked a broad-based effort by people of color to redefine and reshape the modern environmental movement, expanding the concept to include issues of social and economic justice and the right of *all* people to be protected from environmental degradation.

References

Dorsey, Michael K. 1998. "Toward the Idea of International Environmental Justice." *World Resources 1998–99*. New York: Oxford Univ. Press.

Pellow, David Naguib. 2002. *Garbage Wars*. Cambridge, MA: The MIT Press.

sequence of events that unfolded at Love Canal epitomizes the dangers facing millions of citizens in thousands of communities across the nation as a result of our indiscriminate use and careless disposal of hazardous chemicals.

The Love Canal Story

The origin of the chemical dumpsite that became the focus of worldwide attention in the late 1970s can be traced to the mid-1890s, when William T. Love began construction of a canal intended to serve as a navigable power channel, connecting the Upper Niagara to the Niagara Escarpment about seven miles downstream, thereby bypassing the Falls. At the point where Mr. Love's canal was intended to reenter the river, the intention was to construct a model industrial city that would be provided with cheap, abundant hydroelectric power. Unfortunately for Mr. Love, his development company went bankrupt shortly after construction of the canal had begun; the project was abandoned, leaving a waterway approximately 3,000 feet long, 10 feet deep, and 60 feet wide. For many years, residents of this area on the outskirts of town used the canal for recreational fishing and swimming; in 1927 the land was annexed by the city. In 1942 Hooker Chemical Company (now a subsidiary of Occidental Petroleum), one of several major chemical industries located in Niagara Falls, received permission to dump chemical wastes into the canal, which it proceeded to do from that time until 1952 (in 1947 Hooker purchased the canal, along with two 70-feet-wide strips of land adjacent to the canal on each side). During this time more than 21,000 tons of chemical wastes—acids, alkalis, solvents, chlorinated hydrocarbons, etc.—were disposed of at this site. Only a few homes were present in the area at that time, but old-time residents recall the offensive odors, noxious vapors, and frequent fires that accompanied the dumping.

By 1953 the canal was full and so was topped with soil and eventually acquired a covering of grass and weeds. Hooker then offered to sell the land to the Niagara Falls School Board for the token fee of $1. At the same time, company officials pointedly advised school and city administrators that although the site was suitable for a school, parking lot, or playground, any construction activities involving excavation of the area should be avoided to prevent rupturing the dumpsite's clay lining, thereby allowing escape of the impounded chemicals. In 1955 an elementary school and playground were constructed on the site; in 1957 the city began laying storm sewers, roads, and utility lines through the area, disregarding the warnings received a few years earlier. In the years that followed, several hundred modest homes were built in the neighborhood parallel to the banks of the now-invisible canal. Most of the newer residents had no knowledge of the site's past history and, in spite of occasional chemical odors (not considered unusual in a city where chemical manufacturing was a leading industry), few outward signs of trouble were apparent. Unusually heavy precipitation in the mid-1970s, however, was accompanied by some alarming phenomena. Strange-looking, viscous chemicals began oozing through basement walls, floors, and sump holes. Vegetation in yards withered and appeared scorched. Large puddles became permanent backyard features. Holes began to open up in the field that had once been a dumpsite and the tops of corroded 55-gallon drums leaking chemicals could be seen in places protruding from the soil surface. Complaints and fears expressed by citizens were generally downplayed by local authorities who assured them there was nothing to worry about.

By early 1978, pressure from a local congressman and regular critical coverage of events in the Niagara Gazette prompted the U.S. Environmental Protection Agency to undertake a program of air sampling in the basements of Love Canal homes. New York State authorities also began conducting soil analyses and taking samples of residues in sump pumps and storm sewers. The results of these studies indicated that the area was extremely contaminated with more than 200 different chemicals, including 12 known or suspected carcinogens. Benzene, known to be a potent human cancer-causing agent, was readily detected in the air inside many of the houses sampled. Dioxin was subsequently found in high concentrations in some of the soil samples analyzed. State officials in New York estimated that as many as 10% of the chemicals buried at Love Canal were mutagens, teratogens, or carcinogens. On August 2, 1978, the Health Commissioner of New York publicly proclaimed "the existence of a great and imminent peril to the health of the general public" at Love Canal and advised all pregnant women and families with children under the age of two to leave the area if they could do so. Five days later, President Carter officially declared Love Canal a national emergency.

The months that followed witnessed mass relocation at public expense of residents living closest to the dumpsite, as well as openly expressed fears by those left behind on adjacent streets that their health was similarly endangered. A number of health studies, whose methodology and conclusions remain highly controversial, suggested that Love Canal residents had experienced statistically significant elevated rates of miscarriage, birth defects, and chromosomal abnormalities. Ultimately 1,004 families were evacuated from Love Canal, their homes purchased by the state. Over 300 of the residences closest to the canal were demolished and the area covered with a protective layer of clay and a synthetic liner to exclude rainwater. Most of the remaining homes were boarded up, awaiting a pending EPA assessment of whether they could ever again be inhabited. Trenches were dug around the old canal site to capture contaminated groundwater, which was then pumped to a treatment center for detoxification. Nearby creeks where high levels of dioxin seepage were detected were fenced off to protect children and animals. Combined federal and state expenditures for relocating residents, investigating environmental damage, and halting chemical seepage from the site total $150 million, and an additional $32 million has been spent to clean up contaminated creeks and sewers and to determine the future habitability of the neighborhood. The Congressional Office of Technology Assessment estimated that if Hooker had employed current disposal standards and practices, its wastes could have been safely managed for about $2 million in 1979 dollars (Levine, 1982).

Occidental Chemical, which acquired Hooker in a 1968 buy-out, has paid $20 million in out-of-court settlements to affected residents; a federal district court ruling in 1988 held Occidental liable for the cost of previous, ongoing, and future cleanup of the Love Canal site—a figure approximating $250 million. Two years later, the State of New York sued Occidental for an additional $250 million in punitive damages, claiming that its subsidiary Hooker had "displayed reckless disregard for the safety of others." In the spring of 1994, a federal judge ruled against the plaintiff, saying the evidence in the state's case was insufficient; this decision, however, did not alter Occidental's liability for cleanup costs. In the fall of 1988, after reviewing a five-year habitability study of the affected area, New York State Health Commissioner David Axelrod declared that most of the Love Canal neighborhood could be safely resettled by former residents. While the decision was controversial, with some environmentalists warning that "Love Canal is a ticking time bomb," by the summer of 1990 over 200 people had expressed interest in renovated homes selling for 20% less than the prevailing market price. Reassured by government claims that the area no longer presented any threat, new residents began reoccupying homes in the Love Canal neighborhood, renamed "Black Creek Village." Eventually more than 200 abandoned homes were renovated and sold to new owners and 10 new apartment buildings constructed in the area. In 1995 Occidental Chemical agreed to pay the federal government $129 million to cover costs for the pollution cleanup at Love Canal. Hailing the final agreement concluded by the U.S. Department of Justice, EPA Administrator Carol Browner remarked that it represented "this administration's firm commitment to ensuring that polluters, not the American people, pick up the tab for cleaning up toxic waste dumps." The final chapter in this saga concluded in September 2004 when the EPA officially removed the Love Canal site from the Superfund National Priority List, declaring that all work at the site had been completed and cleanup goals achieved.

The events that transpired at Love Canal cannot be shrugged off as a unique tragedy that unfortunately victimized a few thousand people in western New York State but left the rest of the nation unscathed. Health authorities and environmental agency officials regard Love Canal as but the "tip of the iceberg" in alerting society to the widespread nature of the hazardous waste problem. In 2004 EPA released a report projecting that as many as 350,000 sites across the nation may require cleanup over the next 30 years due to contamination with hazardous wastes or petroleum products. If current remediation standards are maintained, the total cleanup costs could be as high as $250 billion. Little wonder that public opinion polls show citizens ranking hazardous waste management issues among their top environmental quality concerns.

What Is "Hazardous" Waste?

In the 1976 Resource Conservation and Recovery Act (RCRA), Congress legally defined hazardous waste as "any discarded material that may pose a substantial threat or potential danger to human health or the environment when improperly handled." EPA has established a two-tier system for determining whether a specific waste is subject to regulation under current hazardous waste management laws:

1. If the substance in question is among the more than 500 wastes or waste streams itemized in Parts 261.31–33 of the Code of Federal Regulations, it will automatically be subject to regulation as a hazardous waste. Wastes may be placed on the list because of their ability to induce cancer, mutations, or birth defects; because of their toxicity to plants; or because even low doses are fatal to humans. However, the Administrator of EPA can exercise a wide measure of discretion in deciding whether to list a particular waste, so a number of potential carcinogens, mutagens, and teratogens are not yet listed as officially "hazardous."

2. In addition to the wastes listed in the federal code, any waste that exhibits one or more of the following characteristics is defined as hazardous and subject to regulation:

   Toxic—wastes such as arsenic, heavy metals, or certain synthetic pesticides are capable of causing either acute or chronic health problems.

   Ignitable—organic solvents, oils, plasticizers, and paint wastes are examples of wastes that are hazardous because they have a flashpoint less than 60°C (140°F) or because they tend to undergo spontaneous combustion. The resultant fires are dangerous not only because of heat and smoke, but also because they can disseminate toxic particles over a wide area.

   Corrosive—substances with a pH of 2 or less or 12.5 and above can eat away at standard container materials or living tissues through chemical action and are termed corrosive. Such wastes, which include acids, alkaline cleaning agents, and battery manufacturing residues, present a special threat to waste haulers who come into bodily contact with leaking containers.

   Reactive—obsolete munitions, wastes from the manufacturing of dynamite or firecrackers, and certain chemical wastes such as picric acid are hazardous because of their tendency to react vigorously with air or water or to explode and generate toxic fumes.

Two other categories of wastes that might logically be considered hazardous—radioactive wastes and potentially infectious medical wastes from hospitals and clinics—are not presently regulated under the same laws as the groups listed above. Radioactive wastes are managed according to regulations adopted by the Nuclear Regulatory Commission under the Atomic Energy Act, while biomedical waste disposal laws vary from state to state. In 1988, public outrage over incidents of used syringes and other medical wastes washing up on East Coast beaches led to passage of the Medical Waste Tracking Act, which set up a two-year pilot project to attempt regulation of biomedical wastes through a procedure similar in nature to the manifest system currently required for off-site shipments of hazardous wastes. With the expiration of that program, individual states have, for the most part, adopted medical waste management programs of their own involving the manifesting of such wastes shipped off-site and, in several states, requiring that infectious wastes be "rendered innocuous" in specially licensed high-temperature incinerators—a form of disposal considerably more expensive than sanitary landfilling. Many authorities deplore what they regard as exaggerated public fears about the threats posed by medical wastes. Pointing out that wastes generated by hospitals are no more dangerous than many of the items tossed into the trash by householders (e.g., used syringes from home insulin injections, bloody bandages, outdated medications, etc.) and that not a single case of human illness has been traced to contact with infectious medical waste, they question the public health benefit of strict new regulations that significantly increase national costs for health care. Ironically, the highly sensationalized beach littering incidents that provoked the federal legislation, initially attributed to illegal ocean dumping by waste haulers, were subsequently traced to sewer discharges of discarded medical devices from private residences.

Generation of Hazardous Wastes

By the first decade of the 21st century, more than 20,000 U.S. manufacturers were sending approximately 7 million tons of hazardous wastes and wastewaters to commercial hazwaste landfills, incinerators, treatment, or recycling facilities each year (Perket, 2004), a figure that does not take into account wastes managed by the generators on-site. Production of these wastes is not evenly distributed among industries, however. More than 85% of all hazardous wastes are produced by just three major categories of generators: chemicals and allied products, metal-related industries, and petroleum and coal products. Geographic location of these industries, as well as population density, are major determinants of which states are the leading hazardous waste generators.

At the time when new federal waste management regulations went into effect in November 1980, EPA estimated that fully 90% of all hazardous wastes were being disposed of by methods that would not meet government standards. Thanks to what is widely regarded as the most stringent hazardous waste management program in the world, that situation has now markedly improved.

Threats Posed by Careless Disposal

Mismanagement of hazardous wastes can adversely affect human health and environmental quality in a number of ways.

Direct contact. Direct contact with wastes can result in skin irritation, the initiation of serious chronic illness, or acute poisoning—as in the case of two 9-year-old

Tampa boys who were killed in June 1992, while playing inside a municipal waste bin. Subsequent investigations revealed that the bin, located behind an industrial firm, contained toluene- and acetone-contaminated waste, leading officials to conclude the boys had died due to inhalation of toxic chemical fumes.

Fire and/or explosions.   In April 1980, a spectacular blaze destroyed a riverside warehouse complex in Elizabeth, New Jersey, where 50,000 chemical-containing drums had been sitting for almost 10 years. Such accidents are a constant threat when hazardous wastes are in transit, carelessly stored, or roughly handled. Explosions are a particular threat to workers at landfills accepting hazardous wastes. In Edison, New Jersey, a bulldozer operator who inadvertently crushed a container of flammable phosphorus was burned so quickly that his corpse was discovered with his hand still on the gearshift.

Poison via the foodchain.   Biomagnification of toxic wastes discharged into the environment can result in the poisoning of animals or humans who consume the toxin indirectly. The tragic outbreak of methyl mercury poisoning at Minamata, Japan, typifies this sort of situation.

Air pollution.   When toxic wastes are burned at temperatures insufficiently high to completely destroy them, serious air pollution problems can result. Only specialized types of equipment are licensed for the incineration of hazardous wastes, and even these must be carefully monitored while operating to ensure a complete burn.

Surface water contamination.   Accidental spills or deliberate dumping of hazardous wastes can easily pollute waterways. The extent and duration of environmental damage to surface waters varies widely, depending on the size of the water body in

Abandoned hazardous waste dumpsite where hundreds of corroding drums leak their toxic contents onto the ground, endangering drinking water aquifers below the surface. [*Illinois Environmental Protection Agency*]

question and the rate of flow, but short-term damage to aquatic ecosystems can be severe. In Butte, Montana, location of the largest Superfund complex in the nation, several hundred snow geese died in 1995 soon after landing on a lake of toxic waste-water that had formed at an open-pit mine. Post-mortem analyses of the birds revealed acid-burned esophagi, indicating they died from drinking the highly polluted water. Public drinking water supplies also can be endangered by hazardous waste discharges; municipal water intake points occasionally must be closed until the plume of pollution from an accidental spill flows past.

Groundwater contamination. The most common problem associated with poor hazardous waste management is the pollution of aquifers with toxic leachates percolating downward through the soil from landfills or surface impoundments. This type of pollution is particularly insidious because it is seldom discovered until it is too late to do anything about it. Citizens in numerous communities around the nation have discovered to their horror that they had unknowingly been consuming well water contaminated with a variety of toxic chemicals that entered the groundwater supply via seepage from disposal sites.

Methods of Hazardous Waste Disposal

Historically, the largest percentage of hazardous wastes have been disposed of on land, primarily because land disposal, particularly prior to government regulation of hazardous waste management, was by far the cheapest option. During the mid-1970s, for example, almost half of all hazardous wastes, the majority of which were in the form of liquids or sludges, were simply dumped into unlined surface impoundments, techni-cally referred to as "pits, ponds, or lagoons," located on the generators' property. These wastes eventually evaporated or percolated into the soil, often resulting in groundwater contamination. Other wastes, about 30% of the total, were buried in sanitary landfills, easily subject to leaching, and another 10% were burned in an uncontrolled manner. None of these methods would be in compliance with current regulations.

Although many citizens are convinced that no methods exist for the safe disposal of hazardous wastes, a number of new technologies have been developed which avoid most of the shortcomings inherent in past hazardous waste management practices. All such methods, not surprisingly, are considerably more expensive than simply dump-ing wastes in a pit or a municipal landfill, and thus were not widely utilized until strict regulatory action was taken by Congress. A listing of legal hazardous waste disposal options would include the following.

Secure chemical landfill. Generally, the cheapest method of hazardous waste disposal is the so-called "secure" chemical landfill, a specially designed earthen exca-vation constructed in such a way as to contain dangerous chemicals and to prevent them from escaping into the environment through leaching or vaporization. In the past, secure landfills frequently differed from sanitary landfills only in that they were topped with a layer of clay to keep water out of the trenches in which chemical drums had been placed. This of course did not prevent chemical seepage from contaminating water supplies. Under current RCRA standards, a secure chemical landfill must be located above the 100-year floodplain and away from fault zones; it must contain dou-ble liners of clay or synthetic materials to keep leaching to a minimum; a network of pipes must be laid to collect and control polluted rainwater and leachate accumulating in the landfill; and monitoring wells must be installed to check the quality of any groundwater deposits in the area (surface water supplies must also be monitored by the landfill operator). In spite of these precautions, most experts agree that there is no way to guarantee that sometime in the future contaminants will not migrate from the

Figure 16-4 A Secure Landfill

landfill site. Liners eventually crack; soil can shift or settle. Since many chemical wastes remain hazardous more or less indefinitely, serious pollution problems can occur many years after a secure chemical landfill has been closed and forgotten. Many authorities feel that although chemical landfills are legal, they are the least acceptable method of managing hazardous wastes.

Since 1984 when more stringent requirements for groundwater monitoring, minimum technology standards, and financial guarantees for post-closure activities took effect, the number of operating facilities has dropped substantially. By 2003 there were just 26 commercial hazardous waste landfills operating in the United States and 5 in Canada (Perket, 2003), compared to more than 1,000 during the 1970s. Within the past few years, the list of wastes for which disposal in landfills is prohibited has been steadily growing; federal legislation enacted in 1984 and fully implemented by 1990 imposed a ban on the landfilling of virtually all hazardous wastes, unless such materials undergo prior treatment to minimize their toxicity and ability to migrate. The explicit intent of such legislation is to reduce reliance on land disposal and to encourage the use of alternative technologies to the greatest extent possible.

Deep well injection. The use of deep wells for waste disposal dates back to the late 19th century when the petroleum industry employed this method to get rid of salt brine, but its use for liquid hazardous waste disposal began only during the 1940s. A number of industries, most notably petroleum refineries and petrochemical plants, now utilize this disposal method. Commercial deep well injection currently is practiced only in the Midwest and in Texas and neighboring states, although many other injection wells operated by private firms solely for the disposal of their own wastes are widely scattered across the United States. The process involves pumping liquid wastes through lined wells into porous rock formations deep underground, well below any drinking water aquifers. Some critics point out that cracks in the well casing or undetected faults in the earth that intersect the disposal zone could result in outward migration of wastes. EPA contends that deep wells are safe, provided that they are constructed, operated, and maintained in accordance with agency regulations.

Various chemical, physical, or biological treatment processes. Processes that render wastes nonhazardous or significantly reduce their volume or toxicity have assumed major importance in recent years, particularly as more and more **"land bans"** have been implemented, prohibiting the landfilling of untreated wastes. With economic motivation spurring invention, a number of promising new technologies are now in the pilot project phase or fully operational, promising safer, more effective ways of cleaning up past mistakes and ensuring that wastes currently being generated are properly managed.

Physical methods include **evaporation** to concentrate corrosive brines, **sedimentation** to separate solids from liquid wastes, **carbon adsorption** to remove certain soluble organic wastes, and **air-stripping** to remove volatile organic compounds from groundwater.

Chemical techniques involve processes such as **neutralization** to render wastes harmless, sulfide **precipitation** to extract certain toxic metals, **oxidation-reduction** processes to convert some metals from a hazardous to a nonhazardous state, and **stabilization/solidification,** in which the waste material is detoxified and then combined with a cement-like material, encapsulated in plastic, blended with organic polymers, or combined with silica to form a solid, inert substance that can be disposed of safely in a landfill or incorporated into road beds. Another innovative technology is **in-situ vitrification (ISV),** a process that relies on large amounts of electricity (about 750 kilowatt-hours per ton of soil) delivered by giant electrodes fixed at several locations in the soil surrounding the area undergoing cleanup. Suitable for detoxifying soils contaminated with toxic organics (e.g., chlorinated pesticides), heavy metals, or radioactive wastes, ISV actually melts the soil as the electricity flows through it, fusing the toxics into a solid block of glassified material, similar to natural obsidian. The solidified material can simply be left in place, no longer posing any environmental threat (but perhaps causing immense puzzlement among archaeologists five thousand years hence, trying to figure out what kind of cultural artifact that huge chunk of glass could possibly be!).

Bioremediation, based on the ability of microbes, fungi, or plants to break down or absorb organic pollutants or toxic metals, is increasingly used for cleanup of oil spills and remediation of contaminated soil and groundwater. The largest number of projects utilizes various species of naturally occurring bacteria. By far the most widely used method of bioremediation is **biostimulation**, in which oxygen and/or nutrients are added to contaminated material to promote more rapid growth of indigenous microbes, resulting in faster, more efficient metabolism of wastes than would have occurred without human intervention. In situations where resident bacteria are too few in number, even with biostimulation, to degrade wastes effectively or when the microbes naturally present are genetically incapable of breaking down a particular waste, it may be necessary to utilize **bioaugmentation**. In such situations, nonindigenous species are added to "lend a hand," working in concert with the local microbes to accomplish pollutant removal more rapidly and completely. In a quest to create new bacterial strains better able to degrade chemicals under specific environmental conditions, scientists have been working to develop genetically engineered microbes (GEMs) to destroy pollutants that have proven resistant to breakdown by naturally occurring species. In order to avoid any possible risk to human health or the environment, the use of GEMs is strictly regulated under the Toxic Substances Control Act, which requires that they undergo a rigorous safety review prior to approval for field use.

Controlled incineration. Because burning at very high temperatures actually destroys hazardous wastes (as opposed to storing them out of sight underground as is

Box 16-4   Plants vs. Pollution

In the summer of 2004, the Army Corps of Engineers launched an innovative pilot project to clean up wastes contaminating approximately 600 acres of residential and university property near American University in northwestern Washington, DC. The area, used during World War I for testing chemical weapons, is tainted with traces of arsenic from those long-ago experiments and a hazardous waste cleanup operation had been ordered. However, the Corps' conventional remediation project had stalled because residents resisted seeing the lovely old trees in their neighborhood removed or damaged during soil removal operations. Responding to such concerns, the Corps opted to deal with problems remaining on more than 100 private properties by utilizing a relatively new waste treatment method known as **phytoremediation**, planting 2,800 arsenic-absorbing brake ferns (*Pteris vittata*) at three different locations within the affected area. If past experience is any guide, the ferns will pull arsenic out of the soil and accumulate the toxic metal in their stems and fronds, concentrating it to more than 50 times soil levels—and do so without any harm to the surrounding trees. Corps personnel will then harvest the ferns, analyze them for arsenic, and subsequently safely dispose of the plants at a hazardous waste facility if arsenic levels are extremely high.

The ability of brake ferns, a common Southeastern species, to accumulate arsenic was discovered in 1998 when researchers from the University of Florida tried growing 14 different plant species in arsenic-contaminated soil at a lumberyard in central Florida (arsenic compounds from wood preservatives are often found in soils where treated lumber has been stored). While few plants even survive in arsenic-tainted soil (arsenic is an effective ingredient in some weed-killers), the brake ferns thrived in this environment and the U. of Florida scientists proudly announced their discovery of the first plant species able to accumulate arsenic in high concentrations. They subsequently patented their discovery and the so-called "edenferns™" are now sold by Edenspace, a Virginia-based bioremediation company. Edenferns™ are currently being used to remove arsenic from soil and drinking water at various locations across the United States, proving themselves a cost-effective alternative to conventional remediation technologies that typically involve excavation, acid-washing, and landfill disposal of contaminated soils.

Edenferns™ are by no means the only plants to prove their worth in cleaning up chemically contaminated sites. At present, over 440 plant species have been identified as possessing the natural ability to take up quantities of metals such as lead, zinc, cadmium, and uranium from soils and accumulate them in quantities that would kill most other species. Referred to as **hyperaccumulators**, such plants can store as much as 2.5% of their dry weight in heavy metals in leaves without suffering any reduction in yields. Researchers have now identified the gene that produces phytochelatins, the substance that allows plants to detoxify heavy metals and hope to use this information to enhance further the natural ability of hyperaccumulator plants to take up toxic metals. Field studies are currently underway in a number of countries to identify which plants are best suited for phytoextraction purposes.

Among those so identified is Indian mustard (*Brassica juncea*), a hyperaccumulator of lead. At a contaminated DaimlerChrysler site in Detroit, a mixed planting of Indian mustard and sunflowers, another lead-absorbing species, reduced existing soil lead concentrations 43%, bringing contaminant levels below legal limits; the cost of the remediation project was $1 million less than conventional soil excavation would have been and waste from the project consisted merely of a few cubic yards of lead-laden plant material. Indian mustard is also being used to remove selenium from contaminated soils in California's San Joaquin Valley, where toxic selenium in agricultural drainage water has severely disrupted the ecosystem at Kesterson Reservoir. The state has set a high priority on remediating high-selenium soils and on minimizing movement of the chemical from soil to irrigation effluent. Since most of the conventional methods investigated were either very costly or only marginally effective, phytoremediation has attracted considerable interest as an economical, environmentally friendly alternative. Long-term field studies have shown that the top 24 inches of soil experienced nearly a 40% reduction in selenium content when planted with Indian mustard. Most of the selenium taken up was incorporated into plant tissue, while some was biologically volatilized into the air, primarily via the roots. Mustard plants with elevated concentrations of selenium have the potential to become a high-value crop for farmers, as well as a cheap method of soil improvement. Because selenium is an essential trace element for mammals, selenium-containing mustard could be blended with alfalfa and feed to produce nutritious livestock forage— a win-win situation.

For cleanup of soils contaminated with zinc or cadmium, the humble Alpine pennycress (Thlaspi caerulescens) appears to be one of the most promising candidates. The plant has long been recognized in Europe as a good biological indicator of metal ore deposits. Recent studies have shown that pennycress takes up 35 times more zinc than other plant species growing in the same vicinity, concentrating the metal in its shoots.

Sunflowers have proven effective in remediating water tainted with low-level uranium, a situation where other methods either don't work or are prohibitively expensive. An experiment conducted in 1995 on a small radioactively contaminated pond near Chernobyl utilized sunflowers grown on Styrofoam rafts to extract strontium-90 and cesium-137 from the water. With their dense roots dangling in the water, the sunflowers quickly took up radioisotope concentrations several thousand times higher than those in the pond. The uranium taken up by the plants remains localized in the roots, simplifying waste disposal since only the roots need to be managed as low-level wastes, generally by incineration and land disposal of the residual ash.

Another plant successfully employed in wetlands systems to treat wastewaters contaminated by heavy metals is water hyacinth (Eichhornia crassipes). Water hyacinth multiplies rapidly, absorbing dissolved metals and accumulating them in plant tissues, especially the roots. Since E. crassipes floats on the water's surface, the plant can easily be harvested and, following incineration, its toxic metal component either recovered for reuse or land disposed. Water hyacinth is regarded as having good potential for in-situ remediation of hexavalent chromium, as well as a number of other toxic metals contaminating industrial wastewaters or sediments.

Poplar and willow trees are now employed at numerous locations to pump and treat solvent-contaminated groundwater. During the peak of the growing season, each poplar tree takes up more than 15 gallons of water daily, pulling organic contaminants into the root zone where they are biodegraded by soil microbes or by the plants themselves. Poplars planted near landfills or other potential sites of leachate migration can also be effective in capturing migrating pollutants, pulling them out of the ground before they infiltrate aquifers or surface waters.

At a time when the estimated cost of remediating the nation's hazardous waste legacy using conventional technologies exceeds $700 billion, phytoremediation has the potential to revolutionize our approach to cleanups, especially in situations where levels of contamination are low, dispersed, but nevertheless in violation of standards. Phytoremediation's chief drawback is time; reducing concentrations of toxic metals to safe levels may require several years, depending on initial levels of contamination. Researchers hope that in the not-too-distant-future genetically engineered hyperaccumulators capable of accomplishing the cleanup task more expeditiously will be developed. Nevertheless, for nonemergency situations where toxins are not immediately threatening human health, phytoremediation holds great promise as an affordable, effective, nonintrusive way to restore contaminated sites.

References

Banuelos, G. S. et al., 1997. "Phytoremediation of Selenium-Laden Soils: A New Technology." Journal of Soil and Water Conservation 52, no. 6 (Nov/ Dec):426–31.

Revkin, Andrew C. 2001. "New Pollution Tool: Toxic Avengers with Leaves." New York Times, March 6, D1, 7.

Ruder, Kate. 2004. "Ferns Remove Arsenic from Soil and Water." Arsenic Crisis Group (Aug.6).

essentially the case with various land disposal methods), many hazardous waste management experts regard controlled incineration as the best and, in some cases, the only environmentally acceptable means of disposal. In spite of its relatively high cost compared to other hazwaste management options, controlled incineration is assuming increased importance as land disposal regulations grow more restrictive. Waste generators, fearful of legal liability if their wastes migrate from a land disposal site, are increasingly likely to consider a management method that ensures total waste destruction. A controlled incinerator burns at temperatures ranging from 750–3000°F, with wastes, air, and fuel being thoroughly mixed to ensure complete combustion. Afterburners, which are part of the incineration system, destroy any gaseous hydrocarbons that may have survived the initial incineration process, while scrubbers and electrostatic precipitators remove pollutant emissions from the stack gases. In 1999, EPA further tightened nationwide standards for air emissions from hazwaste combustors. The new regulations required all commercial hazardous waste incinerators (15 operating in the U.S. in 2003), cement kilns, and other facilities that burn hazwastes to achieve a 70% reduction in dioxins and furans as well as reductions in mercury and lead emissions up to 86% by 2002. The technologies employed to lower concentrations of these pollutants also reduce emissions of particulates, carbon monoxide, hydrocarbons, hydrochloric acid, and other toxic metals. The stringent requirements were justified as necessary to protect the health and environment of the 37 million U.S. residents living in the vicinity of hazardous waste combustors.

Waste exchanges.   The ideal way to manage hazardous materials would be to recycle them, thus preventing their entry into the waste stream and eliminating the disposal problem. This is the idea that prompted the establishment of waste exchanges, which act as helpful third parties in establishing contact between waste generators and potential waste users. For example, a paint manufacturer, faced with the problem of how to dispose of hazardous sludges from a mixing operation, contacts a waste exchange and is referred to another company which willingly purchases the sludge to use as a filler coat on cement blocks. Thus, the paint manufacturer avoids the high cost of disposal in a secure chemical landfill or controlled incinerator and also makes a modest profit on the sale of the waste. The buyer, too, is pleased with the arrangement because a needed raw material is obtained for a lower price than unused filler would have cost; and society is well served because a potentially hazardous substance has been prevented from entering the environment. The first waste exchange program began in the Netherlands in 1972. The Midwest Industrial Waste Exchange, started in 1975 in St. Louis, was the first U.S. program, the forerunner of approximately 160 waste and materials exchanges throughout the U.S. and Canada, some coordinated by state or local governments, others run by private, for-profit businesses. Although waste exchanges were originally developed exclusively for industrial hazardous waste trading, the concept has now expanded to include many exchanges dealing in nonhazardous waste materials (technically these are referred to as *materials exchanges*, while those dealing in hazardous wastes are termed *waste exchanges*). While some exchanges exist as actual waste warehouses that utilize printed catalogs to advertise their available commodities, many others are strictly Web sites that serve basically as information clearinghouses, connecting buyers and sellers. Subscribers are allowed to post notices regarding materials wanted for purchase of sale and those interested in the posted commodities then contact each other directly. As waste disposal costs increase and familiarity with Internet-based trading expands, utilization of the services provided by materials and waste exchanges will continue to grow.

Box 16-5 Pollution Prevention

Just as municipal waste management strategies emphasize the value of waste prevention as opposed to cleanup, so does national policy for hazardous waste management stress the importance of reducing the amount and toxicity of waste generated—an approach referred to among waste managers as **P2 (pollution prevention)**. P2 is a concept that has gradually been winning adherents for more than 20 years. In its 1984 Hazardous and Solid Waste Amendments to RCRA, Congress decreed that "the generation of hazardous waste is to be reduced or eliminated as expeditiously as possible." EPA was told to issue waste minimization regulations designed to increase awareness among industrial managers of waste reduction possibilities and to encourage voluntary initiatives aimed at lowering the amounts of waste generated. In 1990, pollution prevention became an official environmental policy of the United States when Congress enacted the **Pollution Prevention Act.** Subsequently, under its Waste Minimization Program, EPA has made reduced generation of wastes containing any of 30 "priority chemicals" its top goal, urging manufacturers to employ production methods that minimize, substitute, or completely eliminate such chemicals wherever possible. A national goal calling for a 50% reduction in these priority chemicals by 2005, as compared with 1991 quantities, was exceeded (53%) in 2001; a further 10% reduction by 2008, using the 2001 baseline, has now been set as a supplemental goal.

Although the initial response to such urgings was tentative within a corporate world still focused on traditional, end-of-pipe controls, P2 has now become a buzzword among savvy managerial types who recognize that implementing effective pollution prevention programs is a key to economic competitiveness. Not simply a public-relations ploy to appease the "green faction," corporate policies to reduce waste at the source constitute economically sound business decisions, since in today's highly regulated world it is far cheaper and more efficient to avoid the generation of waste rather than try to clean it up after the fact. Not only can effective P2 strategies save money on pollution abatement costs but by using raw materials more efficiently they also contribute to lower production costs. Fears of potential liability under the federal Superfund program have also been a strong motivating force for the adoption of pollution prevention programs—the fewer wastes shipped off-site for disposal, the less a company needs to fret about being cited as a "potentially responsible party" when a land disposal facility springs a leak!

The opportunities for significantly reducing the industrial waste stream are numerous—and often require minimal capital investment. Methods that can be employed with significant results include:

1. *Changing manufacturing processes.* By switching from an acid spray to a mechanical scrubber using pumice and rotating brushes to clean copper sheeting at its electronics plant in Columbia, Missouri, the 3M Corporation reduced its generation of liquid hazardous wastes by 40,000 lbs. annually. Similarly, the need to reduce generation of lead waste during cab-salvaging operations led Springfield, Ohio-based International Truck and Engine Corporation to replace their use of lead solder with a portable device that pulls dents out of metal, eliminating the need for solder to fill in defects; by doing so, the company not only eliminated a workplace health hazard but also reduced the time required for repairs from two hours to 5 minutes per cab.

2. *Reformulating the product.* In a plastics factory in New Jersey, Monsanto changed the formula for an industrial adhesive it was producing; in doing so, it eliminated the need for filtering the product and thus no longer had any hazardous filtrate or filters requiring disposal.

3. *Substituting a nonhazardous chemical for a hazardous one in the manufacturing process.* In Pennsylvania, American Video Glass Company (AV) instituted a number of innovative strategies to minimize releases of lead while manufacturing TV picture tubes. By replacing lead oxide with zirconium oxide as shielding in the glass panel, AV reduced its lead consumption by 1,800 tons/year and its generation of lead-containing wastes by 125 tons annually. Performance of the new zirconium oxide shielding compares favorably with that of lead shielding;

the substitution of zirconium oxide shielding allowed AV to increase the size of its glass panels, enhancing the company's competitive position and thereby benefiting both the environment and AV's bottom line.

4. *Changing equipment.* Simply by adding a condenser to an existing piece of equipment, a USS Chemicals plant in Ohio was able to capture escaping emissions of cumene, returning them to the phenol process unit. By so doing, the company solved an air quality problem and recaptured a major raw material.

5. *Altering the way hazardous wastes are handled in-plant.* Basically housekeeping changes, efforts at minimizing spills and using chemicals more conservatively can make a considerable difference in the amount of hazardous wastes generated. Segregating wastes to reduce contamination can also have a major impact. In Fremont, California, the Borden Chemical Company reduced the phenol content of its wastewater by 93% simply by separately collecting and reusing rinsewaters used to clean resin-contaminated filters. Formerly the company had allowed this rinsewater to flow into floor drains where it contaminated all the wastewater that flowed from the factory to a sewage treatment plant. American Video prevented accidental release of toxics-contaminated wastewater into city sewers simply by eliminating floor drains.

Not only do the approaches just described reduce the amounts of hazardous waste requiring disposal, they also save the companies that utilize them a great deal of money. The catch phrase "Pollution Prevention Pays," coined by the 3M Corporation, rings true in case after case. In one year after changing its process for cleaning copper sheeting, 3M saved $15,000 in raw materials and in waste disposal and labor costs; International Truck and Engine estimates that its $1,700 investment in the LP-1000 Lenco dent puller saves the company approximately $125,000 annually in labor and materials costs; by recovering 400,000 pounds of cumene after installation of a $5,000 condenser, USS Chemicals saved $100,000 in raw materials.

Until recently, many companies failed to take a comprehensive view of their waste streams—pinpointing precisely where wastes were generated and the exact management cost of each waste. By lumping all waste treatment, disposal, and oversight expenses together, corporate accountants denied themselves the opportunity of identifying specific process control points where considerable savings could be achieved. More recently, assisted and encouraged by state and federal voluntary programs such as EPA's National Partnership for Environmental Priorities, as well as by enlightened self-interest, a growing number of firms are conducting intensive waste audits, instituting cost-accounting procedures, and involving employees at all levels to identify opportunities for pollution prevention. While wholehearted endorsement of P2 principles within conservative corporate boardrooms is not yet universal, the transition is now well underway.

Reference

EPA Office of Solid Waste. 2004. http://www.epa.gov/epaoswer/hazwaste/minimize/about.htm

Siting Problems: from "NIMBY" to "BANANA"

Everyone wants hazardous wastes to be managed in ways that present the least possible threat to health or the environment, but no one wants to live near the site chosen for such storage, treatment, or disposal. Get rid of such wastes in the next county, a neighboring state, out in the desert, anyplace else—but "Not In My Back Yard!" (referred to as the "NIMBY" problem in agency argot). This, in essence, is the siting dilemma which represents one of the most difficult obstacles faced by those trying to deal with municipal or hazardous wastes (not to mention *radioactive* refuse!) in a safe and responsible manner. Certainly waste disposal horror stories from Love Canal and countless other places across the nation have made citizens understandably nervous at the prospect of seeing hazardous waste management facilities locate in their communities. Nevertheless, if society desires to continue using products whose manufacture entails the production of hazardous wastes, improved waste-handling facilities are urgently

Table 16-3 The ABC's of Waste Disposal

(Wall poster seen at the Environmental Protection Agency)

NIMBY	Not In My Back Yard
NIMFYE	Not In My Front Yard Either
PIITBY	Put It In Their Back Yard
NIMEY	Not In My Election Year
NIMTOO	Not In My Term Of Office
LULU	Locally Unwanted Land Use
NOPE	Not On Planet Earth

Source: A Dictionary of Environmental Quotations, Barbara K. Rodes and Rice Odell, eds., Simon & Schuster, 1992.

needed. Inevitably, the best location for some of those facilities will be in someone's "back yard." Responsible decision-making demands that citizens carefully evaluate the pros and cons of a site under consideration before automatically rejecting it. Laws governing the siting of hazardous waste facilities provide for public information and public participation programs during the siting process, though the scope for public input into the decision-making process varies widely from state to state. Before opposing or supporting a proposed facility, citizens should gather information on the following points:

- characteristics of the wastes involved
- nature of the proposed waste management process
- the design and manner of operation of the proposed facility
- the topographical, hydrogeological, and climatic characteristics of the site
- transportation routes to the site
- safeguards to be employed at the facility
- potential for human or ecological exposure to hazardous chemicals released into the air, water, or soil
- location of the site in reference to population centers, farmland, or valuable natural areas (e.g., wetlands, endangered species' habitat, etc.)
- possible uses of site after closure

Public opposition has stymied acquisition of new hazardous waste management sites in recent years, with objectors mobilizing from far beyond the locality directly affected. Indeed, the sentiment prevailing among many activist groups has moved well beyond the familiar NIMBY protests to encompass the ultimate in negative responses: BANANA (Build Absolutely Nothing Anywhere Near Anything!). Unless society is willing to adopt a lifestyle in which no wastes whatsoever are generated (assuming this is even possible), a more reasonable, middle-ground approach to waste management decisions must be adopted. Protection of public health requires a new willingness on the part of citizens to sanction the siting of new facilities when a thorough review of site and operational considerations indicate that such facilities will not present serious environmental health problems.

Hazardous Waste Management Legislation: RCRA

An evaluation of the types of hazardous waste incidents that have occurred indicate that we are basically dealing with two different categories of hazardous waste problems: how to manage the new volumes of chemical wastes being generated daily by American industry and what to do about wastes improperly disposed of years ago.

In order to tackle the first of these issues, the problem of newly created wastes, Congress in 1976 enacted the **Resource Conservation and Recovery Act (RCRA—** pronounced "rickra" in bureaucratese) which mandates that EPA:

- define which wastes are hazardous
- institute a **"manifest system"** to track the movement of hazardous wastes from the place they were generated to any off-site storage, treatment, or disposal facility
- set performance standards to be met by owners and operators of hazardous waste facilities
- issue permits for operation of such facilities only after technical standards have been met (operating licenses specify which types of wastes may be managed at that facility; thus most hazardous waste disposal sites are authorized to accept only certain classes of wastes)
- help states to develop hazardous waste management programs of their own which may be more stringent than the federal program, but which cannot be less so

RCRA took effect in 1980 when EPA finally issued its generator and transporter regulations (i.e., manifest requirements) and marked an important step forward in responsible hazardous waste management. However, it soon became apparent that the 1976 law featured some glaring loopholes that needed to be plugged. There was also mounting sentiment in Congress and elsewhere that land disposal of hazardous wastes is the least desirable method of managing these substances and that legislation should encourage reliance on alternatives. Accordingly, when RCRA came before Congress for reauthorization in 1984, the original legislation was substantially strengthened with the enactment of the **Hazardous and Solid Waste Amendments (HSWA).** Among the key provisions of this law are mandates that (1) significantly reduce the types of hazardous wastes which can be buried in landfills; (2) strengthen requirements for landfill design and operation; (3) bring into the regulatory framework hundreds of thousands of previously exempt "small quantity generators"—those who produce 100 kg (220 lbs.) per month or more of hazardous wastes (under the original law, only those generators producing 1,000 kg or more per month were subject to regulation); and (4) create a whole new program for detecting and controlling leakage of hazardous liquids (mainly petroleum products) from underground storage tanks. Implementation of these new requirements, while making hazardous waste

---

Box 16-6   Underground Storage Tanks

In the early 1980s, as citizens became increasingly alarmed by the widespread scope of hazardous waste problems, people consoled themselves with the assumption that the threat was largely confined to industrial sites, leaky landfills, or out-of-the-way illegal dumps. It came as a shock, therefore, to discover that virtually every community in the land, no matter how small, harbored invisible sources of potential contamination in the form of **underground storage tanks (USTs)** containing petroleum or other hazardous liquids. By 1984 the extent of the problem was regarded as so serious that when Congress enacted the Hazardous and Solid Waste Amendments (HSWA) to the Resource Conservation and Recovery Act, it created a whole new federal program to deal with the situation. **"Subtitle I,"** the Underground Storage Tank Program, required EPA to develop comprehensive regulations to protect public health and the environment from leaking underground storage tank systems. Groundwater pollution was the primary concern, since even small amounts of pollution can render groundwater supplies unusable without expensive treatment.

At the time the new regulations were issued in 1988, EPA estimated the U.S. had over 2 million underground storage tank systems (i.e., underground tanks with their associated piping) at approximately 700,000 locations nationwide. Of those, between 25– 30% were believed to be leaking their contents into the surrounding soil and aquifers; an additional 50% posed a significant threat of leakage and environmental harm. This sorry state of affairs stemmed from the fact that, until the mid-1980s, most tanks were made of bare steel without any form of corrosion protection and hence were subject to gradual deterioration. Subtitle I banned the installation of any new unprotected tanks as of 1985, but the older tanks remained an overwhelming problem.

Today that situation is well on its way to being resolved. Final UST regulations adopted in September of 1988 required that existing tank systems be replaced, upgraded, or closed (i.e., removed from the ground or filled with sand) by 1998. Owners failing to meet this deadline were advised they would face stiff fines for not complying with the law. The regulations further stipulated that all new tanks must conform with minimum standards that require corrosion protection as well as spill and overflow prevention equipment for the great majority of USTs that contain petroleum. In addition, secondary containment (i.e., essentially a double lining) and interstitial monitoring to detect potential leaks are mandated for the estimated 25,000 USTs that contain hazardous substances.

Most tank owners lacked the financial resources to comply with these requirements, since upgrading a tank can cost more than $12,000 while a new one is about $30,000. Simply closing a tank carries a tab of $5,000–11,000. Accordingly, in 1986 Congress created the Leaking Underground Storage Tank Trust Fund, providing funds for cleanups at sites where the owner of a tank is deceased or can't be located, is financially incapable of responding, or in cases requiring emergency action. Many state governments similarly have created special funds to expedite tank removals. By the time the federal deadline expired in December 1998, the majority of tank owners had complied with EPA regulations. During the preceding ten-year period, a million USTs had been closed or replaced, while an additional 600,000 were upgraded to prevent leakage. Four years later, in December 2002, 81% of the remaining 698,000 federally regulated USTs were in compliance with rules pertaining to spill and overflow prevention and corrosion protection; 74% met the requirements for leak detection. These figures mark a vast improvement over the situation a decade earlier, but indicate that problems still remain; accordingly, EPA is focusing on improving compliance with UST regulations. In addition, since a number of releases have been reported from USTs that were in full compliance with existing regulations, the agency is now conducting field investigations and working in partnership with industry and academic researchers to analyze the components and processes of UST systems in order to determine what improvements might be needed.

Tank removal, replacement, and performance evaluation are only partial solutions to USTs' past legacy of pollution, however. Expensive cleanup efforts at thousands of sites where corroding tanks silently leaked their contents into soil and groundwater for years have been underway since the 1990s, yet approximately 143,000 UST-contaminated sites are still awaiting remediation. Recent recognition that MTBE releases at some of these sites poses an urgent risk to groundwater quality (see box 12-2) has prompted EPA to launch a new initiative to speed up the pace of UST cleanups across the country. The task remaining is immense and will likely continue for several decades; nevertheless, notable progress has been made in the 20 years since attention first focused on the "ticking time bombs" buried in every community across the land.

Reference

EPA, 2003. *Introduction to the Underground Storage Tank Regulations and Policy* (March).

Nardi, Karen J. 1995. "Underground Storage Tanks." In *Environmental Law Handbook, 13th ed.*, edited by Thomas F. P. Sullivan, pp. 76–100. Government Institutes, Inc.

management considerably more expensive than it had been previously, gave new impetus to safer, more environmentally responsible waste management strategies.

While confronting the issue of newly generated wastes with an array of regulatory approaches, RCRA does nothing to deal with the serious problem posed by leaking abandoned dumpsites. Even in the relatively few cases where the owners can be found, they often lack the financial resources to clean up the site, making litigation a futile exercise. Since EPA estimates there may be as many as 350,000 abandoned hazardous waste sites in the United States, the potential for future problems is obviously significant.

"Superfund"

Spurred by public demands that something be done to alleviate problems caused by old, leaking dumpsites, Congress in December of 1980 enacted the **Comprehensive Environmental Response, Compensation, and Liability Act (CERCLA,** dubbed the "Superfund"), authorizing the expenditure of $1.6 billion over a five-year period for emergency cleanup activities and for the more long-term containment of hazardous waste dump sites (the legislation, however, did not include funds to compensate victims for health damage incurred by exposure to such sites—an issue which was the focus of considerable debate). EPA, in cooperation with the states, was charged with compiling a **National Priority List (NPL)** of sites considered to be sufficiently threatening to public health or environmental quality to make them eligible for Superfund cleanup dollars. These funds can be used either to remove hazardous substances from the site (a process which may also include temporary relocation of peo-

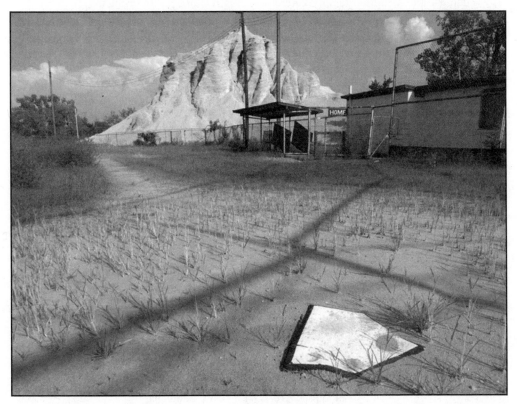

A pile of lead-contaminated waste from a now-closed mine towers over an abandoned ball field in Picher, Oklahoma, home to one of the oldest sites on the Superfund's list of the country's most contaminated toxic waste sites. [*AP photo/J. Pat Carter*]

ple in the area and provision of alternative water supplies) or for remedial measures such as storage and confinement of wastes, incineration, dredging, or permanent relocation of residents. In the years following passage of CERCLA, many states enacted their own "mini-Superfund" laws, aimed at forcing similar cleanups on sites where contamination wasn't bad enough to qualify for placement on the NPL but sufficiently threatening to warrant remediation.

The original federal Superfund bill expired in September 1985, and in spite of public demands for speedy reauthorization so that cleanup work could proceed without interruption, the law was not renewed until late the following year. Extreme congressional dissatisfaction with the excruciatingly slow rate of progress during Superfund's first years led to several significant changes in the 1986 **Superfund Amendments and Reauthorization Act** (SARA). Realizing that 1980 funding levels were inadequate, Congress in 1986 increased Superfund allocations to $8.5 billion to be spent over the next five years and in 1990 allocated an additional $5.1 billion for the program. EPA was given mandatory deadlines for initiating site-specific cleanup plans and remediation activities. Concerned that previous cleanup actions represented little more than moving contaminated wastes from one site to another site, which would itself then become eligible for Superfund status, Congress specified a preference for cleanup actions which "permanently and significantly" reduce the volume, toxicity, or mobility of hazardous substances. This mandate has given a major impetus to development of treatment or disposal technologies (e.g., mobile incinerators that can be moved from one Superfund site to another) which permit hazardous wastes to be destroyed or detoxified on site, thereby avoiding the risks of transporting such wastes to another facility where they might cause future problems.

Several contentious policy issues have provoked heated debate among Superfund supporters and critics since the program's inception. One involves the extent of remediation necessary—How clean is clean enough? While many citizens demand that remediation restore a contaminated site to its original condition, critics complain that it makes no sense to spend millions of dollars to remove every last trace of contamination on a site destined to be paved over for a parking lot. Carol Browner, EPA Administrator during the Clinton administration, acknowledged the validity of such criticism and

---

Table 16-4 "Top 20" Most Prominent Toxic Substances Found at NPL Sites

Lead	Cadmium	Trichloroethylene	DDE
Arsenic	PCBs	DDT	Arochlor 1242
Mercury (metallic)	Benzo(a)pyrene	Arochlor 1254	Dibenzo(a,h)anthracene
Benzene	Chloroform	Hexachlorobutadiene	Hexavalent chromium
Vinyl chloride	Benzo(b)fluoranthene	Arochlor 1260	Dieldrin

Ranking based on: (1) frequency at NPL sites, (2) toxicity, and (3) exposure hazard to humans.

Source: Agency for Toxic Substances and Disease Registry.

Table 16-5 States with the Most Listed NPL Sites (2005)

New Jersey	113	Florida	50	Massachusetts	31
Pennsylvania	94	Washington	46	Ohio	30
California	93	Texas	42	North Carolina	30
New York	89	Illinois	41	Indiana	29
Michigan	67	Wisconsin	38	South Carolina	26

Source: EPA.

Box 16-7   Revitalizing Communities Through "Brownfields" Redevelopment

In cities across America, particularly in the industrial Northeast and Midwest, aging cities are pockmarked by boarded-up gas stations, abandoned factories, and rubble-strewn lots. Although located in close proximity to transportation services, utilities, and a willing workforce, these properties have been bypassed by developers and constitute a visual and economic blight on urban neighborhoods. Known as **brownfields**, these under-used, idled, or abandoned sites are shunned because of actual or suspected environmental contamination. Fearing legal liability for cleanup costs, prospective buyers have chosen to avoid any potential headaches, opting instead for construction on "greenfields" in the suburbs. In doing so, they have thwarted inner-city residents' dreams of economic development, put still-clean lands at risk of future contamination, and exacerbated concerns about urban sprawl. Far from being irrational or discriminatory, developers' decisions have been based on the reality that, under CERCLA's "strict, joint and several" liability provisions, property owners could find themselves responsible for multimillion dollar clean-ups, even though the contamination problems were caused by a previous owner many decades earlier. In addition, a developer's likelihood of being able to obtain financing for construction on a brownfield property was virtually negligible, as lending institutions have been extremely reluctant to finance development for fear that they, too, could incur unlimited liability under Superfund if the property owner were to default or disappear.

This seemingly intractable dilemma was confronted head-on in January 1995, when EPA launched its **Brownfields Action Agenda**. A visionary and aggressive program for restoring blighted properties to productive use while promoting job development and community participation in decision-making, the brownfields initiative has brought entrepreneurial activity and a new sense of hope to urban areas long mired in depression and decay.

The potential scope of brownfields reclamation efforts is immense. Estimates of the number of contaminated sites nationwide range from 350,000 to as many as a million.

On most of these properties levels of contamination are low to moderate; Superfund-type sites that present a serious environmental health risk are not included in the brownfields program. A sizeable portion of brownfields are sites contaminated by gasoline leaking from underground storage tanks. Others may be old dry-cleaning establishments where solvents were dumped on a back lot or abandoned factories with heavy metals contamination. Although most designated sites are urban, brownfields can be found in suburban and rural areas as well.

The Brownfields Action Agenda includes four major initiatives.

1. Grants for brownfields projects comprise the foundation of EPA's program by providing funds for site assessment, remediation, and job training. Federal dollars invested in brownfields projects have had a multiplier effect, leveraging over $6.5 billion from private, state, and local sources for cleanups and redevelopment.

2. Clarification of liability and cleanup issues. Since uncertainty regarding future liability for cleanup at polluted sites has been the main deterrent to restoration of brownfields, several important actions have been taken under this initiative. A major step was EPA's removal of approximately 25,000 locations from the list of potential Superfund sites. The sites deleted were ones already designated by the agency as "no further response action planned," meaning they were not sufficiently contaminated ever to make the NPL. Nevertheless, the fact that they had been retained in the Superfund archives was a deterrent to potential developers, making their deletion from the list a symbolically reassuring action. Equally important was congressional enactment in 2002 of the Small Business Liability Relief and Brownfields Revitalization Act, which limited the potential liability of brownfields purchasers to cleanup costs known at the time of purchase, thereby removing one of the major deterrents to brownfields cleanup. Although a number of states had already enacted similar legislation, passage of the federal law freed developers from any worry that unpleasant surprises discovered later on could entail large, unanticipated expenses for remediation. For those whose property lies above an aquifer contaminated by groundwater flow from an adjacent polluted site, the law guarantees freedom from liability for groundwater cleanup so long as they did not cause or contribute to the pollution.

One of the most critical issues addressed by the Brownfields Initiative was the "How clean is clean enough?" question. Insistence on the near-pristine standards required for remediated Superfund sites would doom the brownfields program by making such ventures cost-prohibitive. Accordingly, EPA and many state environmental agencies have introduced the concept of **risk-based corrective action (RBCA**—referred to in agency jargon as "Rebecca"). Originally applied to the remediation of petroleum-contaminated UST sites, RBCA is a decision-making process in which the required level of cleanup is based on real-life exposure risks, rather than on the assumption that the entire population of an area will be exposed to the maximum level of contamination present. Thus the degree of cleanup is based on the intended future use of a site. For example, a piece of land where trace amounts of lead remain in the soil could be covered with asphalt and used as a shopping mall parking lot without endangering anyone. If the same property were intended for use as a children's playground, higher cleanup standards would be in order.

3. Partnerships and outreach. Every brownfields project aims to establish a cooperative working relationship among federal agencies, states, cities, and community groups. Issues of environmental justice and the empowerment of brownfields area residents, encouraging their participation in decision-making, are key elements in this initiative.

4. Job development and training. A report issued by the Northeast-Midwest Institute categorically stated that "Brownfields and employment problems go together." EPA emphasizes the importance of ensuring that brownfields redevelopment benefits area residents by providing both short- and long-term employment opportunities. To guarantee the availability of a locally based, well-trained labor pool, the Brownfields Action Agenda is establishing partnerships with local educational institutions, striving to develop long-term programs for worker training.

Since 1995 more than 4,800 properties have been assessed and hundreds of brownfields projects have been launched, creating nearly 30,000 new jobs as a result. Geographically, these projects span the nation and include a computer-controlled greenhouse for tomato production in Buffalo, New York; a greenway featuring a bike path linking a series of linear parks in Providence, RI; an upscale shopping and restaurant district in Charlotte, North Carolina; and a community day care facility for more than 200 children on Chicago's West Side. All were built on abandoned, contaminated sites long viewed as worthless.

Brownfields initiatives throughout the country are revitalizing American communities by restoring degraded sites to new uses, increasing property values, stimulating tax revenues, and improving the quality of life in hundreds of low-income neighborhoods. As former EPA Administrator Carol Browner remarked in a press release on the program: "Across the nation, our cities are coming back to life, due in part to the new jobs and new opportunities created by brownfields revitalization."

predicted ". . . there will be different levels of clean." Undoubtedly, the most controversial feature of the Superfund program has been its liability provisions that can hold the owner of a contaminated site (i.e., the **potentially responsible party**) responsible for multi-million dollar cleanup costs, even if that person or company was not directly responsible for the contamination (e.g., a small businessman who unknowingly purchased a property where a former owner, now deceased, dumped hazardous liquids that subsequently contaminated soil and groundwater can himself be held responsible for remediating the site). While business interests demand changes in what they regard as an inherently unfair provision, environmental advocates strongly support the status quo, insisting that concerns about **Superfund liability** alone have caused generators to be much more conscientious about managing their wastes in a responsible manner and have given major impetus to serious pollution prevention efforts.

Since passage of Superfund legislation in 1980, the number of listed NPL sites has grown from an original 400 to 1,242 by mid-2005, with an additional 68 proposed for listing. By the end of 2004, cleanup had been completed at 926 sites, representing 61% of the top priority NPL sites (EPA, 2004). Although most Americans enthusiastically support the concept of cleaning up the nation's hazardous waste mistakes of the past,

Cleanup of hazardous waste dumpsites begins with careful sampling and identification of the abandoned material so that an appropriate disposal method can be chosen. Personnel carrying out the investigation wear protective "moon suits" and respirators to guard against personal injury. [*Illinois Environmental Protection Agency*]

congressional support of the program has waned in recent years. Until the mid-1990s, the lion's share of funding to pay for cleanup of abandoned sites came from a tax on the petroleum and chemical industries—a "superfund" whose creation reflected the prevailing "polluter pays" principle. For obvious reasons, this tax had always been unpopular with the targeted industries and in 1995 federal legislators yielded to corporate pressure and refused to reauthorize the tax. For the next few years EPA continued to finance cleanups with the dollars remaining in the rapidly dwindling Superfund account. Once that source of funding was exhausted, however, the agency became wholly dependent on general tax revenues annually appropriated by Congress. Unfortunately for those living near contaminated sites slated for remediation, Congress has repeatedly failed to allocate sufficient funds to carry out more than a small percentage of cleanups, halting a number of projects underway at some of the nation's most contaminated sites and postponing the ultimate remediation of all NPL sites by many decades.

Household Hazardous Wastes

Comforting references to "Home Sweet Home" are slightly less reassuring today than in years past. The invisible hazards posed by radon and other indoor air pollutants make us wonder if we'd be safer inhaling deeply at a busy intersection than in our paneled family room. More recently, the righteous indignation directed at corporate polluters who disregard public well-being by careless disposal of their toxic by-products is being tempered somewhat by the realization that all of us—whatever our occupations—contribute to the nation's hazardous waste woes through our use, misuse, and thoughtless disposal of hundreds of potentially dangerous household chemicals.

It is estimated that the average American generates about 20 pounds of household hazardous waste each year. Typical examples of such discarded materials include pesticides, paints and varnishes, brush cleaners, ammonia, toilet bowl cleaners, bleaches and disinfectants, oven cleaners, furniture polish, swimming pool chemicals, batteries, motor oil, outdated medicines, and many others. Although these substances may be every bit as toxic, corrosive, flammable, or explosive as the industrial wastes regulated under RCRA, federal and state hazardous waste laws do not apply to the comparatively minor household sources. Nevertheless, the cumulative environmental impact of even small amounts of these materials being carelessly discarded by millions of individuals can be significant.

Household hazardous waste disposal presents a variety of concerns:

1. Stored inside the home, hazardous chemicals pose poisoning risks, particularly for children; some, such as paints and solvents, pose problems of indoor air pollution; others, ammonia and chlorine bleach, for example, can result in highly toxic emissions when inadvertently mixed; still others pose serious fire hazards.

2. The welfare of public employees can be threatened by hazardous household products. Home fires involving hazardous chemicals can result in explosions or the generation of toxic fumes that can kill or seriously injure firefighters. Refuse collectors frequently suffer injury when they throw garbage bags into compactor trucks, unaware that they contain corrosive or flammable materials. In November 1996, a refuse collector in New York was killed when doused with acid from a discarded battery mixed with the trash he tossed into the compacter of his garbage truck; one worker was killed and another critically injured in a fire at a recycling plant caused by aerosol cans fed into a baler (Pellow, 2002).

3. The environment itself can be seriously degraded when householders pour hazardous liquids into drains and flush them down toilets or into septic sys-

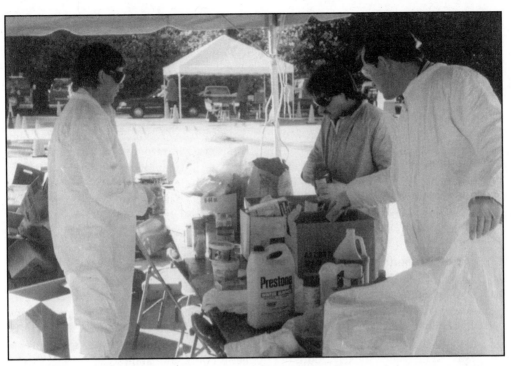

Hazardous household waste collection day: after residents have deposited their old paint cans, motor oil containers, discarded cleaning products, outdated medicine, and the like, workers from the Illinois EPA separate the wastes and prepare them for shipment to a licensed facility for disposal, treatment, or recycling. [*Illinois Environmental Protection Agency*]

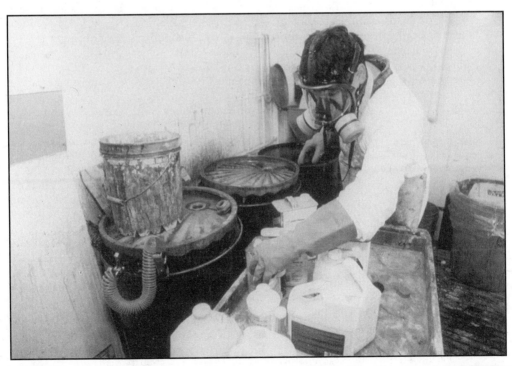

A worker in protective gear examines potentially toxic containers at a hazardous household waste disposal center in Seattle. [© *Steve Schneider/Greenpeace 1994*]

tems. People who pour waste motor oil into storm sewers or dump paint cans in the woods can cause long-lasting damage to ground and surface water supplies. Throwing such hazardous materials in the trash may ultimately result in the threat of contaminated incinerator ash and air pollution or, alternatively, in the formation of toxic leachates at municipal landfills.

In an effort to raise public awareness about these problems and to provide concerned citizens with a safe and responsible way of getting rid of hazardous household wastes, an increasing number of communities, state environmental agencies, and public interest groups have been sponsoring household hazardous waste collection programs in recent years. These events have attracted large numbers of householders who are happy to take advantage of the opportunity to clean out the basement or garage and safely get rid of those old bottles of pesticides, paints—even ammunition—that may have been sitting on a shelf gathering dust for 20 years or more. Once wastes are brought to a collection center, they must be separated by type, packaged, and manifested as RCRA hazardous wastes by trained personnel (usually licensed hazardous waste transporters). They are then taken to a licensed facility for treatment, disposal, or recycling. The cost of running such programs, as well as concerns about legal liability, have limited their more widespread adoption. Nevertheless, these widely publicized efforts have had an impact far beyond the city limits of their sponsoring communities, enhancing public awareness of the fact that each one of us is a part of America's solid waste problem and pointing the way toward safer, more responsible ways of managing the hazardous by-products of our national lifestyle.

References

Berenyi, Eileen Brettler. 1999. "Whither MRF-based Recycling?" *Resource Recycling* 18, no. 4 (April):12–17.

Dufficy, Craig. 2004. U.S. Environmental Protection Agency, Municipal and Industrial Solid Waste Division, Office of Solid Waste, personal communication, Dec. 30.

Environmental Protection Agency (EPA). 2004. "Superfund Progress Contributes to Healthy Communities, Yearly Analysis Shows." News for release: Monday, Nov. 15.

Gitlitz, Jenny. 2004. "Are Bottle Bills Still Relevant?" *Resource Recycling* 23, no. 9 (Sept).

Greczyn, Mary. 1994. "Researchers and Community Reps Call for More Bioaerosol Research." *Environmental Health Letter* 33, no. 7 (March).

Greenhouse, Linda. 1994. "Justices Decide Incinerator Ash Is Toxic Waste." *New York Times,* May 3.

Kaufman, Scott M., Nora Goldstein, Karsten Millrath, and Nickolas J. Themelis. 2004. "The State of Garbage in America: 14th Annual Nationwide Survey of Solid Waste Management in the United States." *BioCycle* 45, no. 1 (Jan).

League of Women Voters Education Fund. 1993. *The Garbage Primer.* New York: Lyon & Burford.

Levine, Adeline G. 1982. *Love Canal: Science, Politics, and People.* Lexington Books, D. C. Heath.

Melosi, Martin V. 1981. *Garbage in the Cities: Refuse, Reform, and the Environment, 1880–1980.* Texas A&M Univ. Press.

Miller, Chaz. 1998. "Profiles in Garbage: Old Newspaper." *Waste Age* 29, no. 8 (Aug):79–80.

Musick, Mark. 2004. "Chlorpyralid Levels Decline, But Controversy Continues." *BioCycle* 45, no. 5 (May).

Pellow, David Naguib. 2002. *Garbage Wars: The Struggle for Environmental Justice in Chicago.* Cambridge, MA: The MIT Press.

Perket, Cary. 2004. "Manufacturers Ship 7 Million Tons per Year to Commercial Hazardous Waste & Wastewater Facilities." *EI Digest, Environmental Information Ltd.* (June 21).

———. 2003. "20th Annual North American Commercial Hazardous Waste & Wastewater Facilities Survey." *E I Digest, Environmental Information Ltd. (Nov. 3).*

Renner, Michael. 2004. "Moving Toward a Less Consumptive Economy." In *State of the World 2004.* New York: Worldwatch Institute/W. W. Norton.

Sheehan, Bill, and Helen Spiegelman. 2005. "Extended Producer Responsibility Policies in the United States and Canada: History and Status." In *The Case of Integrated Product Policy*, edited by Dirk Scheer & Frieder Rubik. Heidleberg, Germany.

Themelis, Nickolas J., and Scott M. Kaufman. 2004. "The State of Garbage in America—Data and Methodology Assessment." *BioCycle* 45, no. 4 (April).

Whyte, Tim. 2003. "The Straight Poop on Diaper Recycling." http://www.the-signal.com (April 20). Accessed 12–11–04.

APPENDIX A
ENVIRONMENTAL AGENCIES
OF THE FEDERAL GOVERNMENT

National policy-making regarding environmental health issues has been delegated among several different federal agencies and cabinet-level departments. Among the more important groups dealing with issues discussed in this book are:

Environmental Protection Agency (EPA)
www.epa.gov

Created by President Nixon in December 1970, the EPA is an independent agency formed to coordinate the administration of a wide range of environmental programs which, prior to that time, had been scattered among a number of governmental agencies and departments, several of which frequently worked at cross-purposes. EPA has been charged with setting and enforcing standards pertaining to air and water pollution, solid and hazardous waste management, noise, public water supplies, pesticides, and radiation (excluding that associated with nuclear power plants). All EPA actions are published in the *Federal Register* as "proposed regulations," with time being allowed for public comment prior to their adoption as legally enforceable "final regulations."

The Administrator of the EPA is appointed by the President of the United States and confirmed by the U.S. Senate. Although EPA headquarters are in the nation's capital, the agency has ten regional offices, each with its own regional administrator, responsible for the states within its region.

The Council on Environmental Quality (CEQ)
www.whitehouse.gov/CEQ

Established by the National Environmental Policy Act signed by President Nixon on January 1, 1970, the CEQ operates within the Executive Office of the president. The CEQ coordinates federal environmental efforts and works closely with agencies and other White House offices in the development of environmental policies and initiatives. The council's chairperson is appointed by the president and serves as principal environmental policy advisor to the president.

Nuclear Regulatory Commission (NRC)
www.nrc.gov

A five-member civilian board, this agency was created in 1974 by the National Energy Reorganization Act, which broke up the old Atomic Energy Commission (AEC) into the research-oriented Energy Research and Development Administration (subsequently absorbed by the Department of Energy) and the NRC. The Nuclear

Regulatory Commission has jurisdiction over the licensing and regulation of nuclear reactors and also over the processing, transportation, and security of nuclear materials.

Office of Science and Technology Policy
www.ostp.gov

Established within the Executive Office of the president, this agency advises the president on scientific and technological considerations involved in a wide range of national concerns, including health and the environment.

Consumer Product Safety Commission
www.cpsc.gov

This independent regulatory agency seeks to reduce unreasonable risks of injury associated with consumer products by encouraging the development of voluntary standards related to consumer product safety, requiring the reporting of hazardous consumer products and, if justified, recalling for corrective action hazardous products already on the market. The commission conducts research on consumer product hazards, can establish mandatory standards, and, if necessary, has the authority to ban hazardous consumer products.

Public Health Service
www.usphs.gov

An office within the Department of Health and Human Services, the U.S. Public Health Service helps states and communities develop local health resources, conducts and supports medical research, and oversees other public health functions. Among the various subdivisions within the Public Health Service, a few are of particular environmental health interest:

Centers for Disease Control and Prevention (CDC)
www.cdc.gov

This agency is charged with protecting public health by providing leadership and direction in the prevention and control of disease. It administers programs related to communicable and vectorborne diseases, urban rat control, control of childhood lead-based paint poisoning, and a range of other environmental health problems. CDC also participates in a national program of research, information, and education regarding smoking and health. The nine major offices of the CDC are those dealing with epidemiology, international health, laboratory improvement, prevention services, environmental health, occupational safety and health, health promotion and education, professional development and training, and infectious diseases.

Food and Drug Administration (FDA)
www.fda.gov

The FDA's activities are aimed at protecting public health against impure and unsafe foods, drugs, cosmetics, and other possible hazards such as radiation. In carrying out its responsibilities, the FDA conducts research and develops standards for food, drugs, medical devices, veterinary medicines, and biologic products. Through its National Center for Toxicological Research, the FDA studies the biologic effects of potentially toxic chemicals in the environment.

Occupational Safety and Health Administration (OSHA)
www.osha.gov

Operating within the Department of Labor, OSHA develops and promulgates safety and health standards and regulations for the American workforce. It conducts investigations and inspections of workplaces to ensure compliance with those regulations and can issue citations and propose penalties for employers who violate such standards.

Fish and Wildlife Service
www.fws.gov

A bureau within the Department of the Interior, the Fish and Wildlife Service has jurisdiction over matters regarding endangered species, certain marine mammals, wild birds, inland sports fisheries, and wildlife research. The bureau carries out biological monitoring for effects of pesticides, heavy metals, and thermal pollution; it maintains wildlife refuges, enforces game laws, and carries out programs to control livestock predators and pest species. The bureau maintains a number of fish hatcheries, conducts environmental education and public information programs, and provides both national and international leadership regarding endangered fish and wildlife species.

Office of Surface Mining Reclamation and Enforcement
www.osmre.gov

Another agency within the Interior Department, this office is charged with assisting states in developing a nationwide program to protect society and the environment during coal mining and reclamation and to reclaim mines abandoned before 1977.

Bureau of Land Management (BLM)
www.blm.gov

The BLM is responsible for managing the nation's 341 million acres of public lands, most of which are located in the Far West. In doing so, the bureau manages the timber, minerals, rangeland vegetation, wild and scenic rivers, wilderness areas, endangered species, and energy resources of these lands. BLM also is involved in watershed protection, development of recreational opportunities, and programs to protect and manage wild horses and burros. The bureau provides for the protection, orderly development, and use of public lands and resources under principles of multiple use and sustained yield. Criticism in recent years has focused on the bureau's overemphasis on permitting exploitation of public resources for private gain and insufficient protection and conservation of these resources.

Natural Resources Conservation Service (NRCS)
www.nrcs.usda.gov

An agency of the Department of Agriculture, the NRCS develops and carries out soil and water conservation programs in cooperation with landowners and operators, land developers, and community planning agencies. NRCS also is active in programs to control agricultural pollution and to bring about environmental improvement.

Appendix B
Environmental Organizations

American Lung Association
www.lungusa.org

Basel Action Network
www.ban.org

Center for Health, Environment and Justice
www.essential.org/cchw/

Center for Science in the Public Interest
www.cspinet.org

Climate Action Network
www.climatenetwork.org

Defenders of Wildlife
www.defenders.org

Ducks Unlimited, Inc.
www.ducks.org

Environmental Defense
www.environmentaldefense.org

Friends of the Earth
www.foe.org

Greenpeace USA, Inc.
www.greenpeace.org

League of Conservation Voters
www.lcv.org

League of Women Voters of the United States
www.lwv.org

National Audubon Society
www.audubon.org

National Environmental Health Association
www.neha.org

National Religious Partnership for
the Environment
www.nrpe.org

National Wildlife Federation
www.nwf.org

The Nature Conservancy
www.tnc.org

Natural Resources Defense Council
www.nrdc.org

Pesticide Action Network North America
www.panna.org

Planned Parenthood Federation of America
www.plannedparenthood.org

Population Action International
www.populationaction.org

The Population Connection
(formerly Zero Population Growth)
www.populationconnection.org

Population Reference Bureau, Inc.
www.prb.org

Rainforest Alliance
www.rainforestalliance.org

Sierra Club
www.sierraclub.org

Union of Concerned Scientists
www.ucsusa.org

The Wilderness Society
www.wilderness.org

Worldwatch Institute
www.worldwatch.org

World Resources Institute
www.wri.org

World Conservation Union (IUCN)
www.iucn.org

World Wildlife Fund
www.worldwildlife.org

INDEX